S0-ANE-377

GASTROINTESTINAL
PAN-ENDOSCOPY

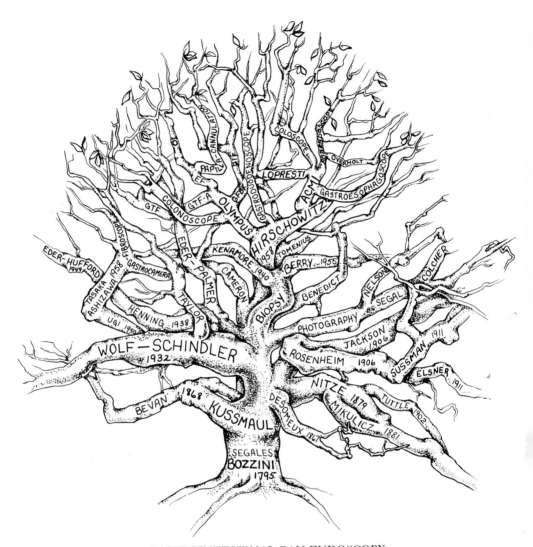

GASTROINTESTINAL PAN-ENDOSCOPY

"Mighty Oaks from Tiny Acorns Grow"
Adapted from Quercus virginiana
Design—L. H. Berry, M.D.   Art Work—Nancy Swan

GASTROINTESTINAL PAN-ENDOSCOPY

ESOPHAGOSCOPY, GASTROSCOPY,
BULBAR AND POSTBULBAR DUODENOSCOPY
PROCTO-SIGMOIDOSCOPY, COLONOSCOPY
AND PERITONEOSCOPY

LEONIDAS H. BERRY, M.S., M.D.

Chief, Gastrointestinal Endoscopy Service
Cook County Hospital
Professor of Gastroenterology and Endoscopy
Cook County Graduate School of Medicine
Clinical Associate Professor of Medicine, Emeritus
University of Illinois
Senior Attending Physician, Provident and
Michael Reese Hospitals
Chicago, Illinois

WITH INTERNATIONAL CONTRIBUTORS

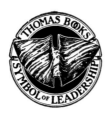

CHARLES C THOMAS · PUBLISHER
Springfield · Illinois · U.S.A.

Published and Distributed Throughout the World by
CHARLES C THOMAS • PUBLISHER
Bannerstone House
301-327 East Lawrence Avenue, Springfield, Illinois, U.S.A.

This book is protected by copyright. No part of it
may be reproduced in any manner without written
permission from the publisher.

© *1974, by* CHARLES C THOMAS • PUBLISHER
ISBN 0-398-02912-1
Library of Congress Catalog Card Number: 73-15562

*With THOMAS BOOKS careful attention is given to all details of
manufacturing and design. It is the Publisher's desire to present books that are
satisfactory as to their physical qualities and artistic possibilities and
appropriate for their particular use. THOMAS BOOKS will be true to those
laws of quality that assure a good name and good will.*

Printed in the United States of America
C-1

Library of Congress Cataloging in Publication Data

Berry, Leonidas H.
   Gastrointestinal pan-endoscopy.

   1. Digestive organs—Diseases—Diagnosis.
2. Endoscope and endoscopy. I. Title.
[DNLM: 1. Endoscopy. 2. Gastrointestinal diseases
—Diagnosis. WI141 B534g 1974]
RC804.E6B47   616.3'3'0754   73-15562
ISBN 0-398-02912-1

CONTRIBUTORS

JONAS ADOMAVICIUS, M.D.
Attending Physician and Endoscopist, Cook County Hospital
Instructor, Gastroenterology and Endoscopy
Cook County Graduate School of Medicine, Chicago, Illinois

ILTIFAT A. ALAVI, B.Sc., M.B., M.R.C.P. (ED.)
Associate Fellow, College of Gastroenterology
Assistant Professor of Clinical Medicine
Chicago Medical School
Attending Physician, Cook County Hospital
Chicago, Illinois
Community Memorial General Hospital, La Grange, Illinois

SOL Z. ALVAREZ, M.D.
Fellow, Philippine College of Physicians
Councilor, International Society of Endoscopy, Asian Zone
Member, International Association for Study of Liver
Assistant Professor of Medicine, University of Santo Tomas
Faculty of Medicine and Surgery, Manila, Philippines
Chairman, Department of Gastroenterology, Santo Tomas University Hospital
St. Lukes Hospital Consultant in Gastroenterology, Makati Medical Center
Chinese General Hospital, Veterans Memorial Hospital
Manila, Philippines

SHINROKU ASHIZAWA, M.D.
Professor, Department of Medicine
Chairman, Division of Gastroenterology
Tokyo Medical College, Japan
Honorary member American Society for Gastrointestinal Endoscopy

JOSEPH P. BELBER, A.B., M.D., F.A.C.P.
Associate Clinical Professor of Medicine, University of California School of Medicine
San Francisco, California
Chief, Gastroenterology Section, Medical Service
Veterans Administration Hospital
Martinez, California
Attending Endoscopist, San Francisco General Hospital
San Francisco, California

LEONIDAS H. BERRY, M.S., M.D., Sc.D. (HON.), F.A.C.P., F.A.C.G.
Professor, Gastroenterology and Endoscopy, Cook County Graduate School
Clinical Associate Professor of Medicine, Emeritus, University of Illinois, Chicago
Senior Attending Physician and Chief Gastrointestinal Endoscopy Service
Cook County Hospital
Senior Attending Physician and former Chairman

Department of Medicine and Division of Gastroenterology, Provident Hospital
Senior Attending Physician, Michael Reese Hospital
Chicago, Illinois, American Society for Gastrointestinal Endoscopy
Member, French National Society of Gastroenterology
Japan Endoscopic Society, Chilean (S.A.) Society of Gastroenterology
Diplomate, The National Board of Medical Examiners
Diplomate, American Board of Internal Medicine
and Subspecialty Board of Gastroenterology

BLAS BRUNI-CELLI, M.D.
Professor of Pathology, Central University
Chief, Pathology Unit, Vargas Hospital
Pathologist "Institute Diagnostico," Caracas, Venezuela

JACQUES CAROLI, M.D.
Professor of Medicine, Saint Antoine Hospital
Paris, France

FONG-MING CHANG, M.D.
Associate Professor of Medicine
China Medical College
Senior Attending Physician, Taipei Gastro-Intestinal Clinic
Taiwan, Republic of China

HENRY COLCHER, B.S., M.D., F.A.C.G.
Associate Clinical Professor of Medicine, College of Physicians and Surgeons
Columbia University, New York, New York
Associate Attending Physician, Francis Delafield Hospital
Assistant Attending Physician, Presbyterian Hospital
Columbia Presbyterian Medical Center, New York, New York
Consultant Lecturer, Department of Medicine, Naval Hospital
St. Albans, New York.

ANGELO E. DAGRADI, A.B., M.D., F.A.C.G., F.A.C.P.
Adjunct Associate Professor of Medicine, U.C. Irvine School of Medicine
Chief, Gastroenterology Section, U.S.V.A. Hospital
Long Beach, California
Consultant Endoscopist, Harbor General Hospital
Torrance, California
Orange County Medical Center

HOWARD J. EDDY, JR., M.D., F.A.C.G.
Associate Attending Surgeon, Community Hospital
Glen Cove, New York
St. John's Hospital, Smithstown, New York
Hempstead General Hospital
Hempstead, Long Island, New York

MITSUO ENDO, M.D., F.I.C.S.
Professor, Department of Surgery
Director of Gastroenterological Surgery
Tokyo Women's Medical College, Japan

NORBERT HENNING, M.D.
Emeritus Professor of Medicine and Director of University Clinic
Erlangen, Nuernberg University, Germany

BASIL I. HIRSCHOWITZ, B.Sc., M.B.B.Ch., M.D., M.R.C.P. (London)
    F.A.C.P. (Edinburgh)
Professor of Medicine, Director, Division of Gastroenterology
Professor of Physiology and Biophysics
Attending Physician, University Hospital
University of Alabama in Birmingham
Consultant Physician, Veterans Hospital
Birmingham, Alabama

PIERRE HOUSSET, M.D.
Attending Physician and Gastroenterologist, Hospital Bichat, Paris, France
Member, the French Society of Gastrointestinal Endoscopy
Honorary member, American Society for Gastrointestinal Endoscopy

RAYMOND J. JACKMAN, M.D.
Consultant in Proctology
Mayo Clinic, Rochester, Minnesota

RAYMOND B. JOHNSON, A.B., M.D.
Assistant Head, Gastroenterology Clinic and Research Branch
National Naval Medical Center, Bethesda, Maryland
Commander (MC), United States Navy
Associate Member, AGA
Member ACP
Associate Fellow, American College of Gastroenterology
Associate Member, American Society for Gastrointestinal Endoscopy

SIR FRANCIS AVERY JONES, M.B., B.S., M.D., F.R.C.P., Lond., M.R.C.S., Eng.,
    C.B.E.
Physician and member, teaching staff, Gastroenterological Department
Central Middlesex Hospital, London, England
Consulting Gastroenterologist to the Royal Navy

ARTURO DOMINGO JORGE, M.D.
Chief, Gastroenterological Department of the Third Cathedra
of the Medical Clinic of the Faculty of Medicine
(Universidad Nacional de Cuyo)
Mendoza, Argentina
Chief, Gastroenterological Department of the Spanish Hospital
Mendoza, Argentina

TATSUZO KASUGAI, M.D., Ph.D.
Chairman, Department of Medicine, Aichi Cancer Center Hospital
Nagoya, Japan

DAVID KATZ, B.S., M.D., F.A.C.P.
Associate Professor of Medicine
New York Medical College
Consultant (GE), USVA Hospital
Montrose, New York
Consultant, (GE) Nyack Hospital
Director (GE) Mt. Vernon Hospital
Mt. Vernon, New York

MAURICE L. KELLEY, JR., M.D., F.A.C.P.
Associate Clinical Professor of Medicine
Dartmouth Medical School
Chairman, Section of Internal Medicine, Hitchcock Clinic
Hanover, New Hampshire

ARTHUR P. KLOTZ, B.S., M.D., F.A.C.P.
Professor of Medicine
Chief, Division of Gastroenterology
University of Kansas Medical Center
Kansas City, Kansas
Consultant in Gastroenterology at Veterans Administration Hospitals
Kansas City, Missouri and Wadsworth, Kansas and
Menorah Medical Center
Kansas City, Missouri

SEIBI KOBAYASHI, M.D., PH.D.
Senior Physician, Department of Medicine
Aichi Cancer Center Hospital
Nagoya, Japan

ROBERT R. LAING, M.D.
Fellow International Academy of Proctology
Associate Fellow, American College of Gastroenterology
Assistant Clinical Professor of Medicine, Kansas University Medical Center
Consultant in Medicine, Kansas City and Wadsworth Veterans Hospitals
Chief, Gastroenterology, Bethany Medical Center
Chief, Department of Medicine
Providence-St. Margaret's Health Center
Kansas City, Kansas

JEAN LAURENT, M.D.
Chief, Digestive Disease Clinic
des hopitaux de Nancy
Member, Cabinet De Groupe De Gastro-Enterologie
Nancy, France

HERWARTH LENT, M.D.
Chief Physician, Department of Internal Medicine
Evangelical Hospital
Bergisch Gladbach, Germany

PHILIP A. LOPRESTI, A.B., M.D., F.A.C.P.
Assistant Professor, Clinical Medicine
New York University School of Medicine
Chairman, Department of Medicine and Division of Gastroenterology
Catholic Medical Center of Brooklyn, New York

WILLIAM M. LUKASH, A.B., M.D., F.A.C.P., F.A.C.G., A.G.A.
Assistant Professor of Medicine, Georgetown University
Washington, D.C.

Rear Admiral (MC) U.S. Navy
Head, Gastroenterology Clinic and Research Branch, National Naval Medical Center
Bethesda, Maryland
White House Physician

RICHARD S. McCRAY, A.B., B.D., M.D.
Assistant Clinical Professor of Medicine, Columbia University
College of Physicians and Surgeons
Associate Attending Physician and Associate Director
Clinical Gastrointestinal Unit, St. Luke's Hospital Center
New York, New York

KIYOMI MIURA, M.D.
Assistant Professor, Department of Medicine
Tohoku University School of Medicine
Sendai, Japan
Assistant Professor, Medical Department of Professor S. Yamagata

JOHN F. MORRISSEY, B.A., M.D., F.A.C.P.
Professor and Vice Chairman, Department of Medicine
University of Wisconsin

ROBERT S. NELSON, B.S., B.M., M.D., F.A.C.P.
Professor, Department of Medicine, University of Texas
General Faculty
Chief, Gastroenterology Section, Department of Medicine
University of Texas
M. D. Anderson Hospital and Tumor Institute
Consultant, Brooke General Hospital
San Antonio, Texas
Consultant, V. A. Hospital
Houston, Texas

YANAO OGURO, M.D.
Chief, Internal Medicine Clinic
National Cancer Center Hospital, Tokyo, Japan

ITARU OI, M.D.
Assistant, Department of Medicine, Division of Gastroenterology
Associate Director of Gastrointestinal Endoscopy
Tokyo Women's Medical College, Japan

ARTHUR M. OLSEN, A.B., M.D., M.S., F.A.C.P.
Professor of Medicine, Mayo Graduate School of Medicine
University of Minnesota
Rochester, Minnesota
Senior Consultant in Internal Medicine and Thoracic Diseases at the Mayo Clinic

RUDOLF OTTENJANN, M.D.
Professor of Medicine and Gastroenterology, University of Erlangen
Nuernberg, Germany

BERGEIN OVERHOLT, M.D.
  Associate Professor of Medicine and Gastroenterology
  University of Tennessee
  Knoxville, Tennessee

EDDY D. PALMER, M.D., F.A.C.P.
  Clinical Professor of Medicine, Rutgers Medical School, Piscataway, N.J.
  Morristown, New Jersey

KODURI R. PRASADRAO, M.B., B.S., M.D.
  Fellow in Gastroenterology, Cook County Hospital
  Chicago, Illinois

ERNESTO J. PULETTI, M.S. (Pharmacology), M.D.
  Assistant Director, Gastrointestinal Research Laboratory
  Franklin Hospital Foundation
  San Francisco, California

JOSEPH ALFRED RIDER, M.D., Ph.D. (Pharmacology), F.A.C.P.
  Director, Gastrointestinal Research Laboratory
  Franklin Hospital Foundation
  San Francisco, California

HANS WOLFGANG ROESCH, M.D.
  Lecturer, Department of Medicine
  University of Erlangen
  Nuernberg, Germany

YOSHIHIRO SAKAI, M.D.
  Associate Director Gastrointestinal Endoscopy, Department of Medicine
  Tokyo Medical College, Japan

TAKAO SAKITA, M.D.
  Professor, Department of Medicine
  University of Tsukuba, Japan

LESLIE JORDAN SANDLOW, M.D., F.A.C.P.
  Assistant Professor, Department of Medicine, University of Chicago
  Attending Physician and Physician in Charge, Clinical Gastroenterology Laboratory
  Deputy Vice President for Professional Affairs, Michael Reese Hospital and Medical
    Center, Chicago

HIROMI SHINYA, M.D.
  Assistant Professor of Surgery, Mount Sinai School of Medicine
  Chief of Surgical Endoscopy Unit, Beth Israel Medical Center
  New York, New York

MITCHELL A. SPELLBERG, M.S., M.D., F.A.C.P., F.A.C.G.
  Clinical Professor of Medicine, Pritzker School of Medicine
  Division of Biological Sciences, University of Chicago
  Senior Attending Physician and Acting Chairman, Division of Gastroenterology,
    Michael Reese Hospital and Medical Center, Chicago

HIROSHI TADAKI, M.D.
Instructor, Department of Medicine
Tohoku University School of Medicine
Sendai, Japan
Instructor and Assistant, Medical Department of Professor S. Yamagata

SACHIO TAKASU, M.D.
Fellow of Japanese Society of Gastroenterological Endoscopy
Chief of Gastrointestinal Department
Kanto-Teishin Hospital, Japan

TADAYOSHI TAKEMOTO, M.D., F.I.S.E.
Professor of the Department of Medicine
Director of Division of Gastroenterology
Tokyo Women's Medical College, Japan

SADATAKA TASAKA, M.D.
Fellow of Japanese Society of Internal Medicine
President of Japanese Society of Gastroenterological Endoscopy
Emeritus Professor of Internal Medicine
University of Tokyo
Director of Kanto-Rosai Hospital, Japan

KENJI TSUNEOKA, M.D.
Professor of the Third Department of Internal Medicine
Nippon Medical School
Tokyo, Japan

JOEL VALENCIA-PARPARCEN, M.D., F.A.C.G.
Professor and Chairman, Department of Gastroenterology
School of Medicine, Central University of Venezuela
Chairman, Gastroenterology Unit, University Hospital
Caracas, Venezuela
Consultant at "Centro Medico de Caracas"

FERNANDO VILLA, M.D.
Member, A.S.G.E., Member, A.C.G.
Associate Professor in Medicine, Loyola University
Chicago, Illinois
Attending Physician, Cook County Hospital
Assistant Director in Gastroenterology, Cook County Hospital
Chicago, Illinois

NOBORU WATANABE, M.D.
Research Fellow of the Third Department of Internal Medicine
Nippon Medical School
Tokyo, Japan

TO

PARENTAL INSPIRATION

AND

THE STIMULATION OF STUDENTS AND ASSOCIATES

PREFACE

D URING THE TRANSITION YEARS between the waning period of semiflexible tube lens gastroscopy and fiberoscopy, there were many inquiries
about the newer technics. My students at Cook County Graduate School of
Medicine and residents at Cook County Hospital frequently requested information regarding endoscopy reference manuals which discussed basic
principles of gastrointestinal endoscopy as well as fiberoptic technics.
Schindler's excellent textbook remained the leading treatise in the English
language on the basic principles of lens gastroscopy and endoscopic pathology of the stomach. However, there was no well known single text which
treated basic principles of upper and lower gastrointestinal endoscopy and
endoscopic pathology. The available texts treated esophagoscopy, gastroscopy and proctoscopy separately and for the most part dealt only with
rigid or semirigid tube technics.

There appeared to be a clear need for a text which would combine the
discussion of basic principles of fiberoptic gastrointestinal endoscopy in
a single textbook for all organs which had been explored. The concept of
pan-endoscopy was clearly on the horizon. The author felt that such a text
should bear heavily on the details of technic and discuss endoscopic pathology as it occurs throughout the alimentary canal. For indeed there is
a basic and fundamental relationship of structure, function, etiological
factors and disease patterns throughout the digestive canal. The idea of
a comprehensive monograph by international contributors was discussed
on a preliminary basis with some of the very active gastroenterologists in
the field whom the writer had known for many years. All of them expressed approval and recognition of the potential value of such a book if
the language barrier could be sufficiently bridged editorially to achieve a
harmonious interrelated monograph.

The idea continued to expand and become firm as the writer talked to
more and more prospective co-authors at various national and international gastroenterology meetings and congresses.

The principal justification of this book lies in the attempt to record a
broad discussion of guidelines and to present a reference manual adequately illustrated with black and white figures and a generous color atlas
for students of gastrointestinal endoscopy. In every technical field, reference manuals and guidelines are used as an essential companion of training and the learning process. In no important technical field, certainly not

those dealing with human life are manuals and guidelines offered as a possible substitute for apprenticeship training.

This undertaking has been its own reward for the senior author and editor and hopefully the same has been true for all of the contributors. The writer feels a special sense of accomplishment in the fact that six of the contributors received their basic training in endoscopy under his tutelage. Doctors Villa, Adomavicius and Alavi are still actively associated as attending physicians with the writer in the Endoscopy Clinic of Cook County Hospital and in research at the Hektoen Institute for Medical Research.

The writing of "Gastrointestinal Pan-Endoscopy with International Contributors" has resulted from a union of professional spirit and trust between men of many nations and cultures. A byproduct has been that experience which goes beyond geography and language, the human sentiment of friendship. My deep and sincere gratitude goes to each of my medical colleagues and friends, the contributors from four major continents of the world.

LEONIDAS H. BERRY

INTRODUCTION

ENDOSCOPY HAS BEEN a very rapidly developing subject since the introduction of the fibre-optic instruments, and the time is opportune for bringing together all the growing points in this field and to assess the contributions that have been made. Progress has been made in a number of countries around the world, and this book is unique in the international representation which is demonstrated by the contributors who come from four continents and ten countries. One of the fascinations of gastroenterology is the geographical variation of diseases. The high incidence of gastric cancer in Japan, for example, has resulted in special concentration of Japanese endoscopy studies of this condition. This has resulted in a much better understanding of the early natural history of the disease and in much improved screening techniques for early diagnosis. In Great Britain and Germany, with their higher risk of carcinoma of the colon, the technique of colonoscopy has been greatly improved. This has resulted not only in more accurate diagnosis, but also as a means for treatment, and the colonoscopist is now beginning to acquire the skills needed for removing polyps, which hitherto would have meant the patient having a laparotomy.

The aim of the authors has been to produce a basic treatise of pathology and background applied physiology relating to endoscopy of the alimentary tract. The techniques involved are all described in considerable detail, and all those who are working in this field of activity will benefit from this concentration of international experience. Many will appreciate particularly the well-written and very interesting account of the history of endoscopy. The extensive and up-to-date bibliography will prove of great help to all serious students and authors.

The older generation of endoscopists will have been brought up on Dr. Rudolf Schindler's *Gastroscopy, the Endoscopic Study of Gastric Pathology*. Although this book remains remarkably interesting, the wider scope of flexible endoscopy has resulted in a number of recent publications, among which this one is the most extensive and certainly the most international. One of the problems of present-day medicine is to narrow the ever-present gap between knowledge and practice, and this book makes a very admirable contribution towards this end. As senior author and editor of this book Dr. Berry has achieved a very worthy successor to Dr. Rudolf Schindler's classic publication.

F. AVERY JONES

London
October, 1973

xvii

ACKNOWLEDGMENTS

THE ROOTS OF the motivation and inspiration to produce this book extend to the beginnings of my entrance into the study and practice of gastroenterology and gastroscopy. I therefore wish to acknowledge those individuals and institutions which played a significant role in the development of the background for the conception of the book as well as for the creation of the book itself.

Chronologically I am indebted to Dr. Homer Wilburn, former Medical Director of Provident Hospital and the co-partnership of this Hospital and the University of Chicago which made possible my specialty training and early practice of gastroenterology and gastroscopy. Next I am indebted to the late Sidney A. Portis who sponsored my training as a Fellow in Internal Medicine and Gastroenterology at the Cook County Hospital and directed my interest into the field of my career in medicine. It was Dr. Portis who introduced me to Dr. Rudolf Schindler who was then Associate Professor at the University of Chicago under whom I was privileged to study the technic and endoscopic pathology of the stomach at Billings and Provident Hospitals. I must acknowledge posthumously the loyal assistance of Dr. T. Jonathan Cole, an early associate at Provident Hospital.

From the time that I first established the Department of Gastroenterology and the Gastroscopy Clinic at Provident Hospital to my present involvement as Chief of the Gastrointestinal Endoscopy Service at Cook County Hospital, I have enjoyed the good fortune and support of excellent nursing assistants. I therefore, wish to express by gratitude to Major Jewel Patterson, R.N., USAF Ret. and Minnie Raines Morris, R.N., my first gastroscopy nurses, long time assistants Juanita Purnell, R.N. and Carrielee Hilton, L.P.N. and recently Anne Smith, R.N. My thanks and deep appreciation must go to my secretaries Cora C. Williams, Delores Davis and Vivian Headen whose dedicated interests were indispenable. Jeffery Williams, art student, and particularly Nancy Swan of the Department of Medical Arts, University of Illinois Medical Center (Professor Hooker Goodwin, Director), are responsible for the art work. We are deeply grateful to Mr. Reinhold Wappler of the American Cystoscope Makers and to the Olympus Corporation of America for their support. Mr. Payne Thomas and Robert Schinneer of the Charles C Thomas Publishing Company were most helpful in the final preparation of the manuscript. The continuing opportunity to teach endoscopy through the administrations of

Deans James Askin, John Neal and Eugene Meyer at the Cook County Graduate School of Medicine for 26 years is gratefully acknowledged. I am also indebted to the Hektoen Institute of Medical Research, Dr. Samuel Hoffman, Director.

The excellent cooperation of all of our contributors from many parts of the world has been most stimulating and my deep and sincere gratitude goes to all of them individually and collectively.

Many other persons made contributions directly and indirectly who cannot be named individually but to whom I am deeply grateful. Finally without the tolerance and understanding of my devoted wife, my role as senior author and editor of this book would not have been possible. For this I am most appreciative and thankful.

L.H.B.

CONTENTS

SECTION I

INTRODUCTORY CONSIDERATIONS IN UPPER GASTROINTESTINAL ENDOSCOPY

Chapter

xxi

SECTION II

ENDOSCOPIC PATHOLOGY OF THE ESOPHAGUS

SECTION III

ENDOSCOPIC PATHOLOGY OF THE STOMACH

SECTION VII

MISCELLANEOUS SUBJECTS OF IMPORTANCE IN UPPER GASTROINTESTINAL ENDOSCOPY

SECTION VIII

PERITONEOSCOPY IN GASTROENTEROLOGY

GASTROINTESTINAL
PAN-ENDOSCOPY

SECTION I

INTRODUCTORY CONSIDERATIONS IN UPPER GASTROINTESTINAL ENDOSCOPY

CHAPTER I

HISTORY OF GASTROINTESTINAL ENDOSCOPY

NORBERT HENNING AND LEONIDAS H. BERRY

INTRODUCTORY STATEMENT

T̲H̲E̲ H̲I̲S̲T̲O̲R̲Y̲ O̲F̲ Gastrointestinal Endoscopy from its primitive and frustrating beginnings to its present state of sophistication has been slow largely because it had to await developments in light sources, light transmission, optics and photography. However, many ingenious devices were used with limited success in the earlier period which laid the foundation of Gastrointestinal Endoscopy.

The history of Gastrointestinal Endoscopy may be looked upon as having developed through three phases: the earliest phase from 1795 to 1932 when the straight rigid tubes were used, the second phase of semiflexible tube endoscopy from 1932 to 1958 and finally the present era of fiberoptic endoscopy, which has continued at a very rapid pace since 1958.

THE EARLY PHASE—RIGID SCOPES
(1795-1932)

Endoscopy probably had its beginnings with the work of Bozzini[1] (Fig. 1-1) in 1795. He constructed an instrument for the examination of the rectum and the uterus and used the candle as the light source. This was followed soon afterwards by Segales of France who presented a modification of Bozzini's instrument before the Royal Academy of Science in 1826. von Desormeaux[2] (Fig. 1-2) in 1853 developed an apparatus for illuminating the endoscope using light obtained from an alcohol and turpentine

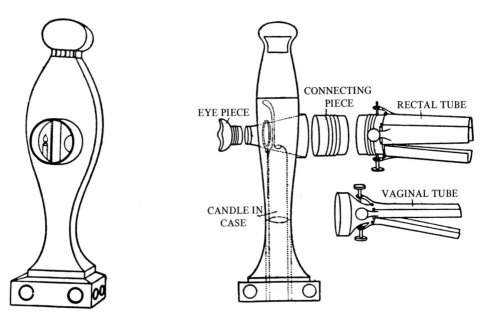

Figure 1-1. (Left) Bozzini Lamp. Note lighted candle. (Right) Endoscope holder with rectal and vaginal tubes.

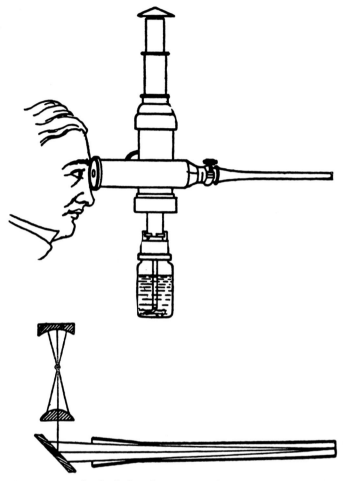

Figure 1-2. Desormeux's alcohol and turpentine lamp with attached endoscope.

lamp. The light after going through a lens system was directed into the endoscope by a forehead reflector. Kussmaul[3] introduced the first gastroscope in 1868 using straight metal tubes with flexible obturators. After watching a sword-swallower, he felt that by introduction of a metal tube it was possible to get the upper dental area and cardia in one straight line. This was the basis of all the rigid gastroscopes that followed. The flexible obturator was passed first and the rigid tube was then passed over the obturator. The obturator was then withdrawn. He used the Desormeaux lamp, but found the illumination to be insufficient and discarded the method.

While some workers were concerning themselves with gastroscopes, others were developing the rigid tube esophagoscope. The first esophagoscope was described by Bevan in 1868.[4] It was used for the extraction of a foreign body and for the examination of tumors and was four inches long.

This was soon followed by Waldenburg's instrument in 1870, which was a single rigid tube with a proximal diameter of 5cm and distal diameter of 1cm. It was modified by using two tubes telescoping into one another and giving an examination field of 12cm length. Concentrated daylight was used as the light source.

Stoerk[5] in 1881 was the first to examine the entire length of the esophagus. His instrument had two movable tubes with a hand grip in the instrument to bring the two tubes into straight line after introduction into the esophagus.

Nitze,[6] using the principles of his cystoscope, developed a gastroscopic instrument in 1879, with an electrically heated platinum wire loop as the light source. This needed a constant stream of water for cooling. It proved impractical and the findings were never published.

An important landmark in the development of the principles of gastroscopy was the work of Mikulicz[7] in 1881. Basing his work on sound anatomical principles, he constructed a gastroscope with an angle of 30 degrees between the distal and the proximal two-thirds. Though he gave up his work due to technical difficulties, his basic ideas contributed to the development of later gastroscopes. Mikulicz should be considered a most important theoretical pioneer before Schindler.

The principle of flexible metal tubes which could be easily introduced and straightened after introduction was developed by Kelling.[8]

It is only natural that scientific curiosity and perhaps urgent necessity had led to attempts to explore the rectum as well as the esophagus and stomach. At the turn of the century when the miniature Edison electric bulb was invented, the first endoscope to be equipped with this source of light was the proctoscope. In 1902, Tuttle[9] made the earliest proctoscope with an electric light carrier (see Chapter 29 for references and description of proctosigmoidoscopes).

Crude surgical procedures on the rectum are recorded in the literature of antiquity and the middle ages. "Epidemic gangrenous rectitis" was described in 1623 by Aleixo d' Abreu.[10] The study and treatment of rectal diseases as a special entity had its beginning with Dr. Fred Salmon's[11] "Fistula Infirmary" in London in 1835. Instruments for use in the rectum were developed along surgical lines. Before the use of tubular instruments for visualization and before the use of anesthetics, hemorrhoids were pulled down with a hook-like instrument known as a velsellum so that they could be well seen and extirpated (Garrison[12]).

As proctology developed, tubal anoscopes and rectal specula were used before proctoscopes and sigmoidoscopes. The rectal speculum with flanges capable of being anchored in place at the desired degree of rectal opening was a favorite for years. Anoscopes with an obturator and a slanting end

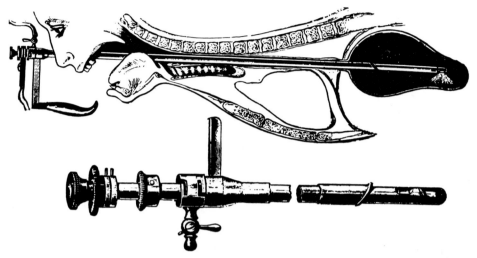

Figure 1-3. Sussman's "flexible" gastroscope which was straightened for "viewing" (1911).

of the Hirschman type are popular, especially with surgeons. Another type bearing the name Brinkerhoff has a sliding panel which exposes a strip of the sidewall of the rectum.

Rosenheim[13] first used the miniature electric lamp for illumination in a gastroscope in 1906. Shortly afterwards, an improved rigid instrument called Bruening's electroscope was used for a few years (Fig. 1-3).

Also during the year 1906, Chevalier Jackson[14] in the United States published his first textbook on bronchoesophagoscopy and with his son, Chevalier L. Jackson, continued a long and distinguished career.[15] He devised bronchoesophagoscopes and special instruments for removing foreign bodies, became world famed, not only for his foreign-body extractions, but also for his writings on inflammations of the trachea, bronchi and the esophagus. He published comprehensive treatises on endoscopy.

Loening and Stieda[16] in 1908 constructed a gastroscope which had an outer tube that was flexible in its lower part and an inner rigid optical tube. However, this still had all the disadvantages of the rigid instruments.

A pioneer in the early twentieth century was Elsner[17] who developed a modified rigid gastroscope which had a rubber finger at its end allowing the safe passage through the lower esophagus and the cardia and the possibility of perforating the distal esophagus was minimized. Schindler's first totally rigid gastroscope was based largely upon the principle of this instrument.

Sussman[18] in 1911 built a metal gastroscope consisting of two segmented concentric tubes. The joints permitted the instrument to be flexible when

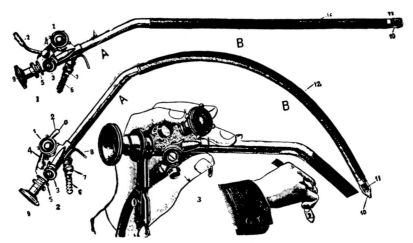

Figure 1-4. Bruening's electroscope. One of the first to use electric illumination (about 1907).

lying in the same plane. When rotated so that the joints were not in the same plane, the tube became straight (Fig. 1-4). This instrument and others of this era remained crude, cumbersome and impractical.

After the advent of the miniature electric bulb, the evolution of a practical gastroscope was on a relatively uninterrupted course for the first time. One European enthusiast was a Doctor Sternberg whose technic of examination raised more controversy than his gastroscope. The successive positions illustrated in Figure 1-5 were viewed with a wide variety of responses from astonishment to compassion. Such was the early crude history of Gastrointestinal Endoscopy.

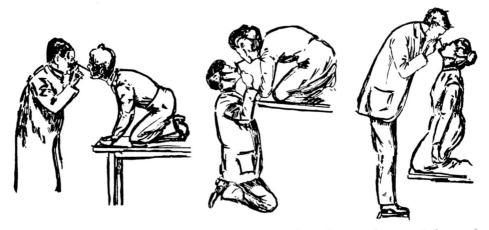

Figure 1-5. Three successive positions used by Sternberg for introduction of the rigid gastroscope (early 1920's).

First Concepts of Gastroscopic Pathology
(1922-1932)

During the decade from 1922 to 1932, there was considerable enthusiasm and work with rigid lens gastroscopes by a few dedicated workers. Among them was Francois Moutier,[19] generally recognized as the father of gastroscopy in France. He published many abstracts, a textbook on gastroscopy and endoscopic pathology of the stomach and an important monograph on gastritis, co-authored with Cornet[20] in later years. Schindler refers frequently to Moutier, Henning and Gutzeit as the significant contributors to the development of gastroscopy during this period.[21] Gutzeit described the clinical value of gastroscopy and Henning wrote a book on endoscopic concepts of gastritis.

Schindler in 1922 introduced his rigid gastroscope which was based on the principle of Elsner's instrument and performed several hundred gastroscopies. While the previous workers had been using the method for the study of isolated lesions, the focus now shifted to the study of endoscopic pathology of the stomach in general. Schindler's "Handbook and Atlas of Gastroscopy"[22] appeared in 1923. In this treatise based on several hundred gastroscopies, he described chronic gastritis, adenomas, myomas, lymphosarcoma, carcinoma and many aspects of the post-operative stomach. His first English article described the aspects of 30 cases of gastric neoplasms in 1923.[23] Schindler and his followers between 1923 and 1932 wrote the first systematic descriptions of gastroscopic pathology in monographic textbooks, the best known being Schindler's book of 1937. Much of this work was carried out with the hazard of rigid tube instruments and helped greatly in generating the demand and the genius for better tolerated and more efficient instruments.

SECOND PHASE—SEMIFLEXIBLE LENS SCOPES
(1932-1958)

Schindler Era of Gastroscopy

With the exploitation by Wolf and Schindler of the principle that it was possible to see through a curved tube with a series of short focal distance lenses, the Wolf-Schindler gastroscope was introduced in 1932 (Fig. 1-6). This was truly the beginning of the era of practical gastroscopy. For the first time there was a real practical breakthrough which made perhaps four fifths or seven eighths of the gastric mucosa adequately illuminated and excellently visualized. In fact, fiberoptic scopes have not excelled the clarity of vision and resolution of semiflexible lens instruments. There was only moderate discomfort in most instances. Because of these new ad-

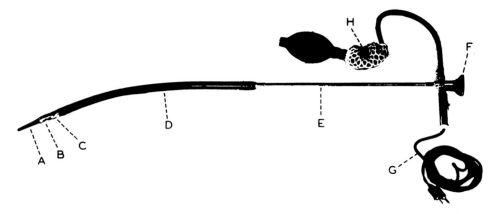

Figure 1-6. Wolff-Schindler instrument. First semiflexible lens gastroscope (1932).

vantages and the remarkable enthusiasm and dedicated work of Schindler, the gastroscopic method began its development as a standard advanced diagnostic procedure. Its spread became international and semiflexible lens gastroscopy was to last for more than a quarter of a century. Schindler truly became the father of gastroscopy. Just two years after the advent of the new instrument in Munich, Germany, Schindler moved to Chicago and remained in the United States until his retirement in 1964, except for a year in Brazil. The thrust of the evolutionary history of endoscopy shifted from Europe for its major development to the United States.

First Semiflexible Lens Gastroscope—Schindler (1932)

The Schindler semiflexible lens gastroscope was built upon the optical principle of Lang who in 1917 had found that an optical image could be transmitted through a curved tube by means of several thick convex lenses and the image would retain its clarity if the curvature was not too great. The Schindler instrument had a soft rubber finger and a prism objective. Near the objective there was a removable eight volt miniature electrical bulb. The gastroscope was a closed tube 78cm (31 inches) long. The flexible portion was 24.5cm in length and 12mm in diameter. The upper rigid portion was 34cm long and 8.5mm in diameter. The flexible and rigid portions contained numerous short focus convex lenses arranged at short distances apart.

Modified Semiflexible Lens Scopes

Many modifications of the Schindler gastroscope were developed. Henning modified this instrument (Figs. 1-7 & 8), with two models—one in 1939, another in 1948. He used a rubber balloon instead of the elastic rubber finger and relocated the optic window high, making it possible to clean

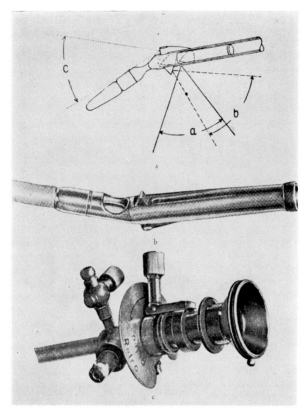

Figure 1-7. (By Dr. Henning) Omniangle semiflexible gastroscope by Henning with prograde, orthograde and maximal retrograde vision, using only one optic shaft or tube (1939).

the optic on the posterior wall when the objective was soiled. The proximal rigid part was also made smaller to 7.5mm and was more comfortable to the patient.

In 1932, Henning[24] introduced esophagoscopy into gastroenterology for diagnostic purposes. Prior to this time, esophagoscopy was exclusively within the province of otolaryngology primarily for removal of foreign bodies. The extraction of foreign bodies was left to the laryngologists. The esophagoscope used by Henning had a diameter of 7.0mm and had a visual angle of 60 degrees. It had an outer tube and two inner optics which could be changed during examination. It was possible also to examine the cardia and the upper gastric mucosa. Henning described the endoscopic view of the esophageal mucosa for the first time and also described the appearance of esophageal varices in their earlier stages. With the help of his camera attachment, Henning was able to take esophagophotograms for the first time.

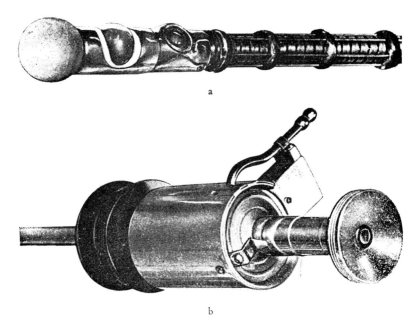

Figure 1-8. (By Dr. Henning) All directions semiflexible gastroscope by Henning without cover (1948).

Herman Taylor[25] of London in 1941 devised a lens gastroscope with a distal flexible portion which could be deflected at the tip, eliminating some portion of the blind areas. However, because of the increased length of the rigid portion, the cardia had to be passed by the rigid part and thereby the chief advantage of the standard instrument was lost. The Taylor instrument had a flexible portion of greater diameter and was not altogether a safe instrument though it was a good adjunct in the hands of expert examiners. Shortly after the Taylor model came the Eder-Palmer Gastroscope (Fig. 1-9), of smaller diameter (9mm) than the Schindler gastroscope. It was designed to be introduced through the Eder-Hufford (see Chapter 5, Fig. 5-1) rigid open tube esophagoscope, but was used more frequently without the esophagoscope. Its tip could be deflected in one direction. It became very popular and virtually replaced the original Schindler lens scope in the United States for a period.

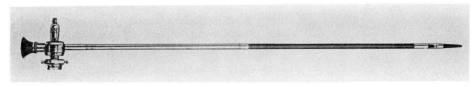

Figure 1-9. The slender (9mm) Eder-Palmer lens scope designed for introduction through the rigid Eder-Hufford esophogoscope.

An important improvement in the technic of endoscopy was made possible by the Eder-Hufford[26] rigid esophagoscope with a flexible obturator (1949). The instrument had a detachable telescope which magnified the image five times. It was passed with the patient lying on his left side in a manner similar to that used in passing the Schindler-type gastroscope.

Cameron developed an "omniangle gastroscope" using the same principle used on the rigid scope by Hohlweg.[27] However the mechanism was more ingenious and consisted of a mirror that could be tilted by a small selenoid which became magnetic on passage of the electric current. However, the blind area was not fully eliminated. The Cameron lens scope was a good instrument and was widely used in the Western Hemisphere.

Hardt[28] introduced a "flexi-rigid" gastroscope in 1944. The instrument had an outer sheath, the lower end of which was flexible. This portion was passed first and a rigid tube containing lenses was then introduced. It had no advantages over the Schindler lens scope.

In 1948 the principle of a built-in biopsy capability was first introduced. This form of gastroscope was devised by ACMI and Benedict.[29] With the provision of an additional canal it was possible to use a biopsy forceps. This *operating* gastroscope was oval and had an excellent lens system. The biopsy specimen was frequently small and inadequate and only a single specimen could be taken at a time, and its construction was hazardous to the patient.

Biopsy and Photography

Eight years before the development of the Benedict biopsy scope, biopsy attachments for existing scopes were being devised. Kenamore[30] in 1940 devised a biopsy forceps which was attached to the Schindler semiflexible gastroscope. It was found to be dangerous and was used very little. Wood[31] and his associates carried out extensive blind biopsy procedures in Australia. They used a simple suction tube not attached to a gastroscope. These studies established the value of suction biopsy in diffuse gastric diseases. It was, of course, impossible to direct the apparatus. Tomenius[32] devised a suction attachment built in a permanent fashion to a Schindler semiflexible lens scope with the help of the Metro-Tec Company of Chicago. It was a useful instrument in certain parts of the stomach, but could not be accurately directed to a small target lesion. Berry[33] with the help of the Eder Instrument Company devised a direct vision suction gastrobiopsy instrument for use with the Eder-Palmer semiflexible lens gastroscope. The instrument was first demonstrated on a patient before the American Gastroscopic Society during a "wet" session of its annual meeting in Chicago in 1956 (further discussion of this instrument in Chapter 28I).

During the Schindler era, there was some progress in the field of photography. Henning and Keilhack[34] had obtained the first satisfactory color photographs through the old rigid scope in 1938. The first successful black and white photographs made with the semiflexible Schindler lens scope were produced by Segal and Watkins.[35] Lange[36] and Meltzing probably devised the first intragastric photographic camera. It was attached to the end of a rubber tube and introduced into the stomach. This effort was made in 1898. Its results were crude and unsatisfactory. Heilpern and Back[37] used the same principle in their gastrophotor in 1929.

Henning[38] made black and white photographs through the Schindler rigid scope which were photographically satisfactory. However, it was obvious that only color photographs would finally meet the needs of gastroscopy. The first color photographs were made by Henning and Keilhack.[34] Segal and Watkins[35] made the first satisfactory color photographs through the semiflexible lens gastroscope (for further discussion of still and cinephotography see Chapter 26).

Ancillary Technics

The most unsatisfactory feature of gastroscopy with the Schindler type semiflexible lens gastroscope was the four *blind* spots which could not be reached in every patient. The most important of these was the prepyloric antral lesser curvature. Another was a narrow strip along the posterior wall at the level of the middle and upper body. Two other blind spots were the fundic area and a small area along the greater curvature, lower body and upper antrum. The movable tips and omniangle mechanism had failed to eliminate these blind areas. Rogers[39] in 1939 had devised a rubber cuff supporting a small balloon which would slide over the shaft of the instrument and when inflated was meant to push away the posterior wall to bring that blind spot into view. It was only partly successful and was soon discarded.

Efforts to improve the *blind* spots continued throughout the Schindler era of gastroscopy. The Eder-Palmer gastroscope was finally manufactured with a recessed lamp and larger window. Schindler states that this method was first suggested by Ould and Daley. This innovation improved the upper posterior wall view in some cases.

It was suggested by Berry[40] that the right-side position on the examining table be used in difficult cases. This improved the visualization of the all important lesser curvature prepyloric *blind* spot. The right-side technic occurred to the author when he had occasion to examine a patient in the standard left-side position which was a case of situs inversus with dextra gastrica. When this patient was examined on his left side, the prepyloric lesser curvature *blind* spot was improved. A number of anatomically normal patients were then comparatively examined on the right and left sides and the findings reported in 1941. The multiple positions technic of examining patients first on the left then dorsal and sometimes right sides (with the instrument *in situ*) was then followed routinely by Berry and others. In 1963, Berry published a report on the "Improved Gastroscopic Diagnosis by the Use of Multiple Positions in Two Thousand Eight Hundred Forty-Three Cases."[41] This technic was readily adopted by the author's students and others through the years. It is still found to be of occasional value, even with fiberoptic instruments (see Chapter 6).

Other ancillary technics to improve diagnoses continued to be devised during the Schindler era, none of them really solving the major problems completely. Various workers in pathology and other fields observed what appeared to be a specific affinity between certain fluorescent dyes and cancer cells. Technics were then devised whereby such dyes were administered to patients with suspected cancer of the breast, brain and other organs and observations for fluorescence under ultraviolet light were carried out. Attempts were made by Berry to apply this principle to gastroscopy. With the assistance of the Eder Instrument Company and A. Vercellati, an electric light bulb engineer of the General Electric Company, a removable head of the Eder-Palmer instrument was equipped with glass window filters permitting the passage of ultraviolet light. The problem of insufficient ultraviolet light in the stomach was not solved. In 1960, Klinger and Katz of Chile, South America, reported the use of ultraviolet light in the examination of gastric washings after tetracycline administration in the diagnosis of gastric cancer. Berk has continued throughout the last decade to further develop these technics and to adapt them to gastroscopy with fiberoptic instruments with some success. In the early fifties, Berry and the Eder Instrument Company constructed an all flexible lens gastroscope. It was not marketed because of its excessive weight, problems of torque and expense.

Gastrocamera

The practical development of a successful intragastric camera was achieved by Uji[42] in 1950 in Japan. At the World Congress of Gastoenterology in 1958 held in Washington, D.C., Tasaka and Ashizawa[43] reported brilliant color photographs taken by this method. Gastrocamera became so successful in Japan, that it virtually displaced the use of the Schindler type lens gastroscope in that country during the 1950s. The use of multiple photographs made during a few minutes after the passage of a tiny instrument which seldom needed local anesthesia was an exciting development for those who used it in Japan (see further discussion in Chapter 14).

Clinical Gastroscopy

The Schindler era of gastroscopy—brilliant in its day—was a period of search for the final perfection of a new and dramatic breakthrough in gastric diagnosis. In relation to modern industrial expertise, the required quarter of a century of semiflexible gastroscopy was not much faster than the crude and painful preceding century of frustrations. There had to be a time of education of gastroenterologists, surgeons and patients. There had to be a time of establishment of the value of the method in a technically advanced society. The Schindler era served these purposes and in the process, a massive body of scientific literature in clinical gastroenterology was also established. Thus, a new diagnostic clinical science supported by new concepts was ready to encompass the next major breakthrough, namely the current era of Fiberoptic Gastrointestinal Endoscopy.

THIRD PHASE—FIBEROPTIC ENDOSCOPES
(1958-   )

The fiberoptic era began with the introduction of the first practical fibergastroscope by Hirschowitz and associates in 1958.[44] The development of this instrument ushered in the third phase in the history of gastroscopy and revolutionary improvements destined to affect endoscopy of all organs where the method had been in use and many undeveloped areas for future explorations.

First Fiberoptic Gastroduodenoscope

The Hirschowitz fiberscope of 1958 was manufactured by the American Cystoscope Makers Incorporated of New York. The technic of introducing the fiberscope was much easier than passing the semiflexible scope for the amateur operator. However, many trained endoscopists could introduce the lens instrument with less discomfort to the patient than that produced by the fiberscope in the hands of an untrained operator. Generally speaking however, the fiberoptic instrument in average hands was considerably less discomforting to the patient. In the earlier years, more injuries were reported by the fiberscope than with the lens scope. This type of unexpected results appears to be changing in the more recent years (see Chapter 32).

The fiberoptic instruments, however, did not solve all of the hazards of endoscopy. This is due partly to the greater use of endoscopes and to the fact that operators with insufficient or no training are inclined to use these instruments. In addition to greater ease of passage, the flexibility of fiberscopes began to solve the remaining *blind* spots of lens gastroscopy. Today, there are practically no blind areas encountered by trained endoscopists for the great majority of patients. Besides these improvements, great strides have been made in photography, biopsy and other refined diagnostic technics (see Chapters 25-27). The progressive development of the various types of instruments are detailed in Chapter Five. However, there are a few points which should be mentioned in the historical development of fiber-optic instruments, since some of these excellent instruments are already obsolete in the wake of amazing and rapid advances.

Types of Fiberscopes

After the development of the first fiberscope by ACMI which was a side-viewing gastroduodenoscope, this company proceeded to develop a forward-viewing esophagogastroscope. This was capable of examining the upper end of the stomach as well as the esophagus and also higher resected stomachs. This was soon followed by similar instruments from Japan.

The Olympus Company had developed an excellent side-viewing gastroscope with precision biopsy and extragastric photographic capabilities. The Olympus Company combined the gastrocamera with a fiberscope in their instrument known as the GFT and later added the movable tip in their instrument known as GFTA. This was a landmark development, for now it was possible to observe a lesion and photograph it under direct vision using up to 32 exposures in a very few minutes. While the photographic technic of these instruments was very simple and the photographs were excellent, other instruments were soon to be preferred by the endoscopists as fiber-optic instruments with new capabilities began to be manufactured rapidly. Excellent biopsy procedures are now carried out wherever mucosa is seen. Cine photography and brush cytology are easily and beneficially performed.

In the last few years, forward-viewing esophagogastroduodenoscopes capable of examining the esophagus, stomach and the duodenum in one sitting have become quite popular. While these instruments are very good, experienced endoscopists realize that the most thorough survey of the stomach is made with the side-viewing instrument. At the present time, side-viewing instruments give little or no visualization in the esophagus. Long side-viewing gastroduodenoscopes are being made by the major manufacturers for the examination of the stomach, bulbar and post-bulbar portions of the duodenum and the cannulation of the papilla of vater. The Eder-Villa instrument was the first to combine side viewing with forward viewing in the same instrument. It was used for a few years, but is no longer on the market.

The Machida Company of Japan during the last year, has introduced a combined side-viewing and forward-viewing instrument with photographic and biopsy capabilities. This instrument seems to have a good future.

It is historically most interesting that so many technics have evolved so rapidly during the last few years.

Colonoscopes

It was inevitable that the fiberoptic instrument would be adapted for the examination of the rectum and colon (see Chapter 30). Three different lengths of this instrument have been manufactured by the major endoscope manufacturers and a number of endoscopists are making satisfactory examinations up to the caecum. In addition to the diagnostic studies by observation and biopsy throughout the great lengths of the colon, the surgical performance of transendoscopic polypectomy is now being carried out. A few endoscopists are also performing satisfactory polypectomy of the stomach (see Chapter 28II).

Television Endoscopy

Symbolic of the rapid strides which have been made during the recent years since the development of fiberoptic examinations is the use of television endoscopy. The equipment for this procedure is still very expensive, but there are a number of institutions in Japan, Europe and the United States where this technic is in use.

ENDOSCOPY SOCIETIES

In 1939, Schindler organized the American Gastroscopic Club in his Chicago home. After World War II, the club became the American Gastroscopic Society and in 1965, the American Society for Gastrointestinal Endoscopy. In the meantime, gastroscopy societies were organized in other countries. Gastrocamera societies were organized in Japan.

In 1970, the European Society for Gastrointestinal Endoscopy was organized. Since then, affiliated or cooperating endoscopy societies have been organized in Britain, Germany, Sweden, Switzerland and other countries of Europe. Similar societies have recently been organized on the Continents of South America, Asia and Africa. In all instances, they are associated with Gastroenterology Societies.

WORLD CONGRESSES OF GASTROINTESTINAL ENDOSCOPY

In 1966, Japanese endoscopists organized and served as hosts to the First World Congress of Gastrointestinal Endoscopy. This was held in Tokyo in connection with a world congress of gastroenterology. The author and co-author of this chapter met for the first time at the Fourth European and Mediterranean Congress of Gastroenterology in Paris, July, 1954, where both workers presented clinical research studies in gastroscopy. Similarly papers were presented at the International Gastroenterology Congresses before and since the First World Endoscopy Congress.

SIGNIFICANCE OF PROGRESS IN ENDOSCOPIC MEDICINE

The history of Gastrointestinal Endoscopy has been much more than the technical evolution of instruments. It has been the progress story of extending physical diagnosis into the innermost recesses of the human body. Part of the net result has been the statistical improvement of the gross diagnosis of gastrointestinal disease. This has led to the observation and analysis of minute gross lesions and the recent Japanese concept of early gastric cancer. Midzonal magnifications and histologic studies of transendoscopic biopsies are improving our concepts of petechial erosions and gastritis. Transendoscopic cannulation of the pancreatic and biliary ducts is only the beginning of the vast possibilities in this field. Definitive therapeutic surgery such as polypectomy is an established fact.

In all of these contributions to medical science, the role of different geographic areas of the world has been an interesting reality. The diffusion of our element of medical culture has been not unlike the history of the diffusion of culture in the arts, industrial technology, the social sciences and the humanities.

It was the destiny of Europe to harbor the long crude century of technical frustrations and human agony which were the roots of progress. The major route of the evolutionary development of endoscopy led westward to America. But, there was an important minor route, eastward to Japan which was destined to overtake the vanguard of progress and show the way of leadership with the rest of the front-running world in gastrointestinal endoscopic medicine. Now there is virtually a pattern of the united nations cooperatively exploring the digestive canal and its diseases. Soon there will be no part of this vast interior which the endoscopist cannot explore without undue risk or undue human discomfort. Indeed the lonely endoscopist with his fixed monocular vision can now share simultaneously the living vistas of the alimentary canal with several or many of his colleagues through the closed circuitry of television. Finally, the zealous pursuit of a common endeavor in science has brought miraculous progress in diagnosis, improved prognosis in human disease and an international camaraderie among scientists with a common goal.

REFERENCES

1. Bozzini, Ph.: Schindler R. Gastroscopy, U. of Chicago Press, 1937.
2. Desormeaux, A. J.: Schindler R. Gastroscopy, U. of Chicago Press, 1937.
3. Kussmaul, A.: About a gastroscopy. *Verh d maturforsch Ges Freiburg,* 5:112, 1968.
4. Bevan, I. A.: Oesophagoscopy. *Lancet,* 1:470, 1868.
5. Stoerk, C.: An examination of esophagus with laryngoscope. *Wein Med Wochenschr,* 25:706-707, 1881.

6. Nitze, N.: Schindler R. Gastroscopy, U. of Chicago Press, 1937.
7. Mikulicz, K.: Gastroscopy and esophagoscopy. *Wien Med Wochenschrift, 12*:1405-1408, 1437-1443, 1473-1477, 1505-1507, 1537-1541, 1573-1577, 1881.
8. Kelling, G.: Having many joints, able to make angle gastroscope with ability to rotate prism of vision. *Munch Med Wochenschr, 45*:1556, 1898.
9. Tuttle, J. P.: A treatise on diseases of the anus rectum and pelvic colon. New York, Appleton & Co., 1905.
10. d'Abreu, Aleixo: quoted in Garrison, F. H.: *History of Medicine,* 4th ed. Philadelphia, Saunders, 1929, p. 272.
11. Salmon, Fred: quoted in Blanchard, C. E.: *The Romance of Proctology,* Youngstown, Medical Success Press, 1938, p. 8.
12. Garrison, F. H.: *History of Medicine,* 4th ed. Philadelphia, Saunders, 1929, p. 272.
13. Rosenheim, T.: About cardia examination and remarks about gastroscopy. *Dtsch Med Wochenschr,* 21, No. 13-15, 1896.
14. Jackson, Chevalier: *Tracheo-Bronchoscopy, Esophagoscopy and Gastroscopy.* St. Louis, The Laryngoscope Co., 1907.
15. Jackson, C. and Jackson, C. L.: Diseases of the air and food passages of foreign body origin. Philadelphia, Saunders Co., 1936.
16. Loening, K., and Stieda, A.: Demonstration of one gastroscope. *Verh Dtsch Ges f Chir,* 1908.
17. Elsner, H. D.: The gastroscope. *Klin Wochenschr, 13*:593, 1910.
18. Sussman, M.: A flexible gastroscope. *Ther Ggw, 52*:433, 1911.
19. Moutier, F.: *Traite de gastroscopie et de pathologie endoscopique de l'estomac,* Paris, Masson, 1935.
20. Moutier, F., and Cornet, A.: *Les Gastrites,* Paris, Masson et Cie. Editeurs, 1953.
21. Schindler, R.: *Gastroscopy—The Endoscopic Study of Gastric Pathology,* 2nd ed. Chicago, University of Chicago Press, 1950. p. 10.
22. Schindler, R.: *Textbook and Atlas of Gastroscopy,* Muenchen, 1923.
23. Schindler, R.: Gastroscopy in 30 cases of neoplasm. *Arch Intern Med, 32*:635, 1923.
24. Henning, N.: About one new esophagoscope for use in the internal medicine clinic. *Klin Wochenschr, 11*:1673-1675, 1932.
25. Taylor, H.: A new gastroscope with controllable flexibility. *Lancet, 240*:281-282, 1941.
26. Eder-Hufford, A. R.: Flexi-rigid optical esophagoscope. *Gastroenterology, 12*:779, 1949.
27. Schindler, R.: *Gastroscopy—The Endoscopic Study of Gastric Pathology,* 2nd ed. Chicago, University of Chicago Press, 1950, p. 65.
28. Hardt, L. L.: Flexi-rigid gastroscope. *Gastroenterology, 3*:508, 1944.
29. Benedict, E. B.: An operating gastroscope. *Gastroenterology, II*:281-283, 1948.
30. Kenamore, B.: A biopsy forceps for the flexible gastroscope. *Am J Dig Dis, 7*:539, 1940.
31. Wood, I. J.; Doigrk, A.; Motteram, R., and Hughes, A.: Gastric biopsy; report on 55 biopsies using new flexible gastric biopsy tubes. *Lancet, 1*:18-21, 1949.
32. Tomenius, J.: Gastroscopi och gastrobiopsi i diagnotiken. *Svensk Lakforsch Tidn,* 53:641, 1956.
33. Berry, L. H.: Direct vision suction gastrobiopsy instrument for Eder-Palmer gastroscopes. Described by Owens, F. J.: in *Brown's Diagnostic Procedures in Gastroenterology,* Chapter 21. St. Louis, Mosby, 1967.
34. Henning, N., and Keilhack, H.: A color photography of gastric mucosa. *Dtsch Med Wochenschr, 64*:1329, 1938.

35. Segal, H. L., and Watkins, J. S.: Color photography through the flexible gastro-scope. *Gastroenterology, 10*:375, 1948.

36. Lange, F., and Meltzing, D.: Inside the stomach photography. *Munch Med Wochenschr, 50*:1585, 1898.

37. Heilpern and Back: quoted by Schindler, R.: *Gastroscopy—the Endoscopic Study of Gastric Pathology,* 2nd ed., 1950, p. 72.

38. Henning, N.: A new apparatus for endoscopic photography of the stomach. *Arch Verdaiuingskv K G, 50*:27-33, 1931.

39. Rodgers, H. W.: Device for increasing field in gastroscopy. *Lancet, 2*:438, 1936.

40. Berry, L. H.: Right-side gastroscopic technic in situs inversus viscerum and visual-ization of "blind spots." *Review of Gastroent,* No. 4, 8:267-272, July-August, 1941.

41. Berry, L. H.: Improved gastroscopic diagnosis by the use of multiple positions in 2843 cases. *Gastroent,* No. 1, *44*:20-24, January, 1963.

42. Uji, T.: The gastrocamera. *Tokyo Med J,* 135, 1952.

43. Tasaka, S. and Ashizawa, S.: Studies on gastric disease using the gastrocamera. *Am Gastroscop Soc Bull,* 5:12, 1958.

44. Hirschowitz, B.; Curtis, L. E.; Peters, C. W., and Pollard, H. M.: Demonstration of a new gastroscope, the fiberscope. *Gastroent,* 35:50, 1958.

CHAPTER 2

ANATOMIC AND TOPOGRAPHIC RELATIONS IN UPPER GASTROINTESTINAL ENDOSCOPY

Leonidas H. Berry and Iltifat Alavi

INTRODUCTORY STATEMENT

THE GASTROINTESTINAL ENDOSCOPIST must be oriented with reference to the gross anatomy of that portion of the alimentary canal with which he is specifically concerned. This includes not only the important mucosal surfaces, but the intraluminal contours, the anatomic subdivisions of each organ, and the relative position of these organs in the neck, the thorax, and the abdominal cavity. Finally, the juxtapositional relationship of contiguous organs and their possible diseases should be thoroughly understood and appreciated by the prospective student of endoscopy.

Knowledge of the anatomy of any organ of the body is incomplete without inclusion of the microscopic or histologic structure. The gastro-intestinal endoscopist must therefore reacquaint himself with the histology of the alimentary canal as a basic requirement for the understanding of endoscopic pathology.

GENERAL BODY CONTOURS

When the endoscopist looks at a prospective patient, he is first concerned with the patient's countenance. The importance of the initial confrontation is discussed in Chapter 6. He should next be concerned with the general body contours as he evaluates indications and contraindications. The length and contours of the patient's neck, the contours of the thoracic cage, and the shape and contour of the abdomen should be quickly observed and evaluated.

If the neck veins are distended or the thyroid gland is grossly enlarged, or if the neck is very short or deformed, the risk of possible injury, whether great or small, must be considered.

The chest is sometimes barrel-shaped, or there may be kyphoscoliosis of varying degree. Abnormal respiration and cardiac impulse may be obvious on general body inspection. The contour and shape of the abdomen should always be noted. The abdomen may be scaphoid, flat, or distended. The extremities may be paralyzed, swollen with arthritis or edema, or deformed in a manner that might directly or remotely risk injury or unusual discomfort to the patient.

MOUTH AND PHARYNX

With the patient on the examining table, the endoscopist's first anatomic concern is the mouth. Its size should be noted, and the presence of open lesions from the lips to the anterior pillars of the fauces should be determined. Teeth that are in a poor state of repair, jagged, or broken may injure the examiner's fingers or the endoscope. Some patients are inclined to bite the examiner's fingers during the introduction of the endoscope, even when they are sedated and the pharyngeal reflex anesthetized. This is often a subconscious reflex action. Very loose teeth associated with chronic gingivitis have been dislodged by the shaft of the instrument, presenting the hazard of swallowing or aspirating the uprooted tooth. Arthritis of the temporomandibular joint or fusion of the joint structure may interfere with wide opening of the mouth. Cleft palate and macroglossia should be readily ruled out or taken into consideration during final inspection of the mouth just before introduction of the scope. Massive enlargement of the tonsils, especially if there is inflammation, may interfere with passage of the endoscope.

The mucous membrane of the mouth consists of stratified squamous epithelium. It may appear pale when there has been blood loss from a lesion in the upper gastrointestinal tract. Seldom are there inflammatory changes of the mouth related to similar changes in the lower gastrointestinal tract. The importance of anatomic abnormalities or pathologic changes in the mouth is primarily in relation to the technic of endoscopy and the risk of injury or undue discomfort to the patient.

The pharynx consists of the nasopharynx, the oropharynx, and the laryngeal pharynx (Fig. 2-1), which lie posterior to the nose, the mouth, and the larynx, respectively. The oropharynx is separated from the mouth by the anterior pillars of the fauces and from the laryngeal part of the pharynx by the epiglottis and the pharyngoepiglottic fold. The pharyngoepiglottic fold is a fold of mucous membrane that extends laterally from each side of the epiglottis to the side wall of the pharynx. It separates the oropharynx from the laryngeal part of the pharynx. Below the fold on each side is the piriform fossa (Fig. 2-1). The piriform fossae are broad above and narrow below and lie at each side of the aperture of the larynx. Below the aperture, the arytenoids and the lamina of the cricoid cartilage are draped over with mucous membrane. The lower part of the pharynx, i.e. the hypopharynx, thus possesses an anterior wall. It is flat, and the posterior wall lies against it, obliterating the piriform fossae as the hypopharynx tapers off, wedge-shaped, into the clasp of the cricopharyngeus muscle.

The location of the piriform fossae at 5 to 6in. (13-15.5cm) below the incisor teeth should be kept in mind because of the importance of avoiding arrest or impingement of the instrument tip in the right or left fossa. The cricopharyngeus sphincter muscle complex begins 1 to 1½in. (2.5-4cm) distal to the fossae, or 6 to 7in. (15.5-18cm) below the incisor teeth. The muscle structure marks the pharyngoesophageal junction and the beginning of the esophagus. This area in the esophagus is of importance to the endoscopist because it remains closed except during the act of swallowing or when its opening is triggered by pressure of a tube or endoscope at the point of closure or upon a nearby *trigger* zone. Such pressure is often accompanied by the act of gagging, which momentarily opens the pharyngoesophageal sphincter complex. The experienced endoscopist will have learned the technic of slipping the scope through during the moment of relaxation. If he misses this moment by advancing the scope too rapidly or too slowly, he may encounter a defensive spasm, which can be sufficiently strong for injury or perforation to occur at this point. Usually, if the endoscopist waits for a few seconds and advances the scope gently, the esophagus will be entered without further difficulty. This is usually the first area where spasm may interfere with the endoscopy. Other areas of

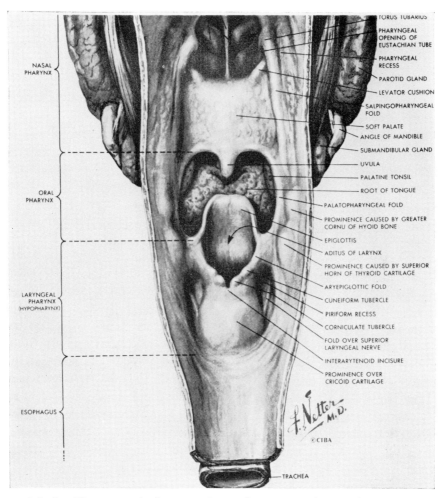

Figure 2-1. Semidiagrammatic drawing of nasopharynx, oropharynx, hypopharynx, and upper part of esophagus. Note particularly the position of the periform sinuses or recesses. (Courtesy of The Ciba Collection, Vol. 3: *Digestive System, Part I.* F. H. Metter (ed.). Boston, Little, Brown, 1959.)

spasm may occur in a hyperspastic individual lower in the esophagus and stomach.

ESOPHAGUS

The esophagus begins about 6½in. (16cm) below the incisor teeth. The esophagus is 10in. (25cm) long and extends from a level of the sixth cervical vertebra and the cricoid cartilage (Fig. 2-1) to the tenth thoracic vertebra. The cervical portion of the esophagus, lying in front of the prevertebral fascia, inclines slightly to the left of the midline. Passing downward through the superior mediastinum, the tube is slightly to the left of the midline posterior to the left main bronchus. The esophagus, which all this time is in contact with the vertebral bodies, now inclines forward with a concavity more marked than that of the vertebral column, passes in front of the descending aorta, in contact with the pericardium, and pierces the diaphragm 1in. (2.5cm) to the left of the midline opposite the body of the tenth thoracic vertebra. Fibers from the right crus of the diaphragm sweep around the esophageal opening in a slinglike loop. The intra-abdominal part of the esophagus varies in length according to the tone of its muscle and the degree of distention of the stomach. It averages about ½in. (1.5cm). In the superior mediastinum, the esophagus is crossed by the arch of the aorta on its left side and the vena azygos on its right side.

The surface epithelium of the mucous membrane of the esophagus is squamous stratified.

For the endoscopist, a few landmarks in addition to those just described may be of importance in the esophagus. One is a shallow impression in the left anterior wall of the esophagus which marks the level of the aortic arch approximately 8in. (20cm) below the incisor teeth and just above the area where the esophagus passes under the left bronchus. The pressure of the aortic arch causes flattening of the esophageal folds and transmission of the cardiovascular pulsation. The pulsation will be exaggerated in the presence of an aneurysm. Another landmark is the hiatus (Fig. 2-2), the opening in the diaphragm through which the esophagus passes. The opening varies in size within certain normal limits. When enlarged, it is frequently the site of gastric herniations of various portions (see Chap. 9). Usually the hiatus is about 14in. (40cm) below the incisor teeth, and usually it opens and closes with respiration.

Another landmark is the zigzag line at the junction of squamous and columnar epithelium (Fig. 2-2). The color of the esophageal mucosa is pale pink, in contrast to the redder gastric mucosa that begins at the zigzag line. Distributed throughout most of the normal esophageal mucosa can be seen tiny streaking blood vessels. There are longitudinal folds, most prominent in the distal esophagus, which change shape and form with respiration or with peristalsis.

The esophagus enters the stomach at the cardiac orifice, which is protected by a functional, not very obvious, anatomic sphincter, although the lower esophagus often shows a thickening of the circular coat (Fig. 2-2). The sphincter mechanism is more physiologic than anatomic and is the subject of great controversy. The variations in the intraluminal pressures in this area is the most definitive evidence of the exact location of the sphincter mechanism.[1]

The sphincter site may be slightly above or below the hiatus, averaging

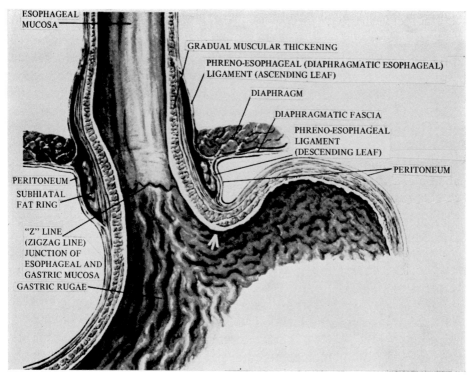

ESOPHAGEAL MUCOSA

GRADUAL MUSCULAR THICKENING

PHRENO-ESOPHAGEAL (DIAPHRAGMATIC ESOPHAGEAL) LIGAMENT (ASCENDING LEAF)

DIAPHRAGM

DIAPHRAGMATIC FASCIA

PHRENO-ESOPHAGEAL LIGAMENT (DESCENDING LEAF)

PERITONEUM

PERITONEUM
SUBHIATAL FAT RING

"Z" LINE (ZIGZAG LINE) JUNCTION OF ESOPHAGEAL AND GASTRIC MUCOSA
GASTRIC RUGAE

Figure 2-2. Semidiagrammatic drawing of frontal section of lower esophagus and upper stomach. (Courtesy of The Ciba Collection, Vol. 3: *Digestive System, Part 1.* F. H. Metter (ed.). Boston, Little, Brown, 1959.)

about 1in. (2.5cm) in length,[2] but varying in different individuals. For further details, see Chapter 13. As the endoscopist views the distal esophagus, he will normally see the sphincter zone closed. As moderate inflation is increased or the tip of the scope approaches the area, the sphincter will be seen to open and close partly or completely with respiration.

The normal direction and course of the esophagus, as well as the intraluminal contours, may be disturbed by skeletal deformities, such as kyphosis, kyphoscoliosis, and ankylosing spondylosis. In addition, compression by the cervical vertebrae, especially in long-necked individuals, mediastinal masses, etc., may deform the normal anatomic relations and make the endoscopic examination more difficult or hazardous.

STOMACH

The gastroscopist must have a fair knowledge of where the stomach lies in the abdominal cavity. Until the turn of the century, the described position of the stomach in the upper abdominal cavity had few variations because our knowledge was based on cadaver studies of the body in the horizontal, supine position. When digestive tract radiology came on the scene, the anatomy of the stomach became a living concept, the description being of the stomach filled with a barium mixture, physiologically active, and in the vertical position. It was soon found that under these circumstances the stomach often reached the pelvis and might have many variations of shapes and contours. A review of the literature on anatomic terminology of the stomach was published by Lewis in 1912.[3] Since the era of gastroscopy, the concepts of the position and shape of the stomach are again based on the horizontal position of the body, but now the living organ is seen in natural color, physiologically active, and filled with the medium of air. The gastroscopist should know the normal endoscopic variations in position and shape of the stomach as a guide in orientation and as a diagnostic aid in the presence of disease.

The stomach is a muscular pouch connecting the esophagus with the duodenum and suspended primarily by the gastrohepatic ligament attached along its lesser curvature and the gastrocolic ligament attached along its greater curvature. The upper part of the stomach is overlapped upon its anterior surface by the sharp, inferior surface of the left lobe of the liver. Elsewhere the anterior surface is in contact with the diaphragm and the anterior abdominal wall. The posterior wall of the stomach lies within the lesser sac and rests on the body of the pancreas and celiac axis. When the stomach is distended with air, the midportion usually lies at the level of the navel or below it. With the patient lying on his left side and the stomach inflated, it can be shown on x-ray that the gastric fundus usually lies in the left hypochondrium and becomes stretched outward, upward, and toward the patient's right. Thus, 75 per cent of the stomach may lie to the right of the esophageal axis.[4]

Gross Contours

Steerhorn—Fishhook

The gross contour and overall shape of the stomach have been described as corresponding to the general body build of the individual. The strongly built, broad-chested individual with a wide sternal angle is called the hypersthenic type and is most likely to have the so-called steerhorn stomach lying obliquely downward from left to right, with the fundus in the left hypochondrium. The slender individual with a chest of narrow transverse diameter and narrow sternal angle is called the hyposthenic type and is most likely to have a fishhook-shaped stomach.[5] Most other normal-shaped stomachs fit into the category between the two extremes. Certainly there are wide variations from this classification made on the basis of x-ray observations. However, there is some gastroscopic usefulness in this broad classification.

Endoscopically, the steerhorn stomach tends to have a shallow incisura angularis, permitting a long tunnel endoscopic view from the cardia to the pylorus. The fishhook type of stomach has more of a sharp, halfmoon-shaped angularis lying at right angles to the lesser curvature. The distal antrum and pylorus in this type of stomach is better seen with a side-viewing gastroscope, although it may be seen by proper tip deflection with a forward-viewing scope.

Subdivisions

It is of definite advantage in gastroscopy to make use of a widely accepted anatomic subdivision of the stomach. The descriptive location of disease is important for follow-up purposes and to determine, for example, whether a certain polyp seen on x-ray is the one also seen by gastroscopy or

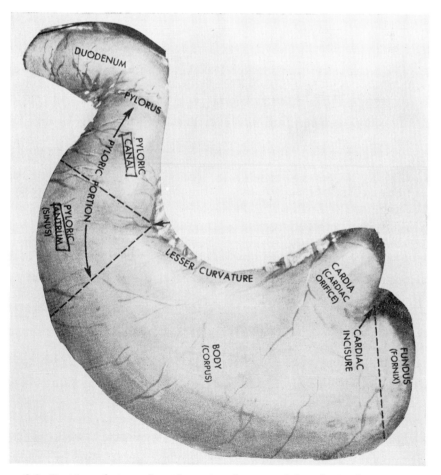

Figure 2-3. Position of stomach with patient lying on left side. Endoscopic position, showing subdivisions. (Courtesy of The Ciba Collection, Vol. 3: *Digestive System, Part I*. F. H. Metter (ed.). Boston, Little, Brown, 1959.)

is an additional one. The descriptive location of a lesion with reference to a subdivision of the stomach may be quite important to an exploring surgeon. The subdivisions of the stomach which are found generally in use by gastroscopists will be described as they are seen through a side-viewing gastroscope with the patient lying on his left side (Fig. 2-3).

Cardia-Fundus

The most cephalad portion of the stomach, that which begins at the cardioesophageal junction and extends distally for 2 or 3cm, is called the cardia. At the level of the cardia the gastroscopist usually sees a transilluminated, deep red curtain, which is the cardiac fold. The cardiac fold corresponds to the cardiac angle or incisura (see Fig. 2-2). It is usually very mobile and is coordinated with respiration. It may be distorted or displaced by carcinoma of the fundus or by hiatus hernia.

The fundus or fornix is that portion of the stomach which lies above the cardiac angle or above the cardiac area. This region, like all the subdivisions, varies with the individual, with the physiologic state of tone, and with whether the stomach is anatomically more fishhooked or steerhorned. In some instances there is very little fundus or area above the level of the cardia. The cardiac orifice and fundic area may be seen best in retroflexed views (see Chapter 6).

Body-Angulus

The body of the stomach is that portion which lies between the cardia and the angulus. It is sometimes further subdivided into upper and lower body. Many gastric lesions occur in this area and, together with lesions more distally located, respond more favorably to surgical intervention than lesions of the cardia and fundus.

The angulus is the endoscopic counterpart of the incisura angularis seen in the x-ray silhouette of the stomach (Plate 1). It has a striking endoscopic configuration. The enface view shows it as an inverted halfmoon-shaped structure which passes horizontally across the lesser curvature, ending in what is described as the anterior pillar on the anterior wall and the posterior pillar on the posterior wall. The anterior pillar of the angulus frequently has a ropelike configuration within its structure. This is due to horizontal muscle fibers which constitute the sphincter muscle of the antrum. It is not seen to be a complete sphincter in the inflated stomach unless there is excessive spastic activity in the pyloric and antral region. The position in space of the halfmoon structure in the view of the endoscopist changes when the patient is rotated from his left side to the back or right side. The musculur sphincter antri is apparently not so well defined under general anesthesia or in the cadaver.

Lesser-Greater Curvatures

The lesser curvature (Plate 2), as seen by the gastroscopist with the patient in the left lateral position, is a longitudinal sweep from the cardia to the pyloric sphincter. It lies in a frontal plane of the patient's body, nearest the right side and in line with the 11 or 12 o'clock position on the ocular dial of the scope. This is the so-called magenstrasse. Many lesions are seen endoscopically along this tract. Benign and malignant prepyloric, lesser curvature ulcers were often poorly seen prior to the advent of fiber-optics and movable tip gastroscopes. A small lesion in this area may still be difficult to see or to biopsy if the examiner is inexperienced.

The greater curvature is the longitudinal area along the outer or left border of the stomach as the patient lies on his left side. It is in the same frontal plane as the lesser curvature and is best seen toward 6 to 5 o'clock in the ocular dial of the scope. Ulcers along the greater curvature are seldom benign. Further orientation of the greater curvature with different types of instruments and in various positions on the examining table is described in Chapter 6.

Anterior-Posterior Walls

With the patient still on his left side, the relatively flat, broad surface of the stomach seen toward the examiner's left through the side-viewing scope is the anterior wall. The largely similar wall toward the examiner's right and the patient's back is, of course, the posterior wall. The anterior wall is best seen throughout its surfaces because the inflated stomach has room to spread out in good viewing distance toward the anterior abdominal wall. The gastroscope descends to a great extent close to the posterior wall, which has relatively little room to expand against the spine and posterior abdominal wall.

Antrum-Pylorus

The gastric antrum (Plates 3 and 4) is a very special organ physiologically and has certain anatomic characteristics of special interest to the gastroscopist. As the motor functional portion of the stomach, peristaltic activity develops in the antrum following inflation and distention. The varying intensity and form of peristaltic waves may have diagnostic meaning. The state of muscular tone may explain why an anatomically normal antrum may appear narrowed on endoscopy or x-ray. Although the antrum is generally tubular, wide variations in shape and contour are within normal limits.

The area dividing the stomach from the duodenum is called the pylorus. Its principal structure is a sphincter muscle, composed chiefly of horizontal muscle fibers. This is normally seen as a complete contractional ring. It opens and closes in response to successive concentric peristaltic waves that traverse the antrum and end with sphincteric contraction (see Plate 5). The structure of the pylorus is somewhat complex. The sphincteric ring surrounds a short pyloric canal. A definite muscular ring can be felt by the surgeon or the pathologist. The surgeon frequently has difficulty in defining the exact point of the ring on the mucosal and serosal sides. Within normal limits, there may be considerable variation in appearance of the sphincteric opening to the endoscopist. In some instances, the pyloric ring may not close completely during a period of observation; at other times, it closes with such intensity that the mucosal coat in the canal herniates back into the prepyloric antrum.

Gastric Mucosa

Gross Structure

The normal gastric mucosa begins at the gastroesophageal junction marked by a gray zigzag line and ends at the pyloric sphincter. It is characterized by a rugal pattern which is recognized by the endoscopic observer as being similar to that seen with the open stomach in the examiner's hands at postmortem or surgery. The size of the folds may be similar to that seen at average reading distance from the eye, or the folds may appear smaller or larger, depending on the angle of vision of a given scope or the distance between the objective and the gastric wall in various parts of the stomach. The flat surfaces between the folds are irregular in shape and are broader on the anterior and posterior walls than along the greater curvature, where the folds are closer together, roughly parallel, and sometimes tortuous. The greater curvature folds are larger than the folds of the anterior and posterior walls (Plate 5). Folds along the narrow strip of the lesser curvature are either scanty or absent. The folds of the gastric mucosa may vary considerably within physiologic limits. The muscularis mucosa is capable of contracting and changing the size and shape of rugal folds. It is for this reason that so-called giant folds on x-ray may appear differently on a different day by gastroscopy.[6]

The normal color of the gastric mucosa is traditionally described endoscopically by the term *orange-red*. The normal color, as seen by the endoscopist, may vary, depending on the intensity or quality of light. The more intense light causes the mucosa to appear paler, and light of low intensity causes the mucosa to appear a darker red. Optical engineers and manufacturers of endoscopes have adjusted lighting mechanisms so that, to a great extent, the working luminations of endoscopes are standardized.

The stomach has a rich vascular network of arteries, veins and lymphatics, with intricate and complicated shunting mechanisms.[7] Standard gastroscopic technics do not visualize blood vessels in the normal stomach except in a small area near the cardia and fundus. There is some difference of opinion about overdistention producing visible vessels (see Chapter 21). When the mucosa is thinned out, as in atrophy of the mucosa, branching arterioles and venules may be seen in the submucosa. Microangiography of fresh surgical segments using opaque suspensions and x-ray has revealed the entire vascular pattern up to the surface epithelium. For the future, gastroscopic study of this vascular pattern and vessel changes will undoubtedly play a role in the early studies of gastric disease. Such studies are already under way and make use of fluorescent dyes and magnifying gastroscopes.

The nerves and lymphatics have a distribution similar to that of the blood vascular system. The question of pathologic changes involving peripheral nerve endings in the gastric mucosa has not been satisfactorily solved. The possible relationship of such changes to the production of symptoms or the absence of symptoms will continue to challenge the gastroenterologist and gastroscopist of the future.

Midzonal

In recent years there has been an increasing interest in the study of the gastric mucosa as it appears under the dissecting microscope. The magnification of the mucosal structure is in the range of 10 times that seen by the unaided eye. Studies at this midzonal level often bring out the details of the polygonal flat-topped islands, the areae gastricae (Fig. 2-4, a and b), divided by slitlike crevices. On the surface of these tiny islands are the openings into the gastric pits, or glands, the foveolae gastricae (Fig. 2-4, a and b). There are those who say that under certain circumstances areae gastricae can be seen by the unaided eye and that this normal gastric pattern or slight variation from normal is what Schindler and earlier gastroscopists described as evidence of hypertrophic gastritis. There apparently are instances of true hypertrophy and hyperplastic changes in some cases, but many workers doubt that this is of inflammatory origin (see Chapter 21).

Microscopic Structure

Microscopically the gastric wall consists of the mucosa, subdivided into surface epithelium; tunica propria; muscularis mucosa; submucosa, muscularis propria, and serosa. The surface epithelium consists of simple columnar cell layers which line the stomach, including the gastric pits as they dip into the lamina propria to receive the branching tubular glands.

The glands are of three types and are distributed mostly in three regions of the stomach. The cardiac glands occur mostly in the region of the car-

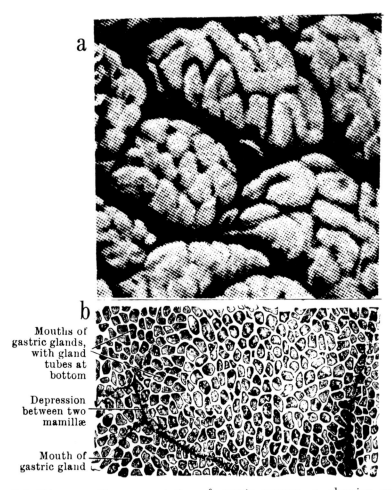

Figure 2-4. Diagrammatic representation of gastric mucosa, *a*, showing polygonal areae gastricae with slitlike crevices. The foveolae gastricae (mouths of gastric glands) are seen on the surface of the areae gastricae. ×25 (Courtesy of Cunningham, D. J.: *Textbook of Anatomy,* 8th ed. New York, Oxford, 1943.) *b,* Foveolae gastricae. ×17 (After Braus, in *Bailey's Textbook of Histology,* 15th ed. Baltimore, Williams & Wilkins, 1964.)

dia. They have short necks and numerous branches, which secrete thick mucus. The gastric and fundic glands occur mostly in the body and fundus. They are the principal glands of the stomach and secrete pepsin from their chief cells and hydrochloric acid from their parietal cells. The third group, the pyloric glands, are located in the pyloric area and secrete a mucus, thinner than that of the cardiac glands. The gastroscopist sees at least two types of mucus. The first is translucent and colorless. It adheres cohesively (forming the main portion of the mucus barrier) and produces the normal degree of glistening highlights. Another type is thick and not

so adherent. It is grayish to dirty gray; the dirty-gray mucus is inflammatory. Occasionally there is a third type, which is white, flaky, and porcelain-
like. In addition there are the secretions which primarily contain the hydrochloric acid, pepsin, and dissolved mucus. The stomach is known to secrete selectively to certain specific stimuli. For example, strong alcohol produces a predominance of mucus, weak alcohol produces acid substances;
histalog, etc., tend to produce a watery secretion containing acid.

The glandular structure of the stomach is primarily in the lamina propria. These glands are intertwined by connective tissue fibers and infiltrated by fibroblasts, histiocytes, and some plasma cells. There are numerous
infiltrations by lymphocytes.[8] There are small lymphocytic nodules or follicles in the lamina propria which occur frequently in the pyloric region.
This concept of normal structure is of special interest to the endoscopist
because these infiltrations are an important part of the histologic picture
of inflammation or gastritis. The difference between the anatomic and the
pathologic as described by many pathologists is largely quantitative. It is
therefore difficult at times to determine where the anatomic stops and the
pathologic begins. It is even more difficult in some cases to correlate the
endoscopic picture of inflammation with the microscopic and finally with
the clinical picture of inflammation of the stomach.

The underlying thin strip of longitudinal and transverse muscle which
can control the shape and form of the rugal folds is the muscularis mucosa.[6] The next layer, the submucosa, contains loosely arranged connective
tissue and the medium-sized blood vessels which send a network of capillaries into the rugal folds and interrugal spaces. The submucosal arterioles
and venules are the principal vessels gastroscopically in the thinned-out
atrophic mucosa.

DUODENUM

Contours and Subdivisions

The duodenum consists of the proximal 10cm of the 7m long small intestines. (Its name is derived from the fact that its length equals approximately 12 fingerbreadths.) It begins at the termination of the pyloric ring
and ends at the duodenojejunal junction, or the ligament of Treitz (Fig.
2-5). Roughly, it forms a horseshoe configuration in the adult and is described as being divided into four parts. The first or superior portion, often called the bulb on x-rays, is about 2in. (5cm) long. It extends slightly
backward, upward and to the right. The duodenum then bends downward
for a distance of 3in. (7.5cm), which is the second and descending portion.
It curves around the right border of the head of the pancreas to form the
transverse or third portion. The short, ascending fourth portion ends at
the ligament of Treitz.

On the medial aspect of the midportion of the descending duodenum lies the papilla of Vater 3 to 4in. (7.5-10cm) distal to the pyloric ring (Fig. 2-5). At the summit of the papilla there is an orifice which is common to the pancreatic duct of Wirsung and the common bile duct. In some instances the pancreatic duct and the common bile duct open separately into the duodenum. Frequently there is an accessory pancreatic duct (Santorini) from the pancreas that enters the duodenum about 1in. (2.5cm) proximal to the papilla (Fig. 2-5).

The surface of the duodenum is characterized by the formation of semicircular (Kerckring) folds (Fig. 2-6), also known as plicae circulares or valvulae conniventes.[8] The folds increase the absorptive surface and retard the transport of the intestinal content. They extend one-half to two-thirds the distance around the circumference. Rarely do they complete the circle. (They contain all layers of the mucosa and submucosa.) These folds are not present in the bulbar duodenum. They begin at about 1in.

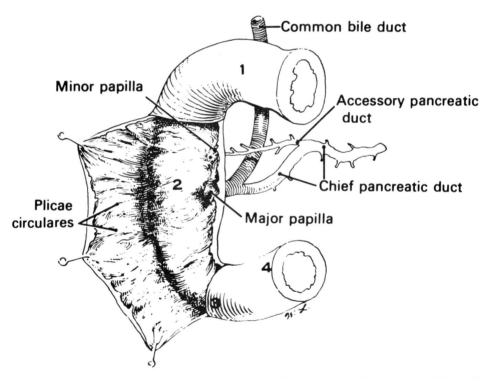

Figure 2-5. The duodenum, its parts and internal structure, and associated bile and pancreatic ducts. *1,* Superior portion (bulb). *2,* Descending portion. *3,* Transverse portion (foreshortened in perspective). *4,* Short, ascending portion at duodenojejunal junction (ligament of Treitz). (Courtesy of Becker, R. F., Wilson, J. W., and Gehweiler, J. A.: *The Anatomical Basis of Medical Practice.* Baltimore, Williams & Wilkins, 1971.)

Openings of the intestinal glands Lymphoid nodule in the submucosa

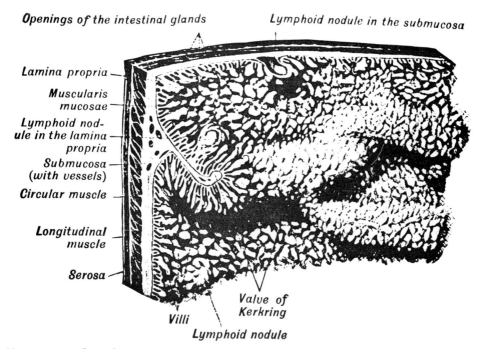

Lamina propria

Muscularis mucosae

Lymphoid nodule in the lamina propria

Submucosa (with vessels)

Circular muscle

Longitudinal muscle

Serosa

Villi

Valve of Kerkring

Lymphoid nodule

Figure 2-6. Three-dimensional reconstruction of part of small intestines drawn with binocular microscope from sections. ×17 (After Braus, in Maximow, A. A., and Bloom, W.: *Textbook of Histology*, 6th ed. Philadelphia, Saunders, 1952.)

(2.5cm) to 2in. (5cm) beyond the pylorus. In the lower descending duodenum, below the ampulla, the folds are very large.

Midzonal

A magnifying lens (10-20×) will disclose the villi (see Fig. 2-6), which are most numerous in the four divisions of the duodenum but are present throughout the small intestine.[8] The villous structure gives an endoscopic velvety and sometimes granular appearance. Electron microscopy shows very vascular microvilli, which further increase the absorptive surface of the organ.[9] Further examination of the surface of the mucosa with the magnifying lens (10-20×) will reveal the crypts of Lieberkühn. These innumerable openings of the intestinal glands may be seen between the bases of the villi. Undoubtedly, magnifying endoscopes will explore these midzonal structures in the future study of physiology and pathologic anatomy of the duodenum.

The villi are leaflike projections with their long diameters in a transverse direction and arranged in longitudinal rows. Between the villi can be seen the tiny openings called the crypts of Lieberkühn. They dip down to the muscularis mucosa, and the spaces between them are wider than the spaces between the glands of the stomach.

Microscopic Structure

The epithelial layer consists of simple columnar cells of three types: (1) cells with striated borders, (2) goblet cells, and (3) argentaffin cells. The epithelium covers the villi and continues to line the crypts or glands of Lieberkühn. The lamina propria surrounds the crypts and extends up to form the core of the villi. The lamina contains a special type of connective tissue and various types of cellular elements, including small lymphocytes and plasma cells. The latter cells increase greatly during digestion. Isolated lymphatic nodules occur in the duodenum but are more numerous and larger in the ileum, where they are known as Peyer's patches.

The muscularis mucosa averages about 38μ in thickness. It consists of an inner circular layer of smooth muscle and an outer longitudinal layer.

The submucosa consists of dense connective tissue, elastic fibers, and occasional adipose lobules. Within this layer for the most part are the characteristic duodenal glands of Brunner. Sometimes the Brunner glands extend a few centimeters into the pylorus. They are arranged in lobules, the terminal portions of which are richly branching tubules that enter the bottom or the sides of the crypts of Lieberkühn. The glands become smaller in size and finally disappear in the distal two thirds of the duodenum.

The two remaining layers of the duodenal wall are the muscularis propria and the serosa, which are quite similar in the remaining small intestines.

REFERENCES

1. Code, C. F., Schlegel, J. F., Kelley, J. L., Olsen, A. M., and Ellis, F. H.: Hypertensive gastroesophageal sphincter. *Proc Staff Meet, Mayo Clin,* 35:391, 1960.
2. Botha, G. S. M., Astley, R., and Carre, I. J.: A combined cineradiographic and manometric study of the gastroesophageal junction. *Lancet,* 1:659, 1957.
3. Lewis, F. T.: The form of the stomach in human embryos with notes upon the nomenclature of the stomach. *Am J Anat,* 13:477, 1912.
4. Palmer, E. D.: *Stomach Disease as Diagnosed by Gastroscopy.* Philadelphia, Lea & Febiger, 1949.
5. Schlosinger, E.: *Die Röntgendiagnosis der Magen und Darmkrankheiten.* Berlin, 1917, pp. 36, 50.
6. Forssell, G.: Studies of the mechanism of the movement of the mucous membrane of the digestive tract. *Am J Roentgenol,* 10:87, 1923.
7. Barclay, A. E., and Bentley, F. H.: Vascularization of human stomach: Preliminary note on shunting effects of trauma. *Brit J Radiol,* 22:67, 1949.
8. Maximow, A. A., and Bloom, W.: *Textbook of Histology,* 6th ed. Philadelphia, Saunders, 1952.
9. Becker, R. F., Wilson, J. W., and Gehweiler, J. A.: *The Anatomical Basis of Medical Practice.* Baltimore, Williams & Wilkins, 1971, p. 577.

CHAPTER 3

INDICATIONS, CONTRAINDICATIONS AND LIMITATIONS IN UPPER GASTROINTESTINAL ENDOSCOPY

Leonidas H. Berry

41

FOR ALL TYPES OF SCOPES
    EXTRINSIC ESOPHAGEAL AND GASTRIC DISPLACEMENTS
    GENERAL SYSTEMIC DISORDERS
    PENETRATING AND PERFORATED GASTRIC ULCER
    BULBAR DUODENAL LESIONS
    POST BULBAR DUODENAL LESIONS
    EXTREMES OF AGE GROUPS AND UNCOOPERATIVE PATIENT
LIMITATIONS

GENERAL INDICATIONS

SCHINDLER,[1] BERRY[2] AND OTHERS[3-6] have described indications from the early years of modern gastroscopy to the present time. As the endoscopic method increased in usage and scope, indications, values and advantages of upper gastrointestinal endoscopy have increased. Upper gastrointestinal endoscopy is indicated in broad terms when there are persistent symptoms individually or in combination with epigastric distress, vomiting, gross or latent hemorrhage, dysphagia or other persistent apparently minor symptoms referrable to the upper gastrointestinal tract. Most patients in these categories will have had or should have had x-ray studies of the upper gastrointestinal canal before endoscopy. Important possible exceptions are cases of acute gross upper gastrointestinal hemorrhage where the aggressive diagnostic approach is employed. Other exceptions might include patients who because of weakness, transportation and upright x-ray studies are not immediately feasible. When upper gastrointestinal x-ray findings are negative, endoscopy has one of its greatest indications. When a positive x-ray lesion is diagnosed or suspected such as ulcer, cancer or esophageal obstruction, endoscopy is indicated for further delineation or conformation of the lesion in its natural state and for photography, biopsy or cytology.

An important general indication for endoscopy is the repeated examination for monitoring the healing of benign ulcer and especially those which by their rate and character of anatomical change may indicate possible malignancy and surgical removal. Other lesions where repeated monitoring may be indicated include cases where more than one possible source of bleeding is found on first examination such as hemorrhagic erosion and esophageal varices with or without gastroduodenal ulcer. Repeated endoscopy may be indicated especially in such cases when the hematocrit after transfusion is persistently low or falling. Repeated endoscopy may also be indicated when first examination by x-ray and endoscopy are negative and symptoms are persistent.

In summary, I would like to emphasize that whatever the apparent or technical indication, endoscopy should be done primarily in the interest of the patient and his individual diagnostic problem. This ethic can be applied broadly enough to include all reasonable controlled clinical research observations. When this is clearly not the case, it is especially important that the informed written consent of the patient be obtained. Certain ulterior motive *indications* for gastroscopy as appropriately emphasized by Brown[7] should be totally unacceptable by the responsible endoscopy community, thus preserving and promoting the ever increasing value and advantages of endoscopic diagnosis.

SPECIFIC INDICATIONS
Esophageal Lesions

Esophagitis and Ulcerations

When there is persistent retro-manubrial pyrosis or pain on swallowing, esophagitis must be considered. When there are symptoms due to diffuse or localized inflammation of the esophagus x-ray is usually negative. Esophagoscopy then becomes the principal diagnostic tool and should be carried out except when there are specific individual contraindications. Ulceration may be an extension of esophagitis or primary as a solitary Barrett's peptic ulcer (see Chapter 9).

Erosions

Primary erosions may occur in the esophagus either independently or in association with other erosions in the stomach and/or the duodenum. They may or may not be sufficient to cause symptoms. Erosion may be associated with localized or diffuse inflammation which characterizes the syndrome of erosive esophagitis.

Varices

Esophageal varices occur commonly with liver diseases and portal hypertension. When upper gastrointestinal hemorrhage occurs in the presence of known or suspected liver disease or chronic alcoholism, esophageal varices must be ruled out. Frequently varices are not demonstrated by x-ray while being easily visualized by esophagoscopy.[8] The esophagoscopist must try to find a site of bleeding or erosions on the varices. When absent, other sites in the upper gastrointestinal tract may be the source of hemorrhage.

Malignant Neoplasms, Primary and Secondary

The most significant neoplasm of the esophagus is the squamous cell carcinoma. It may be primarily polypoid or scirrhous. Endoscopy is indicated when this type of lesion is suspected and not revealed by x-ray. It is also indicated whenever a radiographic filling defect is diagnosed for the purpose of gross confirmation,[8] biopsy and brush cytology. Transendoscopic tissue diagnosis may be more important in esophageal than in gastric neoplasms. This is true because frequently, irradiation and dilatation are the choice forms of therapy rather than surgical resection in esophageal malignancies. Not too infrequently, carcinoma causing narrowing of the esophagus is secondary to invasion from a primary bronchogenic carcinoma. Esophagoscopy and bronchoscopy in such cases are indicated in combination with x-ray to determine whether such a lesion is extrinsic and causing lateral pressure or whether miliary invasion has reached the esophageal mucosa.

CASE HISTORY

Illustrative of the role of esophagoscopy and transendoscopic procedures in such problems is the following case description: A 54-year-old woman was seen with the chief presenting symptom of dysphagia. She was a *chain* smoker and had a *cigarette cough* for a number of years. The dysphagia had become progressively worse for the last few weeks. The physical examination was essentially negative. The complete blood count, FBS, BUN, cholesterol, alkaline phosphatase, amylase, bilirubin, urinalysis and the stool examinations were within normal limits. The x-ray of the esophagus showed narrowing approximately at the level of the bifurcation of the trachea. The esophagoscopic view showed a narrowed lumen and relatively smooth mucosa. Brush smears from the narrowed portion revealed class V cytological changes indicative of malignancy. The biopsy was negative. X-ray and chest tomograms indicated clearly, pressure on the esophagus of an external mass at the level of the carina (Fig. 3-1). Subsequent bronchoscopy with biopsy revealed a positive histologic picture of bronchogenic carcinoma. The subsequent course and follow up of this patient substantiated the diagnosis of secondary malignant invasion of the esophagus from primary carcinoma of the left bronchus.

Carcinoma high in the fundus or cardia may invade or partially block the cardio-esophageal junction and produce symptoms of dysphagia. Side-viewing endoscopy may be contraindicated in such a case but forward-viewing endoscopy in the hands of a skillful endoscopist may be indicated for biopsy or brush cytology.

Benign Neoplasms and Granulomas

Quite uncommonly a tumor of the esophagus may be non-malignant and originate from either mucosa or submucosal tissues (see Chapter 11). The entire gamut of such benign neoplasms which have been found though rarely, in any part of the gastrointestinal canal have also occurred in the esophagus. Most of them have been incidental findings at autopsy. They are usually of clinical importance only if by finding and identifying them malignancy can be ruled out. On rare occasions a cavernous hemangi-

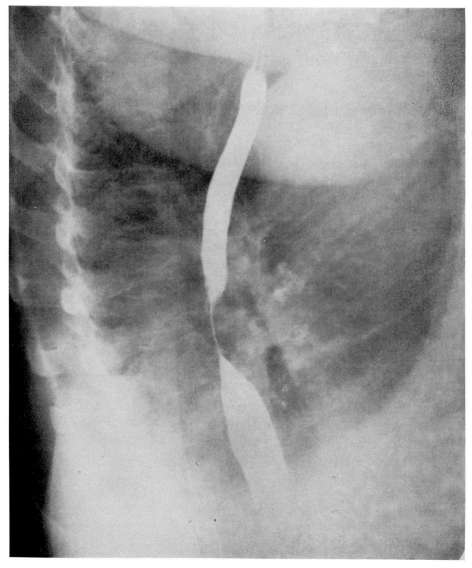

Figure 3-1. Lateral x-ray view of chest showing compression and invasion of esophagus by bronchogenic carcinoma.

oma may be the cause of upper gastrointestinal hemorrhage or as reported by Broders and associates,[9] the bluish discoloration of a cyst-like tumor in the esophageal lumen may be recognized endoscopically as hemangioma.

Granulomatous diseases including tuberculosis, syphilis, Crohn's disease and fungus infections have all been described as occurring in the esophagus. When these diseases appear in other parts of the body associated with dysphagia or other esophageal symptoms, investigation by esophagoscopy is indicated.

Achalasia and Hiatus Hernia

Achalasia or so-called cardiospasm is commonly seen by the gastroenterologist. While there are classical roentgenographic signs of this disorder, the examination is not complete without esophagoscopy. One should rule out scirrhous carcinoma by direct vision and perhaps brush cytology or biopsy. Usually, acute esophagitis is remarkably absent in my experience. Undoubtedly this is because of the protective mechanism of hypersecretion of long glary mucus which cardiospastic patients carry around all day and the increased adherent mucus barrier. Clinically significant, hiatus hernia is sometimes diagnosed by a skillful endoscopist which is not seen on the x-ray film (see Chapter 9). There are both prograde and retrograde fiberoptic technics which may be employed. Among other less common disorders in which esophagoscopy may be indicated are diffuse spasm, Plumer-Vinson syndrome (iron deficiency dysphagia), strictures, "rings," "webs" and other uncommon disorders.

Mallory Weiss Tears

The tears[10] which occur at the cardioesophageal junction occasionally associated with explosive vomiting in acute alcoholism are more definitively diagnosed by endoscopy than by x-ray.[11] The lesion may be seen by forward-viewing endoscopy or by retroflexion with a side-viewing or forward-viewing gastroscope. Upper Gastrointestinal Hemorrhage where the Mallory-Weiss syndrome is suspected is a clear indication for endoscopy.

Neuromuscular or Collagen and Endocrine Disorders

Esophagoscopy is indicated in disorders which fall into these categories because they include such possibilities as dermatomyositis of the esophagus and scleroderma of the esophagus (see Chapter 12) and such changes as may or may not be present in dysphagia associated with diabetes, hypercalcemia of parathyroid disease and other such disorders.

Dysphagia in Psychosomatic Disorders

All gastroenterologists have to deal with the problem of patients complaining of what is variously described as globus hystericus, sour belching or eruction, heartburn, hiccough, substernal pyrosis, aerophagy and esophageal spasm. In most instances, such patients have normal esophagograms. When these symptoms are persistent, fiberoptic endoscopy may be indicated to assist in ruling out organic disease or occasionally to discover the presence of organic changes.

Gastric Lesions

Gastric Ulcer

One of the most important indications for gastroscopy is the possible discovery of healing or early benign peptic ulcer too small or too difficulty placed to be seen by x-ray. The excellent facilities for brush cytology and biopsy in combination with gastroscopy (see Chapter 15), greatly enhance the differential diagnosis of malignant ulcer. Gastric ulcer is sometimes the demonstrable site of gross upper gastrointestinal hemorrhage.

Advanced Cancer

Advanced, so-called Borrmann-type, gastric cancer is often easily demonstrated by x-ray. The indications for gastroscopy include those cases where x-ray filling defects are questionable and biopsy or brush cytology may prove or disprove carcinoma. Biopsy and cytology may also differentiate between carcinoma and radiosensitive sarcomas and lymphosarcoma. Chronic gastritis and other lesions not seen on x-ray also may be disclosed by endoscopy. It is not unusual that the so-called advanced types of gastric cancer may be seen endoscopically and not revealed on x-ray. The relative diagnostic accuracy of x-ray versus gastroscopy has favored gastroscopy[12, 13] through the years, although the use of both methods has been better than either method alone.

Early Gastric Cancer

The Japan Endoscopy Society has developed a unique endoscopic and histologic concept of early gastric cancer. Japanese workers have made a good case for these concepts internationally over the past several years. If gastric cancer can be readily identified while it is still limited to the mucosa and submucosa by combined gastroscopy and transendoscopic biopsy and cytology, the many decades of effort in this field will have been justified. Discussions of this subject in Chapter 18 would seem to make gastroscopy in responsible hands mandatory upon the slightest suspicion of cancer.

Non-Carcinomatous Malignancies

Non-carcinomatous malignancies arise in tissues other than the epithelial cells of the mucosa. Perhaps the two most common types seen by the endoscopist are the leiomyosarcomas and the lymphosarcomas. In this group we will include certain other uncommon neoplasms. These include Hodgkins disease, reticulum cell sarcomas, various subgroups of malignant lymphoma and leukemia. Although these tumors arise in the deep portions of the mucosa, submucosa and muscular layers, they are not usually diagnosed until they bulge into the lumen. They may be of single or multiple origins, part of a generalized disease or primary in the stomach. Gastroscopy combined with biopsy and cytology is indicated when any of these lesions are suspected or when they have to be ruled out because of gross similarities to other lesions. The differential diagnosis and other features of non-carcinomatous malignancies are discussed in Chapter 19.

Benign Tumors and Polyps

Gastric tumors which are benign in nature may not cause any symptoms. This is particularly true of the common adenomatous polyps. They usually cause symptoms only if they bleed or block the pylorus intermittently in a *ball-valve* fashion. The patient may have an associated gastritis or other factors which may account for symptoms. In any event, firm evidence or suspicion of benign gastric tumors on x-ray or on clinical grounds such as hemorrhage are indications for gastroscopy. A detailed discussion of the gastroscopic significance of benign neoplasms appears in Chapter 19.

Post-Operative Stomach

The patient with upper gastrointestinal symptoms shortly after gastric surgery or months, even years thereafter, has an indication for gastroscopy. These are symptoms related to mechanical defects of gastric surgery: recurrent ulcer and carcinoma or indeed of psychosomatic origin which may be clarified by gastroscopy, gastro-jejunoscopy and transendoscopic procedures. Because the gastric stump is often retrocostal, the organ may be difficult to palpate by the fluoroscopist while the area is easily reached by the shorter length, forward- or side-viewing endoscopes. Roentgenography is frequently inconclusive. Endoscopy is an important complementary diagnostic method. This subject is extensively covered in Chapter 20.

Gastritis, Acute and Chronic

One of the most difficult and controversial problems of digestive disorders is gastritis. No diagnostic study of upper gastrointestinal symptoms is complete without consideration of gastritis and it can best be diagnosed by gastroscopy and gastrobiopsy. Gastritis may be associated with upper gastrointestinal hemorrhage, gastroduodenal ulcer and diseases of the biliary tract and pancreas increasing the symptomatic manifestations of these and other disorders. Gastritis must be distinguished from upper gastrointestinal distress due to functional disturbances. Endoscopy for the study of possible acute and chronic gastritis has an important indication. Endoscopic and related histopathologic aspects of this subject are discussed in Chapter 21.

Gastric Deformities

Hour-glass deformity of the stomach is not too uncommon. It characteristically has a prominent incisura across the greater curvature and a lesser curvature ulcer at or near the same level. This "B"-shaped deformity is

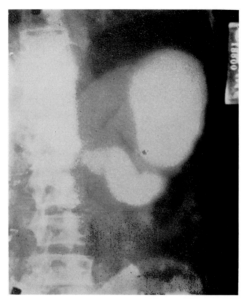

Figure 3-2. B-shaped stomach due to lesser curvature ulcer and benign constriction.

best seen by x-ray (Fig. 3-2). Gastroscopy is indicated to confirm the benignancy of the ulcer or rule out malignancy. The incisura usually persists
for an indefinite period although the ulcer may be found to have completely healed by gastroscopy. If the hour-glass is "V"-shaped, it is more
likely to be a scirrhous carcinoma and gastrobiopsy and cytology are indicated.

Acquired gastric diverticulum-like deformities may occur in the healing
process of a large ulcer. Gastroscopy is indicated because the "diverticulum" may prove to be the ulcer crater itself. Various other types of gastric
deformities especially in the antrum may be related to large diverticula
in which gastroscopy is indicated.[14] The so-called cascade stomach (Fig.
3-3) may present a bizarre appearance to the roentgenologist and the gastroscopist without revealing any mucosal changes. This phenomenon may
prevent visualization of parts of the stomach by x-ray and gastroscopy.
The combined methods are then necessary for best results in ruling out organic disease.

Displacement of the stomach may occur to the right or left anteriorly,
or by tortion, distorting the gastric silhouette by x-ray. External compression may likewise cause deformity of the gastric profile. The cause of
these defects may be enlarged liver, tumors in the pancreas or elsewhere in
the upper abdomen, spinal deformities and other defects. When displacements or deformities are severe, gastroscopy is frequently indicated as a
complementary method with x-ray to rule out intragastric tumors.

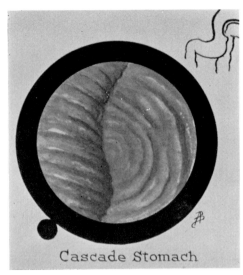

Figure 3-3. Diagram of one variety of cascade stomach as seen by gastroscopy and radiography.

A patient with situs inversus viscerum and dextra gastrica will occasionally be referred for gastroscopy. This defect of visceral rotation may be associated with symptoms, functional or organic. Gastroscopy is indicated especially when this congenital defect is not entirely obvious by x-ray. The gastroscopic examination of a case of situs inversus with dextra gastrica by the author[15] led to the use of "right-side" and "multiple positions" technic[16] in the improvement of "blind spots" with the lens gastroscope. The author still finds indications for "rotation" of the patient on the table and raising or lowering the head of the table in the gastroscopic examination of difficult cases. Volvulus and many other gastric deformities with dyspeptic symptoms may constitute indications for gastroscopy.

Miscellaneous and Rare Diseases

Granulomas, Hodgkins disease, tuberculosis, syphilis and leukemia of the stomach have all been reported or observed gastroscopically. Foreign bodies and bezoars composed of hair,[17] persimmons[18] and other substances have been reported by gastroscopists. Many systemic diseases associated with upper gastrointestinal symptoms have gastric involvement of the disseminated specific disease. Some of these diseases have primary gastric origin. The use of fiberoptic endoscopes for the removal of foreign bodies as a common practice may not be very far into the future.[19]

Bulbar Duodenal Lesions

Duodenoscopy has become more and more a part of routine upper gastrointestinal endoscopy. This is particularly true when the longer forward-viewing scopes are used. Side-viewing scopes are excellent if not preferable for gastric examination. It is also a good instrument for bulbar duodenoscopy and indispensable at present for cannulating the papilla of Vater. Bulbar duodenoscopy is indicated to search for or confirm an ulcer crater when the x-ray shows a deformed bulb, to attempt to prove or disprove a duodenitis when the x-ray shows an irritable bulb or when there are symptoms of duodenal ulcer and a negative x-ray. Duodenoscopy is also indicated when there is a demonstrated or suspected bulbar polyp or suspected erosions, apparent extrinsic pressure deformities or other possible bulbar disorders. Further discussion of this subject appears in Chapter 23.

Post Bulbar Duodenal Lesions

Post-bulbar duodenoscopy is indicated when there are questionable or definitive x-ray lesions in this portion of the organ, x-ray or other findings indicating probable disease in the biliary system or pancreas. Some of these disorders are ulcerative, scirrhous or polypoid carcinoma originating in the duodenum or at the papilla of Vater. Visualization and study of the biliary tract and pancreatic ductal system by cannulation of the papilla of Vater and the combined use of x-ray have become an ever increasing indication for post-bulbar duodenoscopy, choledocho-cholangiography and pancreatograms.

CONTRAINDICATIONS

Contraindications are usually classified as absolute and relative. In these times of rapidly developing *miracle* endoscopes there are very few absolute contraindications for upper gastrointestinal fiberoptic endoscopy which are not very obvious.

Absolute Contraindications

Absolute contraindications would include any case of very severe shock from massive blood loss (until patient is reasonably out of shock), acute coronary occlusion, severe heart failure, hyperpyrexia as in massive pneumonia and other severe infections. Comatose states, presence of acute and subacute crises, as in asthmatic dyspnea, recent epileptic seizure, severe symptoms of emphysema and obstructive pulmonary diseases should be regarded as strong contraindications. Finally, severe states of physical disability from any cause and episodes associated with dementia are contraindications to endoscopy. There are two major anatomical defects which should be especially considered as absolute contraindications. They are aortic aneurysms and large Zenkers' type esophageal diverticulum. The latter defect should be obvious by x-ray and lesions or suspected lesions below such a diverticulum should not tempt the risks of endoscopy.

Relative Contraindications

The discussion of relative contraindications to upper gastrointestinal endoscopy may be divided into two divisions, namely, contraindications for side-viewing scopes, and contraindication for forward-viewing scopes. The construction differentials of the two types of instruments are discussed in Chapter 5.

For Side-Viewing Scopes

Side-viewing endoscopy is relatively contraindicated in all cases of intrinsic or extrinsic obstruction along the passageway of the esophagus. This is true because the standard side-viewing scopes do not adequately visualize the esophagus except in mega-esophagus. Introduction of these instruments including the original lens scopes of the Schindler type depend upon the sense of resistance in the examiner's hands and fingers as the principal guide to passage through the esophagus. In the hands of the skilled endoscopist, however, this type of sensitivity may be more trustworthy than the observing eye. In the not too distant future, improved combined forward and side-viewing scopes or smaller diameter *side eye* scopes may modify the relative contraindications of today.

The principal intrinsic esophageal lesions which may relatively contraindicate side-viewing endoscopy are cancer, partial stricture, persistent spasm, advanced achalasia, small diverticula, massive varices, neoplasms partially blocking the cardio-esophageal orifice, large hiatus hernia with displacement of the upper loculus and recent ingested corrosives.

Extrinsic esophageal lesions which may constitute relative contraindications to side-viewing endoscopy include thoracic lesions which cause pressure on the esophagus such as mediastinal tumors, bronchogenic carcinoma, massive hilar adenopathy, pulmonary neoplasms with massive lung envolvement and extreme spinal deformities.

For Forward-Viewing Scopes

Forward-viewing endoscopes, rigid or fiberoptic are the only endoscopic instruments so far developed which adequately visualize the esophagus. Because esophageal mucosa and the lumen can be viewed ahead of the tip of the instrument, there are few intrinsic contraindications in this type of examination in the hands of a trained endoscopist. There is a relative contraindication to forceful attempts to pass a blunt-nose endoscope through a constricted area of the esophagus. Careful introduction of a transendoscopic biopsy forceps or brush is important to achieve a tissue diagnosis. Inserting the tip of a forceps or brush, however, into a constricted lumen beyond the continuous sight of the operator is perilous and may sooner or later lead to calamity.

For All Types of Scopes

EXTRINSIC ESOPHAGEAL AND GASTRIC DISPLACEMENTS: These displacements may constitute relative contraindications to endoscopy with all types of scopes. When the stomach is displaced or its shape considerably altered due to compression by liver enlargement, pancreatic tumor, spinal deformities or post-operative lesions, forward and side-viewing scopes may fail to enter the upper or lower depths of the stomach. When gentle introduction and manipulations fail to enter any part of the gastric pouch, the examiner must be willing to fail rather than risk forceful projection of the instrument, especially with undaunted tip deflection and rotation.

GENERAL SYSTEMIC DISORDERS: Diseases involving other systems may be severe, moderate or mild. As discussed earlier in this chapter, endoscopy is seldom justified in the presence of severe systemic disorders. If the systemic disorders are of moderate severity, endoscopy may or may not be relatively contraindicated for all types of instruments. Once the endoscope has passed through the esophagus, contraindications are the same for forward and side-viewing instruments.

PENETRATING AND PERFORATED GASTRIC ULCER: Among other relative contraindications to gastroscopy, must be mentioned penetrating and perforated gastric ulcer especially with the inordinate use of air. If there are acute symptoms of penetration or a local area of acute abdominal tenderness suggesting localized peritoneal irritation, endoscopy must be carried out with special caution. The decision of when to withhold or proceed in these cases must be based upon experience and considered judgment.

BULBAR DUODENAL LESIONS: Contraindications to bulbar duodenoscopy must include impending perforation of penetrating duodenal ulcer as made by x-ray and clinical judgment, marked deformity and obstruction as determined by x-ray, clinical judgment and perhaps gentle endoscopy trial and intractable bleeding with hemorrhagic shock.

POST-BULBAR DUODENAL LESIONS: Contraindications in post-bulbar duodenoscopy include all the conditions described above plus the occasional occurrence of congenitally predisposed diverticula near the papilla of Vater.

EXTREMES OF AGE GROUPS AND UNCOOPERATIVE PATIENT: Two other categories must be mentioned in the consideration of contraindications. One is that of age. The very young and the very elderly are likely not be to good choices for endoscopy. Secondly, if the patient is very uncooperative or demented, his reactions may be unpredictable during the course of an endoscopic procedure. When such a history is known or predictable, the examination may be contraindicated. Irrational patients and severe chronic alcoholics must sometimes be considered in this category to avoid injury to the patient and the instruments.

In the final analysis, relative contraindications to endoscopy involve such additional factors as adequate psychological preparation, adequate pre-medication and the relative skill of the examiner.

LIMITATIONS

When one considers the limitations of upper gastrointestinal endoscopy he most frequently thinks of the procedure in terms of comparison with routine x-ray. Schindler warned in the very beginning that gastroscopy should not be regarded as being in competition with x-ray. He rightfully emphasized that the endoscopic method should be regarded as a comple-mentary method. Fiberoptic endoscopy has now firmly established itself as a complementary method to x-ray and in some instances it is indeed fast becoming a competitive method for x-ray. It is competitive in the sense of being equal or of greater relative importance, rather than replacing x-ray.

Through the years on the plus side for x-ray has been its greater con-venience for the patient. X-ray is less discomforting for the patient and the compassionate amateur endoscopist. This is not to malign compassion, for compassion is always a greater virtue than overzealousness in endos-copy. X-ray is less expensive and is less subject to accidents.

For the sake of comparison, let us consider the advantages of x-ray and endoscopy in the three upper organs of the alimentary tract. High-grade constrictions producing a lumen smaller than the diameter of the scope, marked achalasia, large hiatus hernias with partial obstruction and marked distortion of the esophagus by external compression are conditions in which endoscopy would have very definite limitations or no accessibility. X-ray in all these conditions may be diagnostic. In those conditions where x-ray and endoscopy have equal accessibility, endoscopy may have the ef-fect of confirming x-ray opinions or ruling out a false positive or negative x-ray finding and the added advantage of a tissue diagnosis. Thus the lim-itations of endoscopy and x-ray may be similar in instances where both to-gether are quite productive.

With reference to the stomach, endoscopy again may have definite lim-itations if there are severe obstructive lesions, intrinsic or extrinsic. How-ever, these conditions are not very frequent. On the other hand, in the overwhelming majority of cases where intragastric disease is present, gas-troscopy is capable of a definitive diagnosis probably with no *blind spots*. There are many instances where routine x-ray cannot do nearly as well. I refer particularly to the gastritides, small or difficultly placed ulcer and can-cers and other lesions discussed in detail in other chapters in this text.

The addition of x-ray mucosal relief films are always better than routine studies with the barium-filled stomach.

With reference to the bulbar duodenum, added skill is required to consistently enter the bulb after gastroscopy. Still more practice and knowledge are required to properly examine the post-bulbar duodenum and to carry out papilla cannulation procedures, which are well described in Chapter 24.

Finally, in the consideration of all that has been written above it must be remembered that actually a relative contraindication for one operator may be an absolute contraindication for another. The limitations and risks of endoscopy are directly proportional to the training and skill of the endoscopist. It is therefore, of paramount importance that any doctor who wishes to perform endoscopy should have been trained first and preferably in gastroenterology. Otherwise he must be trained as an internist, abdominal surgeon or occasionally as a roentgenologist before entering upon his training as a gastrointestinal endoscopist and coming face to face with the responsible decisions of indications, contraindications and limitations in gastrointestinal endoscopy.

REFERENCES

1. Schindler, R.: *Gastroscopy, Endoscopic Pathology of the Stomach.* Chicago, Univ. of Chicago Press, 1937.
2. Berry, L. H.: Gastroscopy, indications and limitations. *Hospital Medicine,* 5:85-97, 1969.
3. Palmer, E. D.: *Clinical Gastroenterology.* New York, Hoeber, 1957, pp. 44-48.
4. Hillman, H. S., and Parsons, P. J.: Gastroscopy—its uses and limitations. *Med J Aust,* 2:11-13, 1962.
5. Hirschowitz, B. I.: Gastroduodenal endoscopy with the fiberscope. *Bull Gastrointestinal Endoscopy,* 8:15-22, 1962.
6. McGlone, F. B., and Phillips, R. G.: Indications, contraindications and complications of gastroscopy. *Gastrointest Endos,* 14:108-112, 1967.
7. Brown, C. H.: Editorial. Why does one do gastroscopy? *Gastrointest Endos,* 16:110, 1969.
8. Brick, J. B., and Palmer, E. D.: Comparison of esophagoscopy and roentgenography in the diagnosis of varices in cirrhosis of the liver. *Am J Roentgenol,* 73:387, 1955.
9. Broders, A. C., Vinson, P. P., and Davis, P. K.: Hemangioendothelioma of the esophagus: case report. *Arch Otorhinolaryng,* 18:168-171, 1933.
10. Mallory, G. K., and Weiss, S.: Hemorrhage from lacerations of the cardiac orifice of the stomach due to vomiting. *Am J Med Sci,* 178:506, 1929.
11. Dagradi, A. E., Stempien, S. J., Juler, G., Broderick, J., and Wolinski, S.: The Mallory-Weiss lesion, an endoscopic study of thirty cases. *Gastrointest Endos,* 13:18-19, 1967.
12. Berry, L. H.: Analysis of 1400 consecutive gastroscopic examinations. *Proc Inst Med Chic,* 16:237, 1946.
13. Berry, L. H., Villa, F., Adomavicius, P., and Alavi, I.: Comparative endoscopic study of gastroesophageal cancer. (In Press)

14. Bralow, S. P., and Spellberg, M. A.: Diverticula of the stomach: report of 26 new cases. *Gastroenterology, 11*:59-82, 1948.
15. Berry, L. H.: Right side gastroscopic technic in situs inversus viscerum and visualization of "blind spots." *Rev Gastroent, 8*:267-272, 1941.
16. Berry, L. H.: Improved gastroscopic diagnosis by the use of multiple positions in 2843 cases. *Gastroenterology, 44*:20-24, 1963.
17. Valeri, J., and DiBianco, J.: Trichobezoar: an endoscopic study. *Gastrointest Endos, 13*:31-33, 1967.
18. Nelson, R. S.: Gastroscopic observations on the persimmon bezoar. *Bull Gastrointestinal Endoscopy, 10*:9-12, 1963.
19. Kleckner, F. S.: Intragastric magnet for removal of foreign bodies. *Gastrointest Endos, 16*:151, 1970.

CHAPTER 4

PREPARATION AND PREMEDICATION IN UPPER GASTROINTESTINAL ENDOSCOPY

ARTHUR P. KLOTZ AND ROBERT R. LAING

INTRODUCTION

THE FLEXIBLE WOLF-SCHINDLER gastroscope introduced in 1932 established gastroscopy as both a hospital and outpatient procedure. The outpatient examination is preferably performed in the hospital. The patient usually is able to leave following the examination after a brief rest and proceed with his daily routine. Since he must fast for the examination the most convenient time is in the morning.

PSYCHOLOGICAL PREPARATION OF THE PATIENT

Successful endoscopy as clearly pointed out by Berry depends upon preliminary psychological preparation of the patient to dispel anxiety and fear.[1] The endoscopist should personally provide a simple, clear, brief explanation about the procedure. If he acts as a consultant he should visit the patient the day before to establish rapport. At this time he can assess the general personality of the patient, inquire into the history of any drug allergies and ask about medications currently being taken.

PREMEDICATIONS

Ordinarily a hypodermic premedication given 10 to 15 minutes in advance of the procedure followed by the application of a topical anesthetic to the oropharynx is the standard approach. The ideal premedication should 1) allay apprehension and fear, 2) increase pain tolerance, 3) depress the gag reflex, 4) decrease oral and gastric secretions, 5) have minimal side effects, and 6) be of short duration, preferably leaving the patient alert at the completion of the examination.[2, 3]

Few routines meet these criteria. Many sedate the patient for hours thus making them impractical for outpatients. Increased levels of sedation may be detrimental in obtaining optimal results.[4] Any method that sacrifices safety for convenience must be condemned.

Narcotics

Meperidine Hydrochloride (Demerol®) is probably the agent of choice at present and the most popular medication since it is potent, effective and safe.[5] In usual therapeutic doses it has a marked analgesic effect and assists in diminishing apprehension and fear. Some endoscopists suggest that it significantly reduces salivary secretions and possesses spasmolytic sedative qualities. Slight and transient light-headedness and vertigo are the most common side effects. Although many physicians use doses greater than 50mg[6, 7] this amount is probably optimal in the average case since doubling this dose only results in a 25 per cent increase in the pain threshold but a two-fold increase in vertigo and light-headedness.[4, 8]

Fifty to one hundred mg of meperidine intravenously without local anesthetic has been used in a series with some success.[9] However the incidence of serious side effects, particularly respiratory depression is increased thereby limiting this approach. Morphine sulfate has been replaced almost entirely by meperidine in order to avoid nausea and vomiting. Pentazocine (Talwin®) has been used by some but appears to have more side effects.

Anticholinergic Drugs

These decrease salivary secretion and inhibit gastric and duodenal motility and secretion. Atropine is commonly used in combination with meperidine. The usual dose is 0.6mg given 10 to 15 minutes prior to the procedure. Lesser dosages usually do not decrease gastric and salivary secretions and large doses may result in tachycardia as shown by Barowsky et al.[10]

Propantheline bromide (Pro-Banthine®) is similar to atropine. Dosage is usually 6mg. This amount intravenously, or 0.8mg atropine sulfate

I.M.[11] has been shown to produce aperistalsis in 1 to 3½ minutes lasting 5 to 30 minutes.[10] However, propantheline compared to atropine produces fewer and less annoying side effects.

Special premedication consideration must be given to duodenoscopy particularly when it is performed for catheterization of the papilla of Vater and radiological visualization of the pancreatic ducts. Since patients should be well relaxed for this maneuver Japanese authors recommend intravenous tranquilizers and routine use of adequate doses of anticholinergic drugs to decrease motility in the duodenum. This is essential for introduction of the catheter into the duct. As a consequence, the premedication discussed for other routine endoscopic procedures must include larger doses of anticholinergics, plus relaxing tranquilizing medications to allow the endoscopist enough time to accomplish his catheterization maneuvers which may take an additional 30 to 40 minutes.

Radiologic hypotonic duodenography causes relaxation in 5 minutes and lasts 10 to 20 minutes when 30 to 60mg of propantheline is used intramuscularly or intravenously. Such an effect is desirable in duodenoscopy. Tachycardia frequently occurs but is usually of no significance. Propranolol (Inderal®) 0.5 to 1mg I.V. may be used for sinus tachycardia if clinically necessary. Anticholinergics should not be used in patients with glaucoma or bladder neck obstruction nor if antral motility is being evaluated.

Antihistamines and Psychotropic Agents

The antihistaminic agent promethazine hydrochloride (Phenergan®) has a prolonged hypnotic action. In 50mg doses it sedates, decreases oral secretion and potentiates the effect of meperidine.[12] Some authors have suggested that in the elderly and poor risk patient a small dose of meperidine with promethazine may be the combination of choice.[2] Promethazine may also have protective action in the prevention of reactions to local anesthesia.

Tranquilizers such as chlordiazepoxide (Librium®) and chlorpromazine (Thorazine®) in 50mg doses have hypnotic action and potentiate meperidine analgesia. The usefulness of chlorpromazine with meperidine is limited because of a synergistic hypotensive effect. Diazepam (Valium®) in 5 to 10mg doses is moderately effective as shown by Ticktin.[13] It has anticonvulsant properties which may prevent toxic reactions to local anesthetics. Its main advantage is muscle relaxation being five times more potent than chlordiazepoxide.[14] It should be noted, however, that diazepam unlike other tranquilizers sometimes causes central nervous system stimulation.

Barbiturates have been the major psychotropic agents used in premedication for many years. Their anticonvulsant properties were thought to offset toxic reactions to local anesthetics.[2, 3, 15, 16] They are not true analgesics but relieve pain only by impairing consciousness. Overdose may lead to respiratory and circulatory depression and predispose to laryngospasm. In the early years of endoscopy, Dr. Schindler recommended 0.65mg of atropine and 0.13gm of sodium phenobarbital hypodermically one-half to three-quarters of an hour before using local anesthesia.[15] The sodium phenobarbital was used routinely to counteract possible toxic effects of the anesthetic which today is known not to be the case.

Diazepam I.V. is helpful in the extremely anxious patient. Five to ten mg by slow intravenous injection to the point of relaxation allows the endoscopist to perform an adequate examination. Although respiratory depression has been reported, the incidence is quite low.[13, 14] If respiratory depression should occur, the patient's respiration should be assisted by an Ambu bag or a similar device. Such equipment should be permanently available in any room where endoscopy is performed and someone must always be in attendance until the patient is fully recovered.

TOPICAL ANESTHETICS

Some form of oral topical anesthetic is desirable and probably necessary (Table 4-I). It is mainly used to suppress the gag reflex. No unanimity of opinion exists in regard to topical agents. Those most frequently used in

TABLE 4-I

SUGGESTED PREMEDICATION SCHEDULES
(ALWAYS BASED ON INDIVIDUAL PATIENT APPRAISAL)

	Routine	*For the Elderly*
Esophagoscopy and Gastroscopy	25 to 50mgm meperidine I.M. with 0.6mgm atropine I.M. 15-20 min. pre-op, and 5-10mgm diazepam I.V. Immediately pre-op if indicated.*	25mgm meperidine I.M. with 50 mgm promethazine I.M.
Duodenoscopy	50mgm meperidine I.M. with 30-60 mgm propantheline I.V. and 5-10 mgm diazepan I.V. Introduodenal simethicone 5-10 ml or a swallow of Mylicon®.	

Topical Anesthetic: Just before I.V. medication or 5-10 min. pre-op.
1% Tetracaine: Cotton pledget dipped into container with 4-5ml of sol.
1% Dyclonine: Cotton pledget dipped into container with 6-10ml of sol.

* Berry states that in some clinics such as Cook County Hospital, Chicago, 25mgm of meperidine would seldom be sufficient for adequate sedation even in combination with other sedatives in moderate amounts. A frequent schedule there is 50mgm meperidine I.M., and diazepam, 5mgm I.V. or vice versa. In very robust individuals or alcoholics, the doses required are often 75mgm meperidine and 5 to 7½ mgm diazepam. In Japanese clinics much smaller doses of sedatives seem to be required then in many other areas.[34]

the past have been tetracaine hydrochloride (Pontocaine®), hexylcaine (Cyclaine®), lidocaine hydrochloride (Xylocaine®), cocaine and dyclonine hydrochloride (Dyclone®).

Prior to 1943 toxic reactions occurring with endoscopy were not emphasized and only one fatality had been reported.[17] Since that time many non-fatal reactions have been reported as well as occasional reactions which resulted in death.[16, 18, 19] Toxic reactions were originally thought to be due to hypersensitivity. It is now clear that most reactions are actually a consequence of overdose.

In a review of five papers, nine deaths were reported due to the local anesthetic used and where the amount was mentioned all the deaths could be accounted for by an overdose.[17–21] Absorption from the mucous membrane and other highly vascularized areas is more rapid than that observed in perineural tissue accounting for the greater frequency of reactions after topical application compared to surgical nerve blocks. Dr. Schindler advocated the use of 1:1,000 epinephrine solution 1 drop/ml of Pontocaine when 2 per cent Pontocaine was used as the topical anesthetic. This is of historical interest only since it does not decrease absorption.

Evaluations of local anesthetic reactions associated with endoscopy are possible only with large composite series of patients. Palmer and Wirtz in a survey of 307,715 endoscopies noted 42 serious toxic reactions, 38 of which were felt to be related to topical anesthetic use.[22] Of these 38, 18 were pre-treated with barbiturates. In the 38 reactions, 10 resulted in death. The authors concluded that 33 per cent of all endoscopic deaths were due to the local anesthetic. Approximately 25 per cent of all reactions reported were fatal.

Reactions may be divided into *immediate reactions* and *delayed reactions*.[23]

Immediate reactions are the most severe but fortunately are rare. Onset occurs almost immediately after application of the topical anesthetic and usually results in sudden death.

The *delayed reaction* occurs 3 to 20 minutes after the application of the anesthetic. Initial manifestations are euphoria and talkativeness occasionally accompanied by short coughing spells. This may progress to apprehension, restlessness, dyspnea and muscle twitching. If this continues unabated, convulsions and death may follow. Schindler, as noted above, believed that the routine use of barbiturates abolished major reactions. Seevers on the other hand states that "in reality we are living in a fool's paradise since the quantity of barbiturates ordinarily administered for this purpose is entirely inadequate to prevent anything but the most minor manifestations of toxicity from these agents."[24] Weisil reported 19 reactions in 1,000 patients despite the prophylactic administration of sodium luminal.[18]

The addition of a vasoconstrictor such as epinephrine to the anesthetic solution as previously mentioned has been thought to diminish the rate of absorption and to prevent a rapid rise in blood levels. Adriani, however, states that this is only true when the drug is used perineurally or intrathecally.[25] He has demonstrated that epinephrine on mucous membranes does not significantly retard absorption.[26] Because there appears to be no experimental nor clinical justification for the use of epinephrine, we do not employ it nor recommend its use.

The concentration of the local anesthetic is of the utmost importance. If tetracaine is used, the lowest concentration that will give a satisfactory result should be employed such as a ½% or a 1% solution. A 1% solution has been found to give optimal suppression of the gag reflex.[25] The *total dose should not exceed 50mg* whether it is given in a ½% or a 1% solution.[23] A 2% solution of tetracaine is four times as toxic as a 1% solution and 16 times as toxic as a ½% solution. Tetracaine is known to be 2½ times more toxic than cocaine milligram for milligram, however, a 4 to 10% concentration of cocaine is required to produce optimal results. Benzonatate (Tessalon®), a derivative of tetracaine used by some endoscopists, has thus far been found to have a very low incidence of reactions, 1 in 4,000, but anesthesia is not complete.[27] Lidocaine[2, 28] and hexylcaine do not appear to be any less toxic than tetracaine and offer no real advantage.

Dyclonine has been found to be extremely effective.[29, 30] Onset of anesthesia begins in approximately 2 minutes and reaches a maximum intensity in 4 to 6 minutes. Intense anesthesia lasts from 20 to 25 minutes with decreasing anesthesia in an additional 15 minutes.[30] Dyclonine appears to be a safer local anesthetic. Although reactions have been reported the rate is approximately 25 per cent of that seen with the most commonly used local anesthetics.[31]

Several fatalities have been reported. Although we still feel that tetracaine is a satisfactory anesthetic, we prefer dyclonine.

Application for maximum safety is by the use of a cotton pledget on a Sawtelle applicator soaked in the anesthetic solution and applied to the pharynx. Eight to ten milliliters of a 0.5% solution or 4 to 5ml of a 1% solution of tetracaine or 6 to 10ml of a 1% solution of dyclonine are measured into a medicine glass. The cotton pledget is dipped into the solution and pressed dry. The patient is seated comfortably and all loose dentures are removed. A quiet, unhurried atmosphere is desirable. The patient's tongue is grasped between folded gauze and gently pulled forward by the operator. The pledget is placed in the tonsillar fossa or behind the palatine tonsil in the oropharynx at the site of the palatopharyngeal arch. The pledget is held in place for approximately 20 seconds on each side. This is repeated 2 to 4 times or until the gag reflex is adequately suppressed. When the patient no longer gags, anesthesia is satisfactory.

More rapid absorption occurs with an atomized spray or gargle because of the increased surface area covered and absorption of the spray as it is inhaled.[23] Consequently sprays and gargles should in general be avoided. For similar reasons, the solution should not be swallowed.

TREATMENT OF TOXIC REACTIONS
Immediate Reaction

Toxic reactions of the immediate type with sudden and complete collapse of the patient may be cerebral, medullary or cardiovascular (Table 4-II). In such instances, cardiac resuscitation by external cardiac massage should be started immediately and artificial respiration instituted. Electric countershock can be quickly applied for ventricular fibrillation if present and may be added to cardiac massage. Immediately 0.5 to 1.0ml of intracardiac epinephrine 1:1,000 should be given. Thereafter monitoring by EKG and continued artificial respiration must follow.

Delayed Reaction

For delayed reactions consisting of euphoria and talkativeness, placing the patient in the supine position may suffice when the symptoms do not progress. If central nervous system stimulation increases, 2 to 5ml of a

TABLE 4-II

EMERGENCY PROCEDURES FOR ENDOSCOPY DRUG REACTIONS

Immediate Reactions:
  Intermediate cardiac massage. Assistant to obtain EKG monitor with other assistants in room. Establish contact with Anesthesiology Dept. and Cardiac Arrest Team.
  Immediate artificial respiration with oxygen tank and self-inflating (Ambu) bag attached to oxygen mask or mouth to mouth resuscitation.
  Electric countershock for ventricular fibrillation.
  Intracardiac epinephrine 1cc 1:10,000.
  Intravenous sodium pentothal for seizures.
  Place endotracheal tube with laryngoscope and maintain pharyngeal airway. Perform tracheotomy if necessary.

Delayed Reactions:
  Artificial respiration if needed and oxygen by mask.
  Continuous observation with patient in supine position.
  Intravenous barbiturate for CNS stimulation (none if there is CNS depression).

Tachycardias:
  If serious sinus tachycardia use propranolol (Inderal®) 0.5 to 1mgm I.V.
  If P.A.T. try carotid sinus pressure.
  Maintain blood pressure with phenylephrine (Neo-synephrine®) 0.5 to 1.0mgm diluted in 10ml saline intravenously slowly. Maintain B.P. with metaraminol (Aramine®) subcutaneously or I.M. in 3-15mgm dosage.

TABLE 4-III

LOCAL ANESTHETIC REACTIONS

I. Toxic Response in Normal Individuals
  A. CNS effects
    Stimulation or depression
    (a) Cerebral cortex
    (b) Medulla
      1. Respiratory
      2. Vasomotor
      3. Gastrointestinal
  B. Cardiovascular effects
    1. Cardiac arrest
    2. Vasomotor collapse
II. Allergy, Hypersensitivity, Idiosyncracy

2½% sodium pentothal solution should be administered intravenously. Oxygen by machine and mask should also be employed. Caution must be used in the administration of short acting barbiturates because depression from the barbiturates may have an additive effect to the depressive effect of the toxic reaction. Thus when a patient shows signs of central nervous system depression, barbiturates are contraindicated.

Although most reactions are due to anesthetic overdose, a few patients are thought to have allergic reactions (Table 4-III). The clinical separation of these abnormal reactions from toxic responses is difficult but the treatment of both is identical. There is no completely reliable way to pretest for anesthetic sensitivity because patch, intradermal, and conjunctival tests are not valid enough to warrant routine use. Furthermore, a history of the uneventful use of a given anesthetic is no insurance against later sensitivity to the same drug. Fortunately, there is little cross antigenicity between most local anesthetics because of their diverse chemical structures. If a patient has a history of a drug reaction, the local anesthetic may be eliminated or another drug may be substituted. The prophylatic use of

TABLE 4-IV

EQUIPMENT ALWAYS ON HAND FOR ENDOSCOPY PROCEDURES

(Extra *assistants* should *always* be *present*. Liaison with Anesthesiology Dept. always maintained.)

1. Oxygen tank. B.P. apparatus and stethoscope.
2. Bag and mask and pharyngeal airway.
3. Laryngoscope and endotracheal tube.
4. Epinephrine for intracardiac injection for cardiac arrest.
5. Sodium pentothal for intravenous injection for convulsions or CNS stimulation.
6. Phenylephrine (Neosynephrine®) for intravenous injection for P.A.T.
7. Metaraminol (Aramine®) for injection to maintain blood pressure.
8. Propranolol (Inderal®) for intravenous injection for severe sinus tachycardia.
9. Cardioverter for ventricular fibrillation, and ECG monitor readily available.

antihistamines in patients with known allergic tendencies may be advisable.[2]

Since toxic reactions can occur quickly, the endoscopic examining room must always be equipped with oxygen, inhalation apparatus, barbiturates for immediate intravenous use and intravenous epinephrine for cardiovascular depressive emergencies (Table 4-IV). Sufficient help should be present for immediate assistance in the application of cardiac massage and artificial respiration.

GENERAL ANESTHESIA

General anesthesia is unnecessary for routine endoscopy. Reasons given for its use have been (1) lack of patient cooperation, (2) endoscopic anatomical variation, (3) heart disease and (4) better endoscopic visualization. Schindler[15] and Palmer[16] have pointed out that peroral endoscopy under general anesthesia is more dangerous than that conducted with some degree of cooperation from the patient.

We feel that general anesthesia is sometimes necessary for foreign body removal from the esophagus, especially in children.[32]

SPECIAL CONSIDERATIONS

In selected instances alterations in routine premedications are necessary. Monat observed that young adults required more medication than older individuals.[7] As a part of a controlled study, we too have observed that the older individuals on a standard dose tolerated the procedure better than the younger ones.[4]

Prompt endoscopy for diagnosis in patients bleeding from the upper gastrointestinal tract is commonly performed. Patients with acute gastrointestinal hemorrhage may require less premedication because of the hypotensive effect of hypnotics and the increased susceptibility to aspiration during the procedure.[33]

In the past with the use of a rigid or older fiberoptic instrument, gastric aspiration with an Ewald tube was routine before passage of the instrument. With the more refined fiberoptic equipment this approach is required only in situations where outlet obstruction is present. This can best be done by passing an Ewald tube into the stomach with the patient in the sitting position. The patient is then placed in the Trendelenburg position, then on his left side and the stomach drained by dependent drainage or suction. The tube may then be used for rinsing the stomach with water or saline to remove all particles. Unless all retained material is thoroughly removed by lavage endoscopy is usually a failure. Therefore, if persistent rinsing is unsuccessful it is better to cancel the procedure until the stomach can be completely cleansed by giving the patient a clear liquid diet or by the use of continuous gastric suction for several days.

Air bubbles may be a problem. Simethicone is quite useful for this. Dispersion of bubbles is accomplished by having the patient chew and swallow two tablets of simethicone immediately prior to the use of the topical anesthetic. This is particularly helpful and desirable in the post-gastrectomy patient.

Air bubbles may also be a major problem in duodenoscopy. Prior ingestion of simethicone is sometimes of no benefit here. We have found that 5 to 10ml of water with 0.4ml simethicone (Mylicon®) rinsed into the suction port with the tip of the tube in the duodenum is quite effective for this.

CONCLUSION

This chapter has reviewed a number of endoscopy premedication combinations reported in the literature that permit the reader reasonable evaluation and selection. Fortunately there is general agreement on certain precautions and premedications.

The endoscopist should select a premedication schedule and use it critically, changing or adjusting to meet his specific needs. It is his responsibility to establish a sound technic which reduces reactions and complications to an absolute minimum. At the same time he must be prepared with appropriate equipment to treat any emergency. The greatest area of danger is the use of topical anesthetics and control of this consists in limitation of the total dose of topical anesthetic used.

REFERENCES

1. Berry, Leonidas H.: How important is endoscopic premedication? Guest Editorial. *Gastrointest Endosc, 15*:170-171, 1969.
2. Benias, G. B.: Anesthetics and premedication in peroral endoscopy. *Arch Otolaryngol, 70*:758-763, 1959.
3. Lierle, D. M.: II. Topical and infiltration anesthesia. *Trans Am Acad Ophthalmol Otolaryngol, 53*:288-293, 1949.
4. Dunn, G. D., Kubin, R. H., Laing, R. R., Sisk, C. W., and Klotz, A. P.: Double-blind study of endoscopy premedications. *Gastrointest Endosc, 14*:229-230, 1970.
5. Batterman, R. C.: Clinical effectiveness and safety of a new synthetic analgesic drug, demerol. *Arch Intern Med, 71*:345-356, 1943.
6. Dobkin, A. B.: Sedatives, analgesics, antidotes, and their interaction; a review. *Can. Anaesth Soc J, 11*:252-279, 1964.
7. Monat, H. A.: Observations on premedication with various drugs in 3000 gastroscopies. *Am J Gastroenterol, 13*:440-441, 1946.
8. Goodman, L. S., and Gilman, A.: *The Pharmacological Basis of Therapeutics*, 2nd ed, New York, Macmillan, 1956.
9. Hofkin, Gerald A.: Simplified anesthesia for peroral endoscopy. *Gastrointest Endosc, 16*:38-39, 1969.
10. Barowsky, H., Greene, L., and Paulo, D.: Cine-gastroscopic observations on the effect of anticholinergic and related drugs on gastric and pyloric motor activity. *Am J Dig Dis, 10*:506-513, 1965.
11. Barowsky, H., Green, L., and Paulo, D.: The effect of anticholinergic drugs on

pyloric function recorded by cinegastroscopy. *Gastrointest Endosc, 12*:23-26, 1966.

12. Laing, R. R., and Klotz, A. P.: Premedication and anesthesia for gastrointestinal endoscopy. *Gastrointest Endosc, 14*:80-86, 1967.

13. Ticktin, H. E., and Trujillo, N. P.: Evaluation of diazepam for preendoscopy medication. *Am J Dig Dis, 10*:948-979, 1956.

14. Feldman, P. E.: An analysis of the efficacy of diazepam. *J Neuropsychiat* (Supplement), *3*:62-67, 1962.

15. Schindler, R.: *Gastroscopy, the Endoscopic Study of Gastric Pathology,* 2nd ed, Chicago, Univ Chicago Press, 1950.

16. Palmer, E. D.: The risks of peroral endoscopy. *U. S. Armed Forces, Med J, 5*:974-994, 1954.

17. Hansen, F. M., Jr., and Stealy, C. L.: Sudden death following the use of pontocaine as a gargle anesthetic for gastroscopic examination. *Am J Gastroenterol 10*:212-213, 1943.

18. Weisel, W., and Tella, R. A.: Reaction to tetracaine (pontocaine) used as topical anesthetic in bronchoscopy, study of 1000 cases. *JAMA, 147*:218-222, 1951.

19. Palmer, E. D., and Deutsch, D. L.: Sudden death during preparation for esophagoscopy with tetracaine gargle. *Am J Dig Dis, 22*:95-96, 1955.

20. Jones, F. A., Doll, R., Fletcher, C., and Rodgers, H. W.: The risks of gastroscopy, a survey of 49,000 examinations. *Lancet, 1*:647-651, 1951.

21. Lintott, G. A. M.: In discussion, P. E. T. Hancock. The practical application of gastroscopy. *Proc R Soc Med, 32*:533-542, 1939.

22. Palmer, E. D., and Wirts, C. W.: Survey of gastroscopic and esophagoscopic accidents: report of a committee on accidents of the American Gastroscopic Society. *JAMA, 164*:2012-2015, 1957.

23. Sadove, M. S., Wyant, G. M., Gittelson, L. A., and Kretchmer, H. E.: Classification and management of reactions to local anesthetic agents. *JAMA, 148*:17-22, 1952.

24. Seevers, M. H.: I. The preparation of the patient. *Trans Am Acad Ophthalmol Otolaryngol, 53*:281-287, 1949.

25. Adriani, J., and Zepernick, R.: Some recent studies on the clinical pharmacology of local anesthetics of practical significance. *Ann Surg, 158*:666-671, 1963.

26. Adriana, J., and Campbell, D.: Fatalities following topical application of local anesthetics to mucous membranes. *JAMA, 162*:1527-1530, 1956.

27. Deutsch, D. L., and Arneson, L. A.: Tessalon as a local anesthetic in peroral endoscopy. *Bull Gastroint Endosc, 12*:25, 1965.

28. Morse, H. R., and Hartman, M. M.: Topical anesthesia for endoscopy. *Pennsylvania Med J, 68*:39-42, 1965.

29. Adriani, J., Zepernick, R., Arens, J., and Authement, E.: The comparative potency and effectiveness of topical anesthetics in man. *Clin Pharmacol Ther, 5*:49-62, 1964.

30. Harris, L. C., Parry, J. C., and Greifenstein, F. E.: Dyclone—a new local anesthetic agent: clinical evaluation. *Anesthesiology, 17*:648-652, 1956.

31. Merifield, D. O., and Johnson, E. E.: Evaluation of a topical anesthetic—dyclone. *Arch Otolaryngol, 74*:437-440, 1961.

32. Jackson, C., and Jackson, C. L.: *Broncho-esophagology.* Philadelphia, Saunders, 1950.

33. Palmer, E. D.: *Diagnosis of Upper Gastrointestinal Hemorrhage.* Springfield, Thomas, 1961.

34. Berry, Leonidas H.: Personal communications to the authors.

CHAPTER 5

PRINCIPLES OF CONSTRUCTION AND TYPES OF INSTRUMENTS FOR UPPER GASTROINTESTINAL ENDOSCOPY

John F. Morrissey

INTRODUCTORY STATEMENT

Endoscopic instruments can be divided into two general types—those which permit direct visualization and those which examine only by photography, gastrocameras. The viewing instruments can be subdivided into three basic types—those which transmit the image directly through an open tipped tube, those in which the image is passed through a series of lenses and those which transmit images through coherent bundles of glass fibers.

OPEN LUMEN ENDOSCOPES

Open lumen instruments are still used in the majority of bronchoscopic and proctoscopic examinations and despite the widespread use of forward-viewing fiberscopes; they are commonly used for esophagoscopy. These instruments have their greatest appeal to surgeons because the open lumen facilitates operative procedures, such as biopsy and polyp removal. Lighting is usually adequate for viewing, but photography requires elaborate equipment and is rarely used. Many surgeons prefer the open-tipped bronchoscopes and esophagoscopes over the fiber optic instruments because, although examinations with the fiberscopes are better tolerated by the patient, they require significantly more time for their completion. Fiber optic colonoscopes are designed for examination of the colon proximal to the distal sigmoid and at times, may not provide as complete an examination of the rectum as can be obtained with a simple open-tipped instrument. Thus, there is no immediate likelihood that the rigid proctoscope will be replaced for routine sigmoidoscopy by flexible instruments (see Chapters 29 and 30).

The introduction by Hufford and the Eder Instrument Company of an esophagoscope with a flexible obturator (Fig. 5-1) converted esophagoscopy from a surgical to a medical procedure.[1] This instrument incorporates a 2.5 power telescopic lens which greatly facilitates diagnosis and surprisingly, has not been adopted by surgeons for their routine esophagoscopic examinations.

Regrettably, two accessories[2,3] which significantly increase the usefulness of the Eder-Hufford instrument, were not available during the many years when the Eder-Hufford instrument was in widespread use, but were introduced during the past few years as the instrument rapidly was being replaced by the new forward-viewing fiber optic instruments. These accessories significantly improve viewing, photography, and biopsy with the instrument. Both accessories have lens optical systems and fiber optic light guides and one of them has a channel for passage of a biopsy forceps.

The new forward viewing fiber optic instruments are rapidly replacing

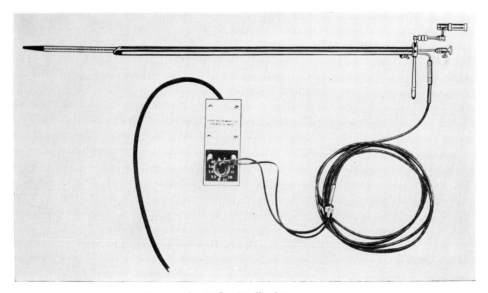

Figure 5-1. Eder-Hufford Instrument.

the rigid esophagoscopes for nearly all the indications for esophagoscopy with the exception of removal of certain foreign bodies. It is only a matter of time until adequate instrumentation is available for use with fiber optic instruments which will permit the removal of essentially all foreign bodies. The latter development is inevitable because so few physicians are being adequately trained at this time in the use of open-tipped instruments.

LENS ENDOSCOPES

The second general type of endoscopic instrument is the lens endoscope. These instruments may be rigid, such as laparoscopes or cystoscopes or semi-flexible, such as the conventional lens gastroscope. Rigid lens systems can transmit images with excellent resolution and faithful color reproduction, but at the expense of a considerable loss of light. Light loss is a major problem in the use of the small semi-flexible lens gastroscopes, such as the Eder-Palmer instrument. Although the human eye can accommodate to low light levels to permit satisfactory viewing, external photography is unsatisfactory. The only lens gastroscopes which permit adequate photography are the French instruments which are equipped with electronic flash.[4] Poor light transmission is a result of the passage of the image through a series of approximately 45 lenses. Each set of lenses focuses the image to a single point, so that some bending of the instrument can take place at each focal point without significantly distorting the image. Great skill is required in order to accurately diagnose more than 40 to 50 per cent of the pathology in the stomach with a lens gastroscope. Modifications were introduced to miniaturize the instrument, provide some degree of tip control, improve close vision, and to provide some degree of biopsy capability. The great shortage of endoscopists who were skilled in the use of the instrument, the inability of these individuals to visualize many rather large gastric lesions because of their location in blind areas, the frequency of diagnostic errors when less skilled physicians attempted to use the instruments, tended to discredit gastroscopy as a diagnostic method within the United States.

FIBEROPTIC ENDOSCOPES

The present advanced era of endoscopy is based upon the development of fiber optics.[5] It comes as a surprise to most endoscopists to learn that the principle that an image could be transmitted by a bundle of glass fibers was known prior to the development of the lens gastroscope. Schindler was aware of the potential of fiber optics, but rejected it in favor of the lens system which he developed with the engineer, George Wolf of Berlin, Germany while working at Munich Schwabing Hospital in Munich. His decision was a sound one because the images transmitted by the early fiber bundles were of poor quality. The transmission of light through a fiber bundle is based upon the fact that a single glass fiber in space will pass a light beam by internal reflection regardless of how the fiber is bent. This occurs because air has a lower refractive index than glass. On the other hand, if a bundle of glass fibers rather than a single fiber is used, light will be lost at each point where one fiber touches another because the glass-air interface has been lost. Thus, the early fiber bundles which were available to Schindler produced poor images because these glass-glass contacts throughout the bundle resulted in excessive light loss. In 1954, Van Heel[6] solved the problem by coating or cladding individual glass fibers with a thin layer of glass of a lower refractive index. Light entering a coated fiber is internally reflected at the glass-glass interface rather than the glass-air interface. There is negligible light leakage from one fiber to another in a bundle made of coated glass fibers.

The image produced by a fiber bundle can be likened to the image of a television screen. In both cases, the image is composed of a series of dots of different colored light. The quality of a television image is dependent on the number of lines which are used to form the image. In a like manner, the quality of a fiber optic image is dependent on the number and size of the individual glass fibers. In addition to the size and number of fibers, image quality is dependent on the ability of the glass fibers to transmit color faithfully. The fiber bundles made in Japan transmit light more faithfully than those made in the United States. The American bundles have always had a loss of red light so that the images tended to be somewhat on the yellow side. This problem is much less now than it was with the very earliest fiberscopes. A second factor in image quality is orientation of individual glass fibers within the bundle. Orientation depends on the technique used to construct the fiber bundle. Fiber bundles are made by winding glass fibers around a large drum—the circumference of which is equal to the desired length of the fiber bundle. The individual fibers are carefully oriented at one point on the drum to form either a round or a square bundle. The fibers are cemented together at that point and the bundle is cut. The cut ends are polished, a powdered lubricant is placed around the free glass fibers to reduce friction between them as the bundle is bent, and the bundle is usually placed in a plastic sheath. Thus, the individual glass fibers are free throughout most of their length permitting the fiber bundles to be flexible. Breakage of fibers was a significant problem in the manufacture of early fiber bundles, but this problem has been corrected to a great extent by the manufacturers.

The Objective Lens

The second feature common to all fiberscopes is an objective lens which focuses the desired image on the distal end of the fiber bundle. Objective lenses are, in many ways, similar to the lenses found in cameras. They may resemble telephoto lenses, such as the lens of the early Hirschowitz gastroscope or they may resemble wide angle lenses, such as the lenses in the more recent forward-viewing fiberscopes. Just as is the case with camera lenses, the telescopic lens has a very shallow depth of field and the wide angle lens has a much greater depth of field. Objective lenses may have a variable focus or a fixed focus, just as camera lenses do. Each lens also has a maximum diaphragm opening or f number which is much larger than the opening provided by the fixed diaphragm. Fiberscopes have not been provided as yet with variable diaphragm settings, such as most cameras have. Since the smaller the diaphragm opening, the greater the depth of field, manufacturers try to set their diaphragm openings as small as possible within the limits of the light provided by their power sources. If the light is adequate and the diaphragm can be set sufficiently small, it may be possible for the manufacturer to use a fixed focus rather than a variable focus objective lens reducing the work of the endoscopist by giving him one less control to deal with. Thus, most colonoscopes and some forward-viewing endoscopes have fixed focus lenses.

Even under ideal conditions, it is not possible to design a lens which has optimal viewing properties throughout the entire range of distances at which it might be used. A manufacturer must select a prime focal distance for each instrument. If an instrument is designed to be used solely within the narrow confines of the duodenum, the prime focal distance can be set quite close, perhaps 1cm. This would permit extremely sharp close-up views of the mucosa and reasonably good views at almost any distance encountered in the organ. A much longer prime focal distance setting would be used in an instrument designed solely for the stomach in order to permit visualization out to perhaps 10cm. The design of a fixed focus lens for a multipurpose instrument built for examining small organs, such as the esophagus and duodenum and also for large organs, such as the stomach, requires some compromises. Thus, the ACMI Poly-directional Forward-Viewing Fiberscope, a fixed focus instrument, permits reasonably sharp views from 8 mm to 6-8 cm. Although this range is adequate for the diagnosis of most of the pathology to be visualized, this instrument cannot provide the extremely sharp close-up views of mucosa which are obtained with the Olympus Model GIF Type D instrument, a variable focus instrument, which permits visualization of the fine capillaries of the gastric mucosa and the villi of the duodenum. As yet, endoscopists have not been able to utilize this dissecting miscroscope type of view of the gastric and duodenal mucosa in order to improve their diagnostic accuracy in the interpretation of gastritis, duodenitis, or other lesions.

The Ocular Lens

A third feature characteristic of all fiberscopes is the presence of an ocular lens which transmits the image from the end of the fiber bundle to the eye or to an external camera. Ocular lenses serve two purposes: First, to magnify the image produced on the end of the fiber bundle and second, to correct for defects in the vision of the endoscopist. These lenses all have an infinity setting which must be used for photographic purposes. The major variable in ocular lenses is that of magnification. Excessive magnification will accentuate the structure of the fiber bundle and provide a distraction to the viewer. This type of distraction is similar to the distraction encountered with the excessively large television screens which were manufactured a few years ago. A second limitation on magnification is the amount of available light which, in turn, is related to the size of the image fiber bundle and to the intensity of the light provided by the fiber light guide in the stomach. Excessive magnification of the image by the ocular lens makes it difficult for external cameras to obtain good photographs. The Olympus instruments incorporate a unique type of ocular lens which can be positioned by an adapter which is attached to an external Olympus Pen camera so that the ocular lens can substitute for the camera lens and focus the image directly on to the photographic film. This provides an economy by eliminating the need for a camera lens and also avoids the additional distortion and light loss produced by passing the image through another lens system. This system has a disadvantage in that the size of the photographic image cannot be varied by changing the focal length of the external camera lens. Lengthening the focal length of the external camera lens will increase the size of the image on the photographic film. It is a common practice to use half-frame cameras for endoscopic photography in order to economize on film costs; and to compensate for the reduction in image size produced by the half-frame camera by using a fairly long 70-100mm lens on the external camera to increase the image size. It should be remembered that doubling the image diameter on a photograph requires a quadrupling of the available light. Most systems are currently designed to provide average exposure times of $\frac{1}{30}$ or $\frac{1}{60}$ of a second, exposures which are just rapid enough to minimize the motion produced by heart action on the photograph.

Illumination

Another variable in fiberscope construction is the source of illumination. All the early fiberscopes made use of tungsten filament bulbs for illumination. The only instruments in widespread use now which make use of tungsten filament bulbs are the gastrocamera fiberscopes. Almost all other instruments make use of an external light source and an integral fiber bundle light guide. The primary reason for shifting from tungsten filament illumination to fiber optic illumination was to provide increased amounts of light for photography with external cameras. In the case of the gastrocamera fiberscopes, photographs are taken with intragastric cameras and there is no need to provide the additional light just for viewing. The external light sources for the fiber optic illumination systems are much more expensive than the simple power sources used for the tungsten filament lamps. The use of fiber optic light guides greatly simplified the construction of the new forward-viewing fiberscopes.

The amount of light delivered by a fiber light guide depends on the size of the fiber bundle and the intensity of the light focused on its proximal end. It is not possible to cut a fiber light guide in two and join it together without a great loss in light, because a large part of the diameter of a fiber bundle is occupied by the spaces between the glass fibers. It is not possible to interrupt a bundle and provide a mechanism for joining it together by which individual fibers match perfectly. This is one reason why all instruments are constructed with a single fiber bundle running from the light source to the tip of the instrument. A second reason is that two fiber bundles would be more costly to make. Instrument manufacturers are taking advantage of the necessary presence of this umbilical cord by including lines for air, water and suction within it. Instruments, in general, make use of a single channel for suction and biopsy. In some instruments, there is only one additional channel which is used for both air and water. In the new Olympus forward-viewing instrument, there are separate tubes for air and water. The disadvantage of having air and water in the same tube is a tendency for a few drops of water to adhere to the inside of the air channel when water is injected into the system and time is wasted getting all the water out of the system in order to produce a clear image.

Tip Deflection

Another consideration in fiberscope manufacture is a mechanism for tip deflection. In recent years, instrument manufacturers have succeeded in providing the endoscopist with increasing degrees of tip control so that the newest ACMI instrument provides over 180° tip deflection in four planes and somewhat lesser degrees of deflection in the intermediate planes between the four primary planes. This ability to maximally deflect the tip of the instrument has been accomplished because fiber bundles have been made sufficiently flexible so that they may be bent in this fashion with a tolerable degree of fiber breakage. Japanese instruments tend to have less tip deflection because their fiber bundles are somewhat less flexible. In order to increase tip deflection, it is necessary to soften the plastic sheath of the tip of the instrument which results in a somewhat floppy tip which makes the instrument more difficult to introduce. A second problem with extreme tip deflection is the difficulty and in some cases the impossibility of passing the biopsy forceps through the instrument in the deflected position. This situation can, in part, be overcome by taking care to curve the instrument so that the biopsy channel follows the outer rather than the inner curvature of the instrument.

Flexibility

The next feature is flexibility. It is possible by altering the construction of the metal sheathing or the plastic covering to greatly vary the rigidity of the connecting tube of a fiberscope. There is definitely an optimal rigidity for a multi-purpose instrument. A more rigid scope is ideal for visualization of lesions in the region of the gastroesophageal junction where the 1:1 response of the tip of such an instrument will permit easy positioning, even in the face of considerable motor activity. On the other hand, when a scope which is too rigid is inserted into the stomach, it will bury itself in the greater curvature and tend to cause an uncomfortable overdistention of the stomach when an attempt is made to pass it toward the pylorus. It is also more likely to cause injury. In contrast, a scope which is too flexible will prove to be very difficult to control in the region of the gastroesophageal junction and will tend to curl and loop back on itself when an attempt is made to pass it into the distal antrum.

The rigidity of the tip has a distinct effect on the function of the tip deflection mechanism. A more rigid instrument will properly maintain the fulcrum at the junction of the connecting tube with the deflecting portion of the instrument. A too flexible scope will tend to fulcrum at the tip of the instrument, thus rendering the deflecting mechanism ineffective. In order to visualize pathology in a deformed pyloroduodenal area, the connecting tube must be rigid enough that deflection of the fiberscope tip will exert sufficient force to move obstructing folds out of the way. The new long forward viewing instruments have optimal flexibility characteristics. This was not the case with some of the older instruments. The earlier Olympus EF-II Fiber Esophagoscope was an example of a too rigid instrument when it was used in the stomach. The Olympus Model JFB Gastroduodenal Fiberscope is an example to a too flexible instrument when it is used to visualize gastric pathology.

TYPES OF FIBERSCOPES

Figure 5-2 shows the Olympus Model GTFA gastrocamera fiberscope.[7, 8] This instrument has a working length of 880mm with a diameter at the tip

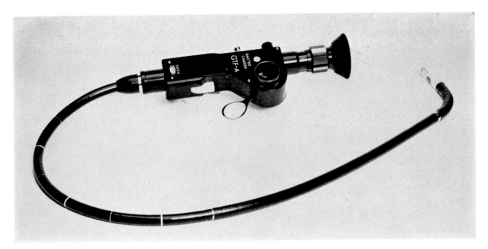

Figure 5-2. Olympus Model GTFA gastrocamera fiberscope.

of 12.7mm. The tip (Fig. 5-3) incorporates a small gastrocamera capable of taking thirty-two 4 × 5mm photographs. The angle of the photographic field is 80° whereas the angle of the visual field is 55°. Objects can be seen from 10-100mm in sharp focus through the 12.5× eye piece. The circular ring on the control unit serves to turn the visual light on and off and to advance the photographic film. A small white knob beneath the ring is the flash button. Tip deflection is 70° upward and downward. Illumination is provided by tungsten filament bulbs. This instrument provides excellent visualization and photography of the entire stomach with the exception of the distal 2cm of antrum and pylorus which will not be well visualized in approximately 10 per cent of cases. The duodenum and esophagus are never visualized with this instrument.

The Eder-Villa Fiberscope[9] was the first fiberscope to attempt by use of a mirror mechanism to provide both forward viewing and side viewing. The development of this instrument was plagued by technical problems and it is no longer being made. The Machida Company has recently introduced a new biopsy fiberscope which also incorporates both forward and side

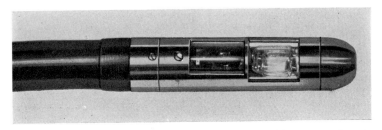

Figure 5-3. The tip of the Model GTFA gastrocamera fiberscope showing the incandescent lamp and the separate lenses for photography and viewing.

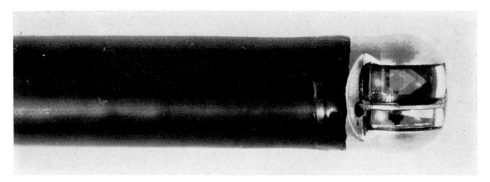

Figure 5-4. Machida two-way scope.

viewing by means of a rotating prism (Fig. 5-4). The disadvantage of these fiberscopes is that the space required for the mirror mechanism has meant elimination of devices for cleaning the lens and a biopsy channel.

Figure 5-5 shows the Olympus Model GIF Type D gastrointestinal fiberscope. This forward-viewing instrument has a working length of 1000mm and a connecting tube diameter of 12.3mm. It has two deflecting mechanisms positioned at right angles to each other to provide 4-way tip control. The proximal angle deflects 150° upward and downward and the distal angle 100° right and left. The variable focus objective lens provides a 75° angle of view with a depth of field from 5mm to infinity. Automatic controls are provided for air, water and suction. Photography requires the use of an external Olympus FIT camera. The suction channel permits the taking of direct vision biopsies and cytologies. Light is provided through an integral fiber light guide from one of four cold light power sources which vary in the intensity of light which they provide and in their automatic features. This instrument permits visualization of the esophagus, stomach and proximal duodenum. The most unique feature of this endoscope is its ability to visualize and photograph mucosa with a greater resolution of detail than is possible with other commonly used endoscopes. Considerable skill is required to make optimal use of this instrument, par-

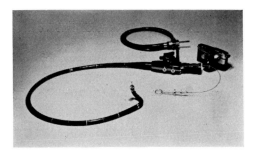

Figure 5-5. The Olympus Model GIF-Type D gastrointestinal fiberscope.

ticularly in order to obtain complete visualization of the proximal lesser curvature of the antrum and cardia.

If the endoscopist wishes to be able to optimally visualize, photograph and biopsy all the lesions which he encounters within the stomach, he must use a side-viewing endoscope, such as the Olympus GF Type B biopsy fiberscope[10] in addition to a longer end-viewing endoscope. The Model GF Type B instrument has a working length of 865mm with a 12mm connecting tube diameter. The variable focus objective lens has an angle of view of 50° and is obliqued 15° forward. The ocular lens magnifies the fiber bundle 12.5×. There is 4-way tip control with 90° up and down and 45° right and left. There is a mechanism to elevate the biopsy forceps 95° into the center of the field of view. Photography is obtained by use of external cameras. Illumination is provided by any one of the cold light supplies used with the Model GIF Type D. The major disadvantage of this instrument is the lack of an automatic air-water-suction mechanism to clean the lens.

Figure 5-6 shows the ACMI Model 7089-P Poly-directional Fiberscope, which is designed for examination of the esophagus, stomach and duodenum. The instrument has an effective length of 105cm with a connecting tube diameter of 12.6mm. It has a forward-viewing 70° wide fixed focus objective lens. Automatic controls are provided for air and suction, and

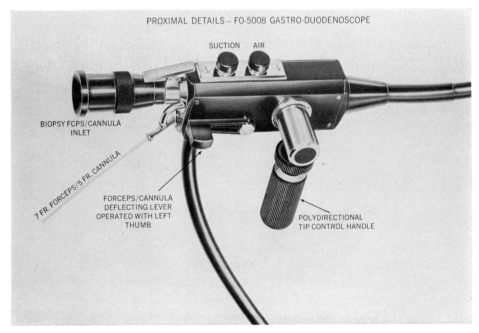

Figure 5-6. FO-5008 Polydirectional Fiberscope. Note the large handle to provide directional control.

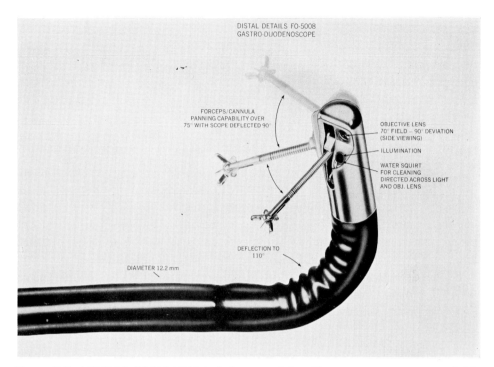

DISTAL DETAILS FO-5008
GASTRO-DUODENOSCOPE

FORCEPS/CANNULA
PANNING CAPABILITY OVER
75° WITH SCOPE DEFLECTED 90°

OBJECTIVE LENS
70° FIELD – 90° DEVIATION
(SIDE VIEWING)

ILLUMINATION

WATER SQUIRT
FOR CLEANING
DIRECTED ACROSS LIGHT
AND OBJ. LENS

DEFLECTION TO
110°

DIAMETER 12.2 mm

Figure 5-7. ACMI Model FO-5008 Polydirectional G.I. fiberscope permits a remarkable 180° curvature of the tip in any of four directions.

water can be introduced by an attached syringe. A unique feature of this instrument is its tip control mechanism which permits a remarkable 180° curvature of the tip in any of four directions (Fig. 5-7). Light is provided by an integral fiber light guide from one of two power sources, the larger of which provides a very bright source of light for photography using a General Electric Mark 300 mercury arc lamp.

An optional recessed tip is preferred by this author over the standard flat tip. The recessed tip keeps the lens away from the mucosa which reduces suction artifacts and prevents loss of view due to *red outs*. This feature is a significant aid in visualization of the duodenal cap and cardia areas. A recessed tip is a standard feature of the Olympus Model GIF instrument.

Very satisfactory results can be obtained with either of the long forward-viewing fiberscopes. It is possible with relative ease to visualize the cardia and fundus in a relaxed patient with the Olympus instrument by deflecting both angles maximally in the same direction. The extra tip deflection provided by the ACMI instrument makes this maneuver much easier. Color transmission of the Olympus fiber bundle is excellent so that the view provides a more natural colored view of the gastric mucosa than that which is seen through the ACMI instrument. Visualization with the Olympus instrument requires the use of a variable focus knob. The need to manipulate an extra control is compensated for by the high resolution of mucosal detail which is obtained.

The average photograph taken by the ACMI instrument tends to be better than what is obtained by the Olympus instrument because of the greater power of its light source, the higher light carrying capacity of its fiber bundles, and the greater depth of field of its fixed focus objective lens. This difference between the instruments is greatest when the object of interest is in motion, making focusing difficult and introducing a motion artifact because of the longer exposure times required for the Olympus fiberscope. On the other hand, when conditions are ideal, the very best photographs in terms of resolution and color rendition will be obtained with the Olympus instrument.

Space does not permit a complete description of all available instruments for examination of the stomach. The instruments which have been described were selected to illustrate various principles of endoscope manu-

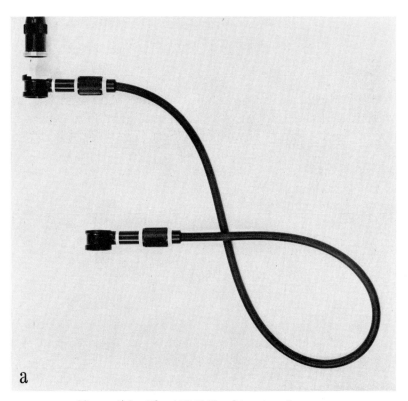

Figure 5-8a. The ACMI Teaching Attachment.

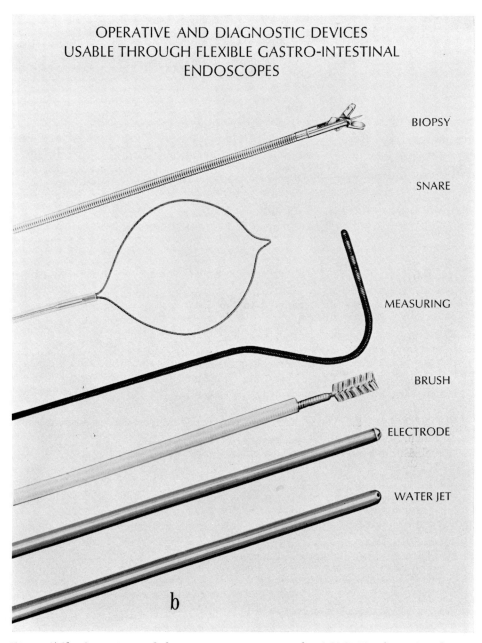

OPERATIVE AND DIAGNOSTIC DEVICES
USABLE THROUGH FLEXIBLE GASTRO-INTESTINAL
ENDOSCOPES

BIOPSY

SNARE

MEASURING

BRUSH

ELECTRODE

WATER JET

b

Figure 5-8b. Operative and diagnostic accessories to the ACMI Teaching Attachment.

facture to assist the endoscopist in the selection of an instrument for his own use. Instrument manufacturers make frequent changes in the characteristics of their instruments, so that the endoscopist must understand the principles behind instrument manufacture if he is to properly evaluate new instruments as they appear on the market. Detailed clinical trials of new instruments are rarely available before instruments are obsolete.

A major advance in endoscopic teaching has been accomplished by the introduction of teaching attachments, such as the ACMI device which is shown in Figures 5-8a and 5-8b. These attachments make use of light splitting prisms which permit approximately one third of the light to reach the endoscopist, one third of the light to reach the student with a loss of approximately one third of the light. The coherent fiber bundles used in these instruments are very similar in quality and cost to the fiber bundles used in the fiberscopes themselves. The quality of view which the endoscopist obtains with these instruments is good enough to permit him to perform essentially all his examinations with the teaching attachment in place, greatly increasing the teaching experience for students in endoscopy.

REFERENCES

1. Hufford, A. R.: Flexi-rigid optical esophagoscope. *Gastroenterology, 12*:779, 1949.
2. Beck, I. T., and Phelps, E.: Esophagoscopic cinematography and biopsy through a new fiberoptic insert adapted to the Hufford esophagoscope. *Gastrointest Endosc, 15*:195-197, 1969.
3. Shipman, J. J.: Illuminated telescope biopsy forceps for sigmoidoscopy or oesophagoscopy. *Lancet, 1*:740, 1965.
4. Colcher, H.: *Gastrophotography and Cinegastroscopy, Progress in Gastroenterology.* Edited by G. B. J. Glass. New York, Grune and Stratton, 1968, p. 97-128.
5. Hirschowitz, B. I.: Fiber optics in modern medicine. *Med Biol Illus, 15*:224-229, 1965.
6. Van Heel, A. C. S.: A new method of transporting optical images without aberration. *Nature, 173*:39, 1954.
7. Cockel, R., and Hawkins, C. F.: Gastroscopy and gastric photography with the Olympus GTF-A. *GUT, 11*:176-181, 1970.
8. Morrissey, J. F., and Koizumi, H.: *The Endoscopic Diagnosis of Gastric Cancer, Sixth National Cancer Conference Proceedings.* Philadelphia, Lippincott, 1970, p. 433-437.
9. Villa, F.: A single scope for the upper GI endoscopic examination. *Gastroenterology, 58*:1078, 1970.
10. Morrissey, J. F.: Gastrointestinal Endoscopy—A review. *Gastroenterology, 62*:1241-1268, 1972.

CHAPTER 6

GENERAL TECHNIC AND ORIENTATION IN UPPER GASTROINTESTINAL ENDOSCOPY

Leonidas H. Berry

INTRODUCTORY REMARKS

T HE DEVELOPMENT OF this chapter must be carried out with the uppermost thought in mind that endoscopy can never be taught in a textbook. Students who hopefully will refer to this manual should thoroughly understand that it is meant to be only a guide and a reference book for those who are receiving or have had practical preliminary training and seriously desire to achieve professional growth and development.

The approach to upper gastrointestinal endoscopy begins with the request for endoscopy consultation. The preliminary interview with the patient then follows to determine the indications and possible contraindications. These decisions are made by the endoscopist himself or his trained assistant, frequently the endoscopy resident. The patient's informed consent and signature are best obtained at this time. The procedure is then scheduled and at the appointed time, the patient is brought into the anteroom for premedication and patient interview.

PREMEDICATION AND PATIENT INTERVIEW

In this room, the examiner and others who will observe should introduce themselves to the patient and review pertinent history, and when necessary pertinent physical examination. At this point the resident will usually present the x-rays of the patient's upper gastrointestinal tract which are observed in shadow-boxes. The questions of indication and contraindication for this particular patient are reviewed. Dialogue is carried on with the patient, he must be impressed with the fact that the examiners are interested in attempting to alleviate his symptoms and his problem and that the procedure about to follow is specifically in his interest. In our clinic, the patient is always addressed as Mr., Mrs., or by other appropriate titles of respect, whether he is a private patient or a so-called charity patient. The rapport established in this interview may determine the success or failure of the entire procedure. If we are dealing with an inpatient he may have had some preliminary premedication before he left his ward. If one is dealing with an outpatient, premedication is given in this anteroom. Intramuscular injection and topical pharyngeal anesthetics are usually given at this point. The details of premedication are discussed in Chapter 4.

EXAMINING-ROOM PROCEDURES

All discussions and examinations of instruments and preparation for the procedure are carried out between the examiner and his associates in the main examining room while the patient remains in the anteroom. It is important to have the instruments to be used in their proper positions. With the cooperation of nursing assistance, everything which is to be used is adequately put in place so that there will be no awkwardness in carrying out this procedure in a professional manner. The anxious patient will be observing every movement of the examining team.

It is most important that a cheerful, relatively quiet attitude should be maintained in the examining room with a major focus of attention on the patient. Orientation with instruments, putting them on easily accessible tables, testing out their working conditions and in some cases, covering them with towels out of the sight of the patient should be carried out before the patient is brought into the examining room.

With the patient on the table, the stomach is emptied or lavaged with an Ewald-type tube if there has been pyloric obstruction or if there is need for lavage cytology. In the early stages of one's experience, it may be desirable to pass the Ewald-tube routinely. This will test out patient's reaction and possibly identify unsuspected obstructive effects. This procedure can be used to collect, measure and test the fasting content for free acid. Otherwise such specimens are collected in a suction trap.

The endoscope is lubricated and introduction time usually begins about five minutes thereafter. The total procedure should be carried out with all deliberate speed and completed in fifteen minutes to a half hour or in exceptional cases, forty-five minutes. If a longer period is required, it may be better to complete procedures such as photographs or even biopsy and cytology at another time. In all instances, the examiner must use individual clinical judgment based upon frequent periodic evaluation of the patient's vital signs and abdominal distension. As the patient lies in the left lateral position on the table, there should be a final check on certain areas of the physical examination. This checkup should include the oral cavity for loose teeth which might be dislodged or jagged teeth which might injure the instrument or the examiner's fingers. Observation should be made of any inflammatory lesions of the lips, tongue, pharynx or deformities of the jaw. Observations should be made also of the presence of a sore arm, especially the left one caused by intravenous procedures, arthritis, etc. which may be painful and require modification of the patient's position on the table.

TECHNIC OF INTRODUCTION (SIDE-VIEWING SCOPES)

Preliminary Statement

The instrument of choice will have been connected to the power units and given a final wiping with an alcohol sponge and lubricated. Usually the introduction of the instrument is carried out with the patient lying on his left side which is the time honored standard position for gastroscopy and flexible obturator esophagoscopy (Eder-Hufford type). From the point of view of safety and patient reaction, introduction of the scope is certainly the most important step in gastrointestinal endoscopy. Since patient reaction during examination may determine the success or failure to find an important lesion, the importance of this phase of the examination is obvious. It is here that the beginner must start to train or educate his fingers to detect varying degrees of resistance at all points of the examination, but especially during introduction through the esophagus. We usually begin training the beginner with the passage of the side-viewing instruments through which the esophagus cannot be observed. If he learns the technic of introduction with this scope, he should have less difficulty with other scopes.

The otolaryngologists who historically passed open rigid tubes into the esophagus more than anyone else accused the early gastroscopists of doing a *blind* introduction. My response has always been that the well trained gastroscopist *sees* with his fingers as he passes the side-viewing scope through the esophagus. Mastering the technic of "seeing with your fingers" is just as important with today's totally flexible fiberscopes. This point is certainly clear with side-viewing gastroscopes and duodenoscopes. The concept may be regarded as untenable with open-tube or forward-viewing scopes. However, I must point out that the operator has two points of concentration as he introduces an endoscope. One, the concentration on what he feels or does with his hands, the other on what he sees or is attempting to see. The beginner is usually "all eyes" once he sees the light reflex and he may forget the always potentially dangerous scope in his hands except for the brutal force required to keep it moving. This is especially true with muscular, not so dexterous and super confident doctors. As one develops his endoscopy skills, there is a greater equalization of concentration on what one feels and what one sees. Eventually, the resistance and maneuverability of the hands and fingers become a delicately trained and conditioned reflex so that the eyes and higher levels of judgment may have major concentration on the search for and recognition of significant endoscopic disease.

There is one important exception in this concept of the technic of introduction. I refer to the well trained endoscopist and certainly, also the not-so-well trained endoscopist who gets in a hurry or who has a certain desire to demonstrate or find a highly suspected lesion, quickly as if by magic. This may be especially for the benefit of certain observers of the examination. Injuries caused in such circumstances are quite possible, but fortunately such errors of procedure are probably not common.

The modern sophisticated individual in medicine may feel that the detailed descriptions I refer to for the technic of introduction are unnecessary with the very flexible fiberscopes in use at this time. To this I must say that it is more difficult to detect with accuracy the degree of resistance which is being exerted during the passage of the fiberscopes than with the semi-flexible lens instruments. Some relatively recent statistics indicate that there are more injuries today with fiberscopes[1-3] than previously with lens structured instruments (see Chapter 32). Undoubtedly this is due partly to the rapid increase of the number of people who are doing or attempting to do endoscopy, but also, in my experience, because the beginner today fells that the fiberscope is entirely harmless and that no technic is especially required in its passage. In undertaking the writing of this book with the assistance of many skilled and experienced endoscopists, it is hoped that we will do as much to discourage doctors who wish to pass endoscopes on patients without previous training, as we hope to do by this carefully written manual to help and encourage qualified doctors who wish to learn under instructors the very valuable but sometimes awesome diagnostic technic of endoscopy.

Regarding the relative ease of passage of fiberscopes as compared with lens scopes, let me say that there still may be occasions when an endoscopist may use a lens structured semi-flexible instrument. I have occasionally

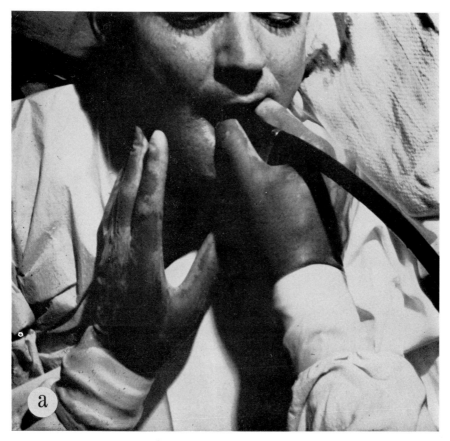

Figure 6-1a. Technic of introduction with right hand only.

reached the stomach with the lens structured Eder-Palmer gastroscope while failing with the fiberscopes. This is true in certain situations such as hiatus hernia with a fairly large thoracic gastric loculus. The same may be true in some cases of narrow cardio-esophageal junctions due to advanced achalasia. There are still occasions for the use of the flexible obturator rigid tube Eder-Hufford esophagoscope. I would say that an individual who learns the technic of Endoscopic Introduction in the manner which we will describe, would feel just as comfortable in passing the semi-flexible instrument as with the fiberscopes and would carry a very limited risk of injury with either instrument.

Passing the Scope

With the nursing assistant attending the patient's head and the patient lying on his left side, the examiner introduces the scope with his right hand. A second assistant, often the resident, supports the proximal end of the scope and stands to the right and slightly behind the examiner. The patient is asked to open his mouth widely and breathe deeply or pant. I never ask the patient to swallow because it is next to impossible for most

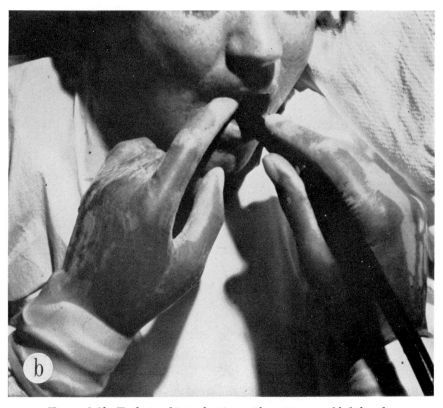

Figure 6-1b. Technic of introduction with assistance of left hand.

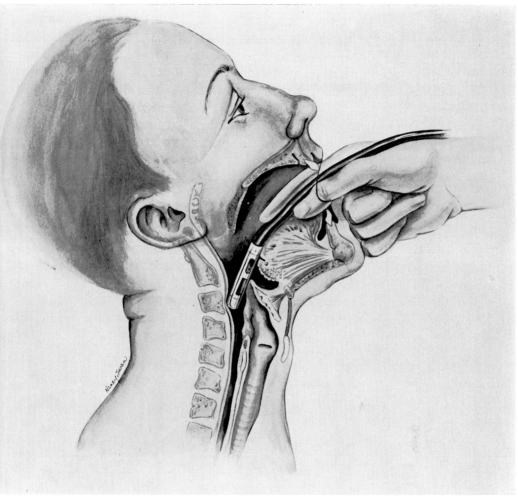

Figure 6-2. Diagram of saggital section through head and neck showing second step in technic of introduction.

people to swallow with the mouth wide open. This is compounded by two or more fingers and the tip of the instrument in the patient's mouth. The examiner holding the tip of the scope as he would hold a writing pen, introduces the scope in the midline over the dorsum of the tongue (see Fig. 6-1a). He may use his left index finger (Fig. 6-1b) to deflect the tip in the direction of the hypopharynx or as I prefer, the tip is "carried" along the midline of the hypopharynx with the thumb and index finger of the right hand (see Fig. 6-2). The assistant examiner must hold the proximal end of the scope lightly and so that it bends naturally at a right angle. To enter the hypopharynx, I prefer that directing the tip at the beginning of the introduction be carried out by the examiner himself without help from the assistant who may be inclined to deflect the tip for the examiner by the hand lever and to "sneak-in" a preview himself, in a kind of tug-of-war with his chief at the other end. With the preferred method, the examiner has the total responsibility for getting the tip into the hypopharynx. While the patient is panting, the scope is introduced or carried into the hypopharynx. The most important maneuver at this point is to prevent the tip from going into the right or left periform sinus and that it hugs the posterior wall of the pharynx to avoid entrance into the trachea. Some endoscopists with much experience and expertise hold the entire instrument during insertion. This is not generally recommended.

ROUTINE INSPECTION AND ORIENTATION

With the side-viewing scope, there is no meaningful visualization at present of the esophagus unless megaesophagus has occurred. The examiner concentrates on his "sense of feel" until the scope traverses the cardioesophageal junction. With some experience, the examiner may detect passage through this point. The light is turned on and a couple of bulbs of air are gently introduced. The scope is then rotated so that the objective points to-

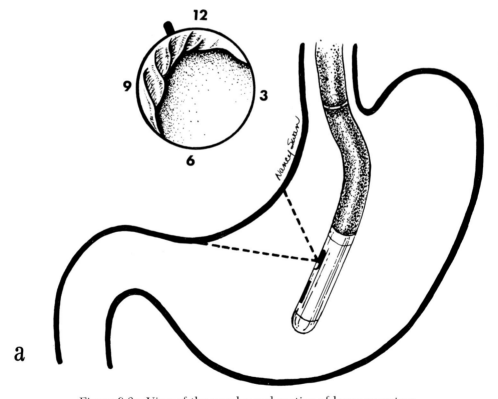

Figure 6-3a. View of the angulus and portion of lesser curvature.

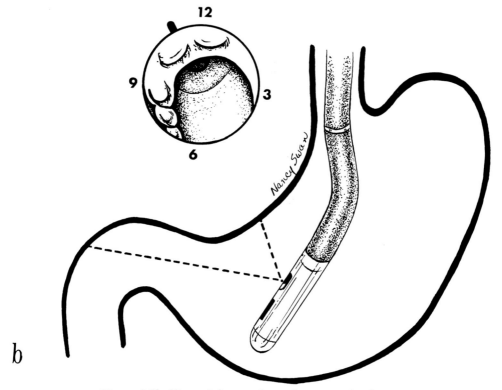

Figure 6-3b. View of the angulus and portion of pylorus.

ward the lesser curvature. This means that the position of the objective is in line with the imaginary point of 11 o'clock on the ocular. The examiner now looks for the angulus by continuing the introduction a few cms distally with little or no rotation. In most instances, the scope follows the curvature of the stomach bringing into view the half-moon shaped angulus (Fig. 6-3a). A few centimeters further forward will also reveal a portion of the pylorus (Fig. 6-3b).

Gastric Motility

By this time, the observer is conscious of one or more rhythmic movements. The gastric field moves and may seem to involve the total organ. The gastric field actually moves distally then proximally and back again. It is synchronous with diaphragmatic respiration. This movement is the Respiration Mobility of the stomach. In many instances, a second movement will be readily seen. This movement is pulsatile being transmitted from an artery in the gastric wall, from the abdominal aorta or elsewhere. Soon after gastric inflation, a third movement is recognized as peristaltic activity (see Plate 3, 4). This movement begins just distal to the angulus and proceeds toward the pylorus. It is usually confined to the antrum. It consists of rhythmic concentric contraction waves which are largest in the upper antrum and become smaller as they progress toward the pylorus to close the sphincter. Infiltrations and filling defects will disturb the rhythm and pattern of these waves. Often the waves become progressively more frequent and more intense or the reverse may be true. Pyloric activity is a most intricate mechanism and fascinating to most observers. When it is intense, bile is often seen to regurgitate into the antrum as mucosal folds appear to herniate from the duodenum. This movement sometimes proceeds while deep contraction waves move forward in a kind of longitudinal circus movement. For a long time, I have had the opinion that spastic hyperactivity of the pylorus as the gastroscopist sees it, may be related to the so-called mucosal prolapse into the duodenal bulb as the roentgenologist sees it.

Spastic activity which is not a part of the propulsive movement may occur in any part of the stomach. It may occur especially during the passage of the scope and during the early period of the examination. Spasm may temporarily prevent entrance of the scope through the cricopharyngeus and into certain other parts of the stomach and account for nonvisualization of lesion seen in x-ray. All patients, especially excitable ones, benefit from words of reassurance and encouragement from the nurse and doctor during the examination. This helps the patient to relax and hyperspastic motility to decrease.

There is a fourth movement which gives the impression of either stiffness or pliability of the gastric wall. It is best observed in relation to respiration. When the normal stomach moves down with inspiration and up with expiration, there is a kind of oscillation or ripple which can be observed in the gastric wall. This is pliability. When this characteristic is absent in a localized or diffused area, it is described as stiffness. This may suggest infiltration and is an important supplementary characteristic in infiltrating carcinoma. The stiff appearance may also occur in lymphosarcoma. Benign hypertrophic gastropathy with its cobble stone pattern appears pliable in contrast to lymphosarcoma and other infiltrating lesions.

Angulus and Mid Body

With the angulus or the incisura angularis as seen on x-ray film in the upper center of the gastroscopic field, the observer views the mid body or middle one third of the stomach along the lesser curvature. If the angulus does not come readily into view at this point, usually about 40 to 50cms from the incisor teeth, the next step usually is to introduce more inflation. If this fails, he will deflect the tip upward toward the lesser curvature or slightly downward until the angulus appears. This is usually the first point at which I use the deflecting mechanism. Sometimes, it may be necessary to move the scope a few centimeters proximally or distally to center the angulus. Periodic replacement of air which has begun to escape through the pylorus or is being belched up is frequently necessary. Only the least amount of air required to keep the area of inspection in good view is used. The angulus serves as a focal point of orientation. It is also very important as the most frequent site of benign peptic ulcer. Most commonly this lesion is just proximal to the angulus. It may dramatically come into view as a circular defect covered by a homogeneous white adherent mucus silhouetted against a background of uniformly normal orange-red mucosa (see Plate 25).

If no ulcer or other obvious defect is seen, one notes carefully the contour of the angulus. If it is smooth, sharp and has a regular inverted half-moon contour, this is normal. If it has an inverted "V" shape, this may foretell the presence of an ulcer just distal to the angulus or a careful concentration may reveal a fine scar of a healed benign ulcer. The inverted "V" is known as the "Henning's Sign."

With the angulus in the upper center of the field at 11 o'clock, routine inspection is continued by rotating the objective clockwise to the 12, 1, 2, 3 and 4 o'clock positions. The objective is thus moved across the posterior

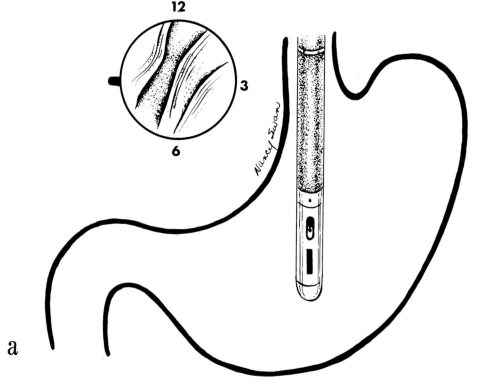

Figure 6-4a. View of anterior wall—mid body.

wall of the mid body from the lesser curvature to a point approximately one-half the distance to the greater curvature. The objective lies close to the gastric wall in this maneuver and so the tip of the scope may need to be deflected away from the wall toward the lumen until the focus is satisfactory. Deflection is more often necessary in the upper half than in the lower half of the passageway because the stomach is held closer to the posterior abdominal wall in its upper half.

I will usually backtrack after reaching 3 or 4 o'clock counterclockwise for a more thorough survey and continue on around thru 12 and 9 o'clock, where the observer sees the mid portion of the anterior wall (Fig. 6-4a). The walls now seem to be at a considerable distance from the objective. This is because the inflated stomach bulges toward the anterior abdominal wall. The normal gastric folds are therefore smaller and spread further apart by contrast with posterior wall (Fig. 6-4b).

Continuing the rotation counterclockwise, the larger and more parallel folds of the greater curvature come into view at 7 and 6 o'clock (Fig. 6-5). As the objective is rotated further around to 5, 4 and 3 o'clock, the tip deflector may again be required because of the proximity of the objec-

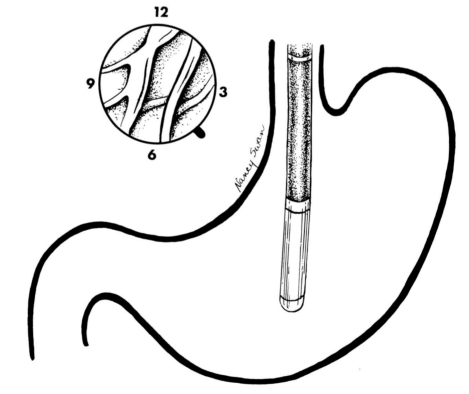

Figure 6-4b. View of posterior wall—mid body.

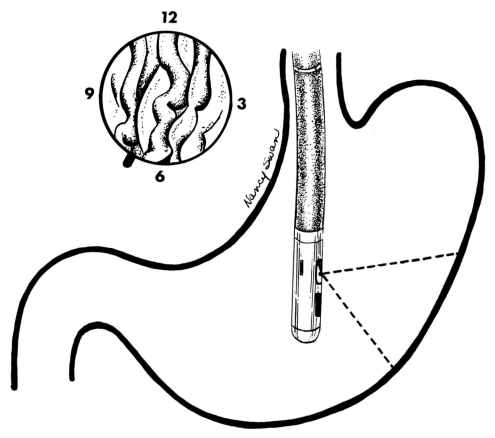

Figure 6-5. View of the greater curvature—mid body.

tive to the posterior wall. One may wish to sweep through the same meridian at the level of the angulus for another good survey and then with the angulus in view proceed downward viewing distally along the lesser curvature to the antrum until the pylorus comes into view. Enroute to the pylorus, the objective is swept "around the clock" every few centimeters.

Antrum

At this level one sees a tunnel view of a wide area at the base of a cone of vision including both walls and both curvatures at the same time (Fig. 6-6) (Plate 2). If peristalsis is normal, concentric waves are seen to traverse the antrum and close the pyloric ring. This is described as a "purse string" or a "tobacco pouch" type closure. The cone of vision decreases in diameter at its base with proportional increased magnification of the area seen as the scope descends and vice versa as it is retrieved. Any variation from the physiologic activity described may be indicative of path-

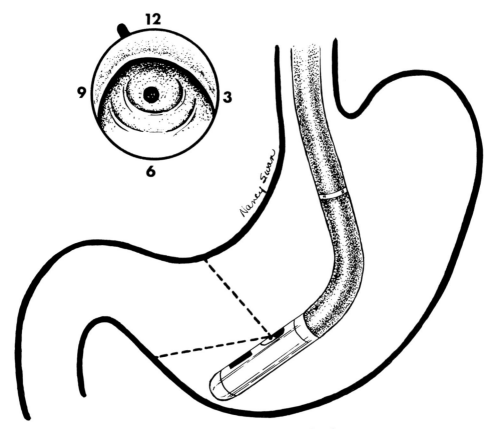

Figure 6-6. Tunnel view of distal antrum and pyloric contraction.

ological change. The waves may be incomplete, semi-circular, rhythmic or absent in the presence of localized or diffuse malignant infiltration, polypoid or ulcerative defects or intramural disease. Disturbance of the pattern of peristalsis may be caused by extrinsic compression of an area of the antral gastric wall or by pulsion defects due to post-operative adhesions.

Upper Body and Cardia

As the stomach is surveyed, any obvious or suspected gross lesions are studied in careful concentrated detail. It should be photographed, biopsied or brushed for cytology as found to be indicated or feasible. The upper body and cardia will have been observed during the downward course of the instrument. I usually do not make an "inch by inch" study of this area on entering the stomach unless a defect is sighted or there is a previous x-ray demonstrated lesion in the upper body. Upon retrieval, however, I again begin at the lesser curvature and rotate clockwise and counterclockwise through frequently selected meridians using tip deflection where needed. I especially like to get an extreme "up" deflection view along the greater curvature high in the upper body for portions of the cardia and fundus. This maneuver is called retroflexion or "U"-Turn.

Retroflexed Views

The next movement in routine inspection, viz, retroflexion, is made by first moving the objective to the mid body. A distant view of the antrum and pylorus is then made for any new developments before proceeding with retroflexion. Sometimes such a view of an antral lesion may show its important relations with surrounding tissue, better than a close-up study. This, however, does not take the place of a close-up study as is sometimes done with forward-viewing instruments. For routine retroflexion, I prefer the dorsal position which will be discussed later. We are now describing retroflexion, using the left side position which is permissible if no contraindications exist. With the objective pointing toward 7 or 6 o'clock, extreme "down" tip deflection is made at the mid portion of the stomach along the greater curvature. While the tip is relatively stationary, the re-

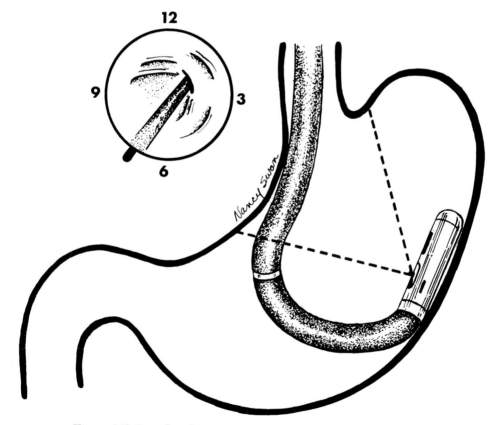

Figure 6-7. Retroflexed view of cardia and gastroesophageal orifice.

mainder of the scope is depressed, until the proximal shaft of the scope comes into view. When properly executed, the protrusion of the shaft through the cardioesophageal junction is easily demonstrated (Fig. 6-7) (Plate 44). I depend greatly upon the feeling of resistance to my fingers and patient reaction during this period to be sure that the tip of the scope is gliding smoothly along the greater curvature and that the "bowing" of the shaft is not obstructed. I am first concerned with whether the gastro-esophageal orifice hugs the shaft of the protruding scope "tightly" or "loosely." When the latter is exaggerated, it is indicative of hiatus hernia. I am next concerned with the occasional occurrence of an ulcer at this point, perhaps overlooked by x-ray (Plate 44). Fundic carcinoma and gastric varices must be ruled out or confirmed with the help of a short "U"-Turn from a higher level (Fig. 6-8). The former by biopsy or brush cytology when feasible. Photographic cataloging should be carried out as often as may be feasible, considering total patient "tolerance-time" and technical capabilities. Time can be saved by the use of teaching attachments, coordinated

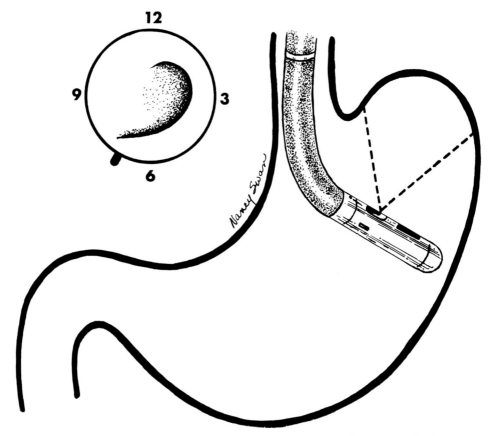

Figure 6-8. High "up-turn" view along greater curvature showing the fundus.

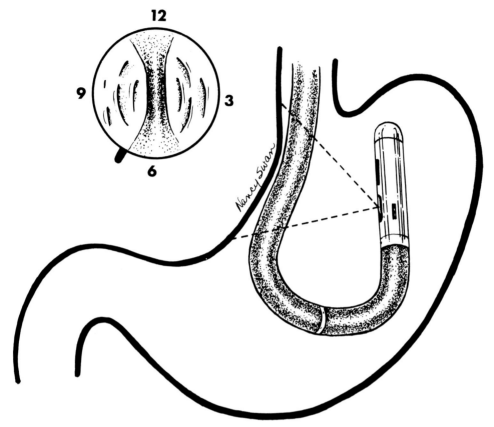

Figure 6-9. Retroflexion—closed U-Turn view of high lesser curvature.

help of a photo technician and limited observation of normal physiology when a lesion is to be studied.

When retroflexion is made at about the mid body with a side viewer, the cardiac area and the protruding scope are seen with a shorter curve than with the forward viewer. As further illustrated in Figure 6-9, the loop may be increased by depressing the scope's shaft distalward, sometimes with external pressure against the left mid abdomen by an assistant. This maneuver deflects the tip toward the lesser curvature while the "U" is further closed, thereby bringing into view the high lesser curvature (Fig. 6-9). I have seen portions of this area in retroflexion which I did not see with straight observation. In one instance a niche was easily seen on x-ray film high on the lesser curvature. Only moderately closed "U"-Turn with left abdominal pressure and focusing on the high lesser curvature brought the ulcer into view. If the "U"-Turn is closed completely or overextended, there will be a retroflexed view back toward the antrum and sometimes the pylorus. This extreme retroflexion is unnecessary and may be dangerous.

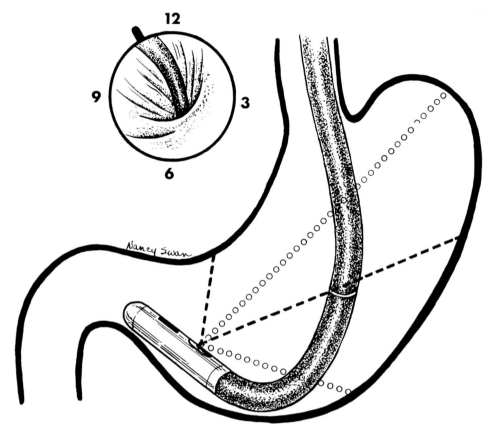

Figure 6-10. Retroflexion with angulation—views of cardia, fundus, lesser and greater curvatures.

Another area should be mentioned where a retroflexed view may occur but unintentionally. When the tip of a gastroduodenoscope reaches the prepyloric area, entering the duodenum may be difficult until the technic is mastered. When the attempt is made too rapidly or without oriented control, the tip may retroflex upon itself bringing an area of the shaft into view (Fig. 6-10). The instrument should then be carefully withdrawn to mid body and the effort to approach the pylorus made all over again.

When retroflexion is made, especially in the area of the fundus, and the tip does not remain in the same plane as the shaft, complete curving of the scope may occur without the shaft becoming visible. Impaction of the instrument in the esophagus and cardiac area has been reported.[4] Retroflexion should always be done with extreme care and only after adequate training and orientation.

TECHNIC OF INTRODUCTION (FORWARD-VIEWING SCOPES)
Preliminary Statement

The most commonly used forward-viewing scope today is, of course, the fiberoptic instrument. It is felt by many endoscopists that the pragmatic approach to upper gastrointestinal endoscopy is to use a panendoscopic or long forward-viewing instrument. Very frequently it is desirable to examine the esophagus, the stomach and the bulbar duodenum, to solve a single diagnostic problem. The only instrument which can be used for this at the present time is the forward-viewing endoscope. If an examiner can have only one instrument, certainly it must be the forward-viewing type; but a carpenter with only one tool can hardly be regarded as an expert craftsman.

The forward-viewing rigid esophagoscope of the Eder-Hufford type still has a place, especially for the removal of foreign bodies, the injection of varices, viewing certain deformities of the esophagus, etc. The lumen, through the esophagus, may sometimes be kept in better view with the rigid esophagoscope. This is probably true because the rigid scope permits less mobility of the esophagus during the passage of the instrument, and there is no "automatic" insensitive curving of the tip as may occur with fiberscopes, especially in presence of spasm.

Passing the Scope

The preferable forward-viewing scope today is the esophagogastroduodenoscope, known also as the panendoscope. It has the disadvantage of being somewhat awkward to handle, if only the esophagus is to be examined. This awkwardness can be overcome with experience. I prefer to introduce this instrument in the same manner described for the introduction of the side-viewing instrument, primarily with the right hand and without help from the left hand as previously described and illustrated (Fig. 6-1a, 1b). When the tip of the instrument is introduced, the examiner should carry out as many of the manipulatory functions as possible by himself. It may be difficult at first to follow the lumen as one proceeds toward the cardio-esophageal junction. This, of course, will improve with practice. I have found with students that the first inclination is to turn all of the levers at once, this usually will get the examiner into difficulty. With patience and concentration, one learns how to keep the lumen of esophagus in view. I seldom find it necessary to deflect the tip in order to follow the esophageal lumen. The view of the esophagus and hypopharynx is frequently better during retrieval than during the introduction of the scope. When in difficulty, retrieve for a few centimeters and start again.

Esophagogastroscopy

As the tip of the forward-viewing scope is introduced into the esophagus, it is important not to start immediately to manipulate the tip deflectors. They had better be used only when necessary. Small squirts of air will bring the mucosa into view. The lumen may appear and disappear. Usually a combination of slight inflation, retraction and progression will keep the view "on target" until the tip of the scope clears the gastroesophageal junction and enters the stomach. Some skill and practice is required to do this effectively and consistently. During the passage through the esophagus, the observer should identify not only pathology, but physiologic activity, coordinated with respiration and normal anatomical landmarks. One should identify the level of the diaphramatic hiatus and the change from esophageal to gastric mucosa at the zigzag line. Normal esophageal folds should be distinguished from varices and superficial traumatic effects should be distinguished from hemorrhagic erosions.

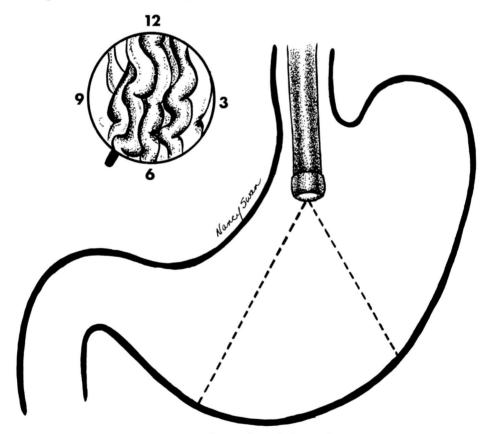

Figure 6-11. Long tunnel view through forward viewing scope.

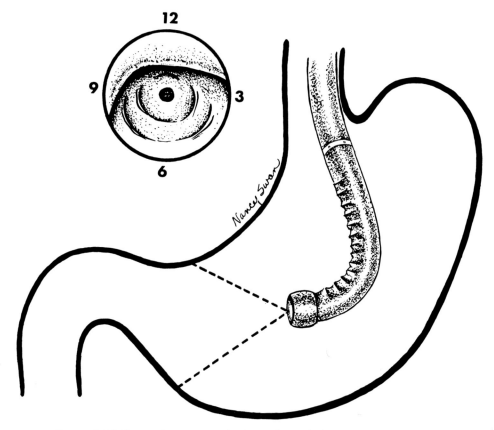

Figure 6-12. View of antrum and pylorus through forward viewing scope.

When the forward-viewing scope passes the gastroesophageal junction, the examiner may see a large sweeping tunnel view of the stomach (Fig. 6-11). In a steerhorn type stomach, he may even see the pylorus in the distance. What he sees at this point and as he moves distally toward the pylorus (Fig. 6-12), is not necessarily all of the stomach. Unfortunately the stomach is not a "bell-bottom trouser" or a long rigid tube. With experience, it is possible to do a fairly adequate examination of the stomach in many instances with forward-viewing scopes. The extreme fishhook stomach or the organ which is deformed or partly displaced by external malcompression or the hyperspastic stomach may be considerably more difficult to examine completely with the forward viewer than with the side-viewing instrument. In earlier years, some examiners found biopsies easier through the forward-viewing instrument. This is no longer true with the perfection of the biopsy mechanism in side-viewing instruments. The four-way deflection capability of the latest forward-viewing scopes, may be of added advantage in seeking out areas which would otherwise remain blind. However, one must know his orientation in the stomach for most effective use of these mechanisms. This includes not only accurate knowledge of intragastric landmarks, but knowledge of the nature and effects of "spasm" and hyperspastic motility.

The newer polydirectional panendoscopes have an extreme tip deflection capability. This should make it possible to view the cardia and fundus without "wide curve" retroflexion (Fig. 6-13a and 13b). However, the tip does not always bend in the same plane as the shaft but obliquely off to the right or left. This makes for inaccurate orientation. Accurate tip deflection indicators should be built into all instruments, especially those with sharp angulation capability. Acute retroflexion for upper body viewing should be made well below the cardia to lessen the risk of "double entry" impaction into the lower esophagus. This type of accident has been reported.[3] The examiner should know the location and the degree of tip deflection at all times for meaningful orientation and maximum safety.

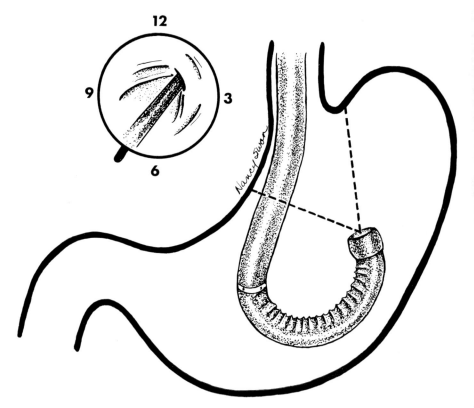

Figure 6-13a. Retroflexed view of cardia and gastroesophageal junction—forward view.

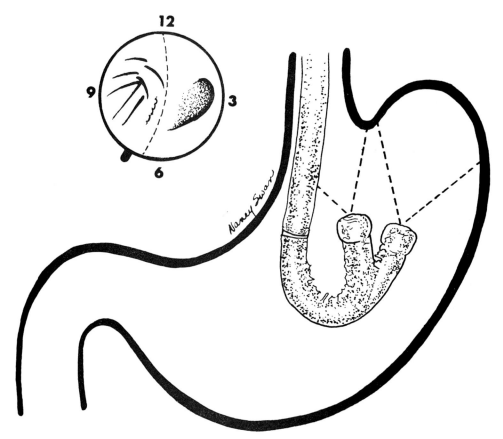

Figure 6-13b. Acute angle visualization—cardia and fundus—forward views.

DUODENOSCOPY

The forward-viewing endoscopes and the side-viewing endoscopes can be introduced from the antrum into the duodenum with equal facility by most gastroscopists.[5] Identification of structure and pathological lesions are carried out with relatively equal facility depending upon the endoscopist and his personal experience. The technics in the second portion of the duodenum involving cannulation of the papilla of Vater, direct cholecystography and pancreatocholangiography can only be carried out satisfactorily with side-viewing duodenoscopes.[6] The detailed discussion of these technics and the pathology of the duodenum are discussed in Chapters 23 and 24.

SPECIAL CONSIDERATIONS IN GASTRIC ORIENTATION

Introductory Statement

The concept of orientation in the stomach is somewhat paradoxical. It is possible for a fairly good examiner to feel quite competent about seeing all areas of the stomach through many examinations, especially with forward-viewing scopes. Experience, however, with careful "inch by inch" systematic surveys and "check backs," with x-ray, repeated examinations and surgery will reveal to the careful, open-minded student that indeed he may not have seen all of the stomach in every case. Orientation is still a continuing learning process in the life history of an endoscopist. The great goal of efficiency is to know when you have seen all areas of the stomach, well, in the individual case.

Blind Spots

The omniangle lens gastroscope by Cameron[7] first utilized two angles of an electromagnetic movable mirror objective to improve blind spots. Herman Taylor[8] of London first utilized a movable tip lens scope and the Eder Instrument Company of Chicago employed a combination of a movable, scanning mirror objective and one-way, tip deflection in a small diameter (9mm) lens scope to improve the problem of "blind spots." This author was the first to add the feature of "Multiple Rotation" of the patient's position on the examining table with the lens instrument *in situ* to eliminate blind spots. Several hundred patients were examined in prospective comparative studies to establish the value of "Multiple Positions" in gastroscopy.[9]

With the introduction of good quality glass fiberoptics and now with four-way deflection, it is said that all "blind spots" are eliminated. To this I must ask the question, in whose hands? And in which individual case? It is one thing to own a three hundred magnum telescopic rifle, it may be quite another thing to bag a lion.

Multiple Positions

The left side position remains standard for gastroscopy (Fig. 6-14a). As previously mentioned, the dorsal position is preferable for retroflexion. The dorsal position is also preferable for the patient with massive ascites, emphysema, cardiac hypertrophy or painful lesions of the left side. The description of orientation under the subject of side-viewing endoscopic technic applies to the left side standard position only. When the patient's position is changed, the orientation with the side-viewing scope changes with each position. The views and orientation to be described will also apply in a general way and in some instances, to forward-viewing scopes with the tip deflected at a right angle.

Dorsal Orientation

With the patient in the dorsal position and the tip of the scope in mid body, the lesser curvature view of the angulus is best seen when the side-viewing objective is in a straight line with the 2 o'clock position on the ocular dial (Fig. 6-14b). The mid posterior wall is at 5 to 6 o'clock and the mid anterior wall is at 11 to 12 o'clock. The contracting pylorus is best seen when the objective reaches the antrum in line with the lesser curvature and in the longitudinal plane with 2 o'clock. At this point, systematic observation is made around the clock to survey the antrum just as was described for the left side position, except that all points of orientation and landmarks in the stomach have shifted 90 degrees clockwise. With this central point and orientation in mind, the instrument is usually retrieved along the lesser curvature for examination of the cardiac and fundic portions. In this area, a sweep around the clock is again carried out.

As previously mentioned, I prefer the dorsal position for retroflexed viewing of cardia and fundus. For this purpose, the tip of the instrument is placed in mid body with the objective pointing towards 8 o'clock, where the greater curvature lies in a longitudinal direction. Extreme down flexion in a proximal direction along the greater curvature. The shaft of the instrument is then depressed gently into the stomach until the upper shaft of the scope comes into view as it protrudes from the esophagus. Further discussion of technic in this area will be found in the earlier pages of this chapter under "Left Side" or "Standard Position." The dorsal position will be found advantageous if a prolonged examination is being carried out in the left-side position. Rotation to the back at this point adds to the patient's comfort and improves relaxation. Frequently I will have my assistant slip a small foam-rubber pillow under the patient's shoulders when he

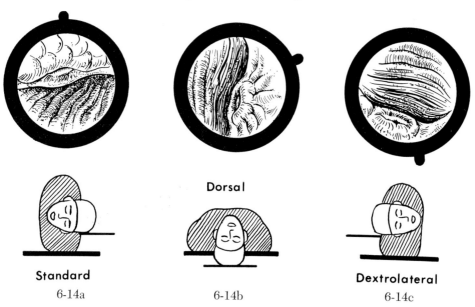

Dorsal

Standard   Dextrolateral
6-14a   6-14b   6-14c

Figure 6-14a, b, c. Gastroscopic view of carcinomatous ulcer at the angulus (artist drawing). a. Standard left-side position; b. Dorsal position; c. Dextra lateral position.

is rotated to the back. This allows for better dorsi-flexion of the head which lessens pressure of the shaft of the instrument on the patient's pharynx, and frequently makes for easier rotation of the scope. The nurse in our clinic monitors abdominal distension during the examination as well as the vital signs. The degree of abdominal distension is determined from time to time by palpating the abdominal wall. This is more conveniently carried out when the patient is in the dorsal position.

Dextra-Lateral Orientation

The dextra-lateral position[10] (Fig. 6-14c) was more frequently used during the era of lens gastroscopy. However, it is occasionally found of advantage with the fiberoptic instruments. Some gastroscopists have found it to be advantageous in entering the duodenum, especially with side-viewing instruments. When the patient is rotated to the right side and with the objective at mid body, the half-moon angulus is seen to be upside down (Fig. 6-15). Its mid point is best seen at 5 to 6 o'clock. The greater curvature is best seen at 11 to 12 o'clock, the mid-anterior wall at 3 o'clock and the mid-posterior wall at 9 o'clock. In this position, the "mucus lake" which accumulates on the greater curvature in the cardiac region with patient in the left-side standard position, is immediately displaced to the prepyloric antrum (Fig. 6-16). I first observed this shift of secretion when I chanced to gastroscope a patient with situs inversus viscerum and dextra-gastrica[10] in the standard left-side position. As the secretions escape slowly

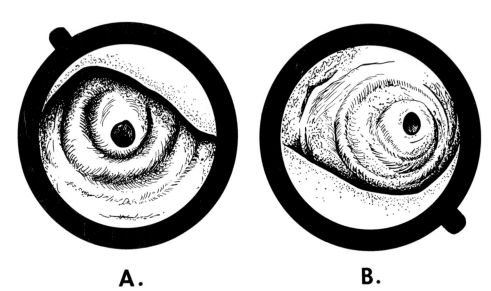

A.   **B.**

Figure 6-15. Comparative gastroscopic views of the angulus in the (A) standard left and (B) dextra lateral position (diagrammatic).

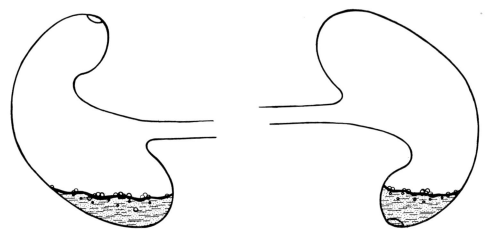

Figure 6-16. Diagram of stomach silhouette in left and right positions showing displacement of "mucus lake" from greater curvature cardiac region to pylorus.

into the duodenum, there is frequently an improved view of the prepyloric lesser curvature without tip deflexion. This was a point of significant importance before the era of fiberoptic-tip-deflexion instruments. The secretions, of course, can now be removed by suction. I have found, occasionally, biopsy easier along the lesser curvature with the patient in the dextra-lateral position, because less deflexion of the tip may be required in reaching the lesion. It is conceivable that retroflexion along the greater curvature from the dextra-lateral position may make biopsy in the cardia region more feasible in some cases.

The dextra-lateral position combined with reverse Trendelenburg has occasionally been found of advantage by the writer. Both for visualization and adequate biopsy of the difficultly placed lesion, adequate visualization in all of the various positions here described must be made with the knowledge of where the objective lies at all times. This depends greatly on the indicators at the proximal end of the instrument. However, adequate orientation is achieved by coordinated knowledge of the regional anatomy of the interior of the stomach. Both criteria must be used for accuracy, especially with four-way deflexion scopes. This is true because four-way scopes have greater flexibility at the tip and will frequently move obliquely from north to south or east to west rather than in the same plane. This is further exaggerated from time to time because of varying pressures exerted on the instrument tip by the gastric wall.

Purposeful Deflation

Before leaving this discussion, I would like to give a word of warning against overdistension of the stomach during prolonged examinations. I have found it of advantage to use what we call Purposeful Deflation. When the abdomen feels distended to the point of discomfort to the patient, it is possible to turn on the suction apparatus for one to two minutes and withdraw most of the air not only from the stomach, but from the proximal small intestines. This can be aided by gentle simultaneous pressure on the abdominal wall. This gives considerable relief to the patient and eliminates a factor of danger. An overdistended stomach may be more easily perforated by the scope (see Chapter 32). Besides the factors of patient comfort and safety, purposeful deflation sometimes improves orientation and may bring into view a lesion or an aspect of a lesion which is not seen except with minimal inflation.

DICTATION OF PROTOCOLS AND RECORDS

It has been my practice through the years to dictate the protocols immediately after the examination. This is taken usually by the resident or an endoscopy student. There are several advantages: Those who have been observing and exchanging opinions with the principal examiner have a chance to listen to the summary concepts and conclusions in each case. The protocol should summarize indications and relative contraindications, clinical and x-ray gastrointestinal diagnoses and associated diagnoses of systemic disease. The protocol form which we use is illustrated in Figure 6-17. We begin the description of the examination with a statement regarding the patient's cooperation. Diagnostic findings are sometimes interpreted in terms of cooperation or the lack of it. Through the years, we have developed standard terminology which for the most part, follows that set up by Rudolf Schindler in his early studies with lens gastroscopy. Certain modifications, of course, have been made in keeping with developments in fiberoptic endoscopy and transendoscopic technics. It is important to describe the approximate size of lesions as well as their contours, shapes and superficial characteristics.

Diffuse disease such as gastritis of the various types are described in summary as localized or diffuse. Gastritis, petechial hemorrhages, erosions and so forth are further described as mild, moderate or severe. When a patient is referred for endoscopy, what the referring doctor really wants as a rule, is a gastroenterology consultation which includes endoscopy. It is therefore appropriate to express an opinion as to whether the endoscopist feels that the findings explain the patient's gastrointestinal symptoms. In some instances, other gastrointestinal diseases may better explain the patient's symptoms, an example of which would be the finding of localized chronic gastritis in a patient who has proven chronic relapsing pancreatitis. Finally, it is well to express in the protocol a recommendation with reference to management, medical or surgical, and whether certain examinations should be repeated, particularly endoscopy or x-ray.

COOK COUNTY HOSPITAL
(ENDOSCOPIC REPORT)

NAME OF PT. . . . . WARD . . . . HOSP. NO. . . . .
DATE . . . . AGE . . . . SEX . . . . REFERRED BY: . . . .
(YES)
RECENT ALCOHOLIC INTAKE: (NO) DATES, AMT. . . . .
(YES)
PREVIOUS ENDOSCOPIES: (NO) DATES . . . .
RECENT ASPIRIN INTAKE: . . . .
OTHER: . . . .
(YES)
RECENT GROSS HEMORRHAGE: (NO) AMT. . . . . . . Hb. . . . . DATE . . . .
CLINICAL DIAGNOSIS: . . . .
G.I.: . . . . + OTHER: . . . .
X-RAY DIAGNOSIS: . . . . DATE . . . .
FREE ACID
FASTING GASTRIC CONTENT: . . . . ML. (TOPFER): + . ., — . . APPEARANCE: . . . . .
(YES)
GASTRIC LAVAGE: (NO)—FOR OBSTRUCTION—FOR CYTOLOGY.
BLOOD . . . ., COLOR . . . ., DATE . . . .
INSTRUMENT: Lo.P   GFB-K   GTF-A   E-V   OTHER
(   )   (   )   (   )   (   )   (   )
INSTRUMENT, COMPARATIVE REGIONS: 1 2 3 4 5 (U⅓, M⅓, L⅓, DUODENUM)
e.g.: 1, 2, etc. . . . .
PROCEDURE: ESOPHAGOSCOPY, GASTROSCOPY, DUODENOSCOPY, COLONOSCOPY
Trendel.,   *Reverse Trendel.*
POSITIONS USED: Lt. Lat.,   Dor.,   Rt. Lat.,   (L, D, R)   (L, D, R)
BEST VIEWS: . . . . REGION . . . .
FINDINGS: BRIEF (ALSO BACK OF SHEET) . . . .
. . . .
(YES)   (YES)
BRUSH: (NO)   *PHOTO:* Still, Cine, No.   *BIOPSY:* (NO) # (   )
IMPRESSION: . . . .
. . . .
. . . .
MEDICAL CONSULTATORY RECOMMENDATIONS: . . . .
. . . .
. . . .
. . . .
SIGNATURE

Figure 6-17. Protocol form used at Cook County Hospital for reporting endoscopic procedures.

With the many procedures being carried out today in endoscopy, it is well to have a systematized method of filing protocols, photographs (still movies and gastrocamera strips). If one is really serious about diagnostic studies with the aid of endoscopic procedure, great care and attention must be given to protocols and records and follow-up studies. Rudolf

Schindler taught me the importance of systematic filing. Following his practice, I have kept a personal consecutive serially numbered protocol for every gastroscopy or endoscopy performed since the beginning of my endoscopic experience. Some have been lost but remarkably few. The number is now close to eight thousand. Many retrospective studies, lectures and publications have had their basis in these detailed records.

POST-ENDOSCOPY PATIENT FOLLOW-UP

I do not consider an endoscopic examination complete without a post-examination follow-up. This follow-up consists of checking the patient's blood pressure, pulse rate and examination of the chest and abdomen up to one hour after the procedure and over a longer period when necessary. This is usually carried out by the endoscopy resident in the case of inpatients. Outpatients must be kept in a recovery area with frequent check of vital signs by the endoscopy nurse. The patient must have recovered from the affects of sedatives and should be discharged to return home with a companion.

SETUP OF ENDOSCOPY UNIT
(ROOMS, TABLES, CABINETS, SUPPLIES)

The Endoscopy Unit should consist of certain minimal facilities and additions as required. Preferably the area should provide for growth and expansion. In some hospitals, endoscopy must be carried out in main operating rooms. In others, the minor surgery unit is used. In either of those arrangements, objections are soon raised by medical house staff who must dress in scrub attire to follow their patients, and others who find such facilities inconvenient and unnecessary. The better arrangement is a separate endoscopy unit (Fig. 6-18). The unit should consist of the main examining room, and anterooms. The latter should include premedication and patient interview room, separate inpatient waiting room for stretchers, outpatient waiting room with sitting facilities, office, fluoroscopy room and nearby toilet facilities. These are the minimal number of rooms. They need not be large but should be adequate for individual hospital requirements. The unit, especially the examining room, should have air conditioning facilities for the comfort of patient and workers.

Examining Room Decor

The examining room should have light colored walls. There should be an orderly arrangement of tables, cabinets, mobile suction units, etc. It should have an orderly, clean appearance including a spotlessly clean light colored flooring. It should be located in a relatively quiet area of the hospital. There should be sufficient and adequate electrical outlets. The lighting should be adequate but capable of being quickly converted into a

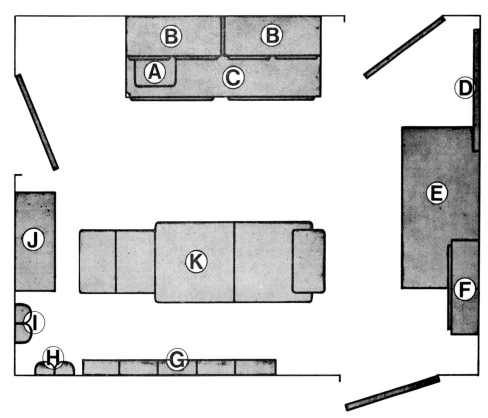

Figure 6-18. Diagram of reasonable adequate endoscopy unit. A. Sink; B. Cabinet unit with refrigerator; C. Bench for endoscopes; D. Bulletin board; E. Cabinet for electrical equipment; F. Anesthetics, emergency, etc.; G. X-ray boxes; H. Suction apparatus; I. Oxygen tank; J. Linen table; K. Motor driven examining table.

darkened room of varying degrees of light or adequately illuminate the patient's position on the table or at times, considerable darkness may be necessary to concentrate on a given field in the stomach and the gastro-intestinal canal. For the beginner, especially, there are times when seeing the long axis of the patient's body and its relationship to the long axis of the scope and the contour of the neck and head may facilitate orientation in the stomach and lower the risk of injury. A local light of the goose-neck type may be convenient for concentrating light, at times, in the area of the patient's head or to make camera readings, etc.

Examining Table and Auxiliary Facilities

The proper examining table is preferably one which is motor-driven but must have the facility for lowering the head and the foot and for raising and lowering the table. It should be properly padded for the comfort of the patient and should have sufficient length for tall individuals. Usually there is an adjustable head-piece which may be used to advantage in the examination.

There must be one principal rectangular shaped table which may be on rollers to be positioned at the head of the examining table. This table is for resting the particular instrument to be used at a given time. Another table or a built-in shelf on the principal table will hold the power units for one or more types of endoscopes. Other supplies such as adequate lubricants, stacks of gauze squares, pharyngeal anesthetizing sprays in atomizers or self-contained receptacles, tongue depressors, specimen jars and other necessary supplies. It is convenient to have a stationary table or preferably a long working table structure extending several feet and connecting with the sink for cleaning instruments etc. This table should contain basins of liquid soap. Another basin should contain clear water, another basin should contain antiseptic solution such as zepherin and there should be a nearby receptable of 70 per cent alcohol.

In the total set-up of the main examining room, there should be one aspirating machine with a y-shaped glass connecting tube leading to two aspirating tubes, one to connect with the instrument, another to a plastic dental aspirating tip for removing saliva from the patient's mouth. If there is room and more available facilities, two aspirating machines for the two functions separately may be of greater convenience. It is always an advantage to have extra cabinets in the room which are nearby for back-up supplies such as analgesics, sedatives, and other drugs of choice suitable for intramuscular and intravenous administration, disposable needles and syringes, bedpans, urinals, etc.

Care of Endoscopes

Used instruments should lay on disposable paper half sheets to be changed between examinations. Doctors, nurses and attendants who handle instruments before and after usage should wash their hands frequently. Failure to maintain a rigid state of cleanliness in all of these procedures is inexcusable. Obviously, there must be available, running hot and cold water, liquid hand soap, preferably with a foot pedal dispenser for liquid soap and antiseptics, fingernail brushes and files, towels and other scrub-up facilities. Small caliber polyethylene tubes are convenient for washing out the biopsy and suction channels of the upper section of some instruments. The tips of suction-equipped scopes should be immersed in water with the suction unit running for cleaning purposes. Liquid soap and water can be used. This should be followed by clear water then by alcohol then air should be forced through with a syringe but never to compressed air jets.

Cleaned instruments at the end of the day's use should be carefully put in their respective cases and carefully stored in security cabinets along with cameras and other expensive items. Biopsy forceps brushes are cleaned, dried and hung full length in a wall rack with their cutting edges specially treated. ACMI has announced a mechanical sterilizer G510.

Photographic Biopsy Facilities

Unused photo films for still and cine camera and miniature intragastric cameras are conveniently stored in the unit refrigerator. Their expiration dates should be watched carefully and checked before loading. There are many chores connected with the care of cameras, films, loading, unloading, codifying, labeling, identifying and filming. In our clinic, we have an Endoscopy-Photography Technician, who is responsible for care of endoscopy properties, photographic technic, filing, recording of photos and assisting with the collection and transportation of biopsy and other specimens. The technicians also assist the Endoscopy Nurse in setting up and managing the endoscopy unit activities.

Emergency Supplies

There should be on hand at all times, cardio-respiratory drugs, antedotes for all medicines used, oxygen, plastic pharyngeal airways or similar emergency instruments, tracheotomy sets, blood pressure cuffs, stethoscope, and a nearby filled oxygen tank or oxygen source from the examining room wall. While speaking of these facilities it is probably appropriate to mention that it is desirable to have a good working relationship with the hospital's Department of Anesthesiology and to have a member of this department to check the emergency facilities of the endoscopy room and to review their use periodically with new residents. Hopefully, emergency supplies and facilities may never have to be used, but the risk of not having them immediately available when needed will not be assumed by an efficient endoscopy team.

REFERENCES

1. Sanders, M. G., and Schimmel, E. M.: Perforation of a gastic remnant following fiber-optic gastroscopy. *Gastrointest Endosc, 17 (4)*:186-187, May, 1971.
2. Rastogi, H., and Brown, C. H.: Pseudo acute abdomen following gastroscopy. *Gastrointest Endosc,* August, 1967, pp. 16-18.
3. Barrett, B.: New instruments, new horizons, new hazards. *Gastrointest Endosc, 16 (3)*:142-143, February, 1970.
4. Braucher, R. E., and Kirsner, J. B.: Case report: Impacted fiberscope. *Gastrointest Endosc, 12 (1)*:20-22, August, 1965.
5. Belber, J. P.: Endoscopic examination of the duodenal bulb; a comparison with x-ray. *Gastroenterology, 61*:55, 1971.

6. Oi, I.: Fiberduodenoscopy and endoscopic pancreatocholangiography. *Gastrointest Endosc, 17*:59, 1970.
7. Schindler, R.: *Gastroscopy—The Endoscopic Study of Gastric Pathology.* Chicago, The University of Chicago Press, 1950.
8. Taylor, H.: A New Gastroscope with Controllable Flexibility. *Lancet, 240*:276, 1971.
9. Berry, L. H.: Improved gastroscopic diagnosis by the use of multiple position in 2943 cases. *Gastroenterology, 44 (1)*:20-24, January, 1963.
10. Berry, L. H.: Right side gastroscopic technic in situs inversus viscerum and visualization of "blind spots." *Review of Gastroenterology, 8 (4)*:267-272, July-August, 1941.

CHAPTER 7

TEACHING OF ENDOSCOPY PART I: THE TEACHING OF UPPER GASTROINTESTINAL ENDOSCOPY

Leonidas H. Berry

INTRODUCTORY STATEMENT

CHAPTER 6, WHICH DEALS with technic in considerable detail, is essentially a discussion of the teaching of endoscopy. This chapter should be interpreted as an extension of the discussion of the learning process in endoscopy.

The training of gastrointestinal endoscopists has a long history of formal individual tutorship. The Chevalier Jackson School in Philadelphia is perhaps the best example of a well-known early approach to teaching this art in esophagoscopy, with only an occasional attempt at gastroscopy. Those were the days of rigid tubes, wheat seed lamps, and no magnifica-

"Commuter" Training Program supported by a research grant from Regional Medical Programs, National Institutes of Health, Bethesda, Md. which is not responsible, nor is the U.S. Government, for opinions expressed in this publication.

tion. Then came the Schindler era of semiflexible lens gastroscopes and flexible obturator Eder-Hufford esophagoscopes with magnifying telescopes. During this period of a quarter of a century or more, roughly from 1932 to 1960, the teaching of gastroscopy and esophagoscopy was also being achieved by formal tutorship and for the most part involved residents in Internal Medicine and Gastroenterology. Usually this meant intermittent, dispersed opportunity and often entailed long intervals of noninvolvement before entering practice.

In the United States, one long existing exception to the general practice of training only residents in gastrointestinal endoscopy has been the program at the Cook County Hospital and Cook County Graduate School in Chicago. Dr. Rudolf Schindler, while stationed at the University of Chicago, gave the first gastroscopy course at the Cook County Graduate School in the late 1930s. This was short-lived, though Dr. Schindler continued his short demonstration courses at the University of Chicago. About 1940, Dr. Leo Hardt, who had his training with Dr. Schindler at Billings Hospital, organized and conducted intensive tutorship courses in gastroscopy at the Cook County Hospital and Graduate School. Eventually, a two-week course was developed, in which practicing internists and gastroenterologists met with the instructor each morning for a *wet* session. In 1946, the writer joined Dr. Hardt at the County Hospital and Graduate School. He had trained with Dr. Schindler at Billings and Provident hospitals and performed more than 1,500 gastroscopies at the latter institution.[1] The two-week intensive gastroscopy courses were continued, each instructor giving one twice yearly. At this time, afternoon sessions were added, consisting of lectures, slide review, and practice on the manikin for 4 to 5 students. In about 1961, after Dr. Hardt's retirement, Dr. Fernando Villa and later Dr. J. Adomavicius, both trained on our service, have continued in association with this writer in the training of postgraduates and G.I. residents in G.I. endoscopy.

The postgraduate students come from all parts of the United States specifically for the two-week courses. Students from other parts of the world, while at other American institutions, have come to Cook County Hospital for this training.

During most of these years, one resident in Gastroenterology at Cook County Hospital has participated in each course as part of his training. For a considerable period there was a standing arrangement between Dr. Harry Segal of Rochester University Medical School and the late Dr. Sara Jordan of the Lahey Clinic in Boston and this writer to give two weeks of basic endoscopic training to their gastroenterology residents. Recent graduates of gastroenterology residencies at other well-known institutions received their basic endoscopy training in our clinic at Cook County Graduate School during the prefiberoptic era.

Nelson has for a number of years given part-time gastroscopy courses for one student at a time one day a week, with satisfactory results.[2] Morrissey has been giving a part-time endoscopy course since 1964 involving one student at a time for two weeks.[3] Other endoscopy teachers in the United States have expressed their feelings of responsibility in passing on the art and science of endoscopy to others.[4, 5]

The intensive daily instruction for two weeks was never regarded as a mechanism for creating an experienced endoscopist. Rather, our experience showed that most of the men learned enough of the gastroscopic technic and endoscopic pathology and orientation to continue their professional growth independently. The courses were evaluated periodically by questionnaire, and the conclusions drwn were the basis for continuing this form of teaching through the years. The writer, through these courses and the residency program, has trained more than 300 endoscopists during the past twenty-five years.

Gradually, since about 1963, with the increasing acceptance of fiberscopes, there have been increasing demands for postgraduate training in gastrointestinal endoscopy. Because there appeared to be few places where qualified specialists in practice could receive practical instruction, we decided to investigate the feasibility of extending opportunities in endoscopy training.

"COMMUTER" TRAINING PROGRAM

The two-week intensive training courses were going well in 1969, with three or four such courses a year being given. Registrations were being made two years in advance. It occurred to us that some of the demand might be met if courses were given for selected students who would spend one day a week for three months in training. It was felt this method should be evaluated on a prospective basis. This led to a two-year funded project in 1970 and 1971, which we called the "Commuter Training Program."[6]

Student Selection and Qualifications

Students were selected primarily from small suburban and inner-city hospitals of Chicago and from smaller Illinois towns within commuting distance. The primary objective in selection was to train men whose hospital services were away from large medical school teaching centers. The endoscopy training opportunities would thus be given to qualified men who otherwise would be less apt to have them. The ultimate goal was to bring to a larger number of patients one of the more recent developments in diagnostic technic and expertise, especially as applied to early diagnosis of upper gastrointestinal cancer.

All selectees were practicing specialists, trained in accredited medical schools and accredited residency programs. All were American specialty board certified or eligible, with an active special interest in gastroenterology or abdominal surgery.

Methodology

During 1970 and 1971 a team of four experienced endoscopists* at the Cook County Hospital undertook on an experimental basis a continuous *commuter* course, with the cooperation of the Cook County Graduate School and the Hektoen Institute for Medical Research. The team included three gastroenterologists and gastrointestinal endoscopists on the regular staff of the hospital and Endoscopy Clinic. The fourth, Dr. Mitaniyama, was a Research Teaching Fellow from Tokyo Medical College, brought here through the cooperation of Professor S. Ashizawa. The Endoscopy Nurse, one Nurse Assistant, and the Endoscopy Technician were important members of the staff. The class was limited to four students, who commuted to Cook County from practical distances.

The course consisted of one all-day session a week for three months, a total of twelve sessions. At the end of each three-month period, the staff would rest for one week and then begin the next course. A morning *wet* session involving three or four patients, was followed by an afternoon session of slide and movie review, lectures, discussions, and practice on a manikin. In order to generate cases, facilities and supporting endoscopy service to patients, the Endoscopy Staff, including a rotating resident, was involved five mornings a week.

"Wet" Sessions

Sessions in which patients were examined by instructor and students were held Wednesday mornings and averaged four hours, sometimes longer. Included were demonstrations in passing the scope and technic of examination. These were followed by passage of instruments by students, under supervision, instruction in technic, and in endoscopic pathology of the esophagus, stomach, and the duodenum.

A variety of the latest fiberoptic instruments was available, including forward-viewing esophagogastroscopes and esophagogastroduodenoscopes. When indicated, side-viewing gastroscopes and gastroduodenoscopes were also used. Fiberoptic teaching attachments were used whenever possible. Occasionally gastrocameras and gastrocamera fiberscopes were employed. Demonstrations and/or individual involvement included endoscopic still and cine-photography, transendoscopic biopsy and cytology technics.

For each patient studied there would be a preliminary review and much correlation of clinical history with physical findings, x-ray and other lab-

---

* Berry, L. H., Project Director, Mitaniyama, A., Villa, F., and Adomavicius, J.

oratory findings. Indications and relative contraindications to endoscopy were reviewed. Special attention was given to psychologic preparation, premedication, and control and prevention of injuries. Gentleness and individual human concern for patients by students were demanded at all times.

The "Dry Run"

It has been found advantageous to have students carry out a set of *trial* and orientation exercises away from the patient. A set of simple procedures we devised during the lens gastroscopy era has been found still useful in teaching fiberoptic endoscopy. The initial awkwardness that most students experience is considerably overcome if the scope can be passed through a simulated oral and pharyngeal canal. It is remarkable to note the differences in dexterity between one candidate and another during the simulated procedure, which we call the "dry run." The procedure is repeated by each student until his introduction is smooth and rhythmic. The maneuver is also carried out a few times before each actual introduction in a patient. The patient is thus saved the discomfort and sometimes terror of the awkward period, and the student learns to rely on the practiced reflexes of his hands while he concentrates on patient reaction and a definite and directed technic.

In the beginning we used an artificial skull, including an *oral cavity* with *teeth* and *pharynx*. Later we found it satisfactory to use the gloved left hand of the instructor, partly closed to simulate the open mouth of a patient lying on his left side. The scope is introduced in three rhythmic steps. The student holds the tip of the scope in his right hand as he would a writing pen and "carries" the tip into the mouth and oropharynx. He sees the tip stay in the midline, avoiding the "piriform sinuses."

A second phase of the "dry run" exercises consists of study of and practice on the "phantom stomach" (Fig. 7-1). This study is carried out with

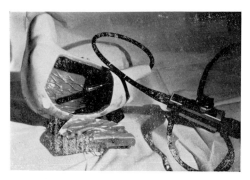

Figure 7-1. Photograph of a "phantom stomach," showing approximate shape and position of inflated organ with patient on left side.

both side-viewing and forward-viewing scopes. The common gastric lesions are built into the phantom or manikin at the sites of predilection.

The simulated stomach is mounted as it would be positioned in the abdomen with the patient on his left side at a 45-degree angle with the examining table. The position of the model is changed from time to time to simulate the dorsal and right-side positions as well. The relative positions of mucosal landmarks to the endoscope objective are identified by the student. This orientation is then translated to the clock-dial indication at the ocular for each patient position on the examining table (see figures on position in Chapter 6).

Slide Review

The afternoon slide review and discussion sessions cover gross and microscopic pathology of all common lesions—and some rare ones—affecting the upper gastrointestinal canal. Collected slides, movies, gastrocamera film strips, biopsy section, and cytology smears of interesting and illustrative cases are presented. Case histories and the problems of clinical gastroenterology are emphasized. It is in these sessions that indications, contraindications, and topographical anatomy are explained in illustrated lectures. Finally, the prevention and management of injuries and the history of endoscopic gastroenterology are presented.

INTENSIVE "ON CAMPUS" TRAINING PROGRAM

As mentioned in the introduction to this chapter, we have been involved in intensive training of endoscopy students for more than a quarter of a century at the Cook County Graduate School. Unlike the "commuter" courses given during the past three years, the intensive courses have always consisted of daily morning and afternoon sessions for two consecutive weeks. This is repeated three to four times a year. Four students are admitted to each class. Forty to fifty endoscopies are carried out in two weeks; thus, each student looks into forty stomachs and passes the scope on an average of ten patients. The students are continuously "on campus" and sometimes spend late afternoons and early evenings in library reading and literature review.

Student Selection

Students selected for the two-week course usually are from out of town. In the twenty-five years the course has been given, almost one half of the states in the United States have been represented. Students have come directly for the courses from Canada, South America and the Caribbean. A number of countries outside the Western Hemisphere have been represented. The educational background and previous training have been of the same high quality as described under the "commuter" course.

Methodology

The methods and technics used in teaching endoscopy have not differed in the "on campus" and "commuter" courses. Because the course has become so broadened as new endoscopic procedures have been introduced, it has become too difficult for one instructor to handle alone. In the past three years, three instructors have been involved with each course.

OBJECTIVES ACHIEVED AND EVALUATION
Prospective Evaluation

During the two-year pilot project, forty-one students were trained. Table 7-I shows the questions asked in a prospective evaluation questionnaire.

TABLE 7-I

QUESTIONS ASKED IN SURVEY OF PROGRESS OF ENDOSCOPY TRAINEES

1. Are you actively doing endoscopy?
2. How many have you done since the course?
3. At what hospitals?
4. If you are not actively doing endoscopy, why?
5. Have you had instances when x-ray missed the diagnosis and endoscopy made the diagnosis? What scopes are you using?
6. Date you took the commuter course.

TABLE 7-II

ACCOMPLISHMENTS OF TRAINEES AND OTHER PERTINENT DATA

1. Total number of trainees from 1970 to March 31, 1972		41
a. Total number of two-week intensive course students	14	
b. Total number of three month "commuter" course students	27	
2. Total number of questionnaires sent to trainees		37
3. Total number of questionnaires received from trainees (as of 4-9-72)		33
4. Specific information (as of 4-9-72)		
a. How many trainees actively doing endoscopy		30
b. How many trainees not actively doing endoscopy		3
(1) Full-time gastroenterologist on staff	1	
(2) No explanation given	2	
c. Number of instances trainees noted that x-ray missed the diagnosis and endoscopy made correct diagnosis proven by surgery		16
5. The specialities of the trainees:		
(1) Surgeon		23
(2) Internist (Gastroenterologist—5)		17
(3) Radiologist		1
6. Total number of endoscopies performed by trainees in three months to one year and nine months following completion of course		809
7. Total number of hospitals involved with trainees		32
8. Total hospitals involved in Chicago		16
9. Total hospitals involved in other cities of Illinois		16
10. Total cities and suburbs involved in Illinois		15
11. Total bed capacity of all involved in Chicago		5,550
12. Total bed capacity of all hospitals involved outside of Chicago, within Illinois		5,520
13. Grand total of hospital bed capacity		11,070

Primarily the concern was whether the trainee began independent endoscopic examinations shortly after completing the course and resuming his hospital practice, in effect launching him into a period of professional growth toward becoming an experienced endoscopist. He was also asked how many examinations he performed in a given period and his analysis of this endoscopic experience. Also tabulated were the geographic locations where each student practiced, his background training, and hospital affiliations, with bed capacities, etc.

Table 7-II shows a breakdown of the accomplishments of the students three months to twenty-one months after their basic training. Of particular interest is the report of a total of sixteen instances during the early post-training period in which endoscopic findings, proved at surgery, were correct and x-ray findings incorrect.

Distances traveled by car pool, private and commercial planes in all types of weather, with only one dropout, is indicative of the interest in the courses. At the end of the teaching project in 1971 there was a backlog of requests for the "commuter" training by well-qualified men.

Retrospective Evaluation

In 1971 questionnaires were sent to students who took the two-week intensive course during the ten years 1959 to 1969. Thirty-nine of the forty-six who answered the questionnaires were doing gastroscopies one to ten years after their training, four had stopped after four or five years, and three had not started for various reasons not related to training.

Most of those answering the questionnaires sent accompanying letters commenting on the benefits of their basic training course. The majority of those trained with lens instruments had changed to fiberoptic scopes and felt the basic training had given them a definite advantage in the change-over.

A retrospective analysis was also made of questionnaires received from students who completed the two-week intensive gastroscopy course at an earlier period. The survey, made in 1963, covered the fifteen years 1948 to 1963. From this group, seventy-nine questionnaires were answered and returned. Data showed that sixty-nine were still doing gastroscopies one to fifteen years after the course; ten trainees were not active at the time of the query. Many letters from these men also commended the adequacy of the basic training they had received.

Comparison of the prospective and retrospective endoscopy training data shows basic similarity in adequacy and effectiveness of these methods of teaching upper gastrointestinal endoscopy. The essential difference in the courses is the important factor of convenience to the student and instructors. In some instances the once-a-week "commuter" course would be more convenient than the two-week intensive course; in other instances the opposite held true.

Evaluation of individual progress of students by the instructors from time to time during the course showed individual variations in dexterity and insight.

RESIDENT TRAINING PROGRAM

The training program in gastrointestinal endoscopy during residency is well established and basic. There should be a better opportunity for correlation of clinical gastroenterology with endoscopy in the residency program. If the program is well organized, as it is in the larger teaching hospitals, the resident should be involved in more endoscopy procedures than students in the intensive short-term courses. There is little difference of opinion among teachers of endoscopy on these points.

At the Cook County Hospital three endoscopists a year, on an average, have been trained through the Gastroenterology Residency program over the past twenty years. The resident has certain built-in opportunities during his period of training. He must evaluate indications and contraindications for endoscopy in every patient considered. He has the opportunity for follow-up to surgery or to postmortem examination. Clinical follow-up after endoscopy can be carried out on inpatients and on outpatients through the clinic. Repeated endoscopies and x-ray examinations and review of photographs and biopsy and cytology specimens offer an excellent training opportunity for residents who are so motivated and can find the time in their busy schedules. Our residents go through the same ritual of training technics described for the intensive courses. One problem raised by some of our residents is the uncertainty of continuity between the end of endoscopic training and beginning of practice or of employment with immediate endoscopy opportunities. This breach in continuity may occur in the residency period itself because of schedules for other important phases of work.

A much greater problem is the need for far more residency programs to meet the legitimate demands for endoscopy training. These unmet needs are a factor in the growing tendency in some areas for physicians to attempt endoscopy without basic training, on a trial-and-error basis. Herein lies a challenge to gastroenterology societies, teaching centers, and manufacturers to supply the demands for gastrointestinal endoscopy training, with the greatest possible protection of patient interests, professional standards, and the integrity of the profession.

REFERENCES

1. Berry, L. H.: Analysis of 1,400 consecutive gastroscopic examinations. *Proc Inst Med Chic, 16*:273, 1946.

2. Nelson, R. S.: Endoscopic training and the fiberscope. *Bull Gastrointest Endosc,* 10:5, 1963

3. Morrissey, John: Personal communication.

4. Hufford, A. R.: The gastroscopist's adaptation to esophagoscopy. *Am J Gastroenterol,* 25:272, 1956.

5. Olsen, A. M.: And gladly teach. *Bull Gastrointest Endosc,* 9:4, 1963.

6. Berry, Leonidas H., Mitaniyama, A., Villa, Fernando, and Adomavicius, J.: "Commuter" training in GI endoscopy; experimental evaluation, funded by Ill. Regional Med. Program, Div. Regional Med. Programs, Nat. Institutes of Health. Bethesda, Md. Grant #OG-8 in press.

TEACHING OF ENDOSCOPY PART II: USES OF CLOSED CIRCUIT TELEVISION IN U.S.A.

J. Alfred Rider and Ernesto J. Puletti[*]

INTRODUCTORY STATEMENT

Historically the credit for developing the first gastroscope goes to Kussmaul in 1868. It was a straight, rigid tube and was passed over a flexible obturator.[1] His subject was a professional sword-swallower.

From that time until 1932, numerous rigid gastroscopes were developed, many of which were passed over flexible tubes. In addition to the difficulty and danger attendant with the induction procedure, the illumination was less than adequate and the mobility of the instruments in the stomach was minimal.

The beginning of modern gastroscopy occurred when Wolf and Schindler[1] developed the first flexible gastroscope in 1932. This instrument, which utilized multiple lenses of short focal distances, produced excellent illumination and moderately good mobility for the individual observer, but not sufficient illumination for photography.

Baird[2] in 1928 showed that optical images could be projected through tiny flexible quartz-glass fibers aligned in bundles, and Hansell[2] in 1930 actually transmitted images in a curved path utilizing similar quartz fibers. But it was not until 1953 that Van Heel[2] by coating individual glass fibers with a substance of lower index refraction than glass (resulting in an internal mirror), was able to project images through a flexible glass bundle.

* We are grateful to Mr. John Landre for cooperation and use of the color videoscope and to Drs. Richard Rider and Pedro Colombini for assistance.

The tools were now available for achieving complete flexibility of the endoscopes, thus increasing markedly the accessibility of the gastrointestinal tract. The way was also open for marked improvement of light transmission.

Since Hirschowitz[3] first reported in 1958 the practical use of a fiberoptic gastroscope, there have been numerous technical advancements which have facilitated still and motion pictures.

First, still black and white pictures were possible, and then intragastric color photography was developed. Although the latter represented a distinct advantage in the technique, it was not totally effective in recording the gastroscopic image. Among the drawbacks were the inability to record actual peristaltic waves, and changes in the size and shape of lesions. Furthermore, considerable time elapsed between the examination and the viewing of the pictures. With the evolution of intragastric color cinematography several advantages were apparent. It was now possible to record peristaltic waves or changes in color, size or shape of lesions; and to observe dynamic anatomy and pathophysiology, including rates of emptying and changes affecting gastric motility. However, this technique also had limitations. Usually several days elapsed between taking and evaluating the films. And, if the quality of the film was unsatisfactory, it was not always possible to repeat the examination. Furthermore, it was impossible for several viewers to simultaneously view the endoscopic image. Therefore teaching the technique resulted in prolongation of the examination, with attendant discomfort to the patient, while each viewer took his turn observing.

ADVANTAGES AND HISTORY OF TELEVISION ENDOSCOPY

The next step of course, was televised recording of the endoscopic image. It was obvious that perfection of this technique would enable an unlimited number of examiners to simultaneously observe the mucosa of the gastrointestinal tract. Immediate discussion and consultation would be available and in cases of controversy, instant playback of the image could be simply accomplished. Historically, television has been applied to endoscopy only in recent years. The first attempts at televised proctoscopy and peritoneoscopy were carried out in black and white and reported in European journals.[4-7] Different types of equipment were used, the Eidophor used by Debray et al.,[8, 9] and a miniature black and white television camera, described by Berci.[10]

Black and white television images are produced in the following fashion: The image passes through a lens and is received by "pick-up" tubes. These tubes in turn translate the image into electronic signals. These signals are further processed, transferred electronically and then finally projected into a receiving tube.

After it was demonstrated that a black and white television image could be obtained, the next step was to develop endoscopic color television. Routine color television images are, however, somewhat more complex.

The lens or objective receives an image. This image is decomposed into three colors: red, green and blue. Each of these color components is carried through individual electron beams; one for each color. These beams are received in the monitor tube where they excite the corresponding three color phosphors. This arrangement is used for routine color television transmission with adequate results, but is not powerful enough to obtain an image from an endoscopic instrument.

Before an adequate color television endoscopic picture is seen, the following requirements must be met: 1) availability of a high intensity external light source; 2) delivery of an adequate fiberoptic cold light to the stomach and back to the observer via a similar bundle; and 3) a color television camera with adequate sensitivity. This last requirement of a suitable camera has been fulfilled by the production of new secondary electron conduction tubes (called SEC pick-up tubes) which were developed first for military night-viewing devices. These tubes were found to be adequate for transmission of gastroscopic images, since they are ten times more sensitive than the conventional lead oxide pick-up tubes, and operate with a minimum illumination, equivalent to only five footcandles.

TECHNIC

We have studied and devised certain technics for the use of closed circuit TV in gastrointestinal endoscopy.[11] The following endoscopes have been used: 1) Hirschowitz Gastroduodenoscope, American Cystoscope Makers, Inc. (ACMI); 2) Panview Mark VII Fibergastroscope, ACMI; 3) Fibergastroscope, Type B, Machida; 4) Fiberduodenoscope, Model L, Machida; and 5) Fibergastroscope GRFA, Olympus.

After routine introduction of the ACMI instrument, a Commercial Electronics, Inc. (CEI) model 4110 fiberscope attachment was coupled with one end to the eyepiece of the gastroscope, and the other to the Color Videoscope™ (CEI) camera (Fig. 7-2). For the other endoscopes we used a special coupling device manufactured by our technicians.

The technical aspects of the equipment in use at the present time in our laboratory are as follows:

1. Three Westinghouse SEC W1-31863 color television pick-up tubes.
2. Filters: Two position filter wheels, one with color temperature-correcting filters and one with neutral density filters.

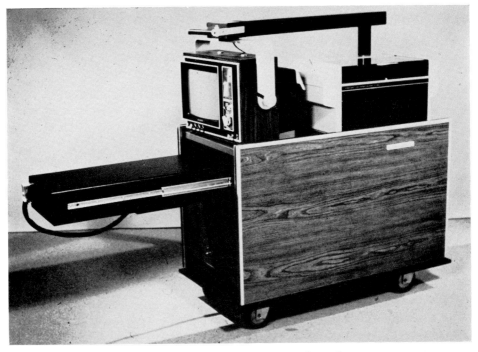

Figure 7-2. Assembled unit of equipment used for color television gastroscopy consisting of camera with fiber bundle, monitor, and video tape recorder.

3. Television system: 525 lines, 60 fields, NTSC (American Broadcasting System, National Television Standardization Committee).
4. Light sensitivity automatic servo control with neutral density wedges.
5. Power requirements: 105-125 volts, 850 watts.
6. Fiberscope attachment: CEI Model 4110, three foot fiberoptic bundle.
7. Monitors: Sony 14″ Model KV-1210U or Sony 7″ Model KV 7010 AU.
8. Tape recording equipment: IVC (International Video Corporation), Color, 1″ recorder.

This assembled unit is portable, and has a height adjustment that is motor-driven. The boom, which has a tiltable monitor, can be adjusted from 32 inches to 46 inches, and rotated 180 degrees. The entire unit, exclusive of video tape recorder, weighs 425 pounds, and has the following dimensions: height, 46 inches to the top of the boom in stowed position; width, 20 inches; and length 42 inches.

This equipment can be operated by the endoscopist and a technician, and the cost of the equipment, not including the endoscopes, is approximately $70,000.

DISCUSSION

We have used the equipment to record representative endoscopic images such as normal esophagus and stomach, hiatal hernias, esophagitis, esophageal neoplasms, gastric ulcers, gastric polyps, and gastric carcinomas. In addition we have been able to record the appearance of the duodenum. The images have been of excellent quality with satisfactory contrast of colors. The original tapes are faithful reproductions of the direct endoscopic image.

In order to be effective, obviously the endoscopist must perform a complete examination. If the examination can be achieved quickly and painlessly it is to the advantage of the patient and will decrease the occurrence of complications.

Since only one person at a time can look through the endoscope examinations can become quite prolonged in teaching situations because of the necessity of demonstrating the gastroscopic scene to referring physicians and students. Furthermore, added time is required if photographs are made of the procedure. Therefore, during routine endoscopic examinations for many viewers with many position changes, frequent interruptions result in order to demonstrate a particular view. (Often by the time the student gets to the eyepiece, the view has changed.) The shortcomings of the routine procedure in these circumstances are evident. Although there is a special teaching attachment through which the gastroscopist and one observer can see the identical scene simultaneously, for live examinations to a large audience, there is no technique comparable to color television endoscopy.

SUMMARY AND CONCLUSIONS

Technically, closed circuit color endoscopic television is accomplished because of: 1) efficient fiber-endoscopes which supply sufficient internal illumination and 2) recent developments in color television cameras which utilize an electron conduction tube sensitive to a minimum of five foot-candles.

Color television has certain advantages over routine endoscopic techniques: it instantaneously makes available the live scene to unlimited observers including other endoscopic consultants and students. The endoscopic scene can be recorded at the time of the procedure, and the tape is available for instant playback so one can review it for the technical accuracy of recording. If adjustments are necessary they can be made immediately, thus eliminating the need for a repeat examination due to technical failure.

The main disadvantage is the expense of the equipment and its bulk which makes it difficult for routine transportation to different locations.

REFERENCES

1. Schindler, R.: Gastroscopy: *The Endoscopic Study of Gastric Pathology.* Chicago, University of Chicago Press, 1937, p. 11.
2. News Release on Fiber Optics, American Cystoscope Makers, Inc., Pelham Manor, New York, May, 1960.
3. Hirschowitz, B. I., Curtiss, L. E., Peters, C. W., and Pollard, H. M.: Demonstration of a new gastroscope, the "fiberscope." *Gastroenterology,* 35:30, 1958.
4. Bruneau, J., Jomain, J., and Dubois de Montereynaurd, J. M.: From Traite Pratique de photographie et cinematographie medicales, Paris, vol. 1.
5. Stoichita, S., and Steclaci, A.: L'endoscopie televisee en blanc et noir et les perspectives de l'endoscopie televisee en couleur en gastroenterologie. *Arch Mal App Dig,* 52:87-93, 1963.
6. Heinkel, K.: Diagnostik und therapie der erkrankugen des Magen-Darm-Kanals. Basel, Verlag S. Karger, 1962 (Supplementun a la revue Gastroenterolgia), p. 309.
7. Henning, N., Heinkel, K., and Landgraf, J.: Die Faseroptik, eine Bericherung der Gastroskopie. *Btsche Med Wschr,* 88:807, 1963.
8. Debray, C., Housset, P., Segal, S., Paolaggi, J. A., and Pette, F.: Etat actuel de la photocinematographie endoscopique digestive en France. Congress International de photographie et cinematorgraphie medicales. *G. Thieme Verlag,* Stuttgart, 1962.
9. Debray, C., Houssett, P., Segal, S., Paolaggi, J. A., and Pette, F.: La photographie et la cinematographie endoscopiques digestives. Etat actual en France. *Sem Hop,* Paris, 37:963-969, 1961.
10. Berci, G.: Endoscopy and television, *Brit Med J,* 1:1610-1613, 1963.
11. Rider, J. A., Puletti, E. J., Rider, R. D., and Colombini, P. N.: Color television gastroscope: A critical analysis. *Gastrointest Endosc,* 18:20, 1971.

TEACHING OF ENDOSCOPY PART III: USES OF CLOSED CIRCUIT TELEVISION IN JAPAN

FONG-MING CHANG AND SHINROKU ASHIZAWA*

HISTORY AND TECHNICS
ADVANTAGES OF TELEVISION IN ENDOSCOPY
FUTURE OF TELEVISION ENDOSCOPY

HISTORY AND TECHNICS

EVER SINCE THE INTRODUCTION of fiber-optics into the field of Endoscopy in 1957, remarkable progress in instruments and technics of Gastrointestinal Endoscopy has occurred. In 1964, Yoshitoshi[1] and his associates in Japan started the employment of closed circuit color television in Gastrofiberoscopy, using a Simultaneous Plumbicon TV Camera and a gastrofiberscope. Unfortunately, the light source from the lamp system of the fiberscope was found insufficient for the illumination of the gastric mucosa with this TV system. However, in 1968, the light guide gastrofiberscope was introduced clinically by which a powerful cold light source was used to make possible image recording and TV viewing of endoscopic images. In 1969, Ikeda[2] successfully employed a Field Sequential Color TV System in gastrofiberoscopy. Meanwhile, Okuda[3] reported a satisfactory result by applying endoscopic TV in Japan. This had the advantage of light weight, high sensitivity, better picture quality, simplified operation and easy maintenance. Most of these TV units have the capacity for still photography, video-tape recording, biopsy, cytology and even for transendoscopic polypectomy, and at present are widely used in the medical teaching institutes of Japan.

The principal and main components of endoscopic TV as used in Japan are illustrated in Figure 7-3. These figures show functions of light source, fiberscope, camera, controller and monitor. The light source constitutes

---

* We are grateful to Mr. S. Hosoi for his kind assistance.

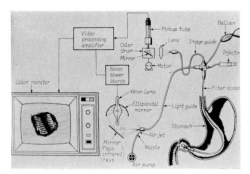

Figure 7-3. The main components of endoscopic television include a light source, fiberscope, camera, controller and monitor as shown above.

one of the most important parts of this equipment and is composed of a power supply, a light concentrating system and a light control system. The color TV systems presently in use in Japan consist of two models, one being a Standard Simultaneous Color TV which is popular among broadcasting stations in the world and the other being a Field Sequential Color TV System (U.S. Columbia Broadcasting Company). The merit of the Simultaneous system is that of being convertible with ordinary related TV systems which are commonly used in the operation room for demonstration

TABLE 7-III

COMPARISON OF FIELD SEQUENTIAL IMAGE ORTHICON CAMERA AND SIMULTANEOUS PLUMBICON CAMERA

	Sequential Type	*Simultaneous Type*
Number of pickup tube	1	3
Construction	Simple	Complicated
Price		
Camera	Low	High
Monitor	High	Low
VTR	High	Low
Functions	No overlapped color	Overlapped three primary colors
	Stable	required. Unstable factors present
Resolution	High	Normal (like broadcasts)
Maintenance	Advantage of using fewer electrical parts	Lasting stability required with use of more electrical parts involved
Color temperature conversion	Either use of conversion filter of color or temperature of filter trimming required	Either use of conversion filter of color temperature of ND filter trimming
Color breakup	Apt to occur in quick moving objects No problem for medical uses	None
System development	High cost and lacking in common use for large system. With special Monitor and VTR involved	Advantage of using ordinary related instruments

of surgical procedures and for teaching programs. The advantages
of the Sequential system are good quality, stable functions, and yet
a simple construction at a low cost in a smaller system. Since both Simultaneous and Sequential systems are available commercially in Japan, comparison of these two systems in the field of Endoscopy is necessary for a
detailed discussion. Table 7-III shows the principal difference between
these two systems.

During the clinical application of endoscopic TV in examination of the
gastrointestinal tract, there are several technical problems to be encountered frequently. For example, during esophagoscopy, because of the narrowed luminal space of the esophagus, the figures shown on the TV monitor often appear strongly contrasted and different from the rather soft
images obtained during conventional esophagofiberoscopy. A similar phenomenon happens during the performance of gastric biopsy in that while
the lesion is close enough for the biopsy forceps to approach the lesion,
the contrast of the images on the monitor increase. In these instances, a
proper distance between the objective lens of the scope and the mucosal
surface is always necessary for obtaining a sharp image and displaying
mucosal details. Color and other electronic problems may cause ill-defined
images and interfere with making an accurate diagnosis.

ADVANTAGES OF TELEVISION IN ENDOSCOPY

Television is applied for four main reasons in the field of Endoscopy.
The first is to permit a group of specialists instead of only one endoscopist
to simultaneously observe the endoscopic examination. The second advantage is the enlarged image permitting a more accurate diagnosis and more
precise biopsy and transendoscopic cytology procedures. The third is an
easier performance of the endoscopic procedure and shortening the examination period and reducing the discomfort for the patient. The fourth
purpose of endoscopic TV is its use in the teaching of Endoscopy. The instructor has the tremendous advantages of showing endoscopic figures
in vivo to the participants in endoscopic teaching programs, and when it
is appropriate even the patient, a family member or others may observe
without distraction from the main purpose of professional service to the
patient. In some instances, a professional group opinion may add to that
service. Video-tape recording is easy and can be made simultaneously for
permanent records, later review and reconfirming suspicious and surgically
proven diagnoses.

FUTURE OF TELEVISION ENDOSCOPY

Future developments in the technical area of endoscopic TV are opti-
mistic owing to an unlimited open field for this approach. As for the field

of development in clinical applications, there is always room for improvement in technics currently employed such as esophagoscopy, gastroscopy, duodenoscopy, colonoscopy, biopsy, cytology and polypectomy. For exciting future development, the following technics undoubtedly will be explored, viz., intestinography, transendoscopic pancreato/cholangiography and other electronic optical variations such as zooming for magnification, vital staining, fluorescent technics, image filtration, ultraviolet or infra-red filtering, etc. Perhaps some of the above mentioned specific technics will open a new era in the future for not only diagnosis but treatment as well in the diseases of the gastrointestinal tract. It is concluded that since the success of color television in the field of Endoscopy in 1968,[4] the current status of this method is that it is very widely and enthusiastically accepted and that it has enhanced the practicability and popularity of Gastrointestinal Endoscopy in Japan.

REFERENCES

1. Yoshitoshi, Y., and Associates: Endoscopic color television. *Gastroenterological Endoscopy,* (Japanese), *11*:72, 1969.
2. Ikeda, S., and Associates: Study on endoscopical television. *Gastroenterological Endoscopy,* (Japanese), *11*:211, 1969.
3. Okuda, S., and Associates: Biopsy under E.T.V. *Gastroenterological Endoscopy,* (Japanese), *11*:212, 1969.
4. Hosoi, S., and Associates: Color television endoscope. *Toshiba Review,* July-August:37, 1968.

SECTION II

ENDOSCOPIC PATHOLOGY OF THE ESOPHAGUS

CHAPTER 8

HISTORY, TECHNICS, VARICES, ESOPHAGITIS, PEPTIC ULCERS AND EROSIONS

Philip A. LoPresti

History and Construction of Esophagoscopes
Preparation and Premedication
Technic of Rigid Esophagoscopy
Technic of Fiberoptic Esophagoscopy
Normal Esophagus
Esophageal Varices
Esophagitis

HISTORY AND CONSTRUCTION OF ESOPHAGOSCOPES

ENDOSCOPIC EXAMINATION OF the esophagus can be performed by three methods: (1) the use of hollow, rigid metal tubes (rigid instruments); (2) the use of flexi-rigid instruments and (3) the use of flexible fiberoptic instruments (flexible instruments).

The rigid instrument was first introduced into medicine in the late nineteenth century and popularized by the Philadelphia Broncho-Esophagological Clinic under Chevalier Jackson. The passage of the instrument under direct vision was made relatively safe by developing the proper control of patient's head, cervical and dorsal spine while the endoscopist threaded the lumen. With skill, the incidence of accidental cricopharyngeal and hiatal region perforations were reduced to a minimum.

The introduction of flexi-rigid instruments by Boros[1] in 1947 and by Hufford[2] in 1949 made the procedure easier and safer. These instruments were designed with suction-light channels, a flexible, rubber-tipped obturator and a four power external telescope (Fig. 8-1). This method encouraged the use of esophagoscopy in the diagnosis of esophageal conditions, further advancing our knowledge of esophageal disease. The instrument had limited photographic capability, however, more recently, Katz[3] had in-

139

troduced a telescopic lens through the lumen of the tube which has extended the photographic capability of the flexi-rigid instrument.

The next major advance in endoscopic examination of the esophagus was made in 1964 when the first successful completely flexible fiberoptic esophagoscope was introduced,[4] further simplifying the technic of esophageal examination. The distal lens system on this instrument was a complex lens (foroblique) allowing forward and oblique viewing of the esophagus. The solid (non-hollow) construction of the instrument necessitated a different endoscopic technic for examining the esophagus, employing air inflation to distend the esophagus, and a separate channel to clear secretions. The proper coordination of air and suction is utilized to obtain a clear view of the esophagus.

Since the introduction of this first instrument, many modifications have evolved.[5-7] Mechanical control of the distal viewing head has allowed the use of a simple lens system. The mechanical method of changing the angle of view as contrasted to the optical methods (complex lens system) has permitted the construction of a shorter distal lens compartment, increasing the flexibility of the viewing end of the instrument. Automatic air inflating and suction devices at the proximal end of the instrument have been incorporated, allowing simpler control of the instrument.

Rigid and flexi-rigid type instruments have been supplanted in the main by fiberoptic instruments for performing medical esophagoscopy. Advan-

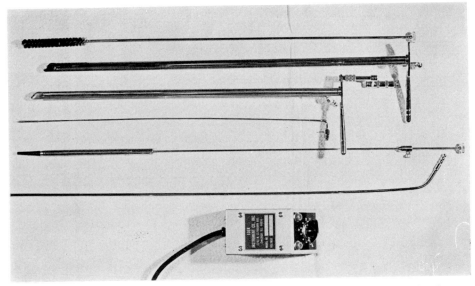

Figure 8-1. Flexi-rigid Instrument. Eder-Hufford Esophagoscope: Two lengths demonstrated, 45 and 55cm. The light carrier, the flexible obturator and the accessory suction tube are demonstrated.

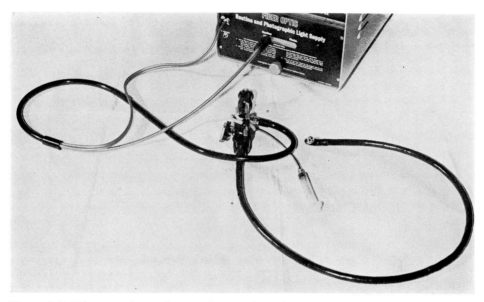

Figure 8-2. Fiberoptic Panendoscope for esophageal, gastric and duodenal examination. Many modifications of this instrument exist. The basic features are: 1) Fiberoptic image transmitting bundle, 2) fiberoptic illuminating bundle, 3) air inflation and suction channel and 4) distal flexion control of the optical field.

tages include comfort to the patient, ease of passage, better and more complete views of the cardioesophageal junction, routine availability of both still and cine photography and the more recent modification of these instruments into pan-endoscopes[8] (Fig. 8-2). These advantages have made fiberoptic instruments more desirable to modern-day gastroenterologists.

Fiberoptic esophagoscopes are more limited in the performance of surgical procedures of the esophagus. The instruments are designed with a small (five to seven French) biopsy channel, through which one can insert a small forceps or a cauterizing device for performing minor surgical procedures. The hollow-type, rigid esophagoscopes are certainly superior for removal of foreign objects or the performance of esophageal dilatation under direct visualization. This limitation of fiberoptic instruments necessitates the preservation of our skill in the use of rigid instruments and underscores the need for continued training in the use of rigid and flexirigid instruments.

PREPARATION AND PREMEDICATION

Preparation of the patient is important for all methods of esophagoscopy. Complete explanation of the procedure to the patient with an honest assessment of the degree of discomfort, in my experience, has been most helpful in obtaining the patient's complete cooperation. Prior instruction is given as to relaxation of the neck and the appropriate moment to swallow. Reassurance is given as to the ability to breathe during the procedure.

Sedation can best be accomplished with intravenous Meperidine Hydrochloride (Demerol®), 50-100mg or Diazepam®, 2-10mg intravenously. The aim of sedation is to achieve a degree of relaxation such that responsiveness is decreased but the ability of the patient to follow instructions is preserved. Topical anesthetics, such as Xylocaine® Viscous (lidocaine) or Dyclone®, are used in selected patients, i.e. they may be used as the only premedication in patients who are examined in a clinic situation where the patient is discharged home after the procedure or they may be used in conjunction with sedation in a patient where the gag reflex is not adequately controlled with sedation. There are a substantial number of patients, who, with proper reassurance, may be examined safely without any premedication. We have not used anticholinergic drugs routinely in premedicating the patient, since we have not found that their use is necessary for the success of the examination.

TECHNIC OF RIGID ESOPHAGOSCOPY

The most widely used rigid instrument is the Eder-Hufford type. These instruments may best be called flexi-rigid instruments since the method of introduction utilizes a flexible obturator for safer passage. It is a hollow lumen tube, 45 or 55cm in length, 7 or 9mm inside diameter with incorporated suction, flexible obturator with a rubber finger and a four power external telescope.

The examination is performed with the patient fasting and all dental prostheses removed. With the patient in the left lateral position, the legs are flexed and the head supported by an assistant, who maneuvers it on command by the endoscopist. The instrument, with the obturator, is introduced into the pharynx with the index finger over the obturator and the neck held in flexion. The right hand guides the instrument, under gentle pressure, with the long axis of the instrument parallel with the patient's spine. The initiation of swallowing or gagging relaxes the upper sphincter; the head is extended with the neck flexed and the instrument advanced when the cricopharyngeal spasm relaxes. As the distal end of the instrument passes the upper sphincter, the obturator is removed and visualization begins. The lumen is kept in view throughout the examination. The patient's head is maneuvered as indicated to keep the lumen in view as the instrument is advanced. Lesions are located in centimeters from the incisor teeth. Advantage is taken of esophageal relaxation during respiratory movements to assist in threading the esophageal lumen. Suction is applied when needed to clear secretions. The central channel of the instrument may further be used for injection of water or inserting accessory suction tubes for further removal of secretion or other debris. Resistance at the upper and lower sphincter is normal and experience is required to attain the proper feeling of what is normal and abnormal resistance. Passing through the sphincters should never give more resistance than that which is felt on most digital rectal examinations. Greater resistance indicates the instrument may be improperly aligned with the esophageal lumen and undue pressure may cause perforation.

The use of a dental aspirator with independent suction, to remove oral secretions, is useful in adding to the patient's comfort during the procedure.

TECHNIC OF FIBEROPTIC ESOPHAGOSCOPY

Today, multipurpose endoscopes are available for examining the esophagus, stomach and duodenum in sequence, with the same instrument, at a single examination. This versatility offers obvious advantages in the investigation of upper gastrointestinal disease of uncertain origin.

Most instruments today incorporate the following basic features: (1) fiberoptic image transmitting bundles approximately 4mm in diameter with proximal and distal lenses; (2) fiberoptic illuminating bundle systems with external light source; the light distally at the examining site is cold; (3) air inflation and suction channels for distending the esophageal lumen and for clearing away secretions. The suction channel also serves as a biopsy channel; (4) distal flexion systems with proximal controls to change the angle of view of the instrument.

The various instruments available today all have good optical systems. They vary in the design of the automated air and suction channels and the degree of mechanical flexion of the distal viewing end. The optical fields give an angle of view of 50 to 75 degrees.

The great degree of mechanical control of the distal viewing end in both the longitudinal and horizontal axis of the instrument is obviously not needed for viewing the anatomically straight esophagus. These features are incorporated for the further examination of the stomach and duodenum.

The introduction into the esophagus of present-day fiberoptic instruments is technically much easier than with rigid and flexi-rigid instruments. This has fostered the attitude by some physicians that little or no training is required for their use. However, before we lapse into a false sense of security as to the safety of these instruments, let us take note of a survey by the Society for Gastrointestinal Endoscopy in 1967.[9] This data, from major United States gastroenterology units, showed that, of 3,211 fiberoptic esophagoscopies performed, there were three perforations for fiberoptic esophagoscopy, an incidence of .093 per cent, compared to .11 per cent for flexi-rigid esophagoscopy. Certainly, this study shows that fiberoptic instruments can be as hazardous as flexi-rigid instruments and there can be no substitute for good training, skill and experience in all types of endoscopy. A major reason for accidents with the early fiberoptic instruments was the plastic cup design of the distal tip. Streamlining of the distal end of the instrument, with discarding of the plastic cup, has made for safer passage through the cricopharyngeal region.

The fasting patient is prepared in the same manner as for rigid esophagoscopy. Explanation of the procedure, reassurance and sedation are used as in rigid endoscopy. The flexibility of the instrument allows examination of the patient in a variety of positions.

The upright position, sitting in a chair, and the left lateral supine position, are most widely used. I prefer the left lateral position with the patient's head supported by a pillow. This position usually allows for better control of the patient's head, which reflexly tends to move backward with the introduction of the instrument. The procedure can be performed without the assistance of a technician. Bedside, emergency procedures are easily performed in patients who are too ill to be transferred to the endoscopy laboratory.

The distal end of the instrument is bent into a gentle curve to approximate the shape of the oropharynx. Upon reaching the cricopharyngeal area, slight resistance is felt. The index finger of the left hand is placed behind the tip of the instrument, resting on the posterior pharynx. The patient is asked to swallow and with the right hand holding the instrument at the oropharynx, gentle forward pressure is applied. A swallowing or gagging action will relax the cricopharyngeal spasm and this is a good time to advance the instrument. Failure to negotiate the esophageal lumen with several gentle attempts may indicate poor position of the tip of the instrument, i.e. placement in the pyriform sinuses. The instrument is then gradually withdrawn and repositioned. Occasionally, the tip of the instrument will lodge against the body of a vertebrae; placing the end of the instrument anteriorally toward the trachea with the left index finger, will serve to dislodge the tip from the body of the vertebrae and allow successful passage. Most esophagoscopists begin viewing as the tip of the instrument passes through the upper sphincter. If it is desired to examine the oropharynx and the region of the vocal chords, good views of this region can be obtained by viewing prior to entering the esophagus. Examination of this region is easier when two endoscopists perform the procedure, one introducing and manipulating the instrument, while the other views the area.

There are few contraindications to esophagoscopy (see Chapter 3). Esophagoscopy may be hazardous in the presence of aortic aneurysm and in patients with severe cardiovascular disease. Deformity of the cervical spine may make it impossible to pass the flexi-rigid instrument. Fiberoptic instruments, because of their flexibility, can be used more safely in cervical spine deformities. Equal caution, as with flexi-rigid instruments, is exercised in patients with severe cardiac, respiratory, or other debilitating diseases. Flexi-rigid and flexible esophagoscopy is contraindicated in an uncooperative patient and when there is high cervical esophageal obstruction. In the latter situation, a safe examination can be performed by starting visualization in the posterior pharynx.

NORMAL ESOPHAGUS

The normal esophageal mucosa is pink in color and smooth in appearance (Plate 6). In the mid-esophagus one can frequently discern a linear bluish vein, the anterior esophageal vein. This is usually flat and can be followed to the lower one third of the esophagus. During peristalsis seen particularly well with fiberoptic instruments, one can observe contractions of the circular and longitudinal muscles. Numerous concentric rings are seen during the initiation of peristalsis terminating in the formation of two to three longitudinal folds. With relaxation of the esophagus, there is complete disappearance of the circular and longitudinal folds. Cardiac pulsations are readily seen in the mid-esophagus.

The lens system of fiberoptic instruments readily visualizes small vessels in the lower esophagus especially at the esophago-gastric junction. The esophago-gastric junction is marked by a change in the normal pink color to the white dentate appearing boundary marking the transition from squamous mucosa to gastric columnar mucosa. The gastric mucosa is reddish-pink in color.

The esophago-gastric junction is most often closed and opens with peristalsis. Passage of the instrument into the stomach is frequently accomplished by blind passage through the closed junction.

ESOPHAGEAL VARICES

The major cause of formation of esophageal varices is intrahepatic portal hypertension due to venous block caused by cirrhosis. The submucous venous tributaries of the upper esophagus drain into the inferior thyroidal vein which empties into the right or left brachiocephalic vein. Tributaries from the mid-esophagus drain mainly to the azygos and right brachiocephalic tributaries. Tributaries from the lower and short abdominal segments drain mostly into the left gastric vein.

The rich network of vessels in the lower esophagus which communicates with the portal system through the coronary vein is normally closed. Increase in pressure in this system causes distension and tortuosity of these poorly supported veins.

Endoscopic examination of non-bleeding esophageal varices is safe providing the patient is cooperative and undue retching is not provoked. In our examination of 600 patients with varices, only two have bled because of instrumentation. Both patients had severe retching induced by the procedure.

The superiority of endoscopy, in the diagnosis of esophageal varices over radiological methods has been documented by many studies.[10] The incidence of esophageal varices, as determined endoscopically, in patients with cirrhosis of the liver is variously reported between 30 to 63 per cent. Medium and large size varices are easily identified by their distended appearance and offer no difficulty to most endoscopists. Small varices present more difficulty and may cause disagreement among experienced endoscopists, particularly in distinguishing small varices from esophageal mucosal folds. Conn et al. have shown that some observer error occurs in esophagoscopic interpretation as in radiologic interpretation, and that training and experience help to reduce this error.[11]

The color of esophageal varices varies with the proximity of the vessels to the mucosa. Varices may be deep, in which event, they have the coloration of the musoca, and then are identified by the tortuosity and elevation of the mucosa (Plate 7). In the lower end of the esophagus, bluish coloration is more common even with small varices (Plate 8). Peristalsis may cause varices to become engorged assuming a larger size and increased tortuosity. With fiberoptic esophagoscopes, a long segment of lumen is visualized, and longitudinal mucosal folds can be differentiated from varices by complete disappearance of folds with the relaxation of the esophagus. In our experience, this method of differentiation has been reliable.

Endoscopically, varices have been graded from one-plus to five-plus by DeGradi[12] according to the longitudinal extent in centimeters, the diameter and size. Grade one varices are blue or red in color. They are usually 2mm in diameter. Grade five varices are grape-like clusters, which occlude the lumen of the esophagus and have cherry red varices on top of varices.

Palmer and Brick[13] grade varices as mild: less than 3mm in diameter; moderate: 3-6mm in diameter, and severe: greater than 6mm in diameter. The longitudinal involvement of the esophagus is recorded. Although it is useful to have some criterion as to the size of varices, agreement on a common grading system has been hard to achieve because of observer variation and the different types of instruments used.

Bleeding from esophageal varices is best determined by direct visualization. Patients who have mild bleeding can be successfully examined with flexi-rigid or fiberoptic instruments, without prior gastric lavage. The examination in massive bleeders is frequently difficult because of the inability to effectively remove blood clots. The use of flexi-rigid instruments, because of their larger central lumen, is more advantageous in massive bleeders than fiberoptic instruments. The ice-water gastric lavage is the most critical step in the preparation of the massive bleeder for esophagoscopy. A large bore 36 French Ewald tube is passed orally into the stomach. Ice-water is repeatedly instilled and withdrawn until the contents return relatively free of blood. With this technique, there is a high percentage of successful examinations.

ESOPHAGITIS

Gastroesophageal reflux generally is held to be the prime cause of esophagitis in man. Long-continued esophagitis may lead to scarring or peptic stricture.

The clinical diagnosis of esophagitis is suspected when there is heartburn aggravated by assuming the supine position. There is generally a poor correlation between the clinical diagnosis and the endoscopic and histologic findings. Siegel and Hendrix[14] studied 25 patients with the clinical diagnosis of esophagitis. Gross and histological evidence of esophageal inflammation did not correlate with the symptoms of heartburn. Eighteen of 25 patients showed inflammatory changes on biopsy while seven had normal biopsies. The esophagoscopic evaluation of mucosal inflammation did not closely parallel the histologic findings. Three of ten patients esophagoscoped in the non-heartburn control group had inflammatory changes histologically.

The poor correlation of histological and clinical symptoms led Ismail-Beigi et al. to re-evaluate the histological criteria for peptic esophagitis.[15] Their study showed that round cell collections are present in many biopsy specimens from normal subjects, and therefore, are of no diagnostic value. The presence of neutrophiles was a rather insensitive indicator of inflammation. The histological feature of basal cell hyperplasia and closeness of the papillae to the epithelial surface correlated well with the presence of symptomatic gastro-esophageal reflux in 85 per cent of their patients. Endoscopy was performed in 34 of their subjects who were symptomatic. In 25 subjects, the diagnosis of esophagitis was made endoscopically. In 22 of them, or 88 per cent, the biopsy was also abnormal by their criteria.

Peters[16] and Sandry,[17] using autopsy and surgical specimens, clearly characterized the inflammatory nature of esophagitis. Sandry states that with erosive esophagitis, there is regeneration of the mucosa with residual submucosal inflammation and scarring. Possibly, the poor correlation between clinical and histological findings may be due to the limitation of the biopsy specimens to adequately reflect the total pathology.

The endoscopic criteria for esophagitis are friability, granularity or ulcerations of the esophageal mucosa. In early esophagitis, the mucosa is redder than normal and covered with a patchy or gray-white exudate, which can be wiped off and bleeds easily (Plate 9). The earliest changes of esophagitis are increased vascularity, 1-2cm above the esophageal gastric junction. As reflux of acid continues, small superficial ulcerations are seen with friability. Ulcerations have been seen involving the upper one third of the esophagus in our alcoholic patients who had severe vomiting (Plate 10). If the process progresses to a more advanced stage, with repeated ulcerations and healing, scar tissue formation may lead to irreversible cicatricial stricture of the lower esophagus. In esophageal stenosis, esophagoscopy reveals a smooth conical narrowing with varying degrees of inflammation depending on the stage of the disease (Plate 11). Visualization beyond the stenotic area is frequently difficult but biopsy may be obtained distally with care and expertise to ascertain whether the process is inflammatory or neoplastic. With fiberoptic instruments, biopsy forceps and special brushes can be advanced through the stricture to obtain gross tissue or cytological specimen. In our patient population, with severe esophagitis, we have been repeatedly disappointed as to the discernible endoscopic improvement after medical therapy even though symptomatic relief may have occurred.

REFERENCES

1. Boros, E.: Esophagoscopy by means of a flexible instrument: A new esophagogastroscope. *Gastroenterology*, 8:427, 1947.
2. Hufford, A. R.: Flexi-rigid, optical esophagoscope. *Gastroenterology*, 12:779, 1949.
3. Katz, D.: Presented at the American Society of Gastrointestinal Endoscopy Meeting, Chicago, Illinois, 1966.
4. LoPresti, P. A., and Hilmi, A.: Clinical experience with a new foroblique fiberoptic esophagoscope. *Am J Dig Dis*, (n.s.) 9:10:690, 1964.
5. LoPresti, P. A., Cifarelli, P. S., Dixit, N., and Kasinathan, M.: A new fiberoptic esophagogastroscope. *Am J Dig Dis*, (n.s.) *16*:1:31, January 1971.
6. Morrissey, J. F., Koizumi, H., Sultari, M. N., and Rockman, S. E.: Clinical use of the Olympus fiberesophagoscope. *Gastrointest Endosc*, 16:207, 1970.
7. Ludwig, R. N., and Sullivan, B. H.: Esophagoscopy and gastroscopy with a single instrument. Experience with a fiberoptic esophagogastroscope. *Gastrointest Endosc*, 17:173, May 1971.
8. American Cystoscope Makers, Inc., Pelham Manor, New York; Olympus Optical Co., Ltd., Tokyo, Japan; Machida Endoscope Co., Ltd., Tokyo, Japan.
9. Katz, D.: Morbidity and mortality in standard and flexible gastrointestinal endoscopy. *Gastrointest Endosc*, p. 134, May 1968.
10. Brick, I. B., and Palmer, E. D.: Comparison of esophagoscopic and roentgenologic diagnosis of esophageal varices in cirrhosis of the liver. *Am J Roentgenol*, 73:387, 1955.
11. Conn, H. O., Mitchell, J. R., and Brodoff, M. G.: A comparison of the radiologic and endoscopic diagnosis of esophageal varices. *N Engl J Med*, 265:160, July 1961.

12. DaGradi, A. E., Stempien, S. J., and Owens, L. K.: Bleeding esophagogastric varices. *Arch Surg, 92:*944, June 1966.
13. Palmer, E. D., and Brick, I. B.: Correlation between the severity of esophageal varices and portal cirrhosis and their propensity toward hemorrhage. *Gastroenterology, 30:*85, 1956.
14. Siegel, C. L., and Hendrix, T. R.: Esophageal motor abnormalities induced by acid perfusion in patients with heartburn. *J Clin Invest, 42:*5:686, 1963.
15. Ismail-Beigi, F., Horton, P., and Pope, C.: Histologica consequences of gastroesophageal reflux in man. *Gastroenterology, 58:*2, 1963.
16. Peters, P.: The pathology of severe digestive esophagitis. *Thorax, 10:*269, 1955.
17. Sandry, R. J.: The pathology of chronic esophagitis. *Gut, 3:*189, 1962.

CHAPTER 9

HIATUS HERNIA, STRICTURES, BARRETT'S SYNDROME, TECHNIC OF STRICTURE DILATATION

Raymond B. Johnson and William M. Lukash*

Introduction
Hiatus Hernia
Corrosive Esophagitis and Dilatation of Benicn Stricture
Barrett's Ulcer
Dilatation of Inoperable Carcinomatous Strictures

INTRODUCTION

THE ROLE OF GASTROINTESTINAL ENDOSCOPY has assumed ever-increasing importance in the evaluation of the numerous varieties of esophageal and gastric disorders. With the constant effort displayed in the manufacture of better and safer instruments, upper gastrointestinal endoscopy has become a part of the *routine* investigation of the gastroenterological patient.

Adequate study of the patient who presents with symptoms of esophageal disease—dysphagia, regurgitation, pyrosis and pain—would certainly be incomplete without the valuable and essential information afforded by endoscopy. We would like to discuss the endoscopic findings in certain of the more common esophageal disorders which are well known to physician and surgeon alike. To be included are hiatus hernia and stricture secondary to reflux esophagitis as well as the strictures associated with caustic ingestion, Barrett's ulceration and malignancy. In addition to the findings noted at endoscopy, the techniques of dilatation of these strictures will be presented.

* We acknowledge the cooperation and assistance of the U.S. Naval Hospital at Bethesda, Maryland. The opinions or assertions contained herein do not necessarily reflect the views of the Bureau of Medicine and Surgery of the Navy Department or the Naval Service at large.

HIATUS HERNIA

The entity of hiatus hernia constitutes one of the most common problems seen by the gastroenterologist. At the present time, there is significant controversy regarding the mechanism in reflux peptic esophagitis. More recent views expressed by Cohen and Harris[1] suggest that more important in symptomatic reflux is the competence of the gastroesophageal sphincter rather than the presence of a hernia itself. Nevertheless, in view of the improved clinical course in many patients following surgical repair of hiatus hernia, the identification of this lesion still seems of importance.

Dependence upon the radiological demonstration of a hiatus hernia may leave the clinician faltering for a definitive diagnosis in a case with symptoms strongly suggestive of this problem. In our experience 40 to 50 per cent of those patients undergoing radiographic examination of the upper gastrointestinal tract will demonstrate hiatus hernias. With the adjunct of endoscopy, however, 70 to 80 per cent of patients will be shown to have hernias, though obviously all are not symptomatic.

In the endoscopic evaluation of a hernia the most important anatomic landmark is the location of the esophagogastric junction where squamous and columnar mucosa join at the Z-Z line and where the pale pink mucosal color of the esophagus contrasts with the reddish-orange color of the stomach (Fig. 9-1). The esophagoscopist often encounters an area of relative narrowing a few centimeters proximal to the esophagogastric junction and the typical hernia with a sac showing characteristic gastric rugae can be noted above the diaphragmatic hiatus. In the more subtle cases, however, the only diagnostic feature is a definite upward movement of the *esophagogastric junction* proximally above the hiatal narrowing with insufflation of air into the lower esophagus. Another helpful maneuver is to have the patient sniff while observing the distal esophagus, watching for similar findings.

Although identification of the hernia is important, a more significant factor is the determination of the presence or absence of reflux esophagitis. The characteristic findings in this entity are presented elsewhere in this text.

Of those patients having persistent symptoms from hiatus hernia, 10 per cent will develop reflux esophagitis. Of these subsequent scarring will result in the ultimate complication of stricture formation in 2 to 3 per cent. Esophagoscopy in these patients will reveal the smooth conical narrowing almost always indicative of benign stricture. There is a tendency for the narrowed lumen to be centrally located. The esophageal lumen may be compromised to varying degrees and the strictures may be soft or very fibrotic (hard). Strictures resulting from reflux esophagitis are usual-

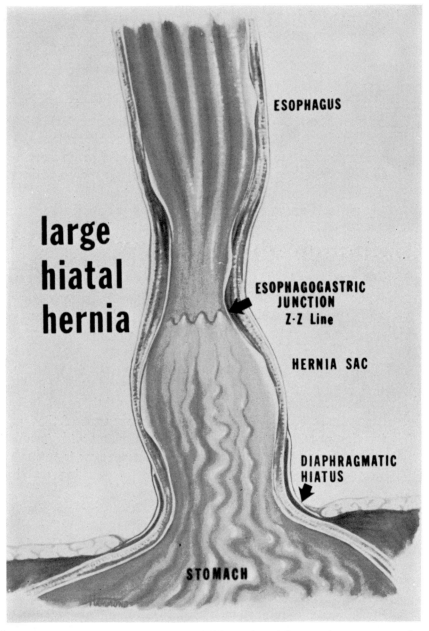

Figure 9-1. Diagrammatic representation of large hiatal hernia showing mucosal color change at Z-Z line.

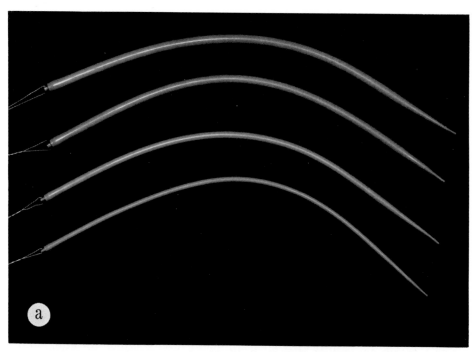

Figure 9-2a. Maloney type mercury-filled tapered bougies showing graduation of sizes.

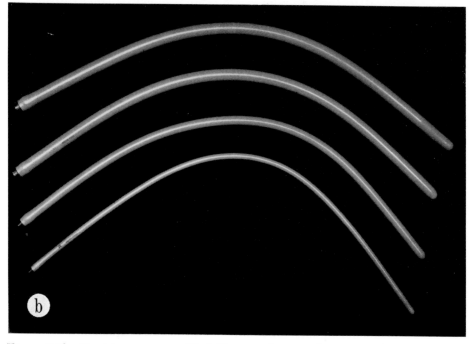

Figure 9-2b. Hurst-type mercury-filled blunt-tip bougies showing graduation of sizes.

ly short in length and involve the terminal segment of the esophagus. Varying degrees of superficial esophagitis will be found at the point of stenosis and proximally, depending on the stage of the problem. Generally, in the hard stricture the overlying proximal mucosa is effaced and the fibrotic response results in a white glistening endoscopic appearance.

Medical management of esophageal strictures secondary to hiatus hernia is accomplished by esophageal bougienage utilizing the mercury-filled Maloney tapered (Fig. 9-2a) or Hurst blunt dilators (Fig. 9-2b). With graduated sizes from 12 to 60 French, 40 French (12mm) usually proves adequate for symptomatic relief. With the patient in the sitting position, the appropriate bougie is introduced through the mouth and passed back and forth through the constricted area two or three times, with larger dilators used as necessary. The frequency and duration of dilatations are dictated by the patient's symptomatic response and may vary from twice weekly to four times yearly for a period of several months to several years.

CORROSIVE ESOPHAGITIS AND DILATATION OF BENIGN STRICTURE

One of the true tests of the skill and care of the esophagoscopist is the examination of the esophagus following the ingestion of a caustic agent. Because of the possibility that such an agent may produce an edematous, necrotic, friable organ, esophageal perforation becomes more than a casual consideration to the endoscopist. And yet, fear of this threatening complication must not deter the examiner from utilizing the only means of determining the presence and extent of esophageal injury. It has been previously well documented that the presence or absence of oral or pharyngeal burns in no way reflects the state of the esophagus subsequent to corrosive ingestion.

The extent of injury to the esophagus covers a wide spectrum. The earliest change is the transitory appearance of hyperemia and passive congestion progressing rapidly to diffuse mucosal edema. Within a few hours, with the concomitant presence of edema and reflex spasm initiated by the corrosive agent, the lumen may be completely occluded. The surface then undergoes a destructive necrosis with the rapid development of erosions and ulcerations and copious amounts of purulent exudate. At twenty-four hours the superficial necrotic layers become detached from the underlying mucosa and slough as a gray-brown membrane in small shreds or as a cast of the esophagus. At this point the organ takes on a violaceous appearance to its surface with ulcerations of various depths and numerous branching small blood vessels.

Edema begins to subside after the third day, though the ulcers continue to enlarge with further sloughing. Destruction comes to an end in about five days, and during the second week, the appearance is dominated by soft granulations. Although active destruction has ceased by the end of the first week, the persistence of acute inflammatory changes in the involved areas produces maximal susceptibility to perforation during the second week. During the third through sixth weeks the esophagus reveals progression of fibrous stricture formation.[2, 3]

If there were one word which would best characterize successful management of caustic injury to the esophagus, it would be prevention—prevention of stricture formation. Yarington[4] has established a simple classification of esophageal burns according to the findings at esophagoscopy, as shown in Table 9-I.

As can be noted, this classification nicely encompasses those changes discussed previously. Most important, however, is that it helps to establish a rational program of therapy. In the superficial burns of the non-circumferential type there is little chance of stricture formation as the muscularis is not involved. With all other types of injury, however, the possibility of ultimate stricture development must be considered as a possible real outcome. In these instances, serial esophagoscopy and dilatation may become necessary.

Although there is little question of the significant role played by the institution of steroids and antibiotics in the reduction of stricture formation, we are of the opinion that these modalities have not replaced the need for esophageal dilatation. Thus, following initial neutralization of the caustic agent, supportive therapy, and institution of antibiotics and steroids, we believe in early esophagoscopy within the first 48 hours, followed by daily dilatations with Maloney or Hurst dilators for four weeks, to prevent the reactive fibrotic changes which may lead to stricture formation.

TABLE 9-I

CLASSIFICATION OF ESOPHAGEAL BURNS ACCORDING TO THE FINDINGS AT ESOPHAGOSCOPY*

Type	Finding
Superficial	Hyperemia, patchy areas of minimal exudate, no bleeding or circumferential burns, and edema
Trans-mucosal	All of the above plus bleeding, erosion of mucosa, exudate and pseudomembrane formation, granulation tissue, and frank ulceration
Full-thickness (First degree)	All of the above plus obstruction of the lumen with inflammatory reaction, lack of peristalsis, loss of muscular tone, persistent narrowing, and failure of mucosal regeneration
Full-thickness (Second degree)	All of the above with mediastinitis and/or perforation

* From Yarington, et al.: *Ann Otol,* 73:1130, 1964.

In the more common case seen by the gastroenterologist the patient has already developed a stricture (Plate 12). In this type of patient we prefer to use the Eder-Peustow dilators because of their greater effectiveness in dilating a chronically scarred area.

With the patient previously premedicated (meperidine, 100mg; pento-barbital, 100mg; and atropine sulfate, 0.4mg intramuscularly), and following a 1 per cent tetracaine hydrochloride oral gargle, a piano wire guide is introduced with the patient in the sitting position. Under fluoroscopic control and with the patient now in a standing position, the wire guide is passed through the stricture into the stomach. This may also be accomplished under esophagoscopic control. With the wire carefully held in place, a metal olive with a diameter smaller than that of the strictured area is then placed on a spiral wand and subsequently passed over the guide wire through the area of stricture. Olives of increasing diameter are then passed until distinct, firm resistance is met or until blood appears on the olive. Both the spiral wire wand with olive and the piano wire guide are then removed. Although dilatations in caustic stricture may be a life-time necessity, a static esophageal lumen usually will be obtained in the first six months.

CASE HISTORY

On July 1, 1968, a twenty-one-year-old man ingested a lye mixture which was mistaken as a pudding. He experienced immediate oral burning, retched and vomited. He sought medical attention that evening but was given only symptomatic treatment for the oral burns. The following day he developed acute dysphagia which cleared over the next 48 hours, when both he and the attending physician felt that he was showing significant improvement. However, two weeks later he returned with significant dysphagia for all solid foods. A barium swallow was obtained and is shown in Figure 9-3. He was subsequently referred to us for further evaluation and management on July 20, 1968. Physical examination was unremarkable. At esophagoscopy a smooth tapering stricture was noted 26cm from the dental margin. The orifice was estimated to be 5 to 6mm in diameter, through which the esophagoscope could not be passed (Plate 13). The chronic esophagitis and narrowing are shown by endoscopic photography. A program of dilatation was initiated with Eder-Peustow dilators because of the fibrous nature of the stricture. Diet was pushed to tolerance. Antibiotics and steroids were not used at this time. Following ten days of daily dilatations, the esophagus admitted a 45 F metal olive. Esophagoscopy was repeated to exclude the presence of other esophageal damage. Dilatations were then continued twice weekly with Maloney dilators, graduating to a 50 F dilator. This program was continued for three weeks. Subsequently, he required three additional dilatations at monthly intervals and reached a static esophageal lumen of 50 F at five months from his initial ingestion. He remains asymptomatic three and a half years after the episode and barium swallow reveals a normal esophagus.

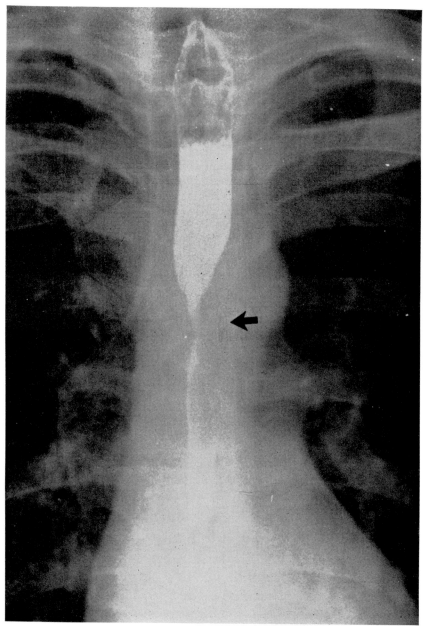

Figure 9-3. X-ray of the esophagus showing stricture in middle third.

BARRETT'S ULCER

Barrett's esophagus, an acquired or congenital disorder, is characterized by the presence of gastric-like columnar epithelium in the lower one third to one half of the esophagus. This type of epithelium replaces the usual

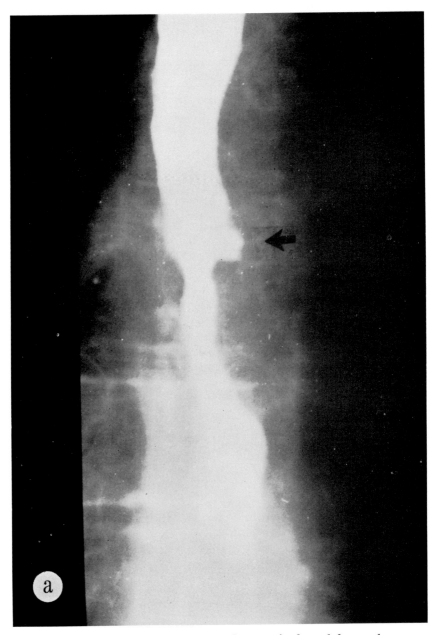

Figure 9-4a. Esophagram of patient with Barrett's ulcer of the esophagus.

squamous epithelium and may contain mucous glands akin to the gastric cardia or, on other occasions, may contain parietal and chief cells.

Because of its resemblance to gastric epithelium, this esophageal columnar epithelium is commonly the site of true peptic ulcer—the so-called Barrett's ulcer (Fig. 9-4a). The ulcer crater will assume the characteristics of a typical gastric ulcer with a sharp, punched-out appearance as opposed to the shallow less discrete ulcerations seen in the squamous-lined esophagus.

The symptom-complex is variable, depending upon the severity and duration of the disease. Generally, however, symptoms will include pain,

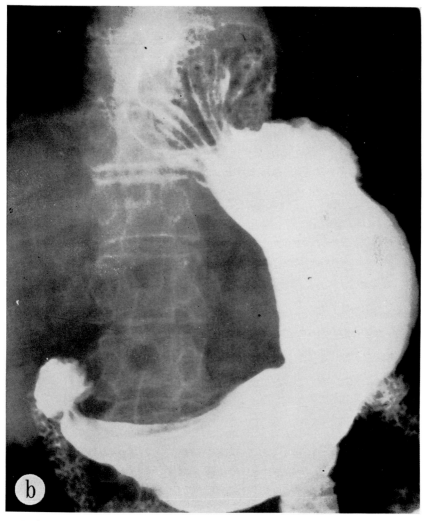

Figure 9-4b. Gastric x-ray of patient with Barrett's ulcer showing co-existing hiatus hernia.

dysphagia, or hematemesis. Pyrosis, indistinguishable from that of peptic esophagitis and hiatus hernia may also constitute a chronic complaint. Figure 9-4b shows the associated large hiatus hernia in the same patient with Barrett's ulcer.

When the ulcer is active, pain and dysphagia may be attributed to associated lower esophageal spasm with subsidence of these symptoms as the ulcer heals. With repeated ulceration, healing and formation of scar tissue at the site, however, a stenosis marked by persistent dysphagia may result. This late symptom may actually be the inciting factor for which the patient seeks medical assistance and, indeed, it is then when the radiographic picture is most typical. A stricture high in the esophagus and distant from the esophagogastric junction, followed by a segment of normal esophagus and then by a hiatus hernia is almost pathognomonic of this condition.

Endoscopically, such a stricture appears as the characteristic smooth, tapered benign stricture with varying degrees of esophagitis. The ulcer may or may not be seen, depending, of course, on the presence or absence of activity at the time. It is essential that biopsies be obtained above, at and below the site of the stricture, searching for the presence of the typical columnar epithelium and helping to exclude the presence of a scirrhous or ulcerative carcinoma. In this latter differentiation, esophageal exfoliative cytology also lends further credence to the definitive nature of the lesion.

Treatment of esophageal stricture secondary to Barrett's ulceration again enlists the aid of dilatation. Satisfactory results can be obtained by utilizing the Maloney, Hurst or Eder-Peustow dilators depending upon the degree of fibrous tissue at the site of the stricture. Dilatation serves the two-fold purpose of relieving dysphagia and facilitating more adequate examination of the esophagus distal to the site of stricture. In addition to this primary form of treatment, dietary alterations and antacid therapy should be utilized to further prevent recurrence of the inciting cause.

DILATATION OF INOPERABLE CARCINOMATOUS STRICTURES

Endoscopic features of malignant esophageal lesions have been discussed elsewhere in the text (see Chapter 11). It should be stressed that whether the lesion is polypoid, fungating, ulcerative or infiltrating, impingement upon the esophageal lumen will invariably lead to dysphagia. In those patients in whom cure can obviously not be achieved, the morbidity and mortality of extensive surgery is usually not justified. These are instances where fistula formation may occur into the bronchi complicating the presence of stricture. This is especially true when the malignancy involves the area of the esophagus as it crosses the left bronchus. In these cases major surgery must sometimes be employed. Prosthetic tubes in these cases have been used with questionable success. Transplants using a segment of bowel is a formidable and rarely successful alternative to careful and selective dilatation and irradiation in malignant disease of the esophagus. In our experience, the use of Maloney, Hurst or Eder-Peustow dilators may relieve symptoms and allow the patient to improve his nutritional status. This treatment on occasions may even better prepare the patient for other forms of more definitive management.

REFERENCES

1. Cohen, S., and Harris, L. D.: Does hiatus hernia affect competence of the gastro-esophageal sphincter? *N Eng J Med, 284*:1053-1056, 1971.
2. Palmer, E. D.: *The Esophagus and Its Diseases.* New York, Hoeber, 1952, pp. 288-305.
3. Terracol, J., and Sweet, R. H.: *Diseases of the Esophagus.* Philadelphia, Saunders, 1958, pp. 358-375.
4. Yarington, C. T., Bales, G. A., and Frazer, J. P.: A study of the management of caustic esophageal trauma. *Ann Otol, 73*:1130-1135, 1964.

CHAPTER 10

DIFFUSE SPASM, ACHALASIA, VIGOROUS ACHALASIA: DIAGNOSIS AND MANAGEMENT

ARTHUR M. OLSEN

DIFFUSE SPASM

Introductory Statement

DIFFUSE SPASM OF the esophagus is physiologically different from achalasia. Diffuse spasm is readily diagnosed by use of manometric studies. Diffuse spasm and early achalasia have much in common, and this led to considerable confusion as to the true clinical findings in achalasia. As early as 1921, Plummer and Vinson[1] recognized that highly nervous patients with pain as their principal manifestation should be grouped separately. However, most early authors failed to differentiate between achalasia and diffuse spasm.

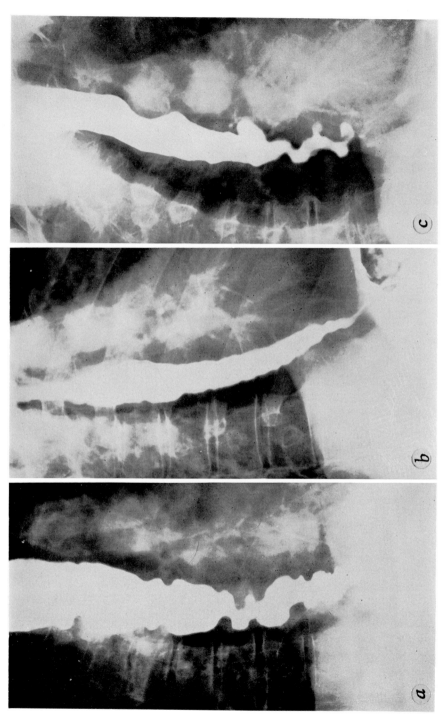

Figure 10-1. Diffuse spasm of esophagus. a) diffuse irregular spasm. b) diffuse constant narrowing. c) pseudodiverticulosis.[6] (By permission of The C. V. Mosby Company.)

Moersch and Camp[2] reported the syndrome of diffuse spasm in 1934 and differentiated this disorder from achalasia. They described roentgenographic findings that were different from the classic findings of achalasia and related these to the clinical findings. Although diffuse spasm may show considerable variation roentgenographically, there are three principal types (Figs. 10-1a, b and c).

Diagnosis

Patients with diffuse spasm tend to be highly nervous and usually have pain as the predominant symptom. Obstructive symptoms are not a constant feature of diffuse spasm. Regurgitation rarely occurs in diffuse spasm, and, when it does, secretions are not retained in the esophagus.

The manometric signs of diffuse spasm are characteristic (Fig. 10-2).[3]

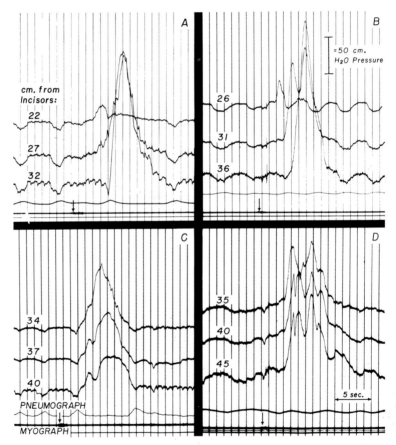

Figure 10-2. Deglutitive pressures from four patients with diffuse spasm, showing variations of abnormal response. Note the simultaneous peaks in each tracing and the simultaneous onset of deglutitive response in *C* and *D*. The abnormally high pressures, the repetitive contractions and their prolonged duration are all apparent.[3] (By permission of The Williams and Wilkins Company.)

Simultaneous and repetitive contractions occur in the smooth muscle portion of the esophagus, and the amplitude of these contractions is invariably greater than normal. Peristalsis is rarely seen in diffuse spasm except in the striated muscle portion of the organ. The amplitude and duration of the resting pressures at both the upper and lower sphincters are normal. The lower sphincter relaxes normally with swallowing. Usually the reaction to the methacholine test is negative in diffuse spasm.

Diffuse spasm must be differentiated from early achalasia and from the syndrome of vigorous achalasia. The distinction is readily made by manometric techniques. There is rarely any difficulty in distinguishing between diffuse spasm and scleroderma. The roentgenographic findings often resemble multiple diverticula of the esophagus (Fig. 10-1c), and diffuse spasm has been designated sometimes as pseudodiverticulosis. Patients who have been successfully treated for achalasia may have roentgenographic findings that are strongly suggestive of diffuse spasm, especially of diffuse, irregular spasm (Fig. 10-1a). Likewise, the tertiary contractions seen in older people commonly called "curling of the esophagus" may produce roentgenographic findings that greatly resemble those of diffuse spasm.

The clinical findings in diffuse spasm may be imitated by the hypertensive sphincter described by Code and his colleagues.[4] The hypertensive sphincter may produce pain similar to that in achalasia; the pain tends to occur most frequently during swallowing. The hypertensive sphincter may be associated with diffuse spasm, and hiatal hernia is occasionally seen with diffuse spasm.

Roentgenographic findings may be normal in some patients with diffuse spasm. Furthermore, some patients with this disorder may have pain totally unrelated to swallowing or any other esophageal symptoms. At times, the pain of diffuse spasm may strongly resemble the pain of coronary artery disease, and because both anginal pain and esophageal pain may be relieved by sublingual use of nitroglycerin, the differentiation is even more difficult. Motility studies, of course, are extremely helpful in differentiating pain of diffuse spasm from pain of cardiac origin. In fact, chest pain is one of the principal reasons for patients being referred to our esophageal motility laboratory.

The diagnosis of diffuse spasm may be suspected from the clinical history and confirmed by the use of roentgen examination and esophageal motility studies. Evidence of extensive thickening of the wall of the esophagus has been found at roentgen examination in some patients with diffuse spasm and is occasionally seen at surgery.[5] The final diagnosis is made after manometric study has been done. Esophagoscopy is frequently done in diffuse spasm to exclude the possibility of associated esophagitis or the unlikely possibility of carcinoma of the esophagus or the cardia.

Treatment

Treatment is difficult because patients with diffuse spasm usually are nervous and often emotionally unstable. The primary problem is psychiatric. Sedatives and tranquilizers, therefore, are usually tried. The pain of esophageal spasm may be relieved by the sublingual use of nitroglycerin. Nitrites in various forms have been tried, with various degrees of success. Generally, the medical management of diffuse spasm has been unsatisfactory.

Esophagoscopy is frequently performed in diffuse spasm, and occasionally the passage of the esophagoscope seems to have some benefit. The passage of bougies into the stomach may be of greater value, especially if the procedure is carried out without anesthesia. Bougies as large as 50 F or 60 F have been used, and at times the results have been striking. Generally, however, endoscopic methods of treating diffuse spasm have not been successful.

The surgeon usually is reluctant to operate in these cases because of the patient's nervousness and emotional instability and because the results of surgical treatment are much less predictable than they are in achalasia. Nevertheless, the surgical treatment of this disorder has been more rewarding than any other approach to the problem. However, long myotomy has been used with considerable success.[5] About two thirds of the patients have favorable results after such a surgical procedure. Unfortunately, the remaining one third not only will fail to benefit from the procedure but also may have their symptoms aggravated, especially if they have signs of gastric reflux.

ACHALASIA

Introductory Statement

Although not a common disorder, achalasia of the esophagus is the most frequent of the neuromuscular disturbances of the esophagus. The condition was first described by Willis[7] in 1674, and his description of the disorder is one of the classics of medical history. Most of the early reports described the condition as a dilatation or enlargement of the esophagus. Zenker and Ziemssen[8] in 1878 referred to the condition as simple ectasia. Mikulicz[9] was the first to recognize a nonorganic obstruction at the esophagogastric junction, and he introduced the term "cardiospasm." Plummer[10] likewise used the term "cardiospasm." For many years, this remained the most common designation for the disorder. Various other terms were used to describe the condition, such as phrenospasm, preventriculosis, mega-esophagus, and fibrosis of the terminal esophagus, depending on the individual's concept of the nature of the disorder.

Although the term "achalasia" was first used by Hertz,[11] Einhorn[12] in 1888 was the first to suggest that failure of relaxation of the lower sphincter was the significant disorder. The term "achalasia" is taken from the Greek and may be translated as "lack of relaxation." Among the various designations for this disorder, achalasia comes closest to describing the condition. Even so, this term is not completely satisfactory, as modern-day manometric techniques with some confirmative endoscopic findings have shown that achalasia is, in truth, a motor failure of the esophagus, accompanied by a failure of the lower sphincter to relax.

Etiology and Pathogenesis

Although achalasia has been attributed to many factors, the cause is still in doubt. Although Chagas' disease produces findings that are identical to achalasia, there is little reason to believe that the achalasia seen in North America is in any way related to trypanosome infection. Chagas' disease not only produces mega-esophagus but also may cause an enlargement of the colon, the ureters, and other viscera. Some authorities have attributed achalasia to trauma, diaphragmatic disease, and particularly psychic disorders. Winkelstein[13] referred to 16 different theories of cardiospasm or achalasia, and he described eight cases in which he believed that the vegetative nervous system was at fault. Although the role of psychosomatic factors in any physical disorder is difficult to assess, one can be reasonably sure that achalasia is not primarily a psychic disturbance.

Degeneration of Auerbach's plexus has long been recognized as a rather constant finding in achalasia. More recently, Cassella and his associates[14] have found abnormalities in the vagus nerve and particularly in the dorsal motor nucleus of the vagus nerve. The manometric studies done by Kronecker and Meltzer[15] in 1883 first suggested that neuromuscular paralysis of the esophagus should be the primary disorder in achalasia. Refined manometric studies in more recent years have demonstrated both the neuromuscular failure and the absence of relaxation at the sphincter. However, there are still no clues as to the basic cause of the condition.

Symptoms and Clinical Course

The early symptoms of achalasia are likely to be intermittent. Most commonly, the patient has a periodic sticking of food in the substernal or subxiphoid region. Occasionally, the patient points to the cricoid region as the site of his obstruction. In the early stages, liquids may cause as much trouble as solid food. Cold food or fluid often tends to provoke the obstructive symptoms.

Pain is not a frequent symptom of achalasia and occurs in less than one third of all patients. Pain is likely to be present in the early stages of the disease and may be either substernal or epigastric. At times it is referred to the neck or to the back, and is particularly likely to be precipitated by drinking cold liquids.

As the disease progresses, regurgitation develops and is almost a constant feature in the more advanced condition. Regurgitation may occur immediately after eating. Some patients may soil their pillows during sleep. Generally, the material that is regurgitated is not sour and consists of typical glairy or stringy esophageal mucus. In advanced cases, the regurgitant material contains recently ingested food. Hemorrhage is uncommon in achalasia, and when it occurs, it should alert the physician to the possibility of a coexisting neoplasm. However, bleeding may result from long-standing retention of food associated with esophagitis. Loss of weight and vitamin deficiency are not infrequent. The pulmonary complications of achalasia are common, especially in the more advanced stages of the disease. Occasionally, the pulmonary symptoms will call attention to the disorder before the patient actually complains of dysphagia. The respiratory symptoms may range from asthmatic attacks to chronic cough and pulmonary suppuration.

The clinical course of achalasia can be divided into three stages. Roentgenologically and endoscopically these are mild dilatation of the esophagus (Fig. 10-3a), diffuse dilatation of the organ (Fig. 10-3b), and extensive enlargement with tortuosity and retention (Fig. 10-3c). Clinically, during

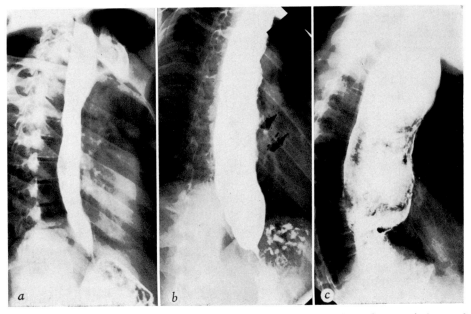

Figure 10-3. Appearance of three stages of achalasia. a) Mild. b) Moderate. c) Severe.[6] (By permission of The C. V. Mosby Company.)

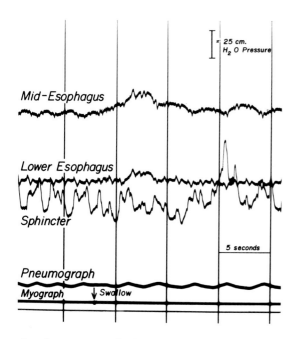

Figure 10-4. Responses to deglutition in a patient with achalasia.[19] (By permission of The C. V. Mosby Company.)

the first stage, before the esophagus has undergone much enlargement, there may be obstruction but no regurgitation. During the second stage, when there is diffuse enlargement, immediate regurgitation is common. During the third stage, when the esophagus is dilated and tortuous, regurgitation is likely to be delayed. There may also be some correlation between the stage and the motility. Although roentgenographic evidence of painless contractions is seen in the early stage of the disorder, activity virtually ceases as the esophagus becomes more dilated. Manometric studies (Fig. 10-4) likewise reveal a profound change in the motor activity of the esophagus. If methacholine is injected, the esophagus may contract vigorously and painfully. Although peristalsis is rare, simultaneous contractions are more likely in the early stages of the disorder than later on when the organ is completely atonic.

Diagnosis

The diagnosis of achalasia may usually be suspected from the history and verified by the use of roentgen examination. Esophagoscopy is useful in excluding other causes of esophageal obstruction. Esophagoscopy is particularly indicated if dysphagia has been present only a short time and if there is the likelihood of carcinoma of the terminal esophagus or upper stomach. Esophagoscopy should be performed if there has been bleeding. Although the chance of carcinoma developing in a patient with advanced achalasia is not great, this possibility should be kept in mind and may make esophagoscopy desirable. At esophagoscopy, one usually finds a dilated, atonic esophagus. However, in the early stages, esophagoscopy may reveal no abnormality, and the esophagoscope will pass into the stomach without any obvious evidence of obstruction. As the esophagus dilates, retained secretions are usually found, and in chronic disease, the esophageal mucous membrane is often inflamed. At the cardia, a mucosal rosette may be seen. In any patient who has had repeated dilatation, esophagoscopy is desirable in order to exclude the possibility of a stricture at the esophagogastric junction. However, more information can be obtained by passage of a bougie over a previously swallowed thread. In typical achalasia, a characteristic but temporary resistance is encountered as a bougie is passed into the stomach, a sign that is virtually diagnostic to the experienced endoscopist. Likewise, passage of a bougie quickly identifies an organic obstruction or a tumor. In fact, the flexible spiral that precedes the sound may pick up material which is suitable for cytologic diagnosis and thus identify a malignant lesion located below the esophagogastric junction and one which could not be detected at esophagoscopy.

As previously indicated, esophagoscopy has its limitations in advanced achalasia. There is so much retained food and often so much tortuosity that esophagoscopy is virtually useless. Even the flexible fiberesophagoscope may have limited value in the sigmoid type of esophagus, as it is very difficult to maintain a clear field of vision. In this situation, lavage with large quantities of normal saline using an Ewald type rubber tube should precede esophagoscopy.

Differential Diagnosis

In the early stages of achalasia, it may be difficult to differentiate achalasia from diffuse spasm. Reference already has been made to the importance of differentiating achalasia from carcinoma of the cardia. Carcinoma may occur in conjunction with achalasia, especially in the advanced stages of the disease. Unless located near either sphincter, the associated carcinoma may escape detection because of the dilatation of the esophagus. The patient will not complain of any change in his obstructive symptoms, and furthermore the radiologist may mistake a tumor for retained food.

At times, benign tumors may produce roentgenographic findings that are almost indistinguishable from those of achalasia. Unless the esophagoscopist already suspects a benign tumor, the lesion may be missed at esophagoscopy because the mucosa covering the lesion is intact.

Pulsion diverticula of the hypopharynx should rarely cause any difficulty in diagnosis. However, pulsion diverticula of the lower esophagus may occur in association with achalasia, and motility studies should be done in all patients with epiphrenic diverticula before any surgical procedure is considered. All too often the pulsion diverticulum of the lower esophagus is an incidental finding when the real problem is achalasia.

Hiatal hernia should rarely cause any problem in differential diagnosis. The symptoms and roentgenographic and endoscopic findings in sliding hiatal hernia usually differentiate the two conditions. The same patient seldom has both hiatal hernia and achalasia.

The postvagotomy syndrome may closely resemble achalasia. In most postvagotomy patients in whom dysphagia develops, the symptoms disappear spontaneously within 3 months.

Scleroderma of the esophagus is another condition that may resemble achalasia. Usually the dermatologic manifestations of this disease are so obvious that there is no problem in differential diagnosis. Occasionally, the typical findings of scleroderma of the esophagus may be found in patients who have Raynaud's syndrome only.

Treatment
Nonsurgical

Obviously, the objective of therapy in achalasia is to relieve the obstructive symptoms. Unfortunately, nothing can be done about the primary motor disturbance in the esophagus. Attention, therefore, must be directed to means of weakening the lower esophageal sphincter. This must be accomplished without permitting reflux of gastric secretions. If the sphincter is destroyed, esophagitis, ulceration, and cicatricial changes may lead to shortening of the esophagus and stricture.

In general, medications of any kind are of little value in the treatment of achalasia. Nitrites and nitroglycerin conceivably may be useful in the very early stages of achalasia but certainly are of no help when the disease is well established. There has been much discussion regarding psychiatric therapy of achalasia. However, if the diagnosis is accurate, psychiatric therapy is of no value in the management.

Achalasia may be treated successfully by either endoscopic or surgical means. To be truly effective, dilatations must be sufficiently forceful to tear the muscles involved in the esophagogastric sphincter.

Daily bougienage was the only method of treatment available until Russel[16] developed the first expanding dilator in 1898. Most instruments that have been developed for forceful dilatation of the cardia have used either air or water to expand a rubber-covered bag after it has been placed across the lower sphincter. However, Starck's expanding metal dilator[17] has also been used successfully for stretching the lower sphincter. It makes little difference which technique is applied provided the lower sphincter is adequately stretched under carefully controlled circumstances.

In my opinion, dilatations are most safely and effectively performed when the dilating instrument is passed over a previously swallowed thread. For many years our group has used the hydrostatic technic devised by Plummer[10, 18] (Fig. 10-5). Air is equally satisfactory for distending the dilator and has been used by many authorities. Although our group prefers passing instruments over a previously swallowed thread, others use mercury-weighted tubes to carry the dilator into the lower esophagus and across the cardia.

During the actual dilation, the amount of pressure must be carefully controlled. The patient can have much pain during the brief time that the sphincter is stretched. Overstretching the sphincter may result in mediastinitis. About 1 per cent of patients who have undergone successful dilation for achalasia can have rather severe reactions although, fortunately, not all will experience rupture of the esophagus. If a "split" occurs, it usually is just above the sphincter and on the left wall of the esophagus. Substernal pain and left pleuritic pain are the usual manifestations of rupture, along with a shock-like state. If there is definite evidence of esopha-

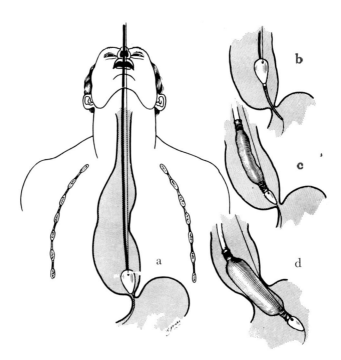

Figure 10-5. Method of performing dilatations. a) Passage of 41 F, olive-tipped bougie to stomach. b) Sound (50 or 60 F), guided by a flexible wire spiral, is passed into stomach. c) Hydrostatic dilator is passed to cardia. d) Distention of hydrostatic dilator across cardia. (By permission of The C. V. Mosby Company.)

geal perforation, immediate thoracotomy is indicated. Less severe reactions usually can be treated with antibiotics and supportive measures.

Our experience has been reviewed from time to time,[18] and we find that about 70 per cent of patients have been relieved of dysphagia for 5 years or more, when dilation has been adequate. Our group does not advocate repeated dilatations unless the initial treatment did not accomplish the objective. If the results of dilatation are temporary, we usually resort to surgery.

Surgical

The only surgical procedure that has stood the test of time is an esophagomyotomy of the Heller type. Manometric studies after successful Heller operations have demonstrated that the subhiatal portion of the sphincter retains its tone. Likewise, manometric studies after successful treatment by hydrostatic dilatation also show a zone of elevated pressure at the lower portion of the sphincter.

Our surgical results with esophagomyotomy have been successful inasmuch as 85 to 90 per cent of the patients who have undergone surgery for achalasia at the Mayo Clinic have had satisfactory or excellent results. Hence, we have been inclined to use the surgical method of treatment more frequently than we used to, and we resort to surgery if forceful dilatation has not been immediately successful. Also we have found that surgical treatment is indicated in most children with achalasia and should also be employed in patients who have associated hiatal hernia. Our experience has indicated that surgical treatment is likely to be unsuccessful in patients who have had repeated forceful dilatations of the cardia. Hence, my surgical colleagues prefer to perform esophagomyotomy as a primary procedure rather than resort to surgery after efforts at dilatation have failed.

SYNDROME OF VIGOROUS ACHALASIA

Introductory Remarks

Sometimes diffuse spasm is difficult to differentiate from early achalasia. Although the symptoms and even the roentgenologic findings may be confusing, results of esophageal motility studies usually clarify the situation. However, a few patients not only have clinical and roentgen features suggestive of both disorders but also have motility signs characteristic of both disorders. This syndrome was first described as "dyschalasia" by Moersch et al.[20] in 1957, and the term "dyschalasia" was also used by Beck et al.[21] in 1966. The condition, however, seems to be a variant of achalasia, and the term "vigorous achalasia" was introduced.[22] Sanderson and colleagues[23] reported a series of 72 patients who had vigorous achalasia.

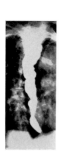

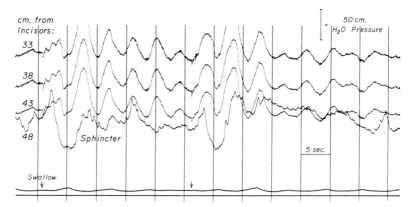

Figure 10-6. Vigorous achalasia. Powerful, simultaneous, repetitive contractions of diminishing amplitude occur in response to swallow. Relaxation of lower sphincter occurs, followed by premature contraction. Note barium swallow at left.[23] (By permission of American College of Chest Physicians.)

Diagnosis

Figure 10-6 illustrates the roentgenographic appearance and motility signs in a representative case of vigorous achalasia. Powerful, simultaneous, repetitive contractions of diminishing amplitude occur, followed by premature contractions. The roentgenographic findings can be mistaken for those of diffuse spasm. The differential diagnosis of achalasia, diffuse spasm, and vigorous achalasia is recorded in Table 10-I.

Kramer and his colleagues[24] have suggested that, in some patients, the diffuse spasm may progress to achalasia. This probably does not occur very often. However, the concept of the syndrome of vigorous achalasia suggests that a transition from diffuse spasm to achalasia is possible. Of the

TABLE 10-I

DIFFERENTIAL DIAGNOSIS OF ACHALASIA, DIFFUSE SPASM,
AND VIGOROUS ACHALASIA[*23]

Symptom or Sign	Incidence According to Diagnosis		
	Achalasia	Diffuse Spasm	Vigorous Achalasia
Pain	Uncommon	Almost always	Frequent
Obstruction	Always	Sometimes	Nearly always
Regurgitation	Common	Rare	Frequent
Retention	Frequent	Never	Frequent
Nervousness	Uncommon	Almost always	Occasional
Roentgenographic findings			
Diffuse dilatation	Common	Never	Occasional
Segmental spasm	Uncommon	Frequent	Common

* By permission of American College of Chest Physicians.

72 patients described by Sanderson et al.,[23] only 12 had no signs of relaxation of the lower sphincter in response to swallowing. In the remaining patients, the relaxation was likely to be poor. Methacholine tests were done in only 16 patients, and the test was positive in 13. Further observation of these patients should lend interesting information on the possible relationship of diffuse spasm and achalasia.

Treatment

Hydrostatic dilatation does not seem to be as successful in this group of patients as in classic achalasia. However, the Heller operation is very successful. Often the surgeon carries the myotomy somewhat higher on the esophagus than he would for classic achalasia. Our experience indicates that a modified Heller myotomy is the treatment of choice.[23]

REFERENCES

1. Plummer, H. S., and Vinson, P. P.: Cardiospasm: A report of 301 cases. *Med Clin North Am,* 5:355, 1921.
2. Moersch, H. J., and Camp, J. D.: Diffuse spasm of the lower part of the esophagus. *Ann Otol Rhinol Laryngol,* 43:1165, 1934.
3. Creamer, B., Donoghue, F. E., and Code, C. F.: Pattern of esophageal motility in diffuse spasm. *Gastroenterology,* 34:782, 1958.
4. Code, C. F., Schlegel, J. F., Kelley, M. L., Jr., Olsen, A. M., and Ellis, F. H., Jr.: Hypertensive gastroesophageal sphincter. *Proc Staff Meet Mayo Clin,* 35:391, 1960.
5. Ellis, F. H., Jr., Olsen, A. M., Schlegel, J. F., and Code, C. F.: Surgical treatment of esophageal hypermotility disturbances. *JAMA, 188*:862, 1964.
6. Olsen, A. M., Harrington, S. W., Moersch, H. J., and Andersen, H. A.: The treatment of cardiospasm: Analysis of a twelve-year experience. *J Thorac Cardiovasc Surg,* 22:164, 1951.
7. Willis, T.: *Pharmaceutice rationalis (sive diatriba de medicamentorum operationibus in humano corpore).* London, Hagae-Comitis, 1674.
8. Zenker, F. A., and Ziemssen, H.: Diseases of the oesophagus. In Ziemssen, H: *Cyclopaedia of the Practice of Medicine.* New York, William Wood and Company, 1878, vol. 8, p. 204.
9. Mikulicz, J. V.: Zur Pathologie und Therapie des Cardiospasmus. *Dtsch Med Wochenschr, 30*:17; 50, 1904.
10. Plummer, H. S.: Cardiospasm, with report of cases. *Minn State Med Assoc Northwestern Lancet, 26*:419, 1906.
11. Hertz, A. F.: Achalasia of the cardia. *Q J Med,* 8:300, 1915.
12. Einhorn, M.: A case of dysphagia with dilatation of the oesophagus. *Med Rec,* 34:751, 1888.
13. Winkelstein, A.: Psychogenic factors in cardiospasm. *Am J Surg, 12*:135, 1931.
14. Cassella, R. R., Brown, A. L., Jr., Sayre, G. P., and Ellis, F. H., Jr.: Achalasia of the esophagus: Pathologic and etiologic considerations. *Ann Surg, 160*:474, 1964.
15. Kronecker, H., and Meltzer, S.: Der Schluckmechanismus, seine Erregung und seine Hemmung. *Arch Anat Physiol, Suppl,* 1883, pp. 328-362.

16. Russel, J. C.: Diagnosis and treatment of spasmodic stricture of the oesophagus. *Br Med J, 1*:1450, 1898.
17. Starck, H.: Die Behandlung der spasmogenen Speiseröhrenerweiterung. *Munch Med Wochenschr, 71*:334, 1924.
18. Ellis, F. H., Jr., and Olsen, A. M.: *Achalasia of the Esophagus*. Philadelphia, Saunders, 1969.
19. Ellis, F. H., Jr., Code, C. F., and Olsen, A. M.: Long esophagomyotomy for diffuse spasm of the esophagus and hypertensive gastroesophageal sphincter. *Surgery, 48*:155, 1960.
20. Moersch, H. J., Code, C. F., and Olsen, A. M.: Dyschalasia of the esophagus. *Coll Papers Mayo Clin, 49*:19, 1957.
21. Beck, I. T., Hernandez, N. A., and Solymar, J.: Dyschalasia: A variant or early phase of achalasia? A review of motor disturbances in achalasia with reference to late relaxation of the lower esophageal sphincter. *Can Med Assoc J, 95*:941, 1966.
22. Olsen, A. M., and Creamer, B.: Studies of esophageal motility, with special reference to the differential diagnosis of diffuse spasm and achalasia (cardiospasm). *Thorax, 12*:279, 1957.
23. Sanderson, D. R., Ellis, F. H., Jr., Schlegel, J. F., and Olsen, A. M.: Syndrome of vigorous achalasia: Clinical and physiologic observations. *Chest, 52*:508, 1967.
24. Kramer, P., Harris, L. D., and Donaldson, R. M., Jr.: Transition from symptomatic diffuse spasm to cardiospasm. *Gut, 8*:115, 1967.

CHAPTER 11

MALIGNANT AND BENIGN TUMORS; DIVERTICULA, FISTULAS, POSTOPERATIVE LESIONS

Tadayoshi Takemoto and Mitsuo Endo

INTRODUCTORY STATEMENT

IN THIS CHAPTER, we will discuss malignant and benign tumors of the esophagus, diverticula, fistula, and postoperative esophageal lesions. Most of these subjects will be illustrated by case histories, and the emphasis will be on endoscopic pathology, correlated in most instances with the x-ray and postoperative findings.

177

MALIGNANT TUMORS
Cancer
Endoscopic Picture

Various classifications of esophageal cancer have been proposed since the introduction of the esophagoscope for diagnosis. This observation method has been improved upon recently by use of an indwelling telescope in the rigid esophagoscope, and the addition of the fiberscope.

Endoscopically, esophageal cancer may be divided into six types: tumor, ulcerative, tumor infiltrating, ulcerative infiltrating, stenotic, and superficial. In the tumor type a tumor mass protrudes into the esophageal lumen. The protrusion has an uneven surface and is reddish or is similar in color to the surrounding tissue. There are two subtypes: one has a smooth mucosal surface and the other has a surface covered by a thick, whitish coating. The ulcerative type consists of a mucosal ulceration that is localized. The margin of the ulcer may be smooth or may be elevated, sometimes forming a tumorous mass. Even when the margin is highly elevated the lesion may be classified in this group if the demarcation is clear. The tumor infiltrating and ulcerative infiltrating types differ from the first two types only by their infiltration into surrounding tissues. The stenotic type shows marked infiltration and narrowing, which makes endoscopic visualization of cancerous tissue impossible. The superficial type is that in which the cancerous invasion remains within the submucosal layer. Clinically, this type is the so-called early esophageal cancer.

The frequency of the various types is shown in Table 11-I. In the 714 cases of endoscopy performed, the ulcerative type and ulcerative infiltrating type constituted 85 per cent of the total.

Clinical Picture

Because of the ease with which radical resection may be accomplished in cancer of the superficial type, we are devoting much attention to the de-

TABLE 11-I

ENDOSCOPIC CLASSIFICATION OF ESOPHAGEAL CANCER
(714 CASES)

Type	*Cases*	*(%)*
Tumor	83	(12)
Ulcerative	372	(52)
Tumor infiltrating	6	(1)
Ulcerative infiltrating	283	(33)
Severe stenotic (nonvisible)	5	(1)
Superficial	10	(1)

tection of these cases. However, we have to date only thirteen cases, of which one is an example of multiple cancer. When we classified topographically our fourteen lesions in thirteen cases, we found one lesion of the cervical esophagus and thirteen lesions of the thoracic esophagus. Of thoracic esophageal lesions, one was in the upper esophagus, six in the middle esophagus, two involved both the middle and lower section and four the lower esophagus.

There were nine males and four females. As for the age distribution, five patients were in their fifties, seven in their sixties and one was 73 years old.

The chief complaints are often of an indefinite and mild nature. Initial symptoms are usually those of an advanced esophageal cancer. If dysphagia alone is considered, some of these small superficial lesions will escape detection. In our series, some patients had only right-sided chest pain as an initial symptom. One patient was asymptomatic and the lesion was detected only during his periodical health examination.

Endoscopically, the protruded types of lesions characteristically are well localized, smooth, nonstenotic, move with the mucosal fold and change form during contraction. In the depressed type with shallow erosion the demarcation from normal epithelium is clear; the erosion is reddish with a granular, uneven whitish coating which bleeds easily on contact. When the lesion covers a large area, differential diagnosis from esophagitis may be difficult and necessitate biopsy. In the depressed type which appears as an ulcer, the margin of ulcer will tend to be emphasized because of the cylindrical form of the esophagus. As a result, the tendency will be to diagnose a more extensive infiltrating lesion than is really present.

TABLE 11-II

SUPERFICIAL TYPE, EARLY ESOPHAGEAL CANCER

Endoscopic Classification	Authors' Cases		Cases in Japan	
Elevated				
Tumorous protruded (S-I)	7	(50%)	14	(58%)
Slightly elevated (S-II)	1	(7%)	5	(21%)
Flat (S-III)	0		0	
Excavated				
Slightly depressed (erosion type) (S-IV)	2	(15%)		
Excavated (ulcerative type) (S-V)	4	(28%)	5	(21%)

The superficial type of esophageal cancer may be divided, according to the endoscopic findings, into three basic types: the protruded type (further divided into tumorous and slightly elevated subtypes), the excavated type

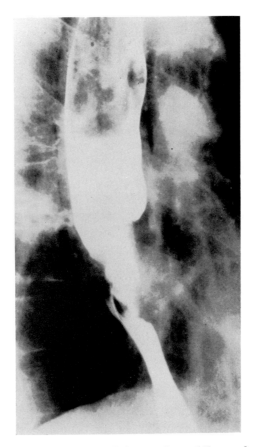

Figure 11-1. Large filling defect in the middle esophagus.

(divided into erosive and ulcerative subtypes), and the flat type. These are shown in Table 11-II.

When we apply this classification to our series of fourteen lesions we find seven cases of tumorous protruded type, one of slightly elevated type, two of depressed erosive type, four of ulcerative excavated type and none of flat type (Table 11-II).

A male patient, aged 65, was hospitalized because of dysphagia. X-ray examination showed a filling defect in the middle part of the esophagus (Fig. 11-1). Esophagofiberscopy disclosed an ulcerative infiltrating type of cancer involving almost the entire circumference (Plate 14).

A male patient, aged 64, was asymptomatic, X-rays showed a filling defect in the middle part of the esophagus (Fig. 11-2). Esophagofiberscopy disclosed a small protruded lesion (Plate 15). The surface of the lesion was reddish and uneven. Biopsy of the lesion revealed a cancerous structure and an operation was performed. In the resected specimen the tumor was 2.2 x 1.8dm in size (Fig. 11-3). The cancerous invasion was limited to the submucosal layer (Fig. 11-4).

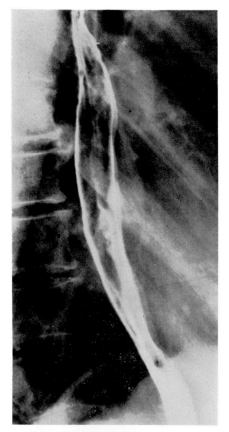

Figure 11-2. Small filling defect in the middle esophagus.

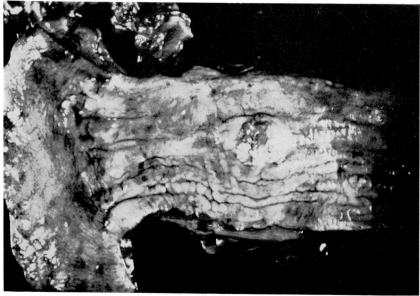

Figure 11-3. The resected specimen contains a tumor 2.2 x 1.8cm.

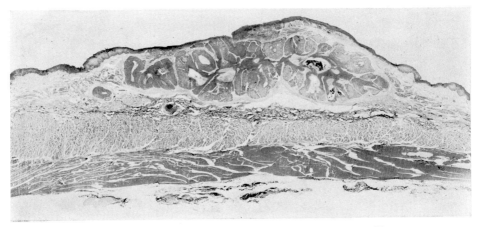

Figure 11-4. The cancer infiltration reaches the submucosal layer.

Sarcomas

Esophageal sarcomas are rare. Jackson (1935) reported seven in 935 esophageal malignant tumors. Goodner (1963) indicated an incidence of 0.5 per cent total esophageal malignant tumors, and Japanese statistics showed 0.1-1.0 per cent. At our hospital the following six cases of esophageal sarcoma were confirmed out of approximately 6,500 esophagoscopic examinations:

4 cases	confirmed by surgical specimen
1 case	confirmed at autopsy
1 case	confirmed by biopsy

and when itemized:

3 cases	leiomyosarcoma
2 cases	malignant melanoma
1 case	carcinosarcoma

Histologically, in Thorek's report (1950) of fifty-eight cases, there were

8	leiomyosarcomas
5	lymphosarcomas
5	melanosarcomas
30	fibrosarcomas
3	rhabdomyosarcomas
7	unclassified

Paulson (1969) stated that leiomyosarcomas were most frequent, but only thirty-six cases were reported in a recent comprehensive review of the world literature. We found in the Japanese literature as many as eight leiomyosarcomas in twenty-one reported esophageal sarcomas; there were four melanosarcomas, four spindle-cell sarcomas and one each reticulo-sarcoma, lymphosarcoma, hemangiosarcoma, rhabdomyosarcoma, and poly-morphocellular sarcoma.

Leiomyosarcoma

Macroscopically, these leiomyosarcomas have been classified by Ewing into ulcerating type and polyp type, by Rainer (1965) into infiltrating type, polyp type and combination type and by Gray (1961) into polyp type protruding into the esophageal lumen and infiltrating type invading the muscular layer.

The 54-year-old man was admitted with dysphagia and a mild degree of precordial pain. X-ray showed an irregular and ulcerating filling defect of about 7cm (Fig. 11-5) and no sign of dilatation in the upper esophagus. At endoscopy

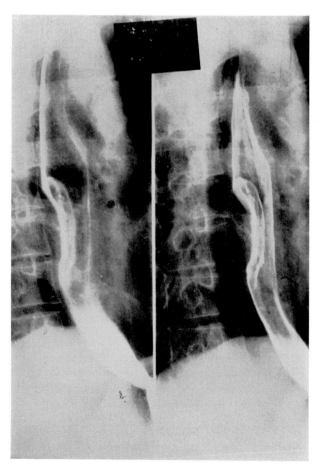

Figure 11-5. An ulcerating filling defect 7cm long.

an ulcerating tumor was found to involve one-half the circumference of the posterior wall at a level of 30cm from the upper incisor teeth. The margin was smooth and not high with regard to the size of the ulcer (Plate 16). The base of the ulcer was irregular and partly covered by a thick white coating. It grew outward as though protruding into the submucosal layer. On biopsy nonepithelial malignant tumor was suspected.

The resected specimen was a 5.5 x 4.0cm ulcerating tumor with a clear borderline; it was infiltrating into the surrounding normal submucosal layer as though protruding into it. Histologic examination revealed leiomyosarcoma.

Endoscopically the leiomyosarcomas in our series consisted of one case of the polyp type in the lower esophagus which protruded into the cavity. The surface showed a small ulceration, together with a white coating and bleeding. The case reported above and another were of the ulcerating type. Both showed a large ulcer involving the lower and middle esophagus. The ulceration was quite characteristic, with apparent erosion into the submucosa. The borderline had a gentle slope compared to the large size of the ulcer.

Neither case showed stenosis in the esophageal cavity. In spite of the large protrusion into the cavity the esophagoscope could easily be passed over the lesion into the distal esophagus.

Malignant Melanoma

The malignant melanoma originating from the esophagus is very rare. Baur (1906) reported it for the first time. Waken (1962) reported an analysis of twenty-two cases and their own additional two cases. We could find only a few cases in Japan.

By macroscopic observation almost all the tumors were described as polypoid and lobulated; many were pedunculated. In our two cases there were no peduncles, but the lesions were large and tumorous, protruding into the esophagus. The endoscopic examination revealed no specific findings on the surface of the tumor and the characteristic blue color observed in some series was found only on the cut surface of the resected specimen.

This patient, 60 years of age, came to the hospital with a complaint of dysphagia. X-rays showed a large filling defect in the middle and lower esophagus (Fig. 11-6). There was a central filling defect which was clearly demarcated. The surface of the tumor exhibited a honey-comb appearance without luminal stenosis at the site of the defect and with no dilatation proximally. Esophagofiberscopy showed a large tumor mass occupying the esophageal lumen (Fig. 11-7). Its surface had a white coating of esophageal epithelium, with some irregular indentations. Biopsy indicated the diagnosis of a sarcomatous lesion. The resected specimen showed a 6.0 x 3.0cm localized protruding tumor with irregular surface and some ulceration (Fig. 11-8). Histologically it was malignant melanoma originating from the esophagus (Fig. 11-9).

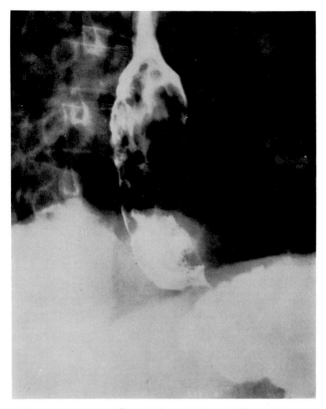

Figure 11-6. Large, tumorous filling defect in the middle and lower esophagus.

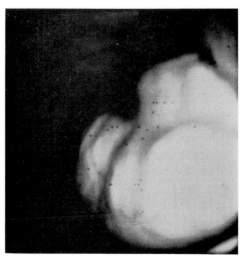

Figure 11-7. Large tumor mass occupies esophageal lumen. Its surface is irregular and covered with white "fur."

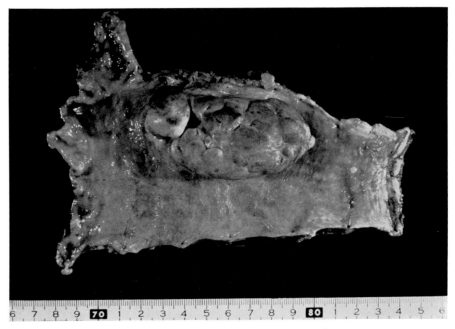

Figure 11-8. Resected specimen reveals the localized protruding tumor 6.0 x 3.0cm.

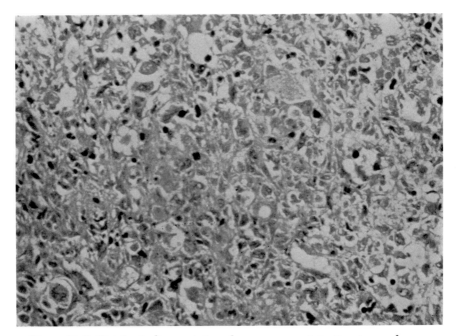

Figure 11-9. Histologic diagnosis is melanosarcoma originating in esophagus.

BENIGN TUMORS

Benign tumors of the esophagus are rare. Moersch and Harrington found forty-four benign tumors of the esophagus in 7,459 autopsies; thirty-two were leiomyomas. Lewis and Maxfield reported that 77 per cent of benign intramural esophageal tumors were myomas. Plachta (1962) recognized 504 cases of esophageal tumors in 19,982 autopsies and reported that 414 were malignant and 90 benign. Benign tumors of the esophagus include leiomyomas, cysts, fibromas, polyps, hemangiomas, fibrolipomas, neurofibromas, fibromyxomas, and papillomas.

Papillomas originate from the mucosal layer of the esophagus. Tumors originating in the submucosal layer are lipomas, cysts, and pedunculated fibromyomas. Leiomyomas, neurofibromas, fibromyomas, and rhabdomyomas are derived from the muscular layer. Those tumors are mostly nonpedunculated. Leiomyomas are the most common.

Esophageal polyps originate from connective tissue of the submucosal layer and protrude like a peduncle in the esophageal lumen, with some interstitial tissue. They commonly occur in the upper esophagus and may have quite a long peduncle.

Leiomyoma

Leiomyomas of the esophagus were reported as 52 per cent of all benign tumors of the esophagus by Plachta and Rose, and as 55 per cent by Japanese colleagues. They are frequently seen in the lower esophagus.

Pathologically leiomyomas arise from one of the smooth muscle coats of the esophagus. Morphologically the tumors are of a solitary, ovoid or spindle shape. Segmental, lobular, or horseshoe types encircling the esophageal cavity have been noted.

> A man, aged 35, had no symptom related to the esophagus. An x-ray film showed a sharply demarcated, smoothly rounded filling defect in the middle part of the esophagus. In the profile view, the contour of the barium column revealed a sharp change in direction where the normal esophageal wall meets the edge of the tumor at an acute angle (Fig. 11-10). These findings suggested submucosal tumor. The endoscopic examination showed a smooth-surfaced tumor protruding into the cavity from the posterior wall of the midesophagus (Fig. 11-11). The mucosa was atrophic and under slight tension but did not show any erosion or ulcer. On resection, a 5.5 x 4.0cm submucosal tumor was found (Fig. 11-12), histologically compatible with leiomyoma.

Papilloma

This is a papillary, small protrusion of the esophageal mucosae, comparatively hard and pale blue in appearance. Histologically, the squamous epithelium shows parakeratosis and hyperkeratosis. Increase of vascular

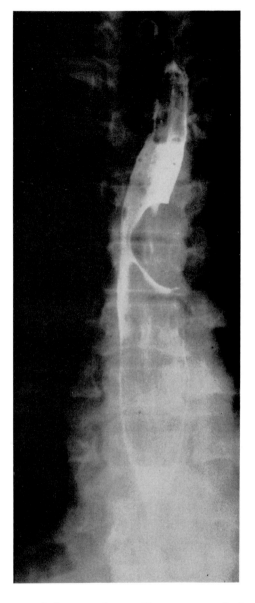

Figure 11-10. A sharply demarcated, smoothly round, filling defect in the midthoracic esophagus.

connective tissues under the submucosal layer of papillary protruded squamous epithelium has been noted.

Cyst

In our series these have been round, smooth, gently sloping swellings without any sign of stenosis. The resected specimens contained a transparent mucous substance.

The pathogenesis of esophageal cyst remains to be settled; there are several theories:

1. Theory of estranged lung bud in the esophageal wall (Fallop 1947).
2. Theory of incomplete fusion and vacuole formation during esophageal development in the fetus (Keith 1933).
3. Theory of inherent esophageal gland obstruction (Laudois 1908).

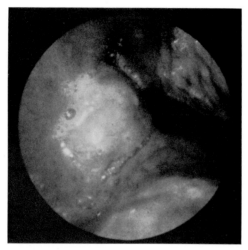

Figure 11-11. A tumor with smooth surface protrudes into the cavity from the posterior wall.

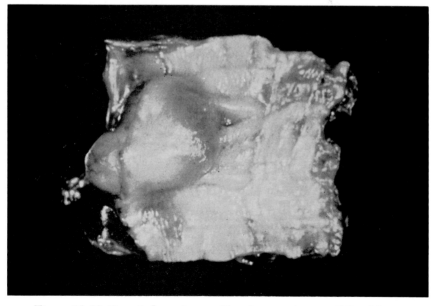

Figure 11-12. Resected specimen with submucosal tumor 5.5 x 4.0cm.

4. Theory of a remnant of a diverticular protrusion originating from the embryonic digestive tract (Lewis & Thyng 1907).

Polyp

These appear as pedunculated and ragged lesions in the lower esophagus, formed of vascular fibroelastic tissue and covered by normal mucosa. The polyp may grow to a very long cylindrical tumor causing swallowing disturbances or pressure symptoms on neighboring organs.

ESOPHAGEAL DIVERTICULA

The esophageal diverticulum is a saccular protrusion of the esophagus which is like a small pouch. It is usually classified into three types: pulsion diverticulum, traction diverticulum and traction-pulsion diverticulum. It may also be classified anatomically according to the site of occurrence as pharyngoesophageal, parabronchial, which occurs near the bifurcation of the trachea, and epiphrenic, which occurs just above the esophageal hiatus.

Mellius found twenty-three cases of diverticula in 1,500 autopsies (1.7%).

With regard to clinical symptoms, when an esophageal diverticulum is associated with other digestive tract disturbances, such as gastroduodenal ulcers, symptoms of the ulcer will dominate. In patients without demonstrable associated diseases, esophageal symptoms concerned with the diverticulum, such as dysphagia or sensation of a foreign body, are noted in 45 per cent of cases. Eighteen per cent are asymptomatic. Patients with small diverticula, from 1cm to 3cm on x-ray examination, may be symptomatic or asymptomatic, whereas those with diverticula larger than 3cm always have some symptoms. Thus the size of diverticulum is an important factor in producing symptoms.

The mechanism of formation of the pharyngoesophageal diverticulum, according to Lahey, is greatly influenced by the innervation of a vulnerable portion of the posterior wall at the pharyngoesophageal junction. This portion is anatomically defined by the inferior constrictor and cricopharyngeal muscles. The former is innervated by both the pharyngeal plexus and the external laryngeal plexus, and the latter is innervated by a pharyngeal fascicle of the recurrent laryngeal nerve. The act of swallowing is performed with the coordination of these nerves. When this coordination is lost, unbalanced contraction of both muscles occurs, resulting in abnormal elevation of pharyngeal pressure. The weak point under such pressure yields progressively from a concave to a saccular form. This diverticulum will be slightly deviated to the left or right as it grows. Moreover, it may enter the upper mediastinum, causing pressure on mediastinal organs, dysphagia, and regurgitation of esophageal contents. The peak age incidence is from 40 to 60 years, and it occurs chiefly in men. During endoscopic examination, the esophagoscope tends to be inserted into the diverticulum, making it more difficult to observe the lumen of the esophagus. Within the diverticulum may be observed food residues, a rough mucous membrane surface and esophagitis. In patients operated on, we found moderate esophagitis within the diverticulum.

A diverticulum seen at the cervical esophagus is essentially different from the pharyngoesophageal diverticulum. Our two cases were on the right side, but it has been reported on the left. According to Brombert the incidence of cervical esophageal diverticula is 3.8 per cent of all esophageal diverticula and its clinical symptomatology resembles closely that of the pharyngoesophageal lesion.

A man, aged 58, had dysphagia on admission and was referred to us with the diagnosis of esophageal cancer. Clinical symptoms of diverticula were not identified. On x-ray examination, a 3cm saccular diverticulum was seen beneath the esophageal entrance on the right side (Fig. 11-13). Moreover, an

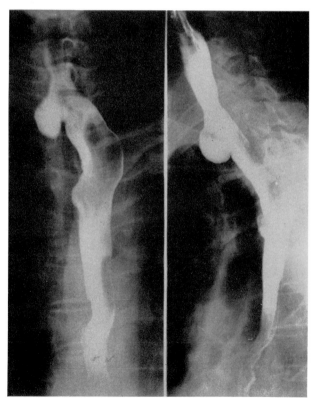

Figure 11-13. Saccular diverticulum is seen beneath the esophageal entrance. In midesophagus there is also an ulcerating carcinoma.

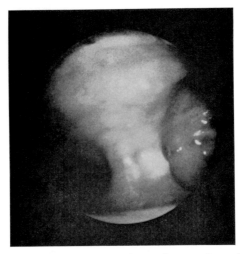

Figure 11-14. Esophagoscopic picture shows diverticulum of the esophagus.

ulcerated filling defect was seen in the midthoracic esophagus. Esophagoscopy revealed a carina-like septum in the esophagus, separating the lumen of the esophagus and the diverticulum (Fig. 11-14). The right side of the picture shows the diverticulum. The mucosal surface lacked luster and was rough at the bottom of the diverticulum though ulcer and erosion were not seen.

Diverticula of the thoracic esophagus are often found around the tracheal bifurcation and endoscopically around the portion depressed by the left main bronchus. In the type with adhesions to surrounding tissues, we naturally did not find the lesion in the posterior wall; thirteen cases were found in the anterior wall, nineteen on the left side, and thirty-six on the right side. The lesion tends to occur slightly more frequently on the right side. By endoscopic examination, the smaller diverticula appear as depressions protruding from the esophageal cavity, and the bigger ones are demarcated by carina-like septa. The latter are best identified by utilizing air insufflation to distend the esophageal cavity.

Some lesions which are clearly identified as diverticular protrusion by x-ray examination of the esophagus are not easily identified by endoscopic examination. These usually are small diverticula with narrow portals of entry and shallow diverticula which can be recognized during esophageal dilatation but are difficult to identify during active contraction because they blend with the neighboring wall during active peristalsis.

Inside the diverticulum inflammatory changes were seldom found in our series. The characteristic findings were those of a transparent capillary network and patches of bluish discoloration, which were most probably the neighboring organs and lymph nodes viewed through the thinned esophageal wall. These findings were also observed when the esophagus and diver-

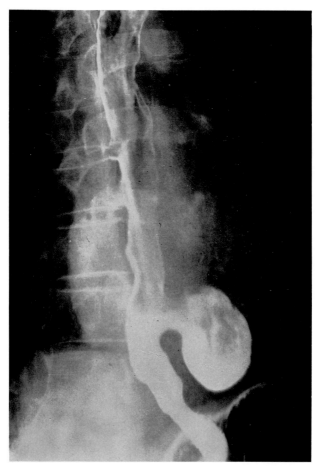

Figure 11-15. An 8cm saccular diverticulum at left side of the middle and lower esophagus.

ticulum were distended by insufflation of air and were not necessarily restricted to anthracotic lymph nodes.

A man, aged 68, came to the hospital with backache and a disturbance at the lower esophagus producing dysphagia. X-ray film (Fig. 11-15) showed an 8cm saccular diverticulum at the left side of the middle and lower esophagus. The contour of the diverticulum was smooth. The endoscopic picture showed a large saccular diverticulum on the left side, 39cm from the upper incisor teeth (Plate 17). A carina-like septum was observed between the esophageal cavity and the diverticulum. The esophageal mucosa around the orifice was almost normal. Food residues were found, as in a mild esophagitis, marked by a rough surface, lack of luster and small areas of granular swelling. Erosion and ulcer were not clearly detected. Diverticulectomy was performed and histologically a moderate esophagitis was found.

A woman, aged 53, was admitted complaining of mild dysphagia. X-ray

Gastrointestinal Pan-Endoscopy

examination showed a saccular diverticulum on the left side above the diaphragm. The contour of the diverticulum was smooth. Endoscopically, we found
a saccular diverticulum separated by a carina-like septum from the esophageal
cavity. No apparent change in the mucosa of the base of the diverticulum was
found. Diverticulectomy was performed through an abdominal incision, the
diverticulum being removed by pulling it into the abdomen. Histologically,
normal mucosa was found.

Operative treatment is rarely indicated for traction diverticulum of the
middle part of the esophagus. Pharyngoesophageal diverticula present a
difficult problem in management. Dysphagia, fetor oris, and reflux are
frequent complaints. In our series of eighty-eight cases, five patients had
operative treatment, one each with pharyngoesophageal diverticulum, cervical diverticulum, and a large diverticulum of the lower esophagus, and
two with epiphrenic diverticulum with severe dysphagia.

ESOPHAGEAL FISTULAS

Fistulas are usually divided into two types, congenital and acquired. In
this section the acquired type of esophageal fistula is dealt with.

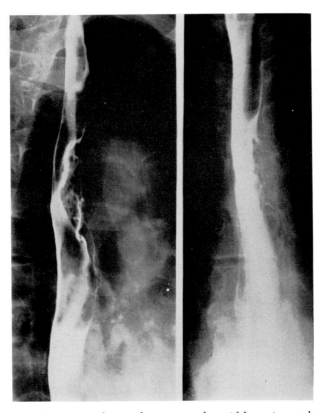

Figure 11-16. Large, ulcerated cancer in the midthoracic esophagus.

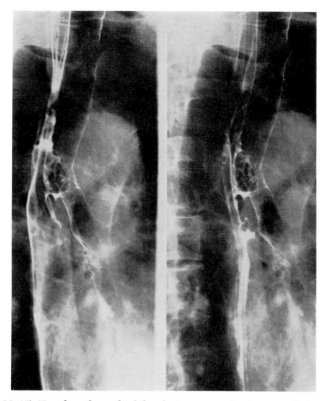

Figure 11-17. Esophagobronchial fistula is seen at the bottom of the cancer.

Fistulas connecting the esophagus with other structures in the thorax are mentioned as complications of various esophageal disorders. The causes of acquired esophageal fistula are thought to be esophageal cancer, peptic ulcer of the esophagus, abscess, foreign body, trauma, instrumentation, tuberculosis, syphilis, diverticulum, benign stricture, and actinomycosis. The commonest cause is cancer of the esophagus. Malignant neoplasms of the trachea and bronchus, mediastinal glands, and thyroid may also result in esophageal fistula. In one large series, Mouserrat found 367 fistulas of cancerous origin, 222 congenital, 41 infectious, and 40 of traumatic origin.

Usually the fistula communicates with either the trachea or a mainstem bronchus. Fistulous tracts leading from the esophagus into the lung, pleura, mediastinum, and pericardium have also been reported. The esophagotracheal or esophagobronchial fistula results from the ulcerating carcinoma of the esophagus in the midthoracic region.

The very tiny fistula may give no symptoms. Respiratory symptoms, such as cough associated with the mixing of blood, mucus and food, dyspnea and dysphagia, should suggest the possibility of a fistula. Respiratory

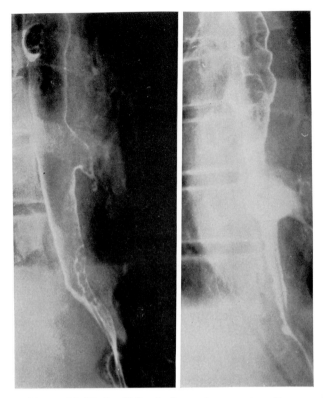

Figure 11-18. Small fistula formation at suture line.

symptoms are usually experienced when the patient swallows liquids. In general, fistula should be suspected when a patient with antecedent dysphagia reports bouts of strangulation after swallowing.

Careful fluoroscopy may demonstrate the fistulous opening. When the presence of esophageal fistula is suspected clinically prior to x-ray examination, it is preferable to avoid giving a barium meal and to use an absorbable oily or aqueous contrast material such as Gastrografin, now commonly used for bronchography. Extension of the contrast medium from the esophageal lumen indicates the presence of fistulous tract.

The prognosis depends upon the etiology of the fistula.

Presenting complaints in a 65-year-old man were dysphagia and productive cough after swallowing. X-rays (Fig. 11-16) showed a large ulcerating cancer in the midthoracic esophagus. After four months of cobalt therapy, the esophagobronchial fistula may be seen at the bottom of the lesion (Fig. 11-17). The barium may be detected flowing into the bronchus immediately thereafter.

A 78-year-old man had a large diverticulum in the lower part of the esophagus. He complained of dysphagia, and diverticulectomy was performed by way of the left thoracic cavity. After operation fistula formation may be seen at the suture line on the x-ray film (Fig. 11-18). Esophagoscopy revealed the fistulas at the suture line to be small in size. Esophagitis and ulceration were not seen near the fistulas.

POSTOPERATIVE LESIONS

There are various methods of reconstruction of the esophagus; there are esophagogastric, esophagojejunal, and esophagocolic anastomoses. The anastomosis may be made in subcutaneous antethoracic, retrosternal, intrathoracic, or intra-abdominal fashion, depending on the preference of the surgeon and the circumstances of the operation. This report deals with anastomoses performed in the thorax and abdomen and studied by endoscopic follow-up examinations. In the past five years, 1,171 postoperative endoscopic examinations were done in our hospital. The endoscopic findings were divided into four categories: normal, reflux esophagitis and ulcer, cicatricial stenosis of the anastomotic stoma, and recurrence. Incidentally we found a few cases with suture remnants (silk) at the anastomosis, foreign bodies in the esophagus from digested foods, and masses of granulation tissue.

Normal Healing

When the healing at the anastomosis is smooth after esophageal reconstruction, the endoscopic finding will be the same whether the anastomosis is to stomach or intestine. The transition of mucosal surface from esophagus to stomach or intestine will be smooth and continuous without denuded granulation tissue. The anastomotic orifice will be larger than 1cm and easily distended by insufflation of air.

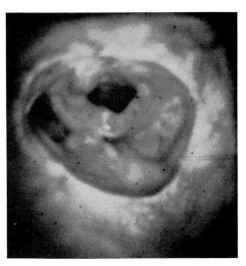

Figure 11-19. Esophagojejunostomy stoma is large and has good distensibility. The mucosa of jejunum can be observed through the stoma.

Woman, aged 63, had esophagectomy and esophagogastrostomy for esophageal cancer. A right intrathoracic approach was used. Fiberoscopy revealed after six months a small cicatricial deformity on the right side of the stoma. The transition of mucosa was smooth, with good distensibility. She had no dysphagia, and the esophagofiberscope could be easily passed over the anastomosis.

A case of cancer of the cardia in a man, 68, was treated by total gastrectomy and abdominal esophagojejunostomy. Figure 11-19 shows no stenosis at the anastomotic stoma after ten months. There is good distensibility, the mucosal surface is smooth, and transition into jejunal mucosa can be seen to be continuous. The jejunal lumen can be observed through the anastomotic stoma.

Reflux Esophagitis and Esophageal Ulcer

The incidence of esophagitis of more than moderate severity—recognizable as erosion on endoscopy—was 8.2 per cent in patients having esophagogastrostomy and 29.3 per cent in patients with esophagojejunostomy. In the esophagojejunostomy group all esophagitis occurred after abdominal anastomosis; not a single case of esophagitis was found in patients with intrathoracic anastomoses. Jejunal interposition between the esophagus and duodenum and Roux-Y anastomoses are associated with the least incidence of esophagitis, followed by the β-type anastomosis. Braun's anastomosis is most frequently associated with esophagitis.

There is poor correlation between endoscopic findings and the patient's complaints (Table 11-III). For instance, the commonest complaint, heartburn, is not necessarily present in every patient with positive endoscopic finding. On the other hand, in the endoscopically normal group, 5 per cent did complain of heartburn.

Endoscopically, esophagitis may be classified as follows: (1) Erythema of the mucosal surface is present without depression. (2) Erosion of various forms is scattered along the longitudinal axis of the esophagus. The surface is depressed, markedly erythematous, with a whitish coating in some areas. (3) The erosive change spreads diffusely to involve half or the entire circumference. (4) A special form with circulatory disturbance is

TABLE 11-III

RELATION BETWEEN CLINICAL COMPLAINTS AND ESOPHAGOSCOPIC FINDINGS

Clinical Complaints	Normal Findings	Esophagitis		
		Slight	Moderate	Severe
No complaints	50	18	17	13
Heartburn	19	36	41	75
Dysphagia	12	27	10	12
Stinging pain	0	0	10	0
Regurgitation	4	0	7	0
Bitter taste	4	9	7	0
Epigastralgia	8	0	4	0

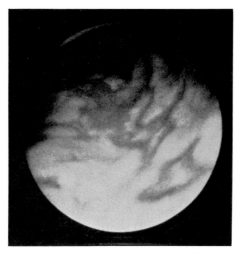

Figure 11-20. In the middle part of the esophagus, well-demarcated, round erosions are scattered along the longitudinal axis.

characterized by diffuse and severe hemorrhagic inflammation throughout the entire esophagus.

Histologically, the first group showed deep ingrowth (so-called papillation) of the lamina propria mucosae into the epithelial layer, with capillary dilatation and hyperplasia at the top of the papilla. Acute inflammatory cellular infiltration is not always prominent, suggesting that the acute inflammatory reaction had already subsided in these cases. The second and third groups showed more definite inflammatory reaction with marked

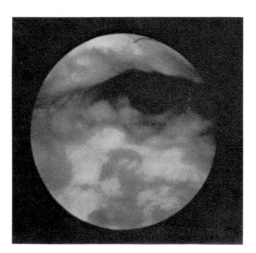

Figure 11-21. Inflammatory changes, consisting of redness, erosion, roughness of surface, and fibrinous mucous membrane are noted over entire circumference.

acute inflammatory infiltration in the interstitial and epithelial layers, not always closely correlated with the endoscopic findings.

A 28-year-old woman had Heyrovsky's operation one year previously for achalasia. She entered our hospital with complaints of heartburn and irritation during swallowing. Endoscopically diffuse erosive changes were found from the upper esophagus down to the anastomotic site, the more proximal being less severe. Near the anastomosis the entire circumference was involved by the erosive change. In the midesophagus, well-demarcated round erosions were scattered along the longitudinal axis (Fig. 11-20). The surface was decidedly reddish; no white coating was found. Result of biopsy was consistent with the diagnosis of esophagitis.

A 65-year-old man, whose chief complaint was heartburn, had total gastrectomy with abdominal esophagojejunostomy three months previously for cancer of the cardia. Endoscopically (Fig. 11-21), inflammatory changes with erythema, erosion, a rough surface and fibrinous mucous membrane were noted throughout the entire circumference, especially in the lower esophagus. The mucosal surface appeared dirty and bled easily.

Cicatricial Stenosis of Anastomosis

Cicatricial stenosis of the anastomosis is found most often after esophagogastrostomy (10%). The incidence after esophagojejunostomy is about 5 per cent. The size of the anastomotic stoma varies from pinhole to 5mm. Not only the size of the stoma, but other conditions of the stoma, such as distensibility, are important factors in producing dysphagia. Thus when a hard, sclerotic stoma becomes softer with passage of time, dysphagia will improve even though the actual stoma size remains almost the same.

A man, aged 28, whose chief complaint was dysphagia, had undergone total gastrectomy with abdominal esophagojejunostomy for gastric cancer two months before. On endoscopy (Fig. 11-22), a markedly stenotic anastomotic stoma (pinhole-sized) and strong cicatricial changes in the surrounding area were found. After one month of bougienage, the stoma was larger and more pliable. Clinical improvement occurred as well.

Recurrence of Cancer

Esophageal and gastric cancer may recur after esophagectomy or total gastrectomy at the anastomosis as a form of local recurrence or may occur in the esophageal wall proximal to the anastomosis as a form of distant metastasis, possibly through lymphatic spread. The latter will be found as scattered, small, nodular elevations of various sizes with a smooth mucosal surface. Generally, the nodular elevations from intramural metastasis vary both in size and color depending on the volume of cancerous mass and the extent of invasion to the epithelial layer.

Total gastrectomy for gastric cancer was done in a woman, aged 45. On periodic postoperative examination she was found to have recurrence. There were no symptoms. The esophagofiberscopic picture showed a smooth, normal

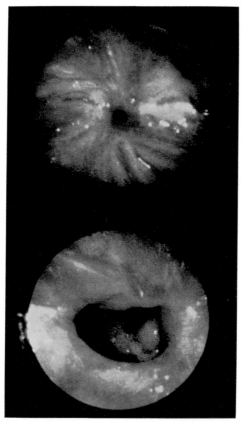

Figure 11-22. *Above,* markedly stenotic anastomotic stoma; *below,* stoma enlarged by bougienage.

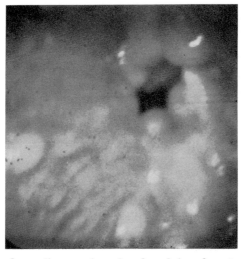

Figure 11-23. Scattered, small, smooth-surfaced nodular elevations of various sizes in the lower esophagus.

anastomosis; however, in the lower esophagus there were scattered, small, well-demarcated, whitish elevations with a smooth surface (Fig. 11-23). Biopsy showed metastatic adenocarcinoma of the same type as the gastric cancer. Cobalt therapy and anticancer chemotherapy were instituted promptly, but the lesion increased in size progressively and finally ulcerated.

MISCELLANEOUS

Besides the aforementioned conditions, we find one or two nonpathologic conditions at the anastomosis, such as inflammatory granulomatous swelling and suture remnants. At present, we use catgut for the inner layer of the anastomosis and silk for the outer layer. This silk may sometimes protrude inside when a continuous suture is used. The presence of such a suture does not always result in formation of an ulcer, but we usually remove it endoscopically provided three weeks have passed after surgery.

A 34-year-old woman noted slight dysphagia two months after total gastrectomy for gastric cancer. Esophagoscopy was performed. The anastomosis showed some stenosis, but the transition of mucosal surface was smooth and there was good distensibility. However, a dangling thread dyed with bile was found at the anastomotic site and was removed endoscopically (Fig. 11-24).

The endoscopic findings of postoperative lesions were divided into four groups. These were normal, reflux esophagitis and ulceration in the neighborhood of the anastomotic stoma, cicatricial stenosis, and recurrence. The flexible esophagofiberscope makes it easier to examine the anastomosis and its surroundings postoperatively. Moreover, the fiberscope makes it possible to observe the circumference of the anastomosis when the stoma is tilted to the left or right side. Endoscopy is the most significant procedure available to reach the exact diagnosis in postoperative lesions.

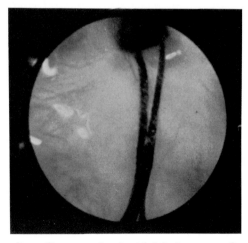

Figure 11-24. Dangling silk suture dyed with bile is seen at the anastomotic site.

REFERENCES

1. Barrett, N.: Benign smooth muscle tumor of the esophagus. *Thorax, 19*:185-194, 1964.
2. Bogedain, W., Carpathios, J., and Akram, N.: Leiomyoma of the esophagus. *Dis Chest, 44*:391-400, 1963
3. Cornell, A.: Cysts of the esophagus: Case report and review of the literature. *Gastroenterology, 15*:260, 1950.
4. Endo, M., Kobayashi, S., Suzuki, H., Takemoto, T., and Nakayama, K.: Diagnosis of early esophageal cancer. *Endoscopy, 3*:61, 1971.
5. Lahey, F., and Warren, K.: Esophageal diverticulum. *Surg Gynec and Obst, 98*:1, 1954.
6. Mellins, R. B.: Acquired fistula between the esophagus and the respiratory tract: Report of a case, review of the literature and discussion of the pathogenesis. *New England J Med, 246*:896, 1952.
7. Mendl, K., and Evans, C.: Congenital and acquired epiphrenic diverticula of the esophagus. *Brit J Radiol, 35*:53, 1962.
8. Plachta, A.: Benign tumors of the esophagus: Review of the literature and report of 99 cases. *Am J Gastroenterol, 38*:639, 1962.
9. Rainer, W. G., and Brus, R.: Leiomyosarcoma of the esophagus: Review of the literature and report of 3 cases. *Surgery, 58*:343-350, 1965.
10. Rettig, J.: Diverticulum of the abdominal portion of the esophagus. *Gastroenterology, 42*:781, 1962.
11. Suzuki, H., Kobayashi, S., Endo, M., and Nakayama, K.: Diagnosis of early esophageal cancer. *Surgery, 71*:99, 1972.
12. Talbert, J. L., and Cantrell, J. R.: Clinical and pathologic characteristics of carcinosarcoma of the esophagus. *J. Thoracic and Cardiovas Surg, 45*:1-12, 1963.
13. Waken, J. K., and Bullock, W. K.: Primary melanosarcoma of the esophagus. *Am J Clin Path, 38*:415-421, 1962.

CHAPTER 12

NEUROMUSCULAR DISORDERS: SCLERODERMA, CONNECTIVE TISSUE DISEASES, OTHER DISORDERS

Maurice L. Kelley, Jr.

Scleroderma
Connective Tissue Diseases Other than Scleroderma
Oculopharyngeal Syndrome
Dysphagia Due to Neurologic Disorders
    Myotonia Dystrophica
    Myasthenia Gravis
    Parkinson's Disease, Amyotrophic Lateral Sclerosis, and Multiple
        Sclerosis
    Diabetes Mellitus
    Presbyesophagus

NEUROMUSCULAR DISORDERS OF the esophagus may be divided into those characterized by *hypo*motility and those in which *hyper*motility is the primary manifestation. The diseases of *hyper*motility, including diffuse spasm and vigorous achalasia, have been covered by other authors. This chapter, therefore, will describe those neuromuscular disorders in which *hypo*motility is the major abnormality.

SCLERODERMA

The type of esophageal motor dysfunction associated with scleroderma is the prototype of motor failure of the esophagus. This abnormality produced by scleroderma with or without Raynaud's phenomenon results in hypotonia and incompetence of the gastroesophageal sphincter and failure of the body of the esophagus to respond to the act of deglutition with an effective contractile response.[1] This results in *double trouble:* not only does the weakness of the gastroesophageal sphincter result in reflux of acid gastric content into the esophagus, but also the organ can no longer respond

204

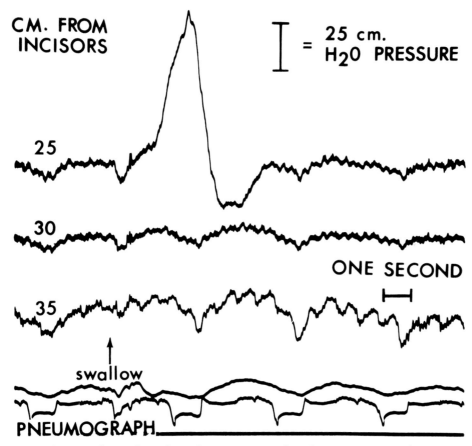

Figure 12-1. Intraluminal esophageal pressure recording from a patient with cutaneous and visceral scleroderma. She complained of severe heartburn and easy regurgitation. Esophagoscopy demonstrated a patulous gastroesophageal sphincter, with reflux and diffuse esophagitis but no stricturing. The three pressure-sensitive units detected a complete absence of esophageal contraction (aperistalsis) following deglutition, except in the upper 6cm of the organ. This is the characteristic motility disturbance seen in about 50 per cent of patients with scleroderma. (Reproduced by permission of Hoeber Medical Division of Harper and Row Publishers.)

with effective secondary contractions to clear itself of regurgitated material. The result is severe reflux esophagitis with all of its attendant complications.

Figure 12-1 shows the poor response of the body of the esophagus to the act of swallowing in a patient with scleroderma, reflux esophagitis, and heartburn. Compare this with Figure 12-2, which is the deglutitive pattern in a subject with cutaneous scleroderma and no visceral involvement.

The endoscopic features of esophageal disease associated with scleroderma are of the utmost importance because they can best illustrate the de-

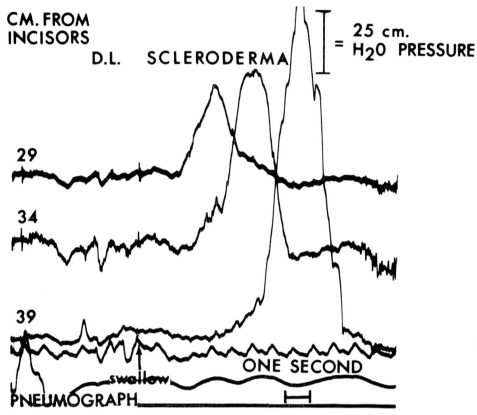

Figure 12-2. Normal deglutitive motor response of the esophageal body recorded in a patient with cutaneous scleroderma (morphea) but no dysphagia or other indication of visceral disease. The contractions are peristaltic and of good amplitude and duration.

structive results of the severe regurgitant esophagitis seen in this condition. The esophagoscopist often sees free reflux of gastric contents into the esophagus; the esophageal mucous membrane is inflamed, friable, edematous, and, if the process has gone on for some length of time, atrophic. Stricture formation eventually develops, and the endoscopist can measure the degree of narrowing and ascertain the amount of inflammatory reaction. Dilatation of the stricture and exclusion of neoplastic disease can likewise be accomplished by the endoscopist.

CONNECTIVE TISSUE DISEASES OTHER THAN SCLERODERMA

Despite the consistency with which disorders of esophageal motor function are found in scleroderma, one would make a mistake to assume that every patient with aperistalsis and absent or decreased gastroesophageal sphincter tone has scleroderma. This motor abnormality is found in patients with other connective tissue disorders, such as periarteritis nodosa and systemic lupus erythematosus, and in subjects with Raynaud's disease, without true sclerodermatous tissue changes.[2] Barium x-ray studies, including cineradiography and intraluminal manometry, are the most sensitive techniques. Endoscopy should be performed to exclude esophagitis, stricture formation, and unsuspected neoplasm, particularly when sticking of food is a major component of the symptoms complex.

Some problems of esophageal motor failure are difficult to diagnose and do not fall into any specific disease category.

CASE HISTORY

A 15-year-old school girl was referred by a pediatrician because since the age of 5 she had had easy regurgitation, particularly while sleeping at night or bending forward. She also noted occasional sticking of food at the midsternal area and had to wash solids down by drinking liquids. In addition, she was subject to what were referred to as "choking spells" during meals.

Upper G.I. series showed a small hiatus hernia without reflux. Otherwise, the study was reported as normal.

Intraluminal manometric studies detected no zone of elevated pressure in the gastroesophageal junctional area. Pressures in the body of the esophagus were slightly higher than those in the stomach, indicating retention of material in the esophagus. With swallowing, no contractions occurred in the body of the esophagus; the few that did develop were weak and simultaneous (Fig. 12-3). The uppermost 1-2cm of the esophagus contracted more powerfully. No good peristaltic sequences were recorded following the act of active deglutition.

Esophagoscopy showed a contraction ring, which had been missed at the time of the x-ray studies, just below the cricopharyngeus. This was dilated, and the instrument introduced into the esophagus. The esophageal mucous membrane was much paler than normal and appeared thin and atrophic. Biopsies showed thinning of the esophageal mucous membrane and low-grade inflammation diagnosed as chronic esophagitis.

Surgical repair of the hiatus hernia relieved all of her symptoms.

COMMENT: The pathophysiology of this patient's major esophageal problem does not fit into a well-defined category and serves to emphasize the importance of endoscopy and intraluminal manometric studies as a supplement to radiography in evaluating obscure causes of dysphagia. She probably had had chalasia (a hypotonic gastroesophageal sphincter with reflux) since infancy, with resultant reflux esophagitis, hiatus hernia formation, and secondary motor failure due to the chronic inflammatory process.

Esophagoscopy was crucial in the evaluation of this patient. An upper esophageal ring, missed by radiography, was identified and dilated and esophagitis due to reflux documented.

OCULOPHARYNGEAL SYNDROME

The so-called oculopharyngeal syndrome consists of ptosis of the eyelids and dysphagia.[3] It occurs almost without exception in French Canadians, probably the descendents of one immigrant who came to the North Ameri-

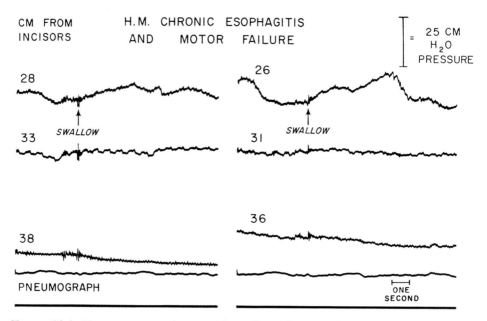

Figure 12-3. Two segments of an esophageal motility tracing from a 15-year-old girl with regurgitation, choking, and heartburn. Three pressure-recording units separated by 5cm intervals are positioned in the body of the esophagus and document weak, inadequate responses to two swallowing efforts. Chronic esophagitis due to a congenitally weak and incompetent gastroesophageal sphincter with hiatus hernia was the presumed pathologic process.

can continent in the 1700s. Severe drooping of the lids develops in mid or late middle age, and difficulty in swallowing, characterized by sticking of food in the pharynx and aspiration, develops shortly thereafter. The major pathologic abnormality is fatty infiltration, fibrosis and degeneration of the musculature of the pharyngoesophageal sphincter. Patients are often thought to have carcinoma of the lower pharynx or upper esophagus and may be referred to the endoscopist because of this possibility.

Barium x-ray studies may be confusing and often are nondescript. The radiologist usually reports a stricture or narrowing in the cricopharyngeal area with aspiration of contrast media into the tracheobronchial tree and suggests a diagnosis of a carcinoma of the pharynx or upper esophagus.

The endoscopic features are those of a nonresilient, narrowed cricopharyngeus through which the esophagoscope passes with considerable difficulty. In some instances a dilator has to be passed blindly through the cricopharyngeus and a small-caliber, rigid esophagoscope introduced over it to visualize the esophagus and the gastroesophageal junction. The treatment is a myotomy of the cricopharyngeal musculature, which sometimes relieves the sticking of food and aspiration pneumonitis.

CASE HISTORY

A 73-year-old French Canadian housewife was referred because of difficulty in swallowing and recurrent aspiration pneumonitis of approximately three years' duration. Barium x-ray studies at other institutions had shown "a stenosis of the upper end of the esophagus at the level of C-7," which impeded passage of barium into the esophagus; the contrast medium was aspirated into the tracheobronchial tree. She had lost about twenty pounds in weight. Seven years prior to being seen at our institution, plastic surgery procedures had been performed to control bilateral ptosis of the eyelids which interfered with her vision. Physical examination showed an emaciated, elderly woman who weighed 80 pounds. Barium x-ray studies showed that the patient had great difficulty in swallowing. There was narrowing in the region of the cricopharyngeus, and most of the contrast media passed into the trachea and bronchi. Roentgenologic impression was "neurogenic dysfunction of swallowing."

Esophagoscopic examination showed a very constricted cricopharyngeal musculature. It was extremely difficult to pass the instrument through the cricopharyngeus, which appeared edematous, solid, and uniformly enlarged through its entire circumference. There was not the usual resiliency of the musculature in the pharyngo-esophageal area. The esophagus and gastroesophageal junctional area appeared normal. It was impossible to perfrom manometric studies, as the pressure-recording tubes always went into the trachea rather than the esophagus.

It was felt that the patient had the oculopharyngeal syndrome with severe dysphagia resulting from the tight, poorly relaxing cricopharyngeus. A cricopharyngeal myotomy was performed. Microscopic examination of tissue from the cricopharyngeus showed a striking infiltration of the muscle by fat, along with an increase in fibrous tissue and atrophy of the muscle fibers. The patient's ability to swallow was considerably improved. Barium x-ray studies five months after the operation showed that barium passed easily from pharynx to esophagus without aspiration into the respiratory tract. The patient gained twenty pounds and felt that she had been much benefited by the surgical procedure.

DYSPHAGIA DUE TO NEUROLOGIC DISORDERS

Myotonia Dystrophica

This is a familial disease, the principal clinical manifestations of which result from myotonia, weakness, and the wasting of voluntary muscles. Frontal baldness, cataracts, testicular tubular atrophy, hypometabolism, and hyperostosis frontalis interna are frequent associated findings. Dysphagia and sticking of food occurring in this disorder were recognized by a number of clinicians, but the cause for the swallowing problem was not specifically characterized until 1964.[4]

Sticking of food is usually intermittent and most often follows the ingestion of poorly masticated solids.

Barium x-ray studies show flaccidity and lack of peristaltic activity. Intraluminal manometric studies in a number of patients with myotonia dystrophica have demonstrated absence of contractions in the body of the esophagus with deglutition. Resting pressures in the gastroesophageal sphincter usually are low, but the sphincter relaxes with swallowing. The pharyngoesophageal sphincter may relax and contract in a relatively normal fashion, although in some subjects relaxation is impaired.

The esophagus does not respond with the tetanic powerful contraction following subcutaneous injection of methacholine chloride as it does in achalasia.

Esophagogastroscopy should be carried out in patients with myotonia dystrophica who have difficulty in swallowing. Endoscopy is the only way to definitely exclude an associated malignancy. It also ascertains whether or not reflux occurs through the hypotonic gastroesophageal sphincter and if there are any indications of esophagitis.

Myasthenia Gravis

Difficulty in initiating the act of swallowing and choking during the process of eating are not uncommon problems in patients with myasthenia gravis. Barium x-ray studies confirm the difficulty the patient has in starting the act of deglutition, and the passage of contrast medium from pharynx to esophagus often is poorly carried out. There are no specific endoscopic findings associated with myasthenia gravis, although the endoscopist may be impressed by weakness of the cricopharyngeus and poor contractility of the body of the esophagus stimulated by passage of the instrument. If the gastroesophageal sphincter is also adversely affected by the neurologic disease, reflux may be documented at the time of endoscopy.

Parkinson's Disease, Amyotrophic Lateral Sclerosis, and Multiple Sclerosis

Dysphagia is not an uncommon complaint in patients with these neurologic diseases. Poor coordination of the complicated reflexes associated with deglutition is the usual cause for this complaint. If sticking of food, heartburn, and substernal pain become a major problem in these individuals, endoscopy should be carried out. There are no specific endoscopic findings, but the procedure is important to exclude or diagnose esophagitis, reflux, stricture formation, or an unsuspected carcinoma. The ease with which esophagoscopy can now be performed utilizing fiberoptic instruments makes one feel much more uninhibited about performing esophagoscopy in these frail, weak, and often depressed and debilitated patients.

Diabetes Mellitus

Esophageal dysfunction associated with diabetes mellitus has now been well documented by both radiographic and intraluminal manometric techniques. Although such patients may have no esophageal symptoms, a certain percentage do complain of difficulty in swallowing, which is related to weak, ineffectual, and at times simultaneous contractions in the body of the esophagus, as well as to impaired relaxation of the gastroesophageal sphincter. Patients with esophageal motor dysfunction usually are those who have diabetic neuropathy and gastroenteropathy, and only a small proportion of these have significant symptoms referable to the esophagus.[5] However, virtually all show striking esophageal motor dysfunction when examined by cineradiographic techniques and manometry. It is well for the clinician to be aware of this, as patients with diabetes mellitus who have dysphagia should be esophagoscoped when the symptoms are of major proportions.

Presbyesophagus

The aging process results in deglutitive abnormalities, which include an increased incidence of nonperistaltic contractions, low amplitude of pressure responses after swallowing, and impairment in the ability of the gastroesophageal sphincter to relax with swallowing.[6]

CASE HISTORY

A 65-year-old housewife, with a huge number of functional complaints, had had burning substernal discomfort and a sensation of sticking of food for six months. Barium x-ray studies of the upper gastrointestinal tract showed poor propulsive activity in the body of the esophagus with holdup and retention of barium in the midesophagus, which was slightly dilated and very irregular. A small sliding hiatus hernia was also identified. The radiographic diagnosis was "motor disturbance with poor propulsive activity of the esophagus and small

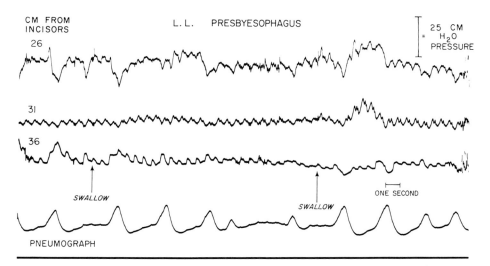

Figure 12-4. Inadequate esophageal contractions after swallowing in a neurotic patient with dysphagia. Objective evidence of a motor disturbance without organic obstruction (presbyesophagus) was of great help in evaluation and management. Esophagoscopy, in addition to manometry, is crucial in studying cases of this type.

hiatus hernia." Intraluminal manometric studies were abnormal, in that no adequate responses to deglutition were recorded in any portion of the body of the esophagus, although the gastroesophageal sphincter relaxed and contracted reasonably well (Fig. 12-4).

Esophagoscopy demonstrated a pale, atrophic lower two thirds of the esophageal mucous membrane through which blood vessels could be easily identified. Esophageal biopsies documented thinning of the mucous membrane but no significant degree of inflammation.

COMMENT: Presbyesophagous was the cause of this neurotic woman's dysphagia. Radiolographic and intraluminal manometric studies proved the diagnosis, while endoscopy excluded tumor and reflux esophagitis. Such objective data in problem cases of this sort are crucial in evaluation and management.

REFERENCES

1. Creamer, B., Andersen, H. A., and Code, C. F.: Esophageal motility in patients with scleroderma and related diseases. *Gastroenterologia, 86*:763, 1956.
2. Stevens, M. B., Hookman, P., and Siegel, C. I.: Aperistalsis of the esophagus in patients with connective tissue disorders and Raynaud's phenomenon. *New England J Med, 270*:1218, 1964.
3. Murphy, S. F., and Drachman, D. B.: Oculopharyngeal syndrome. *JAMA, 203*:1003, 1968.
4. Kelley, M. L., Jr.: Dysphagia and motor failure of the body of the esophagus in myotonia dystrophica. *Neurology, 14*:955, 1964.
5. Mandelstam, P., Siegel, C. I., Lieber, A., and Lieber, M.: The swallowing disorder in patients with diabetic neuropathy—gastroenteropathy. *Gastroenterology 56*:1, 1969.
6. Soergel, K. H., Zboralske, F. F., and Amberg, J. R.: Presbyesophagus. Esophageal motility in nonagenarians. *J Clin Invest, 43*:1472, 1964.

CHAPTER 13

MALLORY-WEISS SYNDROME, LOWER ESOPHAGEAL RING CARDIOESOPHAGEAL LESIONS, JUNCTIONAL IDENTIFICATION

Angelo E. Dagradi

The Mallory-Weiss Syndrome
Lower Esophageal Ring
Cardioesophageal Lesions
Junctional Identification

THE MALLORY-WEISS SYNDROME

L ACERATION OF THE GASTRIC CARDIA as a source for upper gastrointestinal bleeding was originally described in 1929 by Mallory and Weiss.[1] Subsequent reports have demonstrated that this is not a rare disorder; the necessity for considering it in the differential diagnosis of all patients bleeding from the upper gastrointestinal tract has been emphasized.[2]

The laceration is more commonly single, but multiple tears may occur (Plate 18). The individual lesion may be linear, oval, or stellate in appearance and is oriented parallel to the long axis of the stomach. It may be found at any point in the circumference of the cardia. The tear is restricted to the cardiac segment of the stomach and does not extend into the esophagus. It ordinarily penetrates through the mucosa and submucosa; less frequently, the muscular coat is also torn and the lesion extends to, or through, the serosa, resulting in an open perforation. The degree and severity of bleeding are determined by the size and nature of the blood vessels which are ruptured by the trauma.

The gastric mucosa immediately adjacent to the tear is usually edematous and is often hemorrhagic in appearance. A fresh, soft, black clot is seated in and covers the lesion during the early phase of its occurrence. Blood may be seen to ooze from the periphery and trickle downward into the "mucus lake." Rarely, arterial spurting from the laceration is visualized during endoscopy. During the ensuing two days, the clot may be seen to become reduced in size, still adherent to the center of the laceration but leaving the periphery exposed; the latter is coated with a whitish membrane. Still later, the entire clot falls away. The tear now appears as a glistening white, linear ulcer base, the margins of which are still edematous. The lesion usually heals within a period of two to five days (depending upon its original length and depth).

In our experience, an esophageal hiatus sliding hernia has been an invariably encountered abnormality in patients demonstrating this disorder.

The Mallory-Weiss tear is produced by forceful efforts which create a sudden rise in the intra-abdominal pressure. These most commonly involve forceful retching and vomiting; however, blunt abdominal trauma, paroxysmal coughing, straining and lifting, epileptic seizures, and even forceful straining at stool have preceded the manifestation of upper gastrointestinal bleeding. The forceful efforts succeed in jamming the gastric cardia against the relatively rigid and unyielding esophageal hiatus of the diaphragm, with resultant tearing of the gastric wall, the depth of the laceration being variable, as previously noted.

A carefully developed history in a patient who presents with bleeding from the upper gastrointestinal tract should include an exploration for preexisting symptoms suggestive of esophageal hiatus sliding hernia (reflux, regurgitation, heartburn, dysphagia, epigastric distress) in association with the sequence of forceful efforts followed by hematemesis. When such symptoms are present, the Mallory-Weiss lesion should be highly suspect as the source for the patient's bleeding. The characteristic syndrome occurred in only 60 per cent of a series of patients with this disorder reported by us.

A definitive diagnosis during life is made by visualizing the lesion by endoscopy or at surgical exploration. The ordinary upper gastrointestinal radiologic studies may demonstrate an esophageal hiatus sliding hernia but are not conducive to demonstration of the lesion. Visualization by retrograde celiac angiography of radiopaque contrast medium trickling down from the hiatal region along the gastric wall only suggests the location of a bleeding source—not necessarily its nature. Moreover, if angiography is to be of diagnostic assistance, the lesion must be actively bleeding at the time the procedure is performed. Endoscopic examination, however, demonstrates the lesion even when performed at a time when the bleeding has temporarily or permanently ceased. Gastroscopy has been more frequently successful than esophagoscopy in permitting visualization of the lesion.

CASE HISTORY

A 48-year-old, white, chronic alcoholic patient had uncontrollable retching and vomiting the morning after an alcoholic debauch. The vomitus, initially consisting of clear fluid, subsequently became bright red in color. Copious amounts of blood and fresh clots were expelled, and the patient became weak, pale, and diaphoretic. He was brought to the hospital where, following corrective therapy for shock, emergency endoscopic examination was performed, revealing an esophageal hiatus sliding hernia and a fresh, actively bleeding laceration of the gastric mucosa located on the hiatal rim. Bleeding continued and surgery was subsequently performed. A 2cm laceration immediately below the gastric cardia with arterial spurting from its base was identified. The artery was ligated, the laceration repaired, and bleeding was controlled. The patient made an uneventful recovery.

LOWER ESOPHAGEAL RING

A persistent, ringlike constriction of the distalmost portion of the esophagus is observed during radiologic examination in certain patients.[3, 4] These individuals may or may not complain of dysphagia. When present, the symptom is usually chronologically unpredictable, and its occurrence may be frequent or infrequent. Although it is commonly caused by the ingestion of solid food, generally meat or bread, occlusion of the esophagus by the ingested bolus may occur at any time during the course of a given meal or may not occur at all. The obturation is commonly relieved spontaneously by distal progression of the occluding bolus or by its regurgitation. Furthermore, following relief of the obstruction, the patient can usually resume eating the same food without recurrence of dysphagic symptoms.

The transverse diameter of the ring varies from one patient to another, but is remarkably constant in any given patient. The degree of severity of dysphagia can be related to the diameter of the ring; those less than 13mm are almost always symptomatic, those from 13mm to 25mm occasionally produce symptoms, while those in excess of 25mm are asymptomatic.

In all instances, the ring is located at the gastroesophageal mucosal junction and occurs in patients with esophageal hiatus sliding hernia (Fig. 13-1).

During esophagoscopic examination, the ring is usually observed when its diameter is less, or only slightly greater, than the diameter of the instrument being used. It may be of value diagnostically, in some patients, to use an oversized esophagoscope.[5] The characteristic rugose and orange-red (or bright red, if inflamed) gastric mucosa is observable just beyond the ring (this is the mucosal lining of the herniated segment of stomach). Biopsy of a segment of the circumference of the ring demonstrates esophageal mucosa on one side and gastric mucosa on the other.

Treatment of this condition includes dietary instruction and periodic dilatation with bougies. Transesophagoscopic removal of a portion of the circumference of the ringlike structure, using biopsy forceps, may be performed in intractable cases.[5]

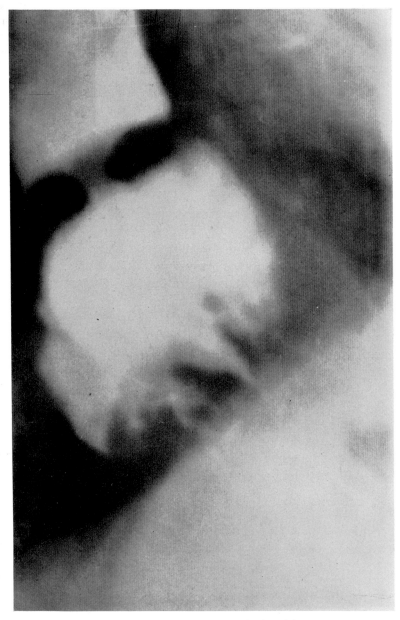

Figure 13-1. Lower esophageal (Schatzki) ring.

CARDIOESOPHAGEAL LESIONS

In the past, when the rigid-tube esophagoscopes and the lens-type gastroscopes were the only available endoscopic instruments, adequate inspection of the cardia was rather unsatisfactory. The area in question frequently was located beyond the reach of the esophagoscope or was not amenable to observation with the lateral-viewing gastroscope.

The development of fiberoptic instruments with controllable tips has permitted adequate visualization of this area. In this regard, the lateral-viewing gastroscopes are more satisfactory than the forward-viewing ones. The objectives of the former can be readily deflected and retroflexed, permitting a panoramic view of the instrument entering the stomach through the esophageal hiatus as well as the gastric cardia and fundus (Plate 19). Thus, lesions such as esophageal hiatus sliding hernia, benign and malignant neoplasms, gastric fundal diverticula, ulcers, varices, extragastric masses, etc., can be viewed.

The forward-viewing fiberoptic instruments with deflectable tips are usually better for visualizing gastric fundal varices and in tracing them proximally into the esophagus. The newest model of this instrument permits a 180-degree deflection of its tip, enabling the examiner to look back at the cardia without retroflexing the instrument itself. The reliability of this instrument for adequate inspection of the cardia remains to be seen. It should be of great value in obtaining biopsy specimens, since it is commonly much more simple and accurate to take a biopsy specimen through a forward-viewing instrument than through a lateral-viewing one.

Malignant neoplasms involving the gastric cardia may create technical problems by partially or completely obstructing passage of the instrument into the stomach.

These lesions usually are readily seen when the forward-viewing instruments are employed. The cardiac orifice in such cases is generally rigid, unyielding, friable, and irregularly outlined; a polypoid mass is frequently apparent just beyond the compromised opening. Definitive diagnosis must, of necessity, depend upon microscopic examination of a biopsy specimen obtained from the lesion. Occasionally, benign stricture of the terminal esophagus, especially when associated with severe inflammatory changes, may be mistakenly interpreted as a neoplasm (Plate 20).

CASE HISTORY

A 54-year-old male was admitted to the hospital because of progressively increasing difficulty in swallowing that had begun three months previously, and a weight loss of 25 pounds.

Radiologic examination demonstrated a narrowing at the gastroesophageal junction, with delayed transit through this region of the ingested barium.

Esophagoscopy disclosed narrowing, deformity, and rigidity of the cardiac orifice preventing entrance of the instrument into the stomach. Biopsy revealed the lesion to be adenocarcinoma.

JUNCTIONAL IDENTIFICATION

The esophagogastric mucosal junction (EGJ) represents the demarcation between the squamous-cell lining of the esophagus and the more distally located columnar-cell lining of the stomach. The mucosae, at this point, are tightly bound to the underlying muscular coat and do not prolapse in a retrograde or proximal direction; the junction, therefore, separates esophagus from stomach. The junction can be observed to move a distance of several centimeters in certain patients with esophageal hiatus sliding hernia ("wandering junction"), being displaced distally during advance of the instrument and drawn proximally as the instrument is withdrawn. This is more commonly observed when the flexi-rigid esophagoscope is used. The movement of the junction occurs in association with similar movement of the underlying layers of esophagus and stomach.

Except when obstructing lesions or anatomic defects interfere, the EGJ should be identified during every esophagoscopic examination. As a corollary, the esophagus cannot be considered to have been adequately inspected unless the EGJ has been identified, since this represents the distal-most boundary of the organ.

The EGJ normally is readily identified. The sharpness of the mucosal color change (yellow-pink of the esophagus to orange-red of the stomach) is characteristic; the velvety appearance of the gastric mucosa contrasts with the smooth lining of the esophagus. The two mucosae interdigitate at the junction, producing an irregular circumferential outline which assumes the form of a smoothly undulating (sinusoidal) curve. Use of the term "Z (for zig-zag) line" applied to the appearance of the junction should be discouraged, since it erroneously implies sharply angular peaks and valleys rather than the smooth outline which is always manifested.

The junction is even more distinct when inflammatory changes affect the esophageal and/or the gastric mucosae. Reddening of either mucosa alone intensifies the junction point. The latter is also clearly apparent in the presence of distal esophagitis, since the erosive component stops abruptly at the junction. On the other hand, junction identification is more difficult when advanced atrophic changes affect the gastric mucosa. In such instances, the pallor and smoothness of the gastric mucosa may closely resemble that of the esophagus, rendering the transition zone less distinct. In such cases, identification of the bright red network of submucosal venules which characterize the gastroesophageal vestibule[6] will assist in establishing the location of the junction point.

REFERENCES

1. Mallory, G. K., and Weiss, S.: Hemorrhages from lacerations of the cardiac orifice of the stomach due to vomiting. *Am J Med Sc, 178*:506, 1929.
2. Dagradi, A. E., Broderick, J. T., Juler, G., Wolinski, S., and Stempien, S. J.: The Mallory-Weiss syndrome and lesion. *Am J Digest Dis,* new series, Vol. *II*, No. 9, 1966.
3. Schatzki, R., and Gary, J. E.: Dysphagia due to a diaphragm-like localized narrowing in the lower esophagus ("lower esophageal ring"). *Am J Roentgenol, 70*:911–922, 1953.
4. Schatzki, R., and Gary, J. E.: The lower esophageal ring. *Am J Roentgenol, 75*:246, 1956.
5. Som, M. L., Wolf, B. S., and Marshak, R. H.: Narrow esophago-gastric ring treated endoscopically. *Gastroenterology, 39*:634, 1960.
6. Dagradi, A. E., Killeen, R. N., and Schindler, R.: Esophageal hiatus sliding hernia: An endoscopic study. *Gastroenterology, 33(1)*:54, 1958.

SECTION III:

ENDOSCOPIC PATHOLOGY OF THE STOMACH

CHAPTER 14

GASTROCAMERA: ITS PAST AND FUTURE

Shinroku Ashizawa and Yoshihiro Sakai

DEVELOPMENTAL HISTORY

THE GASTROCAMERA WAS first developed in 1950 by Uji, Sugiura and Fukami working with engineers of the Olympus Optical Company of Tokyo, Japan.[1] This instrument was an extremely small camera attached to the distal end of a flexible tube. The camera was easily inserted into the stomach and was remotely controlled by an operational panel at the proximal end of the instrument by flashing an intragastric lamp built into the camera. This made it possible to obtain sharp photographs in a wide range of mucosal membrane of the living stomach. This device was soon modified to include recording capability and to reduce mechanical difficulties. A very practical instrument was developed by a series of modifications and reported by Tasaka and Ashizawa[2, 3] before the World Congress held in Washington, D.C., in 1958. This model was the GT-III. It was better tolerated by the patient and had a higher rate of successful gastrophotography than earlier models. This was the first report before a world group. The photographs were enthusiastically viewed and the presentation warmly received.

On the following day, one of us, Ashizawa, accompanied Berry to the Freedman's Hospital in Washington where the first gastrocamera photographs in America were made. A few days later, Ashizawa and Berry performed similar demonstrations in the Gastroscopy Clinic of the Cook County Hospital, Chicago. Following these occasions, Berry continued gastrocamera examinations with the cooperation of Professor Tasaka and the Olympus Company of Japan at the Cook County Hospital, Chicago for

223

several months. Because of very difficult circumstances, at this early period, the project was discontinued. It was four years later that Yoshio F. Hara of the University of Japan, came to the University of Wisconsin and working with Morrissey, carried out the first reportable gastrocamera studies in the United States.

Improved Blind Gastrocamera

In 1960, gastrocamera model GT-V was completed and was found to have the most successful optical system ever developed for clinical use. Gastrophotography examination with this instrument has provided high quality and satisfactory photographs except for the existence of some blind areas. Many endoscopists, namely Tanaka,[4] Fugimori,[5] Okabe,[6] Yoshitishi[7] and Nakayama,[8] modified the GT-V gastrocamera in attempts to improve visualization of the whole stomach.

In 1964, Ashizawa[9] bent the tip of the GT-V gastrocamera upward using an external string. This instrument is known as the model GT-Va gastrocamera. By using this device, one can take pictures of the entire stomach eliminating all blind areas.[10] Sometimes it is difficult to photograph distant views or tangential views of lesions in certain parts of the stomach such as the cardia, fornix and other portions. Model GT-Va in 1965 and GT-W in 1970 have been developed for resolving these problems. The joint-type tilting mechanism is no longer used in these models, several of which are seen in Figure 14-1. In the case of the GT-Va, the instrument can be bent smoothly through an arc of 100 degrees up and down at a point of 10cm from the distal end. The GT-W bends 110 degrees up and down at the tip and 90 degrees from side to side so that four-way tilting is possible (Fig. 14-2). Gastrocamera has been developed to the point that it does all of the things photographically in the stomach which might be reasonably conceived (Plates 21-24). The more advanced improvements include auto-

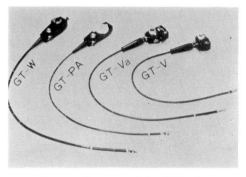

Figure 14-1. Four different models of blind gastrocamera.

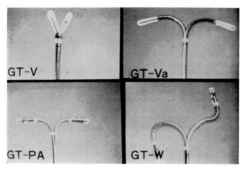

Figure 14-2. Closeup view of the tip of the four models of blind gastrocamera shown in Figure 14-1. Range of mobility in each model is depicted.

matic exposure system, automatic winding mechanism, close-up warning sound and automatic inflation systems.

Gastrocamera With Fiberscope

In spite of the remarkable developments with the gastrocamera, it is still a blind procedure. All other things being equal, it should be more desirable to see the lesion as it is being photographed. During the early years of the development of the gastrocamera, the only practical gastroscope was the Schindler-type lens constructed instrument which is semi-rigid. Because of the greater ease and relative simplicity of the gastrocamera procedure, it became very popular in Japan. At the same time, there was a considerable loss of interest in the Schindler-type lens gastroscope in Japan. On the other hand, interest and development of gastroscopy continued in the United States and Europe. In 1958, at the annual meeting of the American Gastroscopic Society, Hirschowitz and associates[11] introduced the first gastrofiberscope. By 1964, there had been developed in Japan a combined fiberscope and gastrocamera known as the Olympus G.T.F. (Fig. 14-3). This was developed by the Olympus Company working with researchers primarily of the Japan Endoscopic Society and to a great extent under the leadership of Professor Tasaka, its president. This was a remarkable step forward in the developmental history of the gastrocamera. It was not very long before a two-way movable type feature was added to the GTF scope called the G.T.F.-A and its wide use began to spread rapidly throughout Japan[12] and many areas of the world outside of Japan. This instrument is illustrated in Figure 14-3. The GTF gastrocamera with fiberscope had an angle of vision of 60 degrees, an ocular magnification of seven times, an angle of photographic field of 80 degrees and the range of observation was automatic between 1cm and 10cm. The photographic range was from

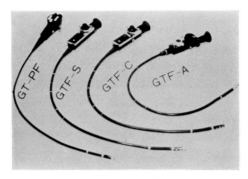

Figure 14-3. Four models of gastrofiberscope with camera.

2cm to 10cm. The GTF-S combined all of the photographic advances of the most advanced gastrocamera with the added feature of being able to see the lesions at the moment of photographing. While all of these features were being developed in Japan, the technics of extragastric photography and transendoscopic biopsy were being developed in the United States and Europe. Paradoxically, in spite of the brilliant developments in gastrocamera fiberscope technics, they have been somewhat overshadowed in some parts of the world by the continued demands for transendoscopic biopsy, brush cytology, polypectomy, etc. Since all of these features cannot as yet be set-up in a single instrument, the major developments have been in the direction of extragastric photography. Nevertheless, the photographic capability and the ease of operation of the gastrocamera and the gastro-camera fiberscope cannot be paralleled by extragastric camera methods.

TECHNIC

As for the clinical application of the gastrocamera as well as the gastro-camera combined with fiberscope, the primary and most important goal has been to obtain excellent photographs in the stomach and to have no blind areas. The technic of the use of both instruments is essentially the same except that one is a blind procedure partly directed by flashing the light through the abdominal wall. The gastrocamera fiberscope on the other hand is operated under direct vision. The following technic is primarily that which is used in the gastrocamera procedures: For obtaining picture in the pyloric antrum, the instrument is inserted deeply, yet gently into the stomach avoiding force. While feeding air gently and turning the objective toward the lesser curvature (11 o'clock position), with the patient on the left side, one can obtain the enface view and photographs of the angulus (Fig. 14-4.1) and the pyloric range as well as close-up views and photographs of the lesser curvature of the antrum (Fig. 14-4.2). The enface figures on the corresponding anterior and posterior walls of the antrum are obtained by rotating the tip of the scope alternately, counterclockwise and then clockwise; although one is not always successful in obtaining the enface view of the greater curvature of the antrum owing to the structure of earlier scopes. The recently devised dual tilting gastrocamera has made possible the obtaining of enface views in the greater majority of cases. As to the body of the stomach, the scope is placed in position with the tip turned slightly down (Fig. 14-4.3) or moderately down (Fig. 14-4.4). By gradually retrieving the instrument and rotating clockwise and counterclockwise, the body of the stomach, for the most part, can be photographed. The enface picture of the greater curvature of the body is best obtained with the objective toward six or seven o'clock with moderately downward angulation (Fig. 14-4.5). In order to obtain an enface view of the posterior wall, the lower U-turn method is essential. In this instance, the objective is faced to the greater curvature and the angulation is made strongly upward to bend the scope in the shape of a "U" (Fig. 14-4.8). Insert the shaft of the scope through the deepest position while keeping the tip relatively in the same "U" shaped position. Several shots are made during this process (see Figure 14-4.9). Finally, photographs of the upper stomach, the fornix and cardia are obtained by an upper U-turn technic. For this purpose, the scope is inserted in a more shallow position with the objective facing the greater

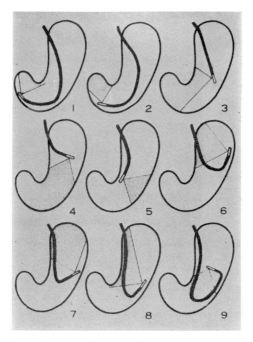

Figure 14-4. Field of visualization of stomach at various portions of gastrocamera in the stomach.

curvature and angulating the scope upward. Pictures of the fornix and cardia are obtained during the angulation, moderately upward positions (Fig. 14-4.7) and slightly upward positions (Fig. 14-4.6). Insufflation of air should be in amounts sufficient for taking photographs at various distances between the wall and the objective. The mucus lake which forms across the greater curvature in the cardiac region with the patient lying on the left side, can be dispersed by raising the head of the table and rotating the patient to the back and then to the right side position.

FUTURE USES

While the trends around the world are emphasizing transendoscopic procedures with extragastric photography, gastrocamera still has a great future. This will be particularly true in high gastric cancer incidence areas such as Japan. It has already played the principal role in the development of the Japanese early gastric cancer concept. If gastric cancer is to be diagnosed anatomically in the earliest stage possible, gastrocamera, which can be used for mass screening with extra technics, probably has the greatest advantage for the purpose of mass screening. Gastrocamera procedures should certainly be used in low gastric cancer incidence areas of the world to correlate epidemiological studies throughout the world.

For mass screening, the gastrocamera model GTP has been developed. This instrument is very slenderized and made softer, making it better tolerated by the patient, in some cases even without pharyngeal anesthesia. A large number of patients can be examined during a short period with this method. An improved mass screening gastrocamera is the GT-PA (see Figures 14-1 and 14-2). Model GT-PF is now on trial. It combines the slender gastrocamera model GT-PA with a fiberscope. Furthermore, a biopsy channel is attached in the GT-PF which allows for forceps and suction biopsy, brush cytology and for transendoscopic polypectomy. This instrument will be a remarkably useful scope in the near future.

REFERENCES

1. Uji, T., Sugiura, K., and Fukami, O.: Studies on photograph of gastric mucosa and its application. *Tokyo J Med* (Jap), *61*:135, 1952.
2. Tasaka, S., and Ashizawa, S.: Studies of diseases using the gastrocamera. *Am Gastroscop Soc Bull,* 5:12, 1958.
3. Tasaka, S.: Gastrocamera—Mechanics and clinical application. Ogata press, Tokyo (Jap), 1959.
4. Tanaka, K.: Photographing blind areas using specific gastrocamera. *Gastroent Endosc* (Jap), 3:154, 1961.
5. Fugimori, A.: Photography of the antrum using modified gastrocamera. *Gastroent Endosc* (Jap) 5:356, 1964.
6. Okabe, H., and Yao, K.: Studies on Cuff-gastrocamera. *Gastroent Endosc* (Jap), 5:380, 1964.

7. Yoshitoshi, Y., Niwa, K., and Hinoshita, Y.: Upper stomach lesions as diagnosed by gastrocamera. *Gastroent Endosc* (Jap), 5:356, 1964.
8. Nakayama, K.: Photography of the cardia using modified gastrocamera model II-N. *Gastroent Endosc* (Jap), 5:355, 1964.
9. Ashizawa, S.: Gastrocamera model Va. *Gastroent Endosc* (Jap), 5:258, 1964.
10. Ashizawa, S., and Oshima, H.: Gastrocamera-Untersuchung. *Zeitschrift fuer Gastroent* (Ger), 5:142, 1967.
11. Hirschowitz, B. I., Curtiss, L. E., Peters, C. W., and Pollard, H. M.: Demonstration of new gastroscope, the fiberscope. *Gastroent*, 35:50, 1958.
12. Utsumi, H., and Kaneko, Y.: Fiberscope and fibercamera. *Gastroent Endosc* (Jap), 7:146, 1965.

CHAPTER 15

BENIGN GASTRIC ULCERS*

RICHARD S. McCRAY

INTRODUCTION

GASTRIC ULCER IS one of the most important lesions for the endoscopist. Whereas in the past x-ray was the primary procedure for diagnosis, now direct gastroscopic visualization is increasingly appreciated. The rapid development of fiberoptic instruments in the past ten years provides complete visualization of virtually the entire stomach. Early endoscopy in the diagnosis of acute upper gastrointestinal hemorrhage demonstrates a number of gastric ulcers not visible to the radiologist.[1-5] With the increase of gastroscopy in patients with peptic symptoms but negative x-rays or radiographically deformed antrums, additional ulcers are demonstrated. Differential diagnosis of gastric ulcer improved significantly with recent advancements in instrumentation and technique. Direct vision biopsy and cytology are the definitive procedures for the diagnosis of gastric carcinoma.[6-9] Finally, the primary purpose of accurate diagnosis and differential diagnosis of gastric ulcer is to provide a basis for appropriate therapy. In the past most surgeons advocated immediate resection of all gastric ulcers[10, 11] because of the fear of cancer; with the development of endoscopic techniques, physicians are willing to take a more rational approach to treatment.[12] This chapter is designed to aid the endoscopist in his complete evaluation of the gastric ulcer and thereby enable him to advise proper therapy.

* Supported in part by a research grant in Endoscopy at St. Luke's Hospital, New York, N.Y. and in part by NIH Training Grant AM 05499.

ENDOSCOPIC PATHOLOGY
Acute and Chronic Ulcer

The endoscopist must learn to evaluate both the acute and the chronic gastric ulcer. Acute ulcers may be quite small and must first be differentiated from traumatic lesions caused by naso-gastric or irrigating tubes. Usually these tubes cause only erosions or abrasions which are red in color and occur either singly or in linear groups corresponding to the multiple openings of some naso-gastric tubes. Generally erosions from tubes are very superficial and cause more difficulty with differentiation from erosive gastritis than from acute gastric ulcer. In our experience, ulcers are distinguished from erosions by the appearance of depth and white exudate. The typical hemorrhagic gastritis caused by alcohol or aspirin is a very diffuse lesion composed of multiple punctuate hemorrhages resembling the exanthem of measles. The erosions may be somewhat larger, looking like the whole gastric mucosa has been scraped with *steel wool.*

Gastric ulcers may be multiple as the so-called *stress ulcers* or associated with the ingestion of gastric irritants such as alcohol or aspirin. These are real ulcers, i.e. they may penetrate into the submucosa or muscularis and are seen as white exudate with surrounding erythema. Superficial ulcers are usually multiple, yet we are impressed with how many acute massively bleeding patients have only single small ulcers. As has been found in all the large series reporting the value of endoscopy in acute hemorrhage,[1, 3–5] we also find a large number of single gastric ulcers too superficial to be demonstrated by x-ray.[2] Eighteen of our last 43 bleeding single gastric ulcers were seen by endoscopy alone. Only one moderate sized vessel must be ulcerated in order to produce significant hemorrhage.

Obviously, acutely bleeding ulcers may be of any size and even the large ulcers may be difficult to diagnose endoscopically. Gastric secretions may be thick and adherent, covering acute ulcers. Blood clots on the surface of the mucosa must be distinguished from those covering acute ulcers; therefore all blood on the surface must be examined closely. Usually white exudate is seen at the edge of a clot which is on an ulcer. The edge of the ulcer can be appreciated by seeing its penetration into the mucosa. Again, there is no substitute for meticulous care in complete visualization of the entire gastric mucosa. In order to distinguish a clot or mucus from a real ulcer, water or saline should be directed across the suspicious lesion. This may either be done through the air-water channel or a polyethylene tube may be passed through the biopsy channel and saline directed onto the suspicious area.

The chronic gastric ulcer presents a less difficult problem in diagnosis than it does in differential diagnosis. In the past, most chronic ulcers were sent for gastroscopy only after diagnosis by x-ray. However, as the value of endoscopy for the diagnosis of patients with peptic type pain and normal x-rays is increasingly appreciated, a number of ulcers are being found in x-ray negative patients. Nine of our last 29 patients with gastric ulcer and only peptic symptoms (i.e. no bleeding) had ulcers too superficial to be demonstrated by x-ray. Size of the ulcer may be very difficult to determine at gastroscopy and distance of the tip of the instrument from the crater is crucial for such determination. Measuring devices are now available which may be used with some experience. We use a flexible rod, calibrated in 2mm markings and passed through the biopsy channel. These devices are particularly useful for following the ulcer on repeated examinations to determine degree of healing.

Benignancy vs Malignancy

As soon as an ulcer is visualized, by x-ray and/or endoscopy, it must be evaluated for benignancy or malignancy. It must always be remembered that endoscopic as well as radiographic diagnosis is only gross diagnosis. A number of characteristics must be carefully evaluated. Size of a gastric ulcer as an indicator of whether it is benign or malignant is debated. Some have found giant gastric ulcers are more likely malignant but others, the opposite.[13] Location has traditionally been thought to be important i.e. benign gastric ulcer found on the lesser and malignant on the greater curvature. However, there are so many exceptions to this that location is no more important a sign than is size.[14]

Both radiographic and gastroscopic appearance of the benign gastric ulcer depend on the underlying pathology and should be considered on the basis of that pathology. A benign gastric ulcer is an inflammatory lesion which displaces the normal gastric wall to varying depths. Some ulcers only penetrate the mucosa whereas others extend into the muscularis. The ulcer base is composed of granulation tissue covered by destroyed gastric and inflammatory cells seen grossly as the exudate. Inflammation composed of edema and acute and chronic inflammatory cells extends to varying distances beyond the edge of the ulcer crater. The junction between exudate and surrounding inflammation is relatively distinct, giving the edge of the ulcer a sharp contour. Just as the depth varies among ulcers, so does the amount of surrounding edema and inflammation. It must be remembered that the surrounding mucosa is just edematous and inflamed and therefore, is soft and pliable and does not interfere with normal gastric fold contour or peristalsis.

These pathologic features produce characteristic x-ray findings (Fig. 15-1). The ulcer crater itself produces the so-called ulcer niche, penetrating to varying depths into the gastric wall. If the ulcer is demonstrated in

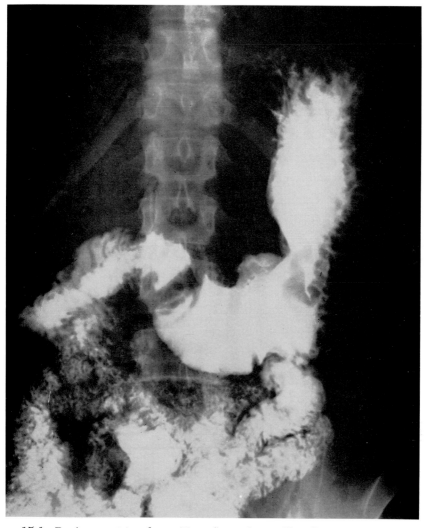

Figure 15-1. Benign gastric ulcer: Note "extra-luminal" collection of barium with radiating gastric folds approaching the smooth edge.

profile by the radiologist, the barium will be seen penetrating beyond the inside edge of the wall of the stomach.[15] One of the most important radiographic signs is then that the ulcer is "extraluminal."[16] Other important radiographic signs are the thin radiolucent "Hampton's line," the somewhat thicker "ulcer collar" or the thicker still "ulcer mound" all thought to be caused by varying amounts of surrounding edema. Edema is the most important variable for the radiologist. When there is significant edema, the benign ulcer may appear radiographically to be "intraluminal" and therefore in a tumor mass (Fig. 15-2). In these ulcers, the

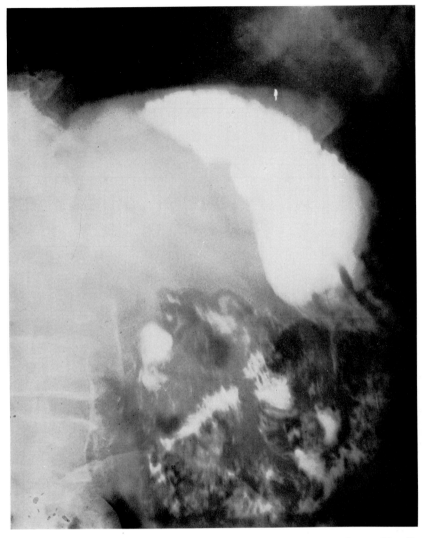

Figure 15-2. (Grossly malignant) benign gastric ulcer: Note "intra-luminal" collection of barium with "overhanging edges" caused by edema surrounding the ulcer.

"shoulders" or edges of the "ulcer mound" must be examined closely for smoothness and peristalsis seen passing over normally appearing folds through the area of the ulcer. Antral ulcers usually cause more difficulty for the radiologist than do ulcers higher in the stomach. Spasm is more of a problem in the antrum as it may produce bizarre configurations. Antral ulcers on the anterior or posterior walls can be very difficult to bring into profile. Finally, the nature of the surrounding mucosa which is so important for differential diagnosis may be best evaluated by the "double-contrast" methods described so well by Japanese radiologists.[17]

Although the gastroscopist has a more direct view of the ulcer, he too may have difficulties in evaluating the benign gastric ulcer. Endoscopically, the benign gastric ulcer has a "punched-out" appearance (Plate 25). Depth varies considerably and may be best appreciated when the ulcer is seen from the side, viewed from above. However, deep ulcers may be missed "on the way down" especially with forward viewing instruments and the tip of the instrument must be turned in order to view the ulcer en fasse. The base of the ulcer covered by inflammatory exudate is classically clean and white but may be somewhat gray in color. If the ulcer has bled recently, varying amounts of blood clot may be seen. The typical benign ulcer is circular but may be somewhat elliptical. More important than shape is the contour of the edges; there is a sharp demarcation between ulcer base and surrounding edge. The smooth, soft, pliable edges may be well appreciated by the endoscopist. Again the surrounding mucosa must be closely examined. Overhanging edges, which cause the radiologist so much difficulty, may be directly examined by the endoscopist. Surrounding mucosa is regularly edematous and often somewhat erythematous but it is smooth and gastric folds, swollen to varying degrees by edema, are seen approaching the edge of the ulcer. Softness and pliability may be appreciated by insufflating air which will flatten even edematous mucosa. Air may reduce spasm in the antrum so that normal surrounding mucosa may be better appreciated by the gastroscopist than the radiologist. The tip of the instrument must be positioned so that the entire edge of the ulcer and surrounding mucosa is examined. Anticholinergic pre-medication may make visualization easier but it has the real disadvantage of reducing peristalsis. Just as the fluoroscopist watches peristalsis closely, so should the endoscopist make sure that normal peristalsis passes through the area of the ulcer.

All of these radiographic and endoscopic criteria are obviously to distinguish the benign from malignant gastric ulcer. The malignant ulcer occurs in a tumor mass, thought to be caused by the tumor outgrowing its blood supply. Therefore the cancer is primary and the ulcer secondary. Cancer replaces normal mucosa as it penetrates into the submucosal layers growing into the lumen of the stomach as well as penetrating into the wall. Tumor growth is disorganized and therefore produces irregular tissue. When the cancer ulcerates it does so in an irregular manner. Thus radiographically the collection of barium is seen within the tumor mass (Fig. 15-3). When the ulcer is seen in profile it appears to be "intraluminal." The edges are not smooth but are distorted by the nodular edge of the tumor. The surrounding mucosa may itself be normal but it is covering tumor and therefore not only irregular, but hard and fixed. Neither normal gastric folds nor peristaltic waves approach the edge of the ulcer but stop at varying distances depending on the size of the underlying tumor mass.

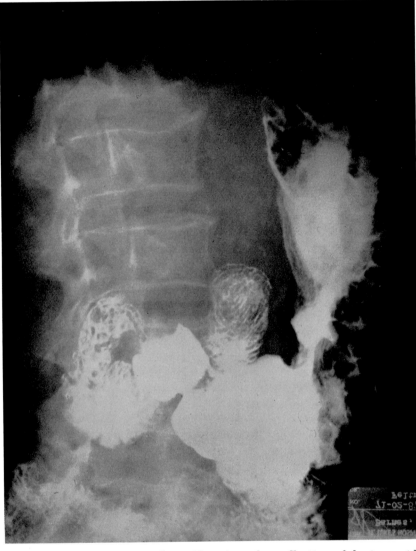

Figure 15-3. Malignant gastric ulcer: Note irregular collection of barium within a large tumor mass in the body of the stomach.

Gastroscopy adds little to the differential diagnosis of large fungating, grossly malignant ulcers. The base of such an ulcer is often described as a dirty grey but color of exudate does not, in our opinion, contribute much to differential diagnosis. The intraluminal nature of the ulcer is easily appreciated gastroscopically as the tumor mass may not be flattened by air. Nodules of tumor tissue, often red in color, may be seen forming the irregular edge of the ulcer. Rigidity of the surrounding mucosa may be well appreciated, again prohibiting normal peristalsis. More subtle changes in smaller tumors may be better evaluated gastroscopically than radiographically. Less marked irregularities in edge contour and superficial plaques of tumor tissue may be appreciated as the lesion is closely examined. The malignant ulcer is further described in Chapters 17 and 18.

Unfortunately, many ulcers do not conform to these characteristics. Edema around a benign ulcer may make it appear to be in a mass both on x-ray and at gastroscopy or even at surgery. Four of our last 45 malignant and 3 of our last 57 benign resected gastric ulcers were erroneously diagnosed grossly at surgery. Lymphosarcoma may be especially difficult to differentiate from benign ulcer with edema.

Another problem with malignant ulcers is obstruction caused by the surrounding tumor. Distal antral cancers may cause so much obstruction that the differential diagnosis of scarring secondary to peptic disease or an obstructing tumor may be virtually impossible on x-ray. These tumors, which are often ulcerated, may grow submucosally, completely obscuring endoscopic visualization of the ulcer (Plate 26). Attempts to diagnose malignancy on the basis of photographic material have apparently not improved overall diagnostic accuracy.

Finally, in our experience most criteria apply to large lesions. Ulcers which appear grossly malignant are unfortunately usually in tumors which have already spread too widely for complete surgical resection. Whereas the earlier Borrmann classification emphasized by Schindler[18] applies to large, usually advanced cancer, the Japan Endoscopy Society has developed a relatively complex system (see Chapter 18) of classification for early gastric cancer.[19] These classifications may be important for prognosis but in our opinion contribute little to diagnosis.

Thus there are special problems even for the gross evaluation of acute and chronic gastric ulcers. It must be remembered that such diagnosis is gross and even the most enthusiastic gastroscopists realize cytology and endoscopic directed biopsy are the most definitive procedures for differential diagnosis. A number of special endoscopic techniques, recently developed, provide both gross and microscopic diagnosis of the acute and chronic gastric ulcer.

The latest Veteran's Administration study of the gastric ulcer found gastroscopy (without biopsy or cytology) added nothing to x-ray for differential diagnosis.[20] However, biopsy and cytology are the two procedures which make gastroscopy indispensable for the differential diagnosis of the gastric ulcer.

Cytology and Biopsy

Gastric cytology is extremely accurate in experienced hands.[7, 8, 19] Some advocate direct vision washing through the gastroscope and others the use of a brush passed through the biopsy channel and applied directly to the ulcer and suspicious surrounding mucosa. Specific instruments have been developed for these procedures. Details of this technic are described in Chapter 27.

Many workers emphasize endoscopic biopsy.[6, 7, 14, 19] We have placed similar emphasis on this technic.

Direct vision gastric biopsy has long been a part of the complete endoscopic examination.[6, 7, 14, 19–22] Forceps were passed through the semiflexible gastroscopes but precise biopsy was nearly impossible until fiberoptic instruments were developed, capable of directing the forceps with *pin-point* control. Japanese workers have found that tumor cells are most likely to be obtained in biopsies of the "inside edge" of the ulcer[6] (Plate 27). If the base of the ulcer is biopsied, usually only necrotic debris or granulation tissue is obtained. The tumor may be covered by normal mucosa so that biopsies of tissue away from the edge of the ulcer often are not deep enough to be positive. In addition, multiple biopsies must be taken from the entire edge, as often, only one side of the ulcer is infiltrated with tumor cells (Fig. 15-4). We have found gastric biopsy our most accurate diagnostic procedure. We have obtained malignant tissue from 63 of our last 64 ulcerated carcinomas. Tumors which are not ulcerated or which cause proximal obstruction are very difficult to biopsy. Biopsies obtained with existing forceps are still relatively superficial and may miss submucosal lesions.

Both cytology and biopsy of ulcers in the presence of significant obstruction warrants special consideration. As discussed previously, ulcers in the distal antrum, either benign or malignant, may cause enough obstruction to either partially or completely obscure gastroscopic visualization (Fig. 15-2). Mucosa over an infiltrating tumor may be grossly indistinguishable from edema surrounding a benign ulcer. We have learned that either cytology or biopsy of this overlying mucosa may not be expected to yield tumor cells. The cytology brush should be inserted into the orifice of the obstruction, rotated and pulled back and forth blindly. The biopsy

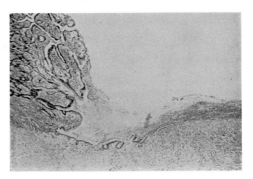

Figure 15-4. Microscopic surgical section of upper edge of malignant ulcer. Note healing margin exhibiting re-epithelialization with no evidence of malignancy.

forceps should also be passed closed through the orifice of the obstruction, then opened with it in the obstructed channel and biopsies obtained blindly. Thus, even if it is not possible to see the ulcer, both cytology and biopsy may be obtained. Reported overall accuracy varies widely among investigators. Furthermore, accuracy should increase significantly with advances in instrumentation. Kasugai[6] emphasized in 1968 that most of his failures were with tumors located high in the body and in the antrum of the stomach. These are the two areas at which recent modifications are directed. Large series will now be needed to obtain accurate evaluation of these most modern instruments. The following case illustrates the importance of such precise biopsy.

CASE HISTORY

F. G., a 68-year-old male, first presented with severe mid-epigastric burning

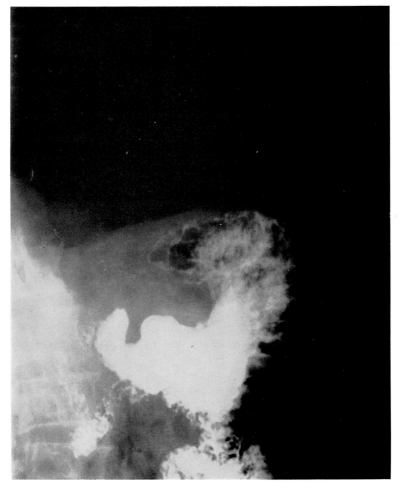

Figure 15-5. Initial ulcer: Note small "extra-luminal" collection of barium on the lesser curvature near the incisura.

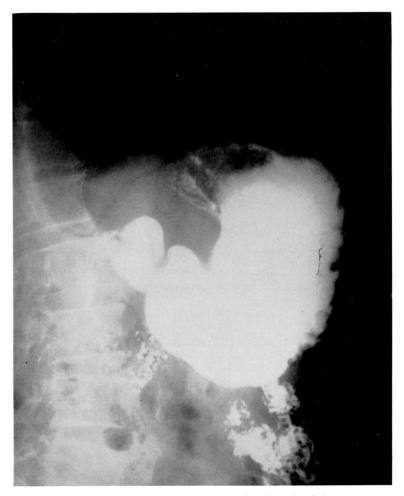

Figure 15-6. Normal x-ray after 3 months of medical therapy.

pain partially relieved by milk and worse at night. He lost ten pounds over the previous year. Past medical history included chronic bronchitis, emphysema, arrested tuberculosis and arteriosclerotic cardiovascular disease with congestive heart failure. Physical examination revealed a well developed, well nourished male with evidence of his cardiopulmonary disease, an enlarged liver and mild mid-epigastric tenderness. He was not anemic and stool guaiac was negative. Upper gastrointestinal roentgenogram revealed an "outpocketing on the lesser curvature consistent with a benign gastric ulcer" (Fig. 15-5). He was given a bland diet, antacids and sedation and a repeat x-ray three months later was normal (Fig. 15-6). He was followed in the outpatient department with chronic pain for the next seven months. He then had his first episode of melena and was admitted to the hospital. Physical examination again revealed signs of chronic lung disease and moderate mid-epigastric tenderness without palpable organs or masses. Hematocrit dropped from 47 to 37 with hydration but transfusion was not required. Stool was 4+ guaiac. Roentgenogram on the day following admission revealed a large ulcer on the lesser curvature measuring 4½cm across its base (Fig. 15-7). The radiologist felt there was no evidence of gastric mass and the stiffness of the lesser curvature surrounding the ulcer crater was interpreted as "due to severe edema of the stomach wall." Maximal histalog stimulation produced 48 mEq H+ per hour. Gastroscopy, performed on the seventh hospital day, confirmed a large ulcer on the lesser curvature just above the angulus. It had "well demarcated borders. The surrounding mucosa appeared reddened." One of 6 biopsies revealed adenocarcinoma (Fig. 15-8).

This patient had a complicated course due to his cardiopulmonary problems and surgery was delayed until the 22nd hospital day. At surgery, a large endurated area with ulceration on the lesser curvature was found. "The pylorous felt thickened and scarred." The post-operative diagnosis was "lesser curvature gastric ulcer with peptic disease and secondary scarring of the pyloric area." Gross pathology revealed "a lesser curvature rhomboidal 11 by 7mm smooth edged ulcer with a depressed crater which had some perceptible radiating ridges. The ulcer crater is subtended by a fan of whitish fibrous tissue, forming the

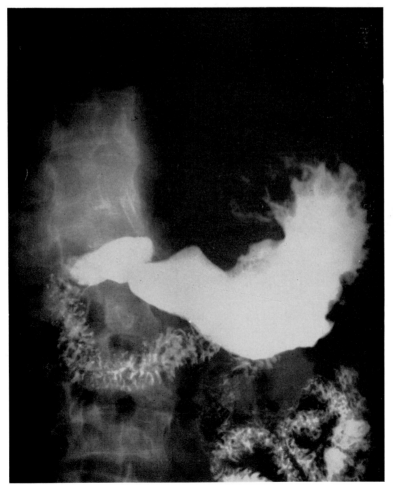

Figure 15-7. F. G. large recurrent gastric cancer, grossly benign: Note "extra-luminal" collection of barium with smooth edges and grossly normal surrounding mucosa.

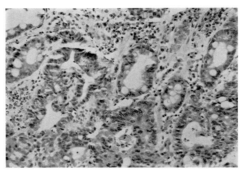

Figure 15-8. Gastroscopic biopsy of intramucosal adenocarcinoma. Note the commingling of intestinal metaplastic and neoplastic glands seen in the superficial mucosa.

posterior wall margin. Contingent to the ulcer was a raised cobbled reddish plaque 13 by 10mm" (Plate 28).

A microscopic section taken through the center of the ulcer illustrates why even deeper biopsies of the ulcer crater often fail to obtain malignant cells. The inflammatory exudate is seen above and the regenerating granulation tissue below. A section through the upper edge of the ulcer shows only regenerating mucosa. A section through the bottom malignant edge shows the intramucosal tumor. Fortunately, one of the six gastroscopic biopsies was taken from this edge and therefore made the correct malignant diagnosis of this benign appearing ulcer.

This patient had acute and chronic lung disease, a classical peptic pain pattern, massive acid secretion and a previous ulcer in the same place with complete radiographic healing one year previously. He almost healed his ulcer (4½cm to 11mm) after three weeks of intensive medical therapy which he received because he was such a poor surgical risk. Without the positive biopsy, surgery probably would not have been considered again. Five years later the patient still has his peptic type pain but does not have any evidence of cancer.

Direct vision gastric biopsy is not only important for the diagnosis of malignant but also benign gastric ulcers. In the past, some have maintained that only malignant biopsies should be considered diagnostic. Of course this is the safest and most conservative position to take. It is difficult not to operate on an ulcer which appears malignant on x-ray and grossly so on endoscopy. Others emphasize the test of healing, expecting at least 50 per cent at three to six week intervals. The case discussed above illustrates the fear of the malignant ulcer that heals with medical therapy. However, with recent advances in x-ray, endoscopic biopsy and cytology, it seems reasonable to follow medically those ulcers diagnosed benign by these procedures. It seems reasonable to re-biopsy any ulcer from which inadequate biopsies have been obtained. Finally, ulcers should be closely followed with repeat endoscopy and biopsy at three to six week intervals until the ulcer is completely healed. We have now biopsied 185 benign ulcers and have had no false positive biopsies.

The following case illustrates the value of endoscopic biopsy for the diagnosis of benign gastric cancer.

CASE HISTORY

S. M., a 67-year-old female, was admitted with her first episode of painless hematemesis and melena. She had some anorexia and *gas* and lost about 15 pounds over the last six months. She had been in good health all her life except for an acute myocardial infarction five years before admission and an adult onset of diabetes mellitus. She denied any other gastrointestinal complaints and had ingested no known gastric irritants. She denied recent emotional stress. Physical examination was normal except for an enlarged heart with a grade 4 systolic precordial murmur and guaiac positive stool. Hematocrit dropped from 30 to 25 with hydration but she did not require transfusion. Upper gastrointestinal x-rays were performed two days after admission and revealed a large, approximately 2cm ulcer on the lesser curvature which appeared intraluminal and therefore "associated either with a large amount of edema or with a tumor mass." Gastroscopy, performed on the seventh hospital day, revealed a "large ulcer in a mass with smooth edges high on the posterior wall" (Plate 29). A lymphosarcoma was seriously considered by the endoscopist. Eight biopsies were obtained from around the inside edge of the ulcer and the surrounding mucosa. The biopsies were consistent with benign gastric ulcer and the patient was placed on a bland diet with sedation in the hospital. Repeat x-ray and gastroscopy on the 22nd and 24th hospital days revealed complete healing. The patient has had no further gastrointestinal complaints for the past 3 years.

This was a 67-year-old woman with painless bleeding and a very suspicious ulcer both by x-ray and endoscopy. Edema surrounding an ulcer was just as much of a problem for the endoscopist as for the radiologist. Although the base of the ulcer appeared clean and the edges were perfectly smooth without any suggestion of nodularity, the edema made the ulcer appear as if it were in a tumor mass. It was suggestive of a lymphosarcoma. Without the biopsies, this patient would certainly have had an unnecessary gastrectomy.

Some of our cases have developed a gastric ulcer while on steroid therapy for arthritis. In one instance, there was a moderately large gross hemorrhage. Plate 30 shows a large steroid ulcer on lesser curvature. Note tiny clots at probable site of gross hemorrhage four hours before. Plate 31 is an example of a case of healing benign prepyloric ulcer, not seen on x-ray. Side-viewing scope left side.

The final case illustrates some of the finer points which must be clearly followed if accurate diagnosis is to be made.

CASE HISTORY

L. S., a 58-year-old female was first admitted with a six month history of mid-epigastric and substernal post-prandial pain and 5 pound weight loss of six months duration. Physical examination was normal as were all blood tests. Upper gastrointestinal roentgenogram revealed a deformed antrum with lesser curvature grossly benign ulcer. Gastroscopy with a lateral viewing instrument failed to visualize the distal antrum. She was treated medically and repeat x-ray was normal 3 weeks later. She was discharged to clinic and was asymptomatic for about 20 months. Her pain then recurred but an x-ray was normal.

Because of continued pain she was readmitted and gastroscopy revealed pyloric and antral deformity and two grossly benign antral ulcers. Three biopsies were obtained which revealed only inflamed mucosa and no ulcer granulation tissue or ulcer edge.

The patient was discharged and followed in clinic where her only complaint was anorexia but she had no weight loss. She refused repeat gastroscopy to follow the ulcers to complete healing. She finally agreed to repeat x-rays 10 months later. The antrum was badly deformed with possibly several ulcers and interpreted as ulcerated carcinoma. Gastroscopy revealed a fixed antrum with two very suspicious ulcers. Biopsies were positive for adenocarcinoma. The tumor was resected and one regional lymph node was positive.

This case illustrates some previous and present problems. Whereas initial x-ray and endoscopic diagnoses were benign, biopsies were not adequate. Her initial ulcer was not even visible with the gastroscope available at that time. That ulcer healed at least radiographically. Upon biopsy of her recurrent ulcers, only 3 specimens were obtained. It is suggested to take a minimum of 5 or 6 biopsies from each ulcer. Neither ulcer granulation tissue nor edge of ulcer were present on the initial biopsies. With inadequate biopsies the patient should have been reexamined and rebiopsied.

A recent report of significant healing of a number of malignant ulcers[22] reemphasizes the necessity for following all ulcers to complete healing. Whereas an occasional malignant ulcer may heal completely, this must be a very rare occurrence. If biopsy and cytology had been performed repeatedly on this patient, the correct diagnosis would probably have been made on the first admission.

SUMMARY AND CONCLUSIONS

Many advances have been made in the last ten years in the endoscopic diagnosis of the gastric ulcer. Ulcers throughout the stomach may be adequately visualized by both forward and lateral viewing instruments. Documentation of findings may be made with excellent photography.[23] These improvements in instrumentation have significantly increased diagnostic accuracy in upper gastrointestinal hemorrhage and in the differential diagnosis of the gastric ulcer. Bleeding ulcers and ulcerations may be visualized in any part of the stomach as part of a complete examination of the esophagus, stomach and duodenum. Direct vision cytology and biopsy add microscopic to gross endoscopic diagnosis of benign and malignant lesions.[24, 25] With such gross and microscopic findings, correct diagnosis may be made in virtually all of these gastric lesions. An increasing number of ulcers may be found endoscopically to account for peptic pain and negative x-rays. Only on the basis of such precise diagnosis of acutely bleeding or chronic gastric ulcers may appropriate medical or surgical therapy be instituted.

REFERENCES

1. Dagradi, A. E., Stempien, S. J., and Lee, E. R.: The indication for endoscopy in acute gastrointestinal hemorrhage. *Gastrointest Endosc, 13*:22, 1966.

2. Gang, M. J., and McCray, R. S.: Emergent endoscopy in a voluntary hospital. *Gastrointest Endosc, 26*:231, 1970.
3. Hedberg, S. E.: Early endoscopic diagnosis in upper gastrointestinal hemorrhage. *Surg Clin N Amer, 46*:499, 1966.
4. Katz, D., Douvres, P., Weisberg, H., McKinnon, W., and Jerzy Glass, G. B.: Early endoscopic diagnosis of acute upper gastrointestinal hemorrhage. *JAMA, 5*:405, 1964.
5. Palmer, E. D.: The vigorous diagnostic approach to upper gastrointestinal hemorrhage. *JAMA, 207*:1477, 1969.
6. Kasugai, T.: Gastric biopsy under direct vision by the fibergastroscope. *Gastrointest Endosc, 15*:33, 1968.
7. Kobayashi, S., Prolla, J. C., Winans, C. S., and Kirsner, J. B.: Improved endoscopic diagnosis of gastroesophageal cancer, combined use of direct vision cytology and biopsy. *JAMA, 212*:2086, 1970.
8. Rubin, C. E., Massey, B. W., Kirsner, J. B., Palmer, W. L., and Stonecypher, D. D.: The clinical value of gastrointestinal cytology. *Gastroenterology, 54*:729, 1968.
9. Weiss, J. B., Gang, M. J., Ekkers, T. J., Gaetz, H. P., and McCray, R. S.: Direct vision gastric biopsy using the Machida FGS-B$_6$ gastroscope. *Gastrointest Endosc, 17*:23, 1970.
10. Raudin, I. S., and Horn, R. C., Jr.: Gastric ulcer and gastric cancer. *Ann Surg, 137*:904, 1953.
11. Zollinger, R. M., Watman, R. N., and Denkwalter, F.: Should all gastric ulcers be treated surgically? *Gastroenterology, 35*:521, 1958.
12. Zollinger, R. M., Morrissey, J. F., Steigmann, F., and Ochsner, A.: Ulcers of the stomach. *Post Grad Med, 50,* 6:82, 1971.
13. Asbury, G. F.: Giant gastric ulcer. *Arch Surg, 89*:488, 1964.
14. Spiro, H. M.: *Clinical Gastroenterology.* London, Collier, Macmillan, 1970, p. 251.
15. Wolf, B. S., and Marshak, R. H.: Profile features of benign gastric niches on Roentgen examination. *Mt. Sinai Hospital Bulletin,* 24.
16. Schatzki, R.: Personal communication.
17. Shirakabe, H.: *Atlas of X-ray Diagnosis of Early Cancer.* Tokyo, Igahu Shoin Ltd.
18. Schindler, R.: *Gastroscopy. The Endoscopic Study of Gastric Pathology.* University of Chicago Monographs in Medicine, 1937, pp. 241-246.
19. Prolla, J. C., Kobayashi, S., and Kirsner, J. B.: Gastric cancer, some recent improvements in diagnosis based upon the Japanese experience. *Arch Int Med, 124*:238, 1969.
20. Fruin, R. G.: Gastroscopy in Veterans Administration cooperative study on gastric ulcer. *Gastroenterology, 61*:632, 1971.
21. Benedict, B.: An operating gastroscope. *Gastroenterology, 11*:281, 1948.
22. Sakita, T., Oguro, Y., Takasu, S., Hisayuki, F., Miwa, T., and Yoshimori, M.: Observations on the healing of ulcerations in early cancer. *Gastroenterology, 60*:835, 1971.
23. Ashizawa, S., and Kidokoro, T.: *Endoscopic Color Atlas of Gastric Disease.* Bunkodo Co., Ltd., Tokyo, Japan, 1970, pp. 136-137.
24. Hampton, A. D.: Incidence of malignancy in chronic prepyloric gastric ulcerations. *Am J Roentgenol, 30*:473, 1933.
25. Baron, J. H.: An assessment of the augmented histamine test in the diagnosis of peptic ulcer. *GUT, 4*:243, 1963.

CHAPTER 16

BENIGN NEOPLASMS, MALFORMATIONS, FOREIGN BODIES

LEONIDAS H. BERRY

INTRODUCTORY STATEMENT

THE PROBLEM of benign gastric tumors is of special importance to the present day gastroscopist from two important points of view. First, diagnosis is becoming more and more endoscopically accurate and refined. Secondly, treatment by transendoscopic polypectomy has become not only a reality but is rapidly growing as a common technique among more progressive endoscopists.

The neophyte endoscopist will begin very early to perform diagnostic biopsy and with some experience may feel challenged to completely extirpate small polyps by the multiple biopsy method. Advanced students of endoscopy may sooner or later wish to remove polyps by the snare and electrocautery method (See Chapter 28-II). Biopsy and extirpation may both be regarded as diagnostic procedures since a negative biopsy never completely ruled out malignancy. For the reasons mentioned and others, gastroscopic consideration of benign neoplasms is taking on an increasing significance at this point in time.

ADENOMATOUS POLYPS

The occurrence of benign adenomatous polyps of the stomach is well known and continues to pose a dilemma for physician and surgeon. They have been observed and studied throughout the era of roentgenography and gastroscopy and are recorded as incidental findings in many postmortem examinations.

Incidence

Schindler[1] reports benign polyps in his early gastroscopic inventories as having an incidence of about 2 per cent in all patients gastroscoped. In our own series of 5,858 gastroscopies reported at the Second World Congress of Gastrointestinal Endoscopy, there were 106 gastroscopic diagnoses of benign polyps, or 1.9 per cent.[2] Only a few of these cases were confirmed by gastrobiopsy. There have been other gastroscopy series which reported about the same incidence of adenomatous polyps prior to the availability of improved routine gastrobiopsy. Ariga, et al.[3] at Nihon University, Japan, reported 1.87 per cent benign polyps in 4,172 cases from their out-patient department, using the gastrocamera. It appears that the incidence of adenomas of the stomach is quite similar among patients who are gastroscoped in the U.S.A. and Japan. Eklof, et al.,[4] reviewed 1,100 tumors of the stomach and duodenum reported by x-ray and found 111 or approximately 10 per cent of benign epithelial tumors.

There is great disparity between the reported incidence of adenomas and other benign tumors by autopsy, surgery, x-ray and gastroscopy. There is considerable evidence that adenomatous polyps are more frequently seen by gastroscopy than by x-ray. It is not unusual in our experience to have one small gastric polyp reported on x-ray and find several by gastroscopy. The gastroscopist must always be careful that the polyp which he observes and one seen by the roentgenologist is the same lesion. In general, adenomatous gastric polyps, once thought to be quite uncommon, are being observed with increasing frequency by x-ray and gastroscopy.

Gastroscopic Features

The gastric epithelial tumor commonly known as benign adenomatous polyp varies in size from a few millimeters in diameter up to a few centimeters. Gastroscopically, they usually appear as smooth, spherical masses protruding into the gastric lumen. However, they may be oval, or finger-like projections. They may be sessile or pedunculated. A sessile appearing polyp may reveal a pedicle if the patient's position is shifted on the examining table, for example from the left side to dorsal and the Trendelenburg position.

The color of an adenomatous polyp is usually orange-red and similar to that of the surrounding mucosa. However, the polyp may be pale against the redder background of surrounding mucosa. Not infrequently, the polyp is normal orange-red and the surrounding mucosa is pale pink or gray with atrophic gastritic changes.

Some polyps are covered partly or completely with adherent gray or whitish mucus or their reddish surface may be granular resembling a strawberry. The surface of the polyp may show tiny blood vessels. They are frequently solitary. In the case illustrated by Plate 32, the polyp protruded from the overhanging gastric wall. It was not seen by x-ray. Adenomatous polyps are frequently multiple, discrete, spherical protrusions between or on the crests of gastric folds (Plate 33). Multiple adenomatous polyps may vary from a few in number to innumerable defects. They may appear in any or all areas of the stomach. Statistically, they are more frequently seen in the lower ⅓ of the stomach. Grafe[5] and associates found 21 of 33 adenomas in the antrum, 10 in the cardia and 2 in the fundus.

When polyps occur in large numbers and irregular size, widely distributed in the stomach, the condition has been described by pathologists since the era of Menetrier in the late 19th century, as "Polyadenomes Polypeux."[6] Students of this problem have referred to the occasional finding of at least one malignant polyp in these multiple lesions,[7] which emphasizes the importance of the decisions of diagnosis and treatment of these cases.

The case history of one of our patients will serve to illustrate the ramification of this problem.

A CASE HISTORY

A. F., a 65 year old male passenger railroad worker had been seen off and on for a period of ten years with dyspeptic symptoms. Clinical and laboratory evaluations, including several complete gastrointestinal x-ray studies had classified the patient as having an irritable bowel syndrome. The patient returned for a checkup just before retirement after an interval of a number of years. He had no abdominal complaints, having had a negative gastric x-ray series seven years before. The current UGI series was reported by the roentgenologist as polypoid carcinoma of the stomach. Gastroscopy, utilizing multiple positions on the examining table revealed multiple smooth polyps of varying sizes, some of them coalescing. Many of them had demonstrable pedicles. Endoscopic biopsy revealed normal adenomatous tissue. At surgery, inspection revealed twelve polyps, several with definite pedicles. Frozen section of representative polyps revealed benignancy. Complete polypectomy rather than gastric resection was performed, particularly because of the wide distribution of the polyps. Fifteen of varying sizes were removed. All polyps were serially sectioned and all proved to be benign adenomas (Pl. 34). A clinical follow-up of five years has revealed that the patient is living and well in retirement.

A pedunculated polyp in the antrum may be swept into the pylorus and produce an intermittent "Ball-Valve" obstruction, causing periodic vomiting. This phenomenon is illustrated by Plate 35. In some instances a small antral polyp with long pedicle may swing into the first portion of the duodenum with a wave of peristalsis and simulate a polyp of bulbar origin. Polyps in this relationship have occasionally been found histologically to be of Brunnerian origin.

Transendoscopic biopsy is frequently performed in these days of sophisticated instruments. The histologic structure of a true adenoma may be readily identified as glandular epithelial tissue without the usual differentiation of normal mucosa into chief, parietal and argentaffin cells (Fig. 16-1).

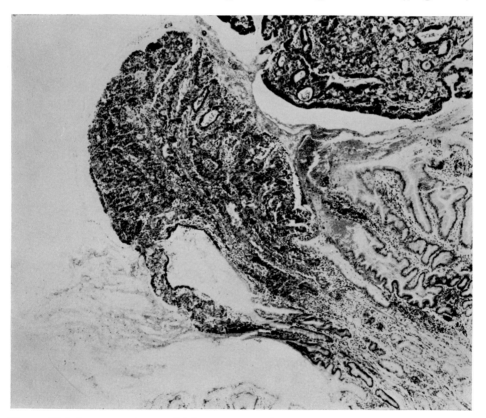

Figure 16-1. Low power view of Adenomatous Polyp projecting from the gastric mucosa with irregular gland spaces. High power view showed goblet cells and absence of normal pattern of gastric epithelium. (Read by Dr. Dorothy Eshbaugh, Michael Reese Hospital)

Relations to Carcinoma

The most important clinical significance of the adenomatous gastric polyp is its possibility of being malignant or its potential for becoming malignant. Some observers have emphasized the long period during which benign gastric adenomas have remained benign showing no sign of malignant change with x-ray and gastroscopic control. Iriga, et al.[3] point to fifteen cases of adenomatous polyps observed gastroscopically for five years, after benignancy had been determined and showing practically no changes. One of these cases increased in size and became more irregular while being followed up gastroscopically for seven years. The patient was therefore subjected to gastrectomy and the lesion found to be entirely benign. The followers of this school of thought have increasing confidence in the facilities of gastroscopy, gastrocamera, gastrobiopsy and cytology in the detection of early gastric cancer. They also have a reluctance to prescribe gastrectomy with its risks and after affects until proven necessary.

Advocates of the other extreme point of view are represented by the reports of McNeer, et al.[8] They reported an analysis of surgical material consisting of 38 benign and 24 malignant gastric polyps. There were 14 instances of benign adenomatous tissue at both ends of a section through malignant polyps. They further reported atypical histologic changes bridging the gap between benign adenoma and cancer in 65 per cent of the cases. These observations suggest a high incidence of malignant transformation. A middle-ground position is probably nearest the truth at this stage of our knowledge of the problem.

There are certain hard facts which will aid the gastroscopist in distinguishing benign from malignant gastric polyps. The Japanese criteria for early gastric cancer (See Chapt. 18) have confirmed an earlier opinion that a polyp of 2 cm in diameter or smaller is likely to be benign while those larger than 2 cm in diameter are more often malignant. Irregular surface and sessile position in the gastric wall are characteristics more likely to indicate malignancy. McNeer and associates[8] report that carcinomatous changes occur in only 6.8 per cent of polyps measuring less than 1.5 cm in diameter and 73.7 per cent of those more than 3 cm in diameter. Measuring sticks and other methods for determining size have been devised by the instrument manufacturers. With some experience size of polyps can be estimated by comparison with folds, degree of inflation and deflation, x-ray films, etc.

It has long been held that the more pedunculated the gastric polyps, the more likely they are to be benign. Stout[9] found that malignancy is 2½ times more frequent in sessile gastric polyps than in pedunculated ones. That pedunculated polyps are very likely to be benign has also been confirmed by our experience and others. Irregularity of the surface contour is a secondary characteristic in favor of malignancy.

Relations to Other Lesions

The presence of gastric atrophy or atrophic gastritis surrounding a polyp increases the statistical chance of malignancy. This has been established by Stout[10] and others. Madeline Brown[11] reported as far back as 1934 that benign polyps frequently occur in the stomachs of pernicious anemia patients. Rigler and Kaplan[12] found fifteen benign tumors in 211 pernicious anemia patients for an incidence of 7.1 per cent.

It is well known that pernicious anemia patients have gastric mucosal atrophy. The high incidence of benign adenoma in the soil of gastric atrophy does not justify complacency with regards to malignant potential. In fact, there is a long and continuing suspicion that atrophic gastritis predisposes to malignancy, and again Rigler's studies have shown that carcinoma occurs twelve times more frequently in the stomach of pernicious anemia patients than in non-pernicious anemia patients. This would seem to add up to the conclusion that if there is atrophic gastritis, pernicious anemia and polyps, there must be a high index of suspicion of malignancy or malignant potential.

Benign adenomatous gastric polyps are occasionally associated with polyps of the colon and other organs, especially the endocrine glands. This has led to the hormone theory of the origin of polyps. In rare instances there is an association of multiple polyps in the intestinal canal and pigmentation of mucosal surfaces in the so-called Puetz-Jegher's Syndrome.

Clinical Features

Benign adenomatous gastric polyps are notorious for the absence of associated symptoms, which can be attributed to the polyps. In our own experience, a great majority of these small excrescences have been symptomless. When the patient has epigastric distress, it is usually due to an associated gastritis or other causes. The exception would be the large benign tumors, 6 or more cm in diameter, or a large number of smaller polyps. Usually, these adenomas give symptoms when they bleed or if they intermittently obstruct the pylorus and cause vomiting.

PSEUDOPOLYPS

This term was used by Schindler to describe certain polyps associated with chronic gastritis which are regarded as compensatory excrescences in response to inflammatory reactions. Inflammatory pseudopolyp has also been used to describe some *puckering,* inflammatory changes sometimes seen at the stoma of postoperative stomachs.

In some instances in the presence of vigorous peristalsis, the gastroscopist will observe a *knuckle* defect along the course of a rugal fold which appears to be a polyp. As peristalsis relaxes or if the *defect* is observed at different angles, or with different degrees of inflation it may become obvious that the apparent defect is a pseudopolyp. This type of pseudopolyp is illustrated in Plate 36.

The term hyperplastic polyp has been used to describe papillomatous changes in the gastric mucosa. The same changes have been described as giant hypertrophic gastritis.

SUBMUCOSAL TUMORS

Benign tumors originating in the gastric wall are of mesenchymal origin and of definite interest to the gastroscopist. Frequently, they will have been observed by x-ray. If they are small, their intramural location may be questionable by x-ray. If they are large, the x-ray evidence of intramural location is often very evident. The tumor may grow centripetally toward the gastric lumen or centrifugally away from the lumen and toward the serosa. In the latter instances, they are not seen by the gastroscopist, but important information may be gained by the peritoneoscopist.

When submucosal tumors grow toward the lumen they may be seen by the gastroscopist as smooth, polyp-like projections with a broad base. These benign tumors may be leiomyomas, fibromyomas, myomas, lipomas, neuromas, vascular tumors, and even osteomas. Most of them are quite rare and the smaller ones are seen only at autopsy as incidental findings.

Rigler and Ericksen[13] observed 47 benign as compared to 187 malignant tumors in a series of 6,743 necropsies for a relative incidence of 26 per cent. They found 11 per cent benign tumors among 239 gastric tumors diagnosed by x-ray. Marshall[14] reported that of 1,700 gastric tumors removed at operation at the Lahey Clinic 4.8 per cent were benign including leiomyomas, adenomatous polyps, lipomas and hemangiomas. Palmer[15] made an interesting review of benign intramural tumors in 1951. It is obvious that statistics will necessarily vary depending on whether they are based upon autopsies, surgery, x-ray or gastroscopy. It may be very difficult to distinguish by gross gastroscopy the different types of benign submucosal tumors, except with the aid of transendoscopic biopsy and brush cytology.

Leiomyomas

Gastric leiomyomas originate in the smooth muscle tissue of the muscularis mucosae or the muscularis propria. The characteristic whorled configuration of the cut surface is readily seen. Histologically, the smooth muscle cells are well defined.

Incidence

The leiomyoma is by far the most common of submucosal benign gastric tumors. We will, therefore, discuss this lesion first. Rieniets[16] reported 43 valid leiomyomas during a careful study of 200 unselected autopsies. Most of these were very small and would not have been seen gastroscopically. While very important gastroscopically and clinically, leiomyomas are rather uncommon among total gastroscopic lesions. Prior to 1958, only 20 leiomyomas and 15 leiomyosarcomas had been seen gastroscopically out of 1,017 tumors.[17] Many more have been diagnosed gastroscopically since 1958 with fiberoptic instruments and improved biopsy facilities.

Gastroscopic Features

For the most part, the gastroscopic findings for leiomyomas are similar to those for all tumors of submucosal origin. As the tumor grows towards

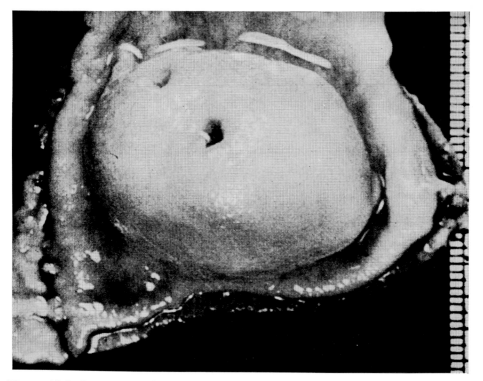

Figure 16-2. Leiomyoma showing *bridging folds* at lower left and upper left areas. Central ulcer also shown. (From Buckstein Roentgenology G.I. Tract, Lippincott)

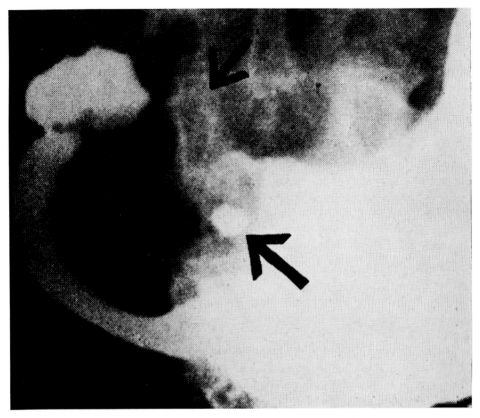

Figure 16-3. X-Ray view of intramural tumor showing ulcer *fleck*. Same case as Figure 16-2.

the lumen, it stretches the overlying mucosa and produces a smooth, round-ed, orange-red surface. In most instances when the tumor becomes 2 or more cm in diameter, one or more *bridging* folds (Pl. 38) can be seen stretching from the upper surface down to the level of the surrounding mucosa. This should always be referred to as the "Schindler sign," since Rudolf Schindler was the first to describe it. As growth continues, an um-bilication or ulcer may develop at its summit (See Fig. 16-2 and Pl. 38). The central ulcer may be seen also by x-ray as illustrated in Figure 16-3.

These tumors have broad stalks. If the smooth surface shows some irregu-larity, multiple petechiae or tiny superficial erosions, leiomyosarcoma may be suspected. Biopsy and brush cytology may help in the differentiation between the benign and the malignant forms. Here is where the addition of clinical evaluation of the patient may be the deciding factor in making the diagnosis and determining the management of the patient.

The gastroscopist must always keep in mind the possibility of a polypoid carcinoma simulating a submucosal tumor. I have had one case of a smooth nodose tumor with *bridging folds* without ulceration, diagnosed leiomyosarcoma but the transendoscopic biopsy showed carcinoma which was confirmed at surgery. A carcinoma may occasionally burrow first into the submucosa and then stretch the overlying mucosa as it grows toward the lumen.

Apparent leiomyomas may show malignant characteristics in that they may be atypical histologically and tend to metastasize by the venous route. These tumors are called leiomyoblastomas.[18]

Clinical symptoms of submucosal tumors when present are nonspecific and most students of endoscopy will be well acquainted with them. I should mention that the principal symptom which should always be kept in mind is Upper GI bleeding, which frequently is unassociated with other symptoms.

Other Benign Tumors

Practically all benign neoplasms that occur elsewhere in the body have also been found in the stomach. As was previously mentioned seldom will the gastroscopist be able to distinguish grossly one benign intramural tumor from another beyond a statistical guess. There are a few benign tumors other than leiomyomas which should be mentioned because of certain special features.

Neurofibromas in rare instances have been found in the stomach associated with generalized von Recklinghausen's disease. Equally rare has been the association of a gastric benign vascular tumor with *hemangiomas* of the skin and elsewhere.

There has been some special interest in the occasional finding of *pancreatic rests* in the gastric wall. There have been reports of symptoms due to pancreatitis within the heterotopic tissue or to obstructive manifestations. The rests are usually small protrusions from the wall with a central umbilication which may have an aberrant ductal structure.[19] A possibility of benign pancreatic nodules in the gastric wall should be kept in mind by the gastroscopist to avoid unnecessary wide gastric resection when confused with cancer.

Adult *hypertrophic pyloric stenosis* is a benign tumefaction which the gastroscopist may see occasionally. It poses the problem of differentiation from annular, Napkin ring, carcinoma and other prepyloric annular deformities.

MALFORMATIONS AND DEFORMITIES

For the sake of convenience, certain malformations and deformities which the gastroscopist must keep in mind are included in this chapter with benign tumors. These defects and processes are in fact *benign* and most of them have the possibility of being confused with benign neoplasms.

Extragastric Masses

External compression of the stomach may be diagnosed if after complete inflation of the organ, a bulging mass covered by normal mucosa is seen to protrude into the gastric cavity. When the stomach is partially deflated, the bulging may disappear. External compression may be caused by the spleen, liver, pancreas, by different segments of the intestine or by pathology in these organs. Schindler gave considerable significance to bulging from the posterior wall of the antrum due to tumors of the pancreas. If a malignancy of the pancreas or other organ infiltrates the serosal surface of the stomach without breaking through to the mucosal surface, the protuberance becomes fixed and differentiation from submucosal mesenchymal neoplasms may be difficult. If the tumor penetrates the mucosal surface of the stomach, differentiation from primary gastric malignancy may be very difficult or impossible. Observation of a lobulated or irregular nodular area at the summit of a bulging posterior wall has been described as carcinoma of the pancreas infiltrating through the gastric wall. Postoperative adhesions may deform the gastric pouch and raise the differential diagnostic problem of neoplasm of the gastric wall. Further significance of gastroscopy and extragastric tumors is discussed in Chapter 3.

Cascade Stomach

Another type of deformity seen occasionally by the roentgenologist and the endoscopist is the cascade stomach. The cascade stomach defect is often characterized by pressure like defect against the posterior wall and greater curvature and usually slightly below the cardiac area. The defect is such as to produce an upper gastric segment so that the gastric content passes over a ridge. This action as seen by the fluoroscopist has been called the cup and spill defect. The defect is usually congenital and may be without symptoms. In some instances, however, gas may be entrapped in the upper loculus and give rise to the so-called Magenblase syndrome. The endoscopist may be concerned with what appears to be a ridge across the posterior wall resembling a neoplasm. The overlying mucosa is usually normal. The defect may interfere with normal visualization of the lower portion of the stomach.

Volvulus and Duplication

There are other uncommon malformations which the gastroscopist may encounter. It is important to have them in mind in order to distinguish them from more common or more serious disorders. Among these are volvulus, most common in childhood but may be seen in adults, particularly, it may be associated with disorders such as diaphragmatic hernia, eventration and status post-phrenisectomy. It has been associated with cancer and ulcer. Essentially, it is a condition of torsion of the stomach on its long axis and may give a bizarre appearance to the gastroscopist. A duplication of the stomach may occur occasionally and may resemble a heterotopic cystic formation.

Hourglass Stomach

Under certain circumstances contour of the gastric pouch is deformed to produce an hourglass shape. Usually this is due to an incisura across the greater curvature and a benign ulcer on the lesser curvature at or near the same level. This is thought to begin as a spasm and later the spastic incisura becomes infiltrated with connective tissue, which may remain as a permanent defect. In the meantime the ulcer crater on the lesser curvature may heal permanently or recur. Endoscopy at this time may be concerned with a differentiation of an infiltrating neoplasm with or without ulcerations. This type of hourglass deformity is frequently referred to as "B" shaped (See Chapt. 3, Fig. 3-2A), and is usually benign. If the hourglass deformity is "V" shaped, it is more likely to be a case of infiltrating carcinoma.

Diverticula

The gastroscopist must be concerned with other malformations and deformities in the stomach. Another of these deformities is that of gastric diverticulum (Pl. 23 and Pl. 37). These defects may be congenital or acquired. The congenital diverticulum occurs in all sizes and may be harmless unless it is large or the mucosal lining becomes inflamed. Otherwise, diverticula are important from the point of view of possible rupture if their stomas are large enough to permit the entrance of the tip of the gastroscope. Acquired diverticula occur usually as a result of a disease. One of the most important is that of a large gastric ulcer, which in the process of healing under medical management may have so deformed the stomach as to produce a diverticulum. These are most common in the antrum. Occasionally, a deformity of this kind appears to be a congenital diverticulum, but actually proves to be on the basis of a large so-called walled-off penetrating ulcer.[20] In many of these cases, the combination of x-ray and gastroscopy is necessary for the proper delineation of such lesions.

FOREIGN BODIES

Bezoars

Bezoars may appear as large irregular accumulations of hair or vegetable material swallowed by the patient. Trichobezoars consist of swallowed hair and are sometimes found in the stomachs of children or mentally deranged adults who habitually swallow their own hair. For some unknown reason the hair ball is not passed through the pylorus when it is small and therefore may grow to such a size that it fills the stomach completely. On gastroscopic examination a small bezoar appears as an irregular, friable, stringy mobile tumor, but when it has grown to the size where it makes a complete cast of the stomach, gastroscopic visualization becomes very difficult. Granulomatous changes may occur in relation to bezoars and simulate a neoplasm.

Phytobezoars are composed of vegetable fibers. One of the most common are the vegetable substances seen in the persimmon.[21] Severe gastritis may accompany these bezoars.

OTHER FOREIGN BODIES

Many large foreign bodies are swallowed accidentally, especially by children. Usually if these objects pass through the esophagus they will continue through the alimentary canal. Some of them remain in the stomach especially in the presence of pyloric stenosis. Some of these foreign bodies have been removed during the last few years by modified fiberoptic gastroscopy techniques.

The first gastroscopic examination which this writer witnessed was performed by Dr. Rudolf Schindler on a patient who proved to have a huge ulceration on the posterior antral wall. The base of this ulcer was formed by a large wandering gallstone, which had fistulated from the biliary tract and became implanted to the wall of the stomach. The diagnosis was not clear gastroscopically and was proven only at surgery.

REFERENCES

1. Schindler, R.: Incidence of the various types of gastric diseases as revealed by gastroscopic study. *Am J Med Sci, 197:*509, 1939.
2. Berry, L. H., Alavi, I., Mitaniyama, A., and Adomavicius, J.: Analysis of 6,000 consecutive fiberoptic and lens gastroscopies. Advances in Gastrointestinal Endoscopy, Proc 2nd World Congress G.I. Endoscopy, Rome and Copenhagen, PICCIN, Padava (Italia), Med Books, 1970.
3. Ariga, Kaizo, Honda, Toshio, and Koizumi, Hajime: Studies on the Endoscopic Findings of Gastric Polyps, Proc 1st Congress Inter Soc Endoscopy, 347-350, Tokyo, 1966.
4. Eklof, O., Eriksson, E., and Sahlin, O.: Benign epithelial tumors of stomach and duodenum, diagnosis and treatment. *Acta Chir Scand. (Suppl.), 255:*1-32, 1960.
5. Grafe, W., Thorbjarnarson, B., Pearce, J. M., and Beal, J. M.: Benign neoplasms of the stomach. *Am J Surg, 100:*561, 1960.
6. Menetrier, P.: Les Polyadenomes Gastriques et leurs Rapports Avec le Cancer de l'Estomac. *Arch Physiol Norm et Path,* 4 series, Tome I, pp. 33 et 236, 1888.
7. Perry, T., and Shekarchi, K.: Polypoid adenomas of the stomach. *Am J Surg, 101:*440, 1961.
8. McNeer, G., Jolly, D. S., and Berg, J. W.: *Neoplasms of the Stomach.* Lippincott, Philadelphia, 1967, p. 4.

9. Stout, A. P., in discussion of Berg, J. W.: Histologic aspects of the relations between gastric adenomatous polyp and gastric cancer. *Bull NY Acad Med, 36*:483-487, 1960.
10. Stout, A. P.: Gastromucosal atrophy and carcinoma of the stomach. *NY J Med, 45*:973-977, 1945.
11. Brown, M. R.: Gastrointestinal pathology in pernicious anemia etc. *N Eng J Med, 210*:473, 1934.
12. Rigler, L. G., and Kaplan, H. S.: Pernicious anemia and the early diagnosis of tumors of the stomach. *JAMA, 128*:426, 1945.
13. Rigler, L. G., and Ericksen, L. G.: Benign tumors of the stomach; observations on their incidence and malignant degeneration. *Radiology, 26*:6-15, 1936.
14. Marshall, S. F.: Gastric tumors other than carcinoma. *Surg Clin North Am, 35*:693, 1955.
15. Palmer, E. D.: Benign intramural tumors of the stomach. A review with special reference to gross pathology. *Medicine, 30*:81, 1951.
16. Rieniets, J. H.: The frequency and pathologic aspects of gastric leiomyomas. Proc Staff Meet. Mayo Clinic, 5:364-366, 1930.
17. Skandalakis, J. E., Gray, S. W., and Shepard, E.: Smooth muscle tumors of the stomach. *Int Abstr Surg, 110*:200-226, March, 1960.
18. McBee, J. W., and Aboumrad, M. H.: Leiomyoblastoma of the stomach. *Gastrointest Endosc, 17*:1, August, 1970.
19. Lukash, W. M., Johnson, R. B., and Bishop, R. P.: Aberrant pancreas in the stomach: Radiographic and gastroscopic findings. *Gastrointest Endosc,* Vol. XVI, No. 3, Feb. 1970.
20. Bralow, S. P., and Spellberg, M. A.: Diverticula of the stomach: Report of 26 new cases. *Gastroenterology, 11*:59-82, 1948.
21. Nelson, R. S.: Gastroscopic observations on the persimmon bezoar. *Bull Gastrointest Endosc, 10*:9-12, 1963.

CHAPTER 17

GASTRIC CARCINOMA—
BORRMANN'S CLASSIFICATION*

LEONIDAS H. BERRY, ILTIFAT ALAVI AND FERNANDO VILLA

INTRODUCTORY STATEMENT

G ASTRIC CARCINOMA AS the term will be used in this chapter, is interchangeable with gastric cancer. During the last few years, resulting
largely from great strides in fiberoptic endoscopy but also in health education, the frontiers in the early diagnosis of gastric cancer have receded
considerably in many parts of the world. There may be a significant difference between the early diagnosis of gastric cancer and the diagnosis of
early gastric cancer. Early diagnosis of gastric cancer suggests getting the
patient to the doctor and to definitive diagnostic facilities at an early period after the onset of symptoms.

The diagnosis of early gastric cancer literally means finding the cancer
lesion when it is in an early stage of development. The two concepts are
not the same although they point toward a common goal, the eventual
eradication of gastric cancer.

* Supported in part by a grant from Regional Medical Programs, against Heart Disease,
Cancer and Stroke, National Institutes of Health, Bethesda, Md. and Hektoen Institute of
Medical Research, Chicago.

In recent years, Japanese workers have approached this problem with a definitive anatomical concept. It is now widely known as the Japanese concept of early gastric cancer. By broad definition, it is gastric cancer which has not extended beyond the mucosa and the submucosa.[1] This subject is discussed in detail by the authors of Chapter 18. In most parts of the world, and especially in areas of low gastric cancer incidence, the diagnosis of early gastric cancer is still an elusive goal. The kind of gastric cancer which is seen most widely throughout the world, including Japan, is that described by the Borrmann's classification. This consists of four types of cancer according to gross shape and configuration with no limitation with reference to size or extent of involvement of the gastric wall or lumen. This is considerably different from the Japanese classification of early gastric cancer developed by the Japan Endoscopy Society, which has definite limitations of size and extent of penetration into the gastric wall and lumen.

Before discussing the pathology of carcinoma of the stomach, we will review the important subject of symptomatology and epidemiology as it exists in many parts of the world today.

SYMPTOMATOLOGY

One of the most insidious of all diseases affecting mankind is gastric cancer. In most parts of the world where mass screening for gastric cancer is not well developed, the patient comes to the doctor because of symptoms. Most endoscopists will not be on the search just for cancer. They will be about the business of explaining symptoms. In America and other areas of the world, many patients will have functional distress and no organic disease will be found. The very first symptoms may be noticeable weight loss. This may be due to the inherent nature of the disease or minor gastric upsets may interfere with appetite sufficiently to result in weight loss. Inlaw et al.[2] found weight loss present in 88 per cent of gastric cancer patients at the Mayo Clinic. Sakita et al.[3] of Japan reports that the great majority of early gastric cancer patients found by mass screening have some symptoms at the time of examination. Careful anamnesis often elicited hunger pains or vague epigastric distress even though the patients were not seeking medical care. Usually when persistent pain develops, the disease is already advanced. If one must have cancer, it may be advantageous to have it deep in the antrum, where vomiting due to partial pyloric obstruction may develop early. When a gastric lesion is found, a well trained gastroenterologist will always ask himself the question, does the finding adequately explain the symptoms. Clinical considerations in diagnosis will remain an important approach until medicine becomes an exact science, if such a possibility exists.

There comes to mind, the case of a forty-year-old man who had a typical benign lesser curvature ulcer with a shallow niche seen on x-ray and gastroscopy. The moderately severe pains which at times radiated to his back seemed out of proportion to the small uncomplicated ulcer which was gradually decreasing in size with treatment. This opinion was so stated and further studies were advised. Pancreatic function tests revealed dysfunction and other studies supported the additional diagnosis of chronic relapsing pancreatitis which was confirmed by surgery and clinical course.

Upper gastrointestinal hemorrhage or the pain of penetrating ulcer are more often the symptoms of benign disease than malignancy. A carcinoma high in the fundus may have dysphagia as the first symptom. Such a lesion is often missed by routine x-ray and until the relatively recent development of retroflexed fiber gastroscopy, such a lesion was often missed also by the endoscopist. A *napkin ring* scirrhous carcinoma near the pylorus can produce the *five gallon* decompensated stomach more often associated with benign cicatricial stenosis of a channel ulcer. The pattern of pain, the course and weight loss should alert the astute clinician to search further, particularly with biopsy and cytology for a more definitive diagnosis. In uncommon instances, a diffuse scirrhous carcinoma with leather bottle stomach may produce gastrogenic diarrhea as a presenting symptom.

Several investigators have found that the average delay between the onset of symptoms and definitive treatment in gastric cancer varies from six months to a year.[4] The total picture of gastric cancer at this time would seem to indicate that a careful elicitation of symptoms can be a major factor in case finding for early diagnosis. Many recent studies indicated that there is a need for prompt endoscopy by competent endoscopists for the mildest type of dyspepsia if major progress in the diagnosis of early gastric cancer is to be universally achieved.

EPIDEMIOLOGY

The gastroenterologist and the gastrointestinal endoscopist must have an interest in the epidemiology of gastric carcinoma. The wide variations in incidence throughout the world regardless of ethnic and cultural differences and within similar ethnic groups in different geographic areas, emphasize the overwhelming importance of environmental factors in this disease. Food, contaminants and pollutants of land, sea and air must be considered in relation to individual habits and occupation in evaluating probable causes and distribution of gastric carcinoma.

Mortality statistics show a remarkably low figure for carcinoma of the stomach in the United States as compared with the figures from some other countries[5] (Table 17-I). In twenty years, gastric cancer incidence in the United States has fallen to half its rate twenty-five years ago. This is true

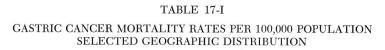

TABLE 17-I

GASTRIC CANCER MORTALITY RATES PER 100,000 POPULATION
SELECTED GEOGRAPHIC DISTRIBUTION

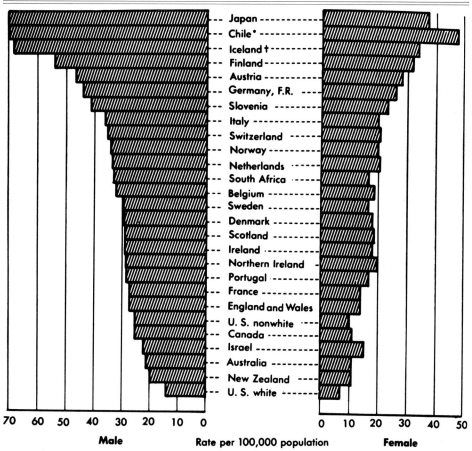

From Eynder et al. in *Cancer, 16*:1461, 1963.

in spite of the increasing life span during this period. As longevity increases, more people reach the age of high cancer incidence. In the United States the paradox of low gastric cancer is seen by the following statistics.[5] The population over age forty-five years was 13 million in 1900, 39 million in 1948, 50 million in 1958, 59 million in 1968. Age alone should always increase cancer incidence, yet gastric cancer incidence has dropped by one-half its sex-age adjusted rate per 100 thousand population in approximately twenty years (1947 to 1962).[5] While carcinoma of the stomach is decreasing in the United States, carcinoma of the lungs is increasing remarkably.[6]

Cancer of the colon is now the leading malignancy of the gastrointestinal tract in the United States having increased by 15 to 18 per cent from 1945 to 1962 in Connecticut and New York. Cancer of the esophagus remains about the same with a slight decrease for the period 1945 to 1962.[6]

The very high incidence rates of carcinoma of the stomach in such widely separated areas as Japan, Chile, South America, Iceland and Finland are a challenge to all cancer workers, epidemiologists and gastroenterologists all over the world. The gastrointestinal endoscopist must play an increasing and important role in case finding in the early diagnosis of carcinoma of the gastrointestinal canal.

It should be emphasized that low statistical incidence does not justify any let up in the continuing search for early gastric cancer or possible precursor lesions. In fact it is our opinion that correlated studies between low incidence and high incidence gastric cancer areas may offer the best opportunity for ultimate discovery of significant causative factors and preventive measures in the control of gastric cancer.

PATHOGENESIS

Because of the eternal search for cancer causes, etiological concern is inherent in every gastroscopic examination. The benign appearing gastric polyps are almost always looked upon as possibly malignant or premalignant. The question of the cancerous potential of benign gastric ulcer has been researched and debated for decades. One of the most important indications for gastroscopy is the possible differential diagnosis of benign and malignant ulcer.

Charles Mayo, great clinical and surgical authority in the pregastroscopy era contended that cancer never occurred in the healthy stomach. Konjetzny[7] and Faber[8] were historically very concerned with the subject of cancer precursor lesions. Authorities worldwide continue to be suspicious of chronic gastritis and especially the atrophic form as being a condition which may predispose the stomach to cancer development. Reports from the high cancer incidence area of Japan indicate that chronic gastritis is very high in incidence and severity in cases of gastric cancer.[9] Intestinal metaplasia or goblet cell transformation of gastric epithelium is an important characteristic of the atrophic gastric mucosa. Ming and Associates[10] in their studies of histogenesis of gastric carcinoma found the occurrence of intestinal metaplasia in 98 per cent of cases.

If proven, stigmata of precancerous changes could be found associated with questionable cancer, this could be supportive evidence of early gastric cancer. The smaller the cancer lesion or the earlier it appears, the greater the chance for negative biopsy and the greater the importance of supportive diagnostic evidence.

This brings us to the point of raising the question, what is early gastric cancer? The Japanese workers have defined it anatomically as being that carcinomatous lesion which has not penetrated beyond the mucosa and submucosa (see Chapter 18) yet, a small percentage of these patients died of metastatic cancer from the gastric primary before the end of the five year survival period.[11] A significant number of patients with large cancer lesions fitting into the category of the Borrmann classification which the Japanese and others would now call advanced, have survived for five years and longer in the United States.[12] This has also been true through the years in Japan and other parts of the world.

To illustrate that patients with so-called advanced gastric cancer or large cancer lesions may survive postoperatively much longer than some patients with so-called early gastric cancer, the following case history is presented:

CASE HISTORY

A housewife, age 49, was first seen in 1949 in the private office of one of us, Berry, complaining of epigastric distress, nausea and periodic vomiting. There had been 5 to 10 lbs. weight loss during 3 or 4 months and her symptoms had occurred for a period of 4 to 5 weeks. The physical findings were essentially negative. All laboratory findings were within normal limits except the barium meal x-ray which showed an antral deformity with questionable diagnosis, but healing ulcer of the posterior antral wall was suggested. Lens gastroscopy confirmed the deformed antrum which blocked the view of the pylorus and the immediate prepyloric area. The mucosa above showed extensive hypertrophic gastritis (gastropathy) (Plate 39). The patient refused surgery for a long time. During this period she was given aggressive medical therapy. At first, the symptoms improved, but finally worsened and the patient agreed to surgery.

The gross specimen (Plate 39) revealed Borrmann's Type II carcinomatous ulcer with extensive hypertrophic gastropathy. The patient recovered after Billroth II gastric resection and continued a useful life for a remarkable twenty-three years. The patient expired on May 10, 1972, because of malignant pleurisy with effusion. The cytological examination of the fluid revealed a class V by the Papanicolau method. There was also a questionable mass in the abdomen. A barium meal x-ray at this time revealed evidence of a four-fifths Billroth II gastric resection and no evidence of recurrent malignancy of the stomach. Autopsy was refused on religious grounds; therefore, it could not be determined whether the terminal malignancy was a metastatic spread from the original gastric cancer or a new primary cancer. At any rate, this was a case of a twenty-three year survival after a four-fifths gastric resection of a Borrmann's Type II carcinomatous ulcer.

ENDOSCOPIC PATHOLOGY

Carcinoma of the stomach as seen by the gastroscopist, covers the entire gamut from multinodular fungating masses to the questionable punched out solitary ulcer. It appears to serve a useful purpose if carcinoma of the stomach is classified according to gross characteristics. Universally gastroscopists have used the classification appropriated by Schindler and originally suggested by Borrmann.[13] The endoscopic descriptions and illustrations to follow will utilize the Borrmann classification.

Types of Lesions

The Borrmann classification consists of four types of lesions.[14] Type I is the polypoid form of gastric carcinoma. Type II, ulcerating non-infiltrating carcinoma. Type III, ulcerating infiltrating carcinoma, and Type IV, scirrhous carcinoma localized or diffuse (Table 17-II).

Type I, Polypoid

Polypoid gastric carcinoma or Type I occurs most frequently in the distal one half of the stomach, but may occur in any part of the organ. It usually arises from a single small lesion, but sometimes it may be multicentric in origin. Its surface becomes irregular and multinodular as it grows (Plate 40). Its color may be similar to the surrounding mucosa, normal orange-red, hyperemic or pale and commensurate with blood loss. The surfaces are often friable and easily traumatized. There may be small superficial erosions or larger ulcerations of its surfaces. In some instances adherent white mucus (Plate 41) is present and has been likened to the frosting on a cake. The surrounding mucosa very frequently shows associated gastritis. It is often superficial or atrophic, but in some instances, it may be hypertrophic gastropathy.

Longer polypoid carcinomas in the majority of instances are easily diagnosed by x-ray. The addition of gastroscopy in these cases sometimes shows additional areas of involvement or a larger primary mass than was seen on x-ray film. In other cases, a significant portion of the filling defect of x-ray is found to be due to spasm when gastroscopy is performed. Ulcerations of polypoid masses are seen by both methods, but a better evaluation is usually made by gastroscopy (Plate 42).

TABLE 17-II

271 GASTRIC CARCINOMAS
GASTROSCOPIC CLASS (BORRMANN)

Type 1 (Polypoid)	104
Type 2 (Non-infiltrating CA. ulcer)	33
Type 3 (Infiltrating CA. ulcer)	44
Type 4 (Infiltrating) scirrhous	86
Total	271

Distribution and classification of gastric carcinoma in 5,858 gastroscopies.[14] In a two year period (1970-71) a total of 713 gastroscopies were performed. In 39 patients, a diagnosis of gastric cancer was made on endoscopy, four of which, on follow-up, proved benign of the 35 confirmed gastric cancers. Fourteen were Borrmann Type I, 7 were Type II, 6 Type II and 8 Type IV.

Polypoid carcinoma must sometimes be differentiated from submucosal tumors. The most common benign submucosal tumor of the stomach is leiomyoma and this must sometimes be differentiated from sarcomas. The typical submucosal tumor usually of muscle tissue origin has a relatively smooth surface and classically may have bridging folds (see Chapters 16 and 19 and Plate 34) at its margin. Some of these tumors have a central umbilication or round ulcer at its summit. This is due to a centrifugal growth and stretching of the mucosal covering of the tumor. The leiomyosarcoma in addition to the above characteristic is likely to be irregular or somewhat nodular and may or may not be associated with hyperemia, friability and tiny erosions or petechiae. The leiomyoma does not have this surface irregularity or nodularity of the polypoid carcinoma or of the leiomyosarcoma. It may be very difficult to distinguish between the leiomyosarcoma and the polypoid carcinoma if bridging folds are not identified, adenomatous polyp, single or multiple must be differentiated from polypoid carcinoma (see Chapter 6). In the final analysis, a biopsy may settle the issue and should be tried in all instances where possible.

Type II, Ulcerating Non-Infiltrating

The ulcerating non-infiltrating carcinoma is known as a Borrmann Type II. It is characterized by a solitary ulcer formation surrounded by a raised wall sometimes said to resemble the hole in a doughnut (Plate 43) (also see gastroscopic drawings in Chapter 6, Fig. 6-17). This type of carcinoma can test the diagnostic acumen of the most experienced gastroscopist. It is sometimes described as an ulcerating plateau. The concept being that it was originally a mound which became widely and deeply ulcerated, so as to resemble the crater in a miniature volcano. It is very probable that many of these lesions begin as ulcers. The ulcerating non-infiltrating carcinoma of the Borrmann Type II is frequently two centimeters or more in diameter. The raised circular wall is its most prominent feature. It is often hyperemic and nodular and sometimes friable. It may be pale pink with hemorrhagic erosions and petechiae. The ulcer crater is often covered with adherent necrotic exudate which characteristically may be dull gray, hemorrhagic or multicolored. The ulcer floor can sometimes be seen to be irregular. This type of ulcer has been described as occurring more frequently on the greater curvature than on the lesser and more frequently in the prepyloric than in the body or cardia. Comfort et al. of the Mayo Clinic in Minnesota, found the lesser curvature as the more common site of predilection for benign and malignant ulcers.[15]

The surrounding mucosa is likely to appear pliable with normal peristaltic activity. There may or may not be gastritic changes in the remainder of the stomach. The x-ray may show this type of tumor as a niche with a surrounding area of translucency known as the meniscus sign of Carman. Lavage or brush cytology is often positive for malignancy in this type of lesion. Transendoscopic biopsy may also be positive and these aids to gross gastroscopy should be used whenever possible.

Two cases will now be described to illustrate endoscopic pathology and the relative diagnostic value of gastroscopy and x-ray in carcinomatous ulcer, Borrmann Type II.

CASE HISTORY

High Posterior Wall Carcinomatous Ulcer Not Seen by X-Ray—Correctly Diagnosed by Gastroscopy.

A 60-year-old woman complained of epigastric distress immediately after meals. The discomfort was mild and intermittent for about two months. The distress occurred immediately after and sometimes during meals, but had not been relieved by milk or antacids. She was occasionally nauseated but there was no vomiting. She had noticed no black stools. She was a known hypertensive for which she had received medication during the last several years. There were no other significant symptoms.

Physical examination revealed a middle-aged well nourished woman. BP 170/100. Pulse 80. Respiration 20. Weight 165 lbs. Height 5'2". The head and neck were normal. Heart and respiratory sounds were normal. The abdomen slightly protuberant with mild epigastric tenderness. The significant laboratory findings were Hgb 11gms, benzidine positive stools, and x-ray of upper G.I. tract negative. Gastroscopy revealed an indurated ulcer about 1.5cm in diameter high on the posterior wall.

The patient was hospitalized for surgery. Gastroscopy was repeated and carcinomatous ulcer confirmed. A repeat x-ray study by a different roentgenologist, mainly for hospital records, was ordered. Meanwhile, the patient was put on the operative schedule for gastric resection. On the day before incision time, an x-ray report of negative stomach was received. The surgeon preferred to defer the operation and await a third x-ray of the stomach. The report for the third time was negative stomach. A third gastroscopy was then performed with the roentgenologist observing. He was convinced of the rather large carcinomatous Borrmann Type II ulcer with a raised irregular circular wall and a relatively shallow crater (see surgical specimen Plate 44).

All observations were made with the Eder-Palmer gastroscope using multiple positions technic. Attempts to biopsy the ulcer crater with the Berry Suction biopsy assembly resulted in a histologic report of chronic gastritis. The patient finally had a high gastric resection including one inch of esophagus. Gross examinations of the surgical specimen revealed a firm almost cartilaginous ulcer base. This undoubtedly accounted for failure to get a biopsy bit deep enough to retrieve carcinomatous tissue. Histological section through the ulcer floor of the surgical specimen revealed carcinoma. The broad relatively shallow ulcer high on the posterior wall could not be demonstrated by x-ray.

CASE HISTORY

Carcinomatous Ulcer Seen by X-Ray and Gastroscopy—Diagnosis More Definitive by Gastroscopy—"Partial Healing" on Medical Management.

A 45-year-old war veteran complained of epigastric pain coming on shortly after meals, partially relieved by soft food and antacids. There were periods of intermittent distress off and on for the previous six months, but occurring every day for the previous two or three weeks. There was nausea but no vomiting or melena. He had lost about 10 pounds during the last year. The history was otherwise noncontributory.

The physical examination revealed a young appearing man apparently in good nutrition. The blood pressure was 130/90. Pulse 80. Temperature 98.6. Respiration 20. Weight 155 lbs. Height 5′9″. The head, neck, heart, lungs and extremities were essentially negative. The abdomen was flat, moderately tender in the epigastric region with no abnormally palpable masses.

Laboratory test revealed 11gm Hgb; normal urine and electrolytes. Upper G.I. x-ray reported a large probably benign ulcer on the lesser curvature. Gastroscopy revealed a large ulcer approximately 2cm in diameter. Ulcer on the lesser curvature just proximal to the angulus, with a raised serrated border around its entire circumference (Plate 45). The base of the crater was covered by a smooth grayish adherent mucus. A diagnosis of carcinomatous ulcer Type II was made with the Eder-Palmer scope. Biopsy attempts with the Berry Biopsy Assembly was unsuccessful.

The patient rejected immediate surgery and pleaded for continued ulcer management. This was carried out rigidly for two months with partial symptomatic relief. At this time, the contraction of the crater with failure of re-epithelialization was seen and surgery was finally accepted at a veteran's hospital where malignancy lesions with metastasis were found. Patient expired after about 18 months following surgery. This case dramatically illustrated correct endoscopic diagnosis against questionable x-ray diagnosis and failure of a rigid "therapeutic test" to re-epithelialize the crater and very significant failure to completely relieve symptoms.

Type III, Ulcerating Infiltrating

The so-called ulcerating infiltrating carcinoma of the Borrmann classification may be difficult to differentiate from the Type II variety. The principal differentiating feature is the absence of the high wall on some portion or all portions of the circumference of the Type III ulcer. One might very well regard Types II and III together as ulcerating, in fact this is done by many postmortem pathologists. However, the separation of the two types of ulcer in accordance with the Borrmann's classification, is well entrenched in the gastroscopic literature.

The raised wall of the ulcer is regarded as delimiting the carcinoma. It is the portion of the circumference without the raised wall which often appears stiff and infiltrated. This portion appears as flat and level or *blended* with the edge of the crater. This flattened area may extend around the ulcer circumference for only a few millimeters. The characteristic flattening or *blending* was an important feature of Schindler's early gastroscopic descriptions. The occurrence of this feature and the difficulty of its evaluation are demonstrated in a patient of Schindler's[16] who refused surgery for four years. During this period, the patient had twenty gastroscopic observations and fourteen x-ray studies of her lesser curvature ulcer. X-ray was indeterminate from the first examination. Gastroscopy diagnosed Type III carcinoma on the first examination because of the *blended* or infiltrated appearance of one edge of the lesion. Both x-ray and gastroscopic opinions by the same examiners equivocated from time to time until eventually the patient agreed to surgery when the lesion was found to be malignant, probably during the entire four-year period of observation.

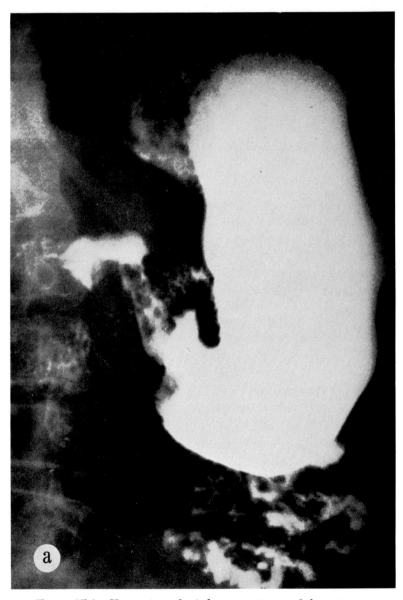

Figure 17-1a. X-ray view of scirrhous carcinoma of the antrum.

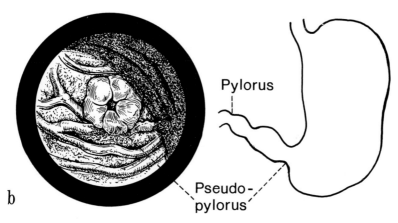

Figure 17-1b. Artist drawing. Gastroscopic view and diagram of same case as in 17-1a. Showing "Psuedo pylorus."

The chronic callous ulcer with firm appearing punched out configuration even with irregular undetermined edges is usually benign. If one edge is raised, or an area near the ulcer border appears stiffened, irregular or nodular, it is probably malignant. If it bleeds easily near the margin, or if it has *blunted* radiating (Plate 46) folds from its margin, it is malignant. If serial gastroscopic observations show a decreasing diameter without re-epithelialization it is malignant (Fig. 17-1a, b). If radiating folds up to an ulcer are spear shaped or pointed, or if there is a uniform narrow ring of hyperemia around the ulcer and if the mucosa around the ulcer close to its margin are smooth, uniformally orange-red and appears soft and pliable, the ulcer is probably benign.

Type IV, Scirrhous, Local, Diffuse

The Borrmann's Type IV carcinoma is the scirrhous form of carcinomatous infiltration. It may involve a very extensive area of the stomach by the time it is first seen. This is the so-called linitis plastica or leather bottle stomach. When the infiltration is very extensive, it is difficult for the gastroscopist to examine the stomach because the patient will rapidly belch up the air used for inflation. Scirrhous carcinoma is a sclerosing lesion where anaplastic malignant cells invade the gastric wall and is followed by extensive overgrowth of connective tissue. The sclerosing process sometimes involves only an annular segment causing the so-called *napkin ring* deformity. This usually occurs in the antrum. In some such cases, the pyloric narrowing may cause symptoms of pyloric obstruction and simulate the cicatricial stenosis of benign gastroduodenal ulcer. In which case, the gastroscopic picture may be that of a relatively normal orange-red mucosa with normal pattern of gastric folds in the upper body (Fig. 17-1a).

When the *napkin ring* scirrhous deformity of the distal antrum develops, the narrowed lumen is seen on x-ray and by gastroscopy as well. As the gastroscopic observation continues, symmetrical peristaltic waves are seen to move distalward, but the narrowed opening which appears to be the pylorus fails to close completely. As peristaltic activity continues, the diameter of the narrowed antral opening remains the same. The mucosa immediately adjacent to the opening may be entirely smooth. This is the typical picture of the "pseudo pylorus" (Fig. 17-1b) with the absence of normal physiologic activity and stellate configuration seen at the pyloric ring. Sometimes, the mucosa adjacent or surrounding the normal antral opening is irregular or nodular which is more characteristic of the proximal end of scirrhous antral carcinoma.

In diffuse scirrhous gastric carcinoma prior to excessive narrowing, the gastroscopic view may be that of a normal appearing orange-red color, but the affected area will appear stiff and non-pliable. Peristaltic waves may move toward but may not pass through the area. Or they may pass through slowly and asymmetrically. The area of involvement is often nodular resembling hypertrophic gastropathy, but the nodules may be irregular in size. If there are gastric folds in the area, as in the body of the stomach, they may be somewhat irregular in size and thickened. If there is a caterpillar-like segmentation of folds, the segments may be irregular in size. If the area resembles benign hypertrophic gastropathy, there may be a striking absence of the velvety, non-glistening appearance usually seen in benign hypertrophic gastropathy. Instead of the decrease or absence of highlights, the latter may be moderately increased in scirrhous carcinoma and there may be mild to moderate hyperemia.

It may be impossible to distinguish infiltrating or scirrhous carcinoma from diffuse lymphosarcoma by gastroscopic survey. The characteristic difference would be that a lymphosarcoma may have all of the characteristics described for scirrhous except that the affected area may appear soft and pliable. Local areas of superficial and atrophic gastritis may appear in areas not directly affected by these malignant changes. There may also be tiny superficial erosions and petechiae particularly in the malignant areas. In any case where the x-ray and endoscopic pictures indicate scirrhous, carcinoma biopsy and brush or lavage cytology should be carried out whereever possible.

In rare instances, scirrhous carcinoma of the stomach must be differentiated from Hodgkin's disease, which may occur as a primary lesion or as a part of the generalized disorder.

CASE HISTORY

A middle-aged woman was seen at the Cook County Hospital because of fever and enlargement of glands in groin and axilla. A biopsy of a femoral gland revealed Hodgkin's disease. The patient was followed for several weeks and eventually developed epigastric distress, nausea and occasional vomiting. Barium meal x-ray studies were carried out and a diagnosis was made of gastric carcinoma. The roentenologist did not know about the finding of Hodgkin's lesion prior to the x-ray examination. The patient was then gastroscoped and, although this examiner knew about the findings and the lymph node, he was unwilling to consider the lesion of Hodgkin's disease to explain the lesion which was found. Instead it was called scirrhous carcinoma with multiple hemorrhagic erosions. The patient became too ill for surgery. Gastrobiopsy was negative, but brush cytology revealed Class V cells typical of malignant lymphoma.

A post-mortem examination was made and the diagnosis of Hodgkin's disease involving the stomach was confirmed.

Superficial Spreading, Carcinoma

Attention should be called to a type of ulcerating carcinoma being reported more frequently in recent years known as superficial spreading carcinoma. This form of malignancy may be closely related to depressed or excavated early gastric cancer of the Japanese classification. Primarily it is a spreading linear or serpiginous ulcerating lesion. Its base may be covered by adherent white mucus, or it may be hemorrhagic. In some instances, the lesion may show tiny nodules. The first case is said to have been described in 1937 by Stout. Thirty-one cases were collected by Golden and Stout between 1937 and 1947 at the Presbyterian Hospital in New York.[17] Microscopically, the carcinoma does not penetrate below the mucosa for a long time. Meanwhile, it may spread within the mucosa for a considerable distance. It may cause some of the gastric folds to be enlarged. In other instances, the folds are flattened. Some of the cases were associated with hypertrophy of the pyloric muscle. Spreading gastric carcinoma has been divided into subgroups by some authors,[18] namely A) superficial spreading type and B) linitis plastica type. The latter spreads beneath the mucosa through the muscle areas and the submucosa. It does not destroy the mucosal epithelium. The superficial spreading carcinoma was also described by Gutman of France in 1939. Eleven of the thirty-one cases collected by Golden and Stout were gastroscoped.[18] One case examined at intervals on three different occasions showed tiny erosions of the antrum which tended to disappear. The latter developments consisted of tiny nodules on an atrophic mucosa. These were regarded as carcinomatous. X-ray examinations had shown persistent antral narrowing in some of these cases which was interpreted as *antral* gastritis.

The antral narrowing phenomenon is worth noting by the student of gastroscopy because of the frequency with which it is seen particularly on x-ray. Radiologists frequently refer to smooth gross narrowing of the antrum as *antral* gastritis in which the gastroscopist sees nothing which would fit into the category of gastritis. The grossly narrowed configuration may be seen to be present for an indefinite period on repeated x-ray examination. When gastroscopy continues to be essentially negative, most of these cases are probably due to a state of spastic contraction of the musculature of the stomach. Superficial spreading carcinoma with spastic antral contraction is also described. A unique spastic phenomenon of superficial spreading carcinoma is the appearance of one to three small spastic incisurae on the greater curvature of the antrum (according to Gutman et al.).[19]

Relative Value of Gastroscopy and Gastroscopy Directed Biopsy

In a large number of series reported in the literature, the gross diagnoses of the gastroscopist have been consistently more correct than routine x-ray as proven by surgery and postmortem.

In more recent years, the improved technic of gastrobiopsy has made possible a histologic diagnosis of gastric cancer prior to laparatomy. This is excellent when the specimen is adequate and positive for cancer. Structural changes demonstrated microscopically have been regarded in the past as the *sine qua non* of malignant disease. Yet studies in electron microscopy and histochemistry are beginning to show that microscopic changes are but *sign posts* of much more definitive evidences of specific disease.

It should be noted that the addition of gastrobiopsy has not always improved diagnostic accuracy. Our recent prospective endoscopic study of gastroesophageal cancers proven at surgery (Table 17-III) showed 57 out of 58 cases or approximately 98 per cent correct for cancer by endoscopy and 24 out of 58 cases or 14 per cent correct for cancer by gastrobiopsy. These results certainly do not condemn gastrobiopsy. The high percentage of endoscopic accuracy undoubtedly reflects the long experience of the attending endoscopists involved who personally performed or closely supervised every examination. It also undoubtedly indicates two and sometimes three biopsy bites from attempted selective sites were not as effective as the six to eight bites reported by other workers. We believe that if endoscopy is well established in an institution and always carried out by or closely supervised by experienced endoscopists, the additional services of gastrobiopsy or brush cytology may not immediately raise an already very high accuracy rate as indicated in the analytical Table 17-III. It may not be reasonable to ask of any method an improvement on 98 per cent accuracy.

Yet, we believe that gastrobiopsy and brush cytology should be carried out in every case where it is feasible. We feel just as strongly that a thorough gross endoscopy survey by an experienced endoscopist should be performed in every case where it is feasible and that this input must be included equally in every diagnostic evaluation.

TABLE 17-III

ANALYSIS OF A PROSPECTIVE ENDOSCOPIC STUDY OF 78 CASES OF
GASTROESOPHAGEAL CANCER CONFIRMED BY SURGERY

The analysis shows 98 per cent diagnostic accuracy for gross endoscopy and 43 per cent diagnostic accuracy for endoscopy-directed biopsy alone.

CONFIRMED CANCERS — 58

BIOPSY	GASTROESOPHAGOSCOPY +	±	−	Not Done	Total
+	24	0	0	0	24
±	1	0	0	0	1
−	13	0	0	0	13
Not Done	19	1	0	0	20
Total	57	1	0	0	58

PROVED BENIGN — 16

BIOPSY	GASTROESOPHAGOSCOPY +	±	−	Not Done	Total
+	0	0	0	0	0
±	0	0	0	0	0
−	4	3	0	0	7
Not Done	8	1	0	0	9
Total	12	4	0	0	16

LOST TO FOLLOW UP — 4

We deplore what appears to be a trend among some workers toward the concept that the only value of endoscopy is to direct a set of forceps toward a suspicious target in the alimentary canal. In our opinion, not enough of the reports describing the advantages of gastrobiopsy and brush cytology list the experiences which include:

1. The bite that's too superficial and shows only fragments of mucosal tissue.
2. The superficial bite that shows only gastritis or esophagitis.
3. The scirrhous tissue that's too hard to bite.
4. The *near miss* bite by a few millimeters.
5. Human considerations and the lack of surgical courage to take eight or ten bites in every case.

THE GASTRIC DIAGNOSTIC PROFILE

In our diagnostic study of the stomach when cancer is suspected, a battery of tests may be utilized, arranged in a convenient time, scheduled for the convenience and minimum discomfort to the patient.

Frequently, the x-ray examination is carried out first. If there is a large and obvious neoplastic lesion on stomach x-ray which confirms a clinical impression of malignancy, biochemical and other indicated tests are performed, but endoscopic procedures may not be indicated from the patient's point of view before surgery. If the lesion is small on x-ray either as a filling defect or niches or the x-ray is negative when the stomach is clinically suspected, endoscopy is usually indicated. In these borderline cases, we feel that gastrobiopsy and frequently brush cytology are indicated.

In many cases, a patient may have lavage for cytology, endoscopy, transendoscopic biopsy and brushing and photographing all at one sitting. In some instances, preendoscopic lavage may be withheld for special reasons. We have had one case of class V cytology with negative biopsy on first examinations. Other such experiences have been reported. There is always the possibility that only one of these methods may be positive for cancer which will lead to a proven early malignancy and definitive treatment.

It is because of this possibility that the diagnostic gastric profile is used in borderline or suspected early gastric cancer. Carcinoma of the stomach remains a devastating disease which continues to defy the world's best efforts for diagnosis and eradication.

It is recommended that more intense diagnostic studies be carried out in geographic areas of low incidence like the United States to complement the intensive studies in areas of high incidence like Japan for more effective solutions to the problem of cancer in general and cancer of the stomach in particular.

REFERENCES

1. Nakayama, K.: Early detection by a coordinated program of periodic gastric mucosal x-ray studies and gastroscopic and gastrocamera observations. *Surgery,* 65:227, 1969.
2. Inlaw, R. B., Dockherty, M. B., and Priestly, T.: Large gastric cancers, collected papers in surgery. Mayo Clinic and Foundation, 56:9-17, 1965-1967.
3. Sakita, T., Oguro, U., Takasu, S., Fukutomi, H., and Miwa, T.: The development of endoscopic diagnosis of early carcinoma of the stomach. *Japanese Source of Clinical Oncology,* 2:112-119, 1971.
4. Swynnerton, B. F., and Traelove, S. C.: *Brit Med J,* 1:237, 1952.
5. Ackerman, L. V., and DelRegato, J. A.: *Cancer, Diagnosis, Treatment and Prognosis,* 4th ed. Mosby, 1970, p. 427-428.
6. Foote, F. M., Eipenberg, H., and Honeyman, M. S.: Trends in cancer incidence and survival in Connecticut. *Cancer,* 19:573-77, 1966.
7. Konzetzny, G. E.: Beziehungen der chronischen gastritis zum magenearinom. *Verhande d deutsch Gessetsch f Chirurg,* 43. Kong. 1914.
8. Faber, K.: *Gastritis and Its Consequences.* London, Oxford Univ. Press, 1935.
9. Imai, T., Kubo, T., and Watanabe, H.: Chronic gastritis in Japanese with reference to high incidence of gastric carcinoma. *J Nat Cancer Inst,* 47:179-195, 1971.
10. Ming, Si-Chun, Goldman, H., and Freiman, D. G.: Intestinal metaplasia and histogenesis of carcinoma in human stomach: light and electron microscopic study. *Cancer,* 20:1418-1429, September, 1967.

11. Sakita, T.: Report on "Retrospective and follow-up studies of early carcinoma of stomach after surgery." *Committee, Early Gastic Cancer, National Hospital,* Japan, 1971.
12. Remine, W. H., Games, M. R., and Dockerty, M. B.: Longterm survival (10-56 years) after surgery for cancer of the stomach. *Am J Surg, 117*:177-182, February, 1969.
13. Borrmann, R., Henke, F., and Lubarsch, O.: *Handbuch der spesiellen pathologischen anatomine und histologie.* Berlin, Springer, 1926, Vol. 4, pt, km, p. 865.
14. Berry, L. H., Alavi, I., Mitaniyama, A., and Adomavicius, J.: Analysis of 6000 consecutive fiberoptic and lens gastroscopies. Proceedings of the 2nd World Congress of Gastrointestinal Endoscopy, Rome and Copenhagen. Padova (Italia), Piccin Medical Books, 1972, p. 699-703.
15. Comfort, M. W., Gray, H. K., Dockerty, M. B., Gage, R. P., Dornberger, G. R., Solis, J., Epperson, D. P., and McNaughton, R. A.: Small gastric cancer. *Arch. Int Med, 94*:513, 1954.
16. Schindler, R.: Gastroscopy: *Endoscopic Study of Gastric Pathology,* 2nd ed. Chicago. Univ. of Chicago Press, 1950, pp. 310-314.
17. Golden, R., and Stout, A. P.: Superficial spreading carcinoma of the stomach. *Amer J Roentgenology, 59*:157-167, 1948.
18. Robbins, L. L.: *Golden's Diagnostic Radiology, Sec 5: Digestive Tract.* Baltimore, Williams and Wilkins Company, 1969. p. 5.287.
19. Gutman, R. A., Bertrand, I., and Peristiany, T. J.: *Le Cancer de L'estonac au Debut.* Paris, G. Doin, 1939.

CHAPTER 18

ENDOSCOPIC DIAGNOSIS OF EARLY GASTRIC CANCER

Takao Sakita and Yanao Oguro

INTRODUCTION

In 1950, with the cooperation of the Olympus Optical Company Ltd., Doctors Uji, Hayashida and Kidokoro, surgeons of Tokyo University Hospital devised the gastrocamera which made it possible to take intragastric photographs with a camera built into the tip of the instrument.

In 1955, Professor S. Tasaka's group of Tokyo University, Drs. T. Sakita, S. Ashizawa and Y. Utsumi succeeded in adapting this instrument to clinical examination. Since then, further improvements of the gastrocamera have been made and many studies of gastric diseases with this instrument have been performed by a large number of researchers.

In 1962, many cases of early gastric cancer were collected throughout Japanese hospitals and analyzed by Professor Tasaka, the president of the Japan Endoscopic Society. At the same time, a committee was established to make definition and classification of early gastric cancer. This committee consisted of some representatives of endoscopy, radiology, surgery and pathology. After repeated meetings and discussions, the criteria of early gastric cancer was established and their critical report prevails today throughout Japan and the rest of the world. However, there are some problems which still remain to be resolved in spite of numerous investigations with the gastrocamera and the gastrofiberscope.

At the Third World Congress of Gastroenterology and the First Interna-

278

tional Congress of Gastrointestinal Endoscopy in Tokyo in 1966, the Japanese criteria for early gastric cancer were recognized and praised widely by international workers.[1-3]

DEFINITION AND CLASSIFICATION

Early gastric cancer is defined as the cancerous invasion within mucosal and submucosal layers. When cancer extends below the submucosal layer it is called advanced gastric cancer. It is very important clinically that nothing is said in this definition about cancerous metastases (Fig. 18-1).

The macroscopic classification of early gastric cancer is illustrated in Figure 18-2. Early gastric cancer is classified grossly into three groups; Type I is the protruded type, Type II is the superficial and Type III is the excavated type. Especially Type II is subdivided into three groups, that is, Type IIa is a superficial elevated type, IIb is the superficial flat type and Type IIc is the superficial depressed type. The limits of protrusion or depression of Types IIa or IIc, respectively, do not exceed twice the thickness of the mucous membrane. However, the differentiation between I and IIa is sometimes quite difficult. Presently an accepted criterion is that IIa, the superficial elevated type, may extend its roots to twice the thickness of the mucosal membrane. Types I and IIa are summarized as the elevated types of early gastric cancer and IIc, III and their combined types as the depressed types of the early gastric cancer. Variations of the basic classification occur frequently enough to justify a subclassification which we call the combined types. They consist of *IIa + IIc, IIc + IIa, IIb + IIc, IIc +*

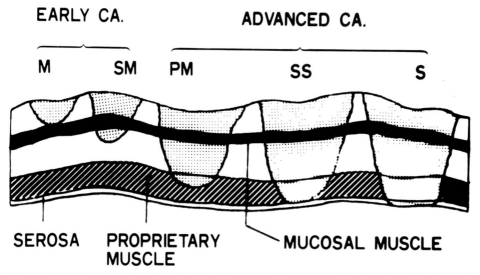

EARLY CA.   ADVANCED CA.

M   SM   PM   SS   S

SEROSA   PROPRIETARY   MUCOSAL MUSCLE
          MUSCLE

Figure 18-1. Diagram showing depth of invasion of gastric wall of early and advanced carcinoma.

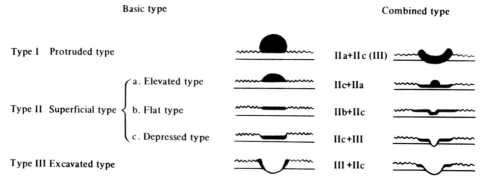

Figure 18-2. Diagrammatic illustration of macroscopic classification of early gastric cancer.

IIb, IIc + III and *III + IIc*. These combinations are described as follows: Type *IIa + IIc* is a low elevation (IIa) with central depression (IIc). Type *IIc + III* is a rather wide and shallow depression (IIc) with central excavation (III). Type *III + IIc* is a rather large excavation (III) with surrounding narrow and shallow depression (IIc).

THE INCIDENCE AND ENDOSCOPIC ACCURACY

According to the statistics of the Japanese Ministry of Health and Welfare, the total number of deaths from all malignant disease in Japan in 1971 were 122,768 (68,407 males, 54,361 females). These mortality figures were second only to the mortality figures of neurovascular diseases. Of the total deaths due to malignancies, nearly half were due to gastric cancer, that is, 49,421 deaths (29,897 males, 19,542 females) in 1971. It is believed that the ratio of limited gastric cancer cures by surgery has greatly increased in recent years due to the newer concepts and earlier diagnoses of gastric cancer. More definitive studies of these data are being made clinically by Japanese workers.

Table 18-1 shows the statistical incidence of gastric cancer in the Japanese population over forty years of age detected by mass survey. There is a

TABLE 18-I

INCIDENCE OF GASTRIC CANCER BY MASS-SURVEY, IN JAPAN

Screening Procedure	Workers	Total Examined	Advanced Cancer Cases	%	Early Cancer Cases	%
Miniature film x-ray	K. Ariga	958,702	1,608	0.15	212	0.02
	T. Sakita	109,392	188	0.05	54	0.12
Combination of gastrocamera and x-ray	K. Fujita	6,967	19	0.27	19	0.27
	T. Sakita	8,161	24	0.29	18	0.22

TABLE 18-II

INCIDENCE OF EACH TYPE OF EARLY GASTRIC CANCER IN 500 CASES PROVEN
BY SURGERY (NATIONAL CANCER HOSPITAL, JAPAN)

Grouping by Basic Type			*Basic and Combined Type*		
	Cases	*%*		*Cases*	*%*
Protruded types (I)	68	13.6	I	67	13.4
			I + IIa	1	0.2
Superficial elevated types (IIa)	79	15.8	IIa	33	6.6
			IIa + IIb	3	0.3
			IIa + IIc	43	8.6
Flat types (IIb)	10	2.0	IIb	4	0.8
			IIb + IIc	6	1.2
Superficial depressed types (IIc)	295	59.0	IIc + IIa	2	0.4
			IIc	225	45.0
			IIc + IIb	5	1.0
			IIc + III	63	12.6
Excavated types (III)	48	9.6	III + IIIa	2	0.4
			III	8	1.6
			III + IIc	38	7.6
Total	500	100.0		500	100.0

great difference in statistical results between the various procedures used in the first screening tests. With the miniature x-ray film, the rates of detection of gastric cancer is markedly inferior to the rates with gastrocamera examinations. Special x-ray and gastroendoscopic examinations are regarded as essential for the mass screening detection and correct diagnosis of early gastric cancer at the present time. X-ray examination alone was the principal procedure for the mass detection of gastric cancer for a long time. Gastrocamera examination developed only in the last twenty years has added immensely to the newer concepts of early gastric cancer.

Five hundred cases of early gastric cancer came to surgery in our hospital during the last ten years. The frequency of each type is shown in Table 18-II. Type I encountered in 68 cases or 13.6 per cent, IIa 79 cases or 15.8 per cent and so on as shown in the table. This table also shows that the great majority of early gastric cancers in our series were the depressed or ulcerated types.

Table 18-III shows the comparative accuracy in diagnosis of early gastric cancer in 165 operated cases at the National Cancer Center Hospital, Japan. Analyses of this table showed that GTF examination was the best, gastrocamera examination was the second, x-ray examination with fluoroscopy third and x-ray examination with miniatured film was the worst. According to these studies we believe gastroendoscopic examination should be

TABLE 18-III

COMPARATIVE ACCURACY OF X-RAY AND GASTROCAMERA-FIBEROSCOPY FIRST
SCREENING OF 165 PATIENTS WITH EARLY GASTRIC CANCER, CONFIRMED BY
SURGERY. (NATIONAL CANCER HOSPITAL, JAPAN)

| | | Diagnosis of Each Examination | | |
| | | Benign | Malignant | |
Procedures	Normal	Lesion	Lesion	Total
X-ray, fluoroscopy	16	49	63	128
X-ray, miniatured film	6	18	13	37
				165
Gastrocamera	8	32	70	110
(GTF) Gastrocamera with fiberscope	1	8	46	55
				165

used in first screening together with x-ray for detection and correct diagnosis of early gastric cancer in spite of any findings with x-ray examination
alone.

At the detection clinic in our hospital, both x-ray and gastroendoscopic
examinations are ordered for all patients complaining of upper gastrointestinal symptoms or requesting upper gastrointestinal screening for
cancer.

ENDOSCOPIC PATHOLOGY

Type I—Protruded Type

This form of early gastric cancer is comparable to the polypoid cancer
Type I of the Borrmann classification of advanced gastric cancer (Plate 47).
The primary difference is the depth of its roots into the gastric wall. Early
gastric cancer as previously stated is by definition a lesion which does not
extend below the mucosa and the submucosa. Retrospective studies after
surgery have shown that the protruded portion of Type I is seldom larger
than 2 or 3cm in diameter. Protruded lesions of 4 or 5cm or more in diameter usually have their roots extended below the submucosa into the muscularis and serosal layers. If a protruded lesion is smaller than 2cm in diameter, it is likely to be a benign adenomatous polyp. Our prospective
follow-up studies and retrospective observations after surgery have revealed that size and shape are the primary endoscopic features of early
gastric cancer lesions. Secondary features are such characteristics as unevenness, hyperemia, erosion, bleeding and coating.

The size of protruded or polypoid lesions may be estimated by direct vision when the endoscopist has acquaintance with the optical distance-
magnification ratio of his instrument and the necessary experience in
judging relative size and distance of folds, pyloric ring and other land-

marks. There are other methods which may be more accurate when feasible. The x-ray compression method is sometimes incorrect. The double contrast method is better but sometimes fails to visualize the lesion. The measuring gastrofiberscope or the transendoscopic meter rule are the most accurate and better than the x-ray methods.

Shapes of protruded early gastric cancer lesions are quite important in distinguishing their malignant character from benign lesions. Shapes may be described as horizontal and vertical. Figures 18-3 and 18-4 show the relative diagnostic importance of shapes of elevated or protruded early gastric lesions proven by surgery. If a protruded lesion is sessile, it is more likely to be malignant. If it is pedunculated, especially if it is also less than 2cm

SHAPE	POLYP	EARLY CA. ELEVATED TYPE (I.IIa)	ATP
CIRCLE	113	6	3
GOURD	5	1	2
MULBERRY	0	5	9
OVAL	1	1	0
ROD	0	3	0
WINDING	0	2	1
SIMILAR TO CIRCLE	16	5	0
IRREGULAR	5	21	8
WITH CENTRAL DEPRESSION	0	10	0
TOTAL	141	42	23

Figure 18-3. Diagram of horizontal shapes of elevated or protruded early gastric cancers.

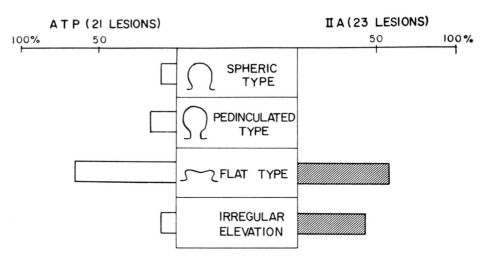

Figure 18-4. Diagram of vertical shapes of elevated and protruded early gastric cancer.

in diameter, it is probably a benign adenomatous polyp. If the polyp is uneven or nodular or irregular in shape and contour, it is more likely to be malignant.

Secondary features of protruded early gastric cancer (Fig. 18-5) such as hyperemia, erosion, bleeding or coating may be significant of malignancy when combined with the malignant characteristics of shape and size. They are less significant of malignancy when combined with benign characteris-

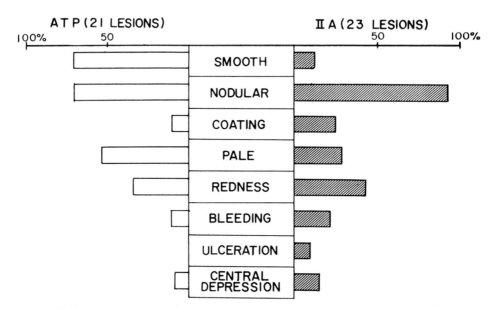

Figure 18-5. Comparative incidence of secondary features in 21 ATP lesions and 23 II A lesions proven by biopsy or surgery.

tics of shape and size. Transendoscopic biopsy or cytology may be of considerable diagnostic significance in any of these cases.

Figure 18-6 shows the relative significance of secondary endoscopic features in protruded early gastric cancer and benign adenomatous polyps proven at surgery. Type I protruded type early gastric cancer must be differentiated from other types of protruded or polypoid tumors. First of all, it should be differentiated from superficial Type IIa and its combined subgroup of early cancer (IIa + IIc) (Fig. 18-2). Note that the differentiation between Type I and IIa is mainly a matter of size. The difference between Type I and Type *IIa + IIc* is a matter of size and shape. More significantly, Type I protruded must be differentiated from benign adenomatous polyp. The latter, as previously stated, is usually less than 2cm in diameter, often pedunculated and less likely to be coated, eroded or nodular. However, a smooth eroded-bleeding polyp has been well described in the context of this discussion as well as summarized in the tables. This lesion and the benign pseudopolyp must be considered in the differential.

Next in frequency and importance comes the Polypoid Advanced Cancer or Borrmann's Type I. Again, the primary difference is in size and shape, the advanced Type I being much larger than early Type I. The advanced Type I is rarely pedunculated, often nodular, hyperemic sometimes ulcerated or coated and easily traumatized. Type I early gastric cancer must also be differentiated from tumors of submucosal origin such as the leiomyomas

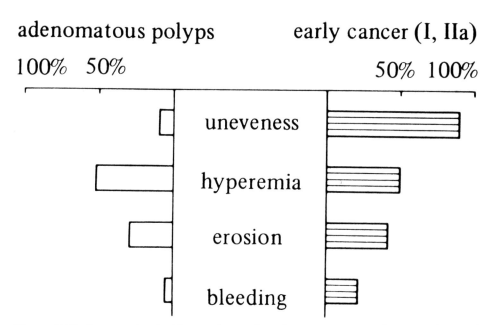

adenomatous polyps   early cancer (I, IIa)

100% 50%   50% 100%

uneveness

hyperemia

erosion

bleeding

Figure 18-6. Comparative incidence of secondary features in proven benign polyps and protruded early gastric cancer.

TABLE 18-IV

DIFFERENTIAL DIAGNOSIS BETWEEN TYPE I EARLY CANCER AND
POLYPOID TUMORS

Type I	Usually larger than 2cm, sometimes sessile, nodular and erosive, often bleeding.
Adenomatous polyp	Less than 2cm, usually pedunculated, and with smooth surface.
Submucosal tumor (leiomyoma, etc.)	Gradual elevation with smooth surface and bridging folds.
Borrmann I type of advanced carcinoma (polypoid)	Larger than type I of early carcinoma, thick coating and sometimes with ulceration.
Leiomyosarcoma	Large tumor with central ulceration, but with gradual elevation.

which are usually larger and with a smooth surface, gradually elevated from
the floor of the mucosa, often leaving *bridging folds.* If a leiomyoma has
become sarcomatous, there is often a central umbilication or ulceration. It
may be more friable and less smooth in contour. Table 18-IV shows a
differential diagnosis between Type I early gastric cancer and other polypoid tumors.

Type IIa—Superficial Elevated Type

This type lesion is smaller than Type I and usually shows a low and sessile elevation like a flat gastric polyp (Plate 48). It is usually easy to identify by an experienced endoscopist. Its combined subgroup *IIa + IIc* should
be considered in the differential (see Table 18-II).

Endoscopists, gastroenterologists and surgical pathologists in the high
gastric cancer incidence area of Japan have observed a benign lesion which
is called A.T.P. or Atypical Epithelium. This lesion has a pale, slightly
nodular or smooth surface. It is soft and hemispherical or oval in shape.
Its diameter is more frequently less than 2cm and must be differentiated
from IIa elevated cancer and combined *IIa + IIc.* Gastrobiopsy is often
the deciding factor in these cases. Benign adenomatous polyps and small
tumors of submucosal origin must also be thought of in this differential
diagnosis. Occasionally xanthomas, which are small benign yellowish elevations, sometimes singular rather than multiple may create a gross diagnostic problem endoscopically.

Type IIa + IIc—Superficial Elevated With Central Depression

The features of this type of early gastric cancer are described and illustrated in Figure 18-2, Table 18-V and Plate 49. Primarily, it has a slight
elevation over a broader central depression. The differentiation from the
varioliform gastritis and the small Borrmann Type II of the advanced
cancer is usually not so easy. The varioliform gastritis is usually multiple,

TABLE 18-V

DIFFERENTIAL DIAGNOSIS OF TYPE IIa and IIc:
ELEVATED TYPE WITH CENTRAL DEPRESSION

Type IIa + IIc ulcer	Nodular elevation with central depression. Smooth marginal swelling, with healing tendency.
Varioliform erosion	Small, smooth, multiple usually at pyloric antrum with hyperacidity.
Type IIa	No central depression.
Type IIc	Some of IIc resemble to IIa + IIc, because of slight marginal swelling of IIc.
Borrmann II type of advanced carcinoma	Large and marked crater.

soft and small lesion and the gastric secretion of acid is usually higher as compared with Type *IIa + IIc*. Although the feature of the varioliform gastritis may vary with its course, the shape of Type *IIa + IIc* is usually stable or only slightly changeable in its short course. The Borrmann Type II of advanced cancer is usually large and shows a marked crater. But, there is sometimes an intermediate lesion hard to be differentiated.

The differentiation from the Atypical Epithelium is sometimes difficult but not impossible for the same reasons as mentioned about IIa. The Atypical Epithelium is sometimes a pale, soft and regular elevation without a central depression, but Type *IIa + IIc* is a rather nodular irregular and not so pale elevation with a central depression. The differentiation from the submucosal tumor is not difficult. Type *IIa + IIc* may be thought to be a kind of penetrating carcinoma and its five-year survival rate after surgical operation is the worst of all the types of early gastric cancer. The differentiation from Type *IIc + IIa* is sometimes difficult in such a case as *IIa + IIc* with incomplete circular elevation. These problems are fairly complicated and now under discussion in Japan; therefore, these are omitted here and will be published in the near future after further clarification.

Type IIb—Flat Type

The flat type (Fig. 18-2) (Table 18-VI) (Plate 50) of early gastric cancer shows neither elevation nor depression so that it is very difficult to be detected. This was subdivided recently as follows: the first is called the "typical IIb" which is very difficult to detect and is found incidentally

TABLE 18-VI

DIFFERENTIAL DIAGNOSIS OF TYPE IIb: FLAT TYPE

Type IIb	Only slight change of color and fading, difficult to detect endoscopically.
Localized atrophy	Often accompanied by scar and with obscure margin.
Type IIc	Very shallow type of IIc is called a similar IIb.

TABLE 18-VII

DIFFERENTIAL DIAGNOSIS OF TYPE IIc: DEPRESSED TYPE

Type IIc	Well-demarcated, step-like and shallow depression, with surrounding, broken converging folds, variegated coating, bleeding and unevenness inside of IIc.
Localized atrophy	As same as, Table 18-VI.
Erosion	Hard to differentiate from small IIc.
Ulcer scar	Regular converging folds.
Reactive lymphoreticular hyperplasia	Complicated shape, very difficult to differentiate.
Borrmann IV type of advanced carcinoma	With stiff and thickening folds.
Malignant lymphomas	Variegated, biopsy is effective.

only by the pathological examination of the operated specimen. The second is the "similar IIb" which shows a very slight depression or elevation and is called a IIc like IIb or a IIa like IIb. The last is an "accompanied IIb," accompanied by or attached to the other type of early gastric cancer. A "single IIb" is not accompanied by any malignant lesion. The accompanied IIb is sometimes found around IIc. Recent endoscopic examination can find out not only the similar IIb but also the single IIb by the features of discoloration, paleness and bleeding, if performed carefully. The similar IIb is found not rarely. Recently, the progress of gastric biopsy has greatly contributed to their detection.

Type IIc—Superficial Depressed Type

The depressed types of early gastric cancer (Fig. 18-2) (Table 18-VII) (Plate 51) which comprise the great majority of all of early gastric cancers, make a group of common yet variable features.

The diagnosis of the typical IIc of early gastric cancer is not so difficult. The order of observation of Type IIc is as follows:

a) Typical features of the inside of the Type IIc.

At the inside of IIc, there are irregularly mixed changes such as erosion, hyperemia or bleeding and fading or discoloration etc. The small elevation called islands can be observed.

b) Characteristic features of the margin of Type IIc (Fig. 18-7).

The margin of the shallow depression, Type IIc, can be traced usually with well demarcated and frequently mouse-eaten edges. Converging folds

TABLE 18-VIII

DIFFERENTIAL DIAGNOSIS OF TYPE III AND TYPE III & IIc

Type III and III + IIc	Similar to ulcer, but irregular margin and broken converging folds. Healing tendency.
Ulcer	Smooth margin, regular converging folds.
Advanced carcinoma with ulceration	Large tumor with deep ulceration, progressive.
Reactive lymphoreticular hyperplasia	Same as, Table 18-VII.

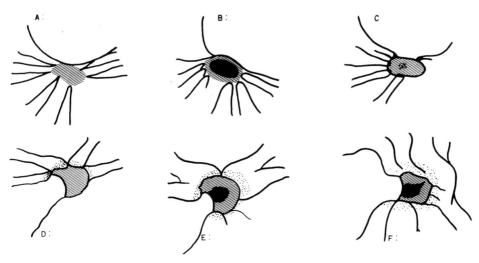

Figure 18-7. Characteristic features of the margins of Type II C, early gastric cancer.

with disruption at the margin are the most typical pattern of Type IIc. In detail description, sudden break, mouse-eaten edge, irregular narrowing, club-like thickening and pick-like thinning, etc. can be recognized at the margin of the mucosal folds. When these characteristic features are observed, the confirmation of the Type IIc is easy. But, in the lesions with more shallow depression, that is, appearance nearly similar to Type IIc, diagnosis is more difficult because those findings become obscure and disappear sometimes. In these cases, biopsy is very effective.

Type III—Excavated Type

The features of the typical Type III of early gastric cancer is only with excavation and without any surrounding elevation or depression (Plate 52). The differential diagnosis of Type III is shown in Table 18-VIII. The cancerous invasion of this type is limited to the margin or the surrounding submucosal layer; therefore, the Type III may be called correctly as *III + IIb*. The recognition of this form of IIb is very difficult endoscopically so that *III + IIb* is almost impossible to distinguish from the benign ulcer without biopsy. Type III may change its characteristics to Type *III + IIc* and then to Type *IIc + III* and at least to Type IIc following the course. Only in these later stages it becomes possible to check malignant signs endoscopically. This is called the malignant cycle which will be mentioned in detail later.

Type III + IIc and Type IIc + III—The Combined Type

The wider the area of the shallow depression IIc around the excavation (III) spreads, the easier becomes the confirmation of the malignancy.

Type *III* + *IIc* and *IIc* + *III* (Fig. 18-2) are from the same origin because Type III may change to Type *III* + *IIc* and then to Type *IIc* + *III* in a short period and at last to Type IIc or Type IIb. This means that the ulceration located in the depressed type of early gastric cancer has the healing tendency in its course as well as the benign ulcer.

LIFE CYCLE AND NATURAL HISTORY
Life Cycle of Malignant Ulcer

The development of gastroendoscopy has been clarifying the course of growth and development of gastric cancer, especially in its early stage. The retrospective study of former gastrocamera films makes possible those clarifications. Growth and course of carcinoma are explained in the following order: Malignant cycle of the depressed cancer, growth of the elevated cancer and then survival rate of the early epigastric cancer after surgery.

The life cycle of the malignant ulcer is shown in the following figure (Fig. 18-8).

The life cycle of the malignant ulcer means that the ulceration located in the depressed type of the early gastric cancer, that is the malignant ulcer at its earliest stage has the same tendency to heal as the benign ulcer by medicament treatment. But the cancerous tissue remains of course. This phenomenon will be illustrated by the schema as shown in Figure 18-8. "A" in Figure 18-8 is the typical Type III of the early gastric cancer (A1 and A2 in Fig. 18-8) and (Plate 49) of which the cancerous invasion is limited to the mucosal layer and which may be impossible to differentiate from

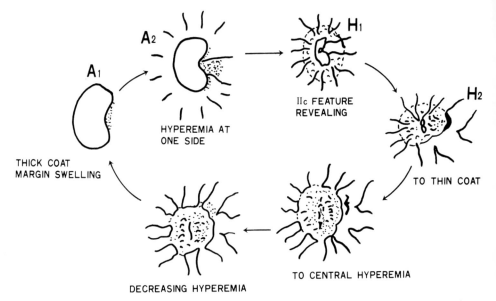

Figure 18-8. Illustration of life cycle of malignant ulcer of early gastric cancer.

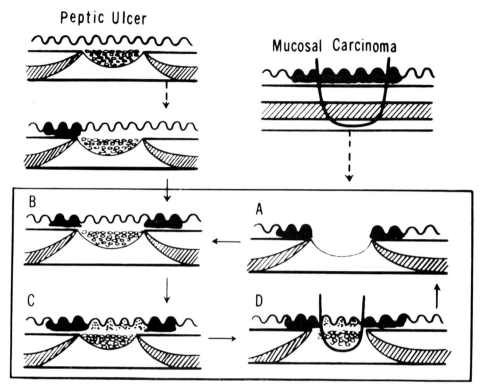

Figure 18-9. Histologic representation of life cycle of malignant ulcer. The black portion represents carcinomatous tissue. There are two theories about the pathogenesis of gastric cancer as shown by dotted arrow and lined arrow. The latter shows the course of malignant cycle.

the benign ulcer. The picture "B" in Figure 18-8 means that the noncancerous tissue around the ulcer covers the base of the ulcer and then the ulcer heals (stage between A2 and H1 in Fig. 18-6 and Plate 50). The figure "C" in Figure 18-8 shows that the marginal cancerous tissue is invading into this scar as shown in Figure 18-8 from H1 to S2. The picture "D" in Figure 18-8 means the ulceration occurred again inside of the same lesion as shown in A1 in Figure 18-6.

This is a schema of a case following the typical course. Practical various courses may be observed. For instance at the phase of the incomplete healing of the ulceration, recurrence of the ulceration is possible. If the size of the recurrent ulceration should be larger than the extent of the early gastric cancer, the cancerous tissue might be completely destroyed and the patient could be cured, especially in case of a small cancer. But it is very difficult to prove this phenomenon. The clarification of the pathogenosis of this phenomenon is one of the important problems to be solved in the field of gastric cancer for the future. Figure 18-9 is a histologic diagram of the life cycle of malignant ulcer.

Course of Elevated Types

The course of the elevated types of early gastric cancer is based upon our analyses of 16 cases of protruded type, Type I and elevated type, Type II, of gastric cancers which were retrospectively observed by gastroendoscopy for more than six months and up to five years. These types of gastric cancers had been increasing in size and height continuously but slowly. The initial features of these lesions had already a slight elevation.

At the initial stage of the Type IIa + IIc some changes were found retrospectively to have occurred at the same place. These changes were very small and sometimes scarcely any except erosions (Case 1, Plate 54 and Plate 49). Type IIa + IIc which we discovered and named in 1968

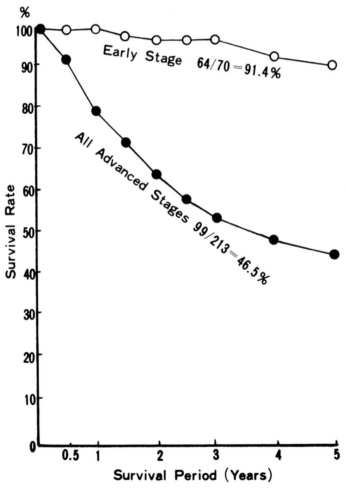

Figure 18-10. Curve of yearly survival rates of gastric cancer radically operated in early and advanced stages, National Cancer Center, Tokyo.

could have developed to the Borrmann Type II of advanced cancer in a year or so.

Follow Up Study After Surgery

According to the committee on early gastric cancer of the National Hospitals of Japan of which Sakita was the chairman, 652 cases of early gastric cancer receiving surgery from 1964 to 1969 were registered. Only 17 cases (2.6%) out of this group died by recurrence of carcinoma. The chief causes of death were liver metastasis—6, peritonitis—4, general metastasis including kidney and brain—2 and others—5.

The five-year survival rates of the operated patients with gastric cancer in our National Cancer Center Hospital (1962-1964) dropped proportionately with the depth of cancerous invasion. The rate at the mucosal level is 96.5 per cent, at the submucosal layer 88.1 per cent, at the muscularis propria layer 51.5 per cent, at the subserosa layer 51.6 per cent and at the serosa layer 36.7 to 25.0 per cent (see Figure 18-10). The curve of early gastric cancer shows a markedly better prognosis than the curve of advanced cancer. These findings are the principal justification and support of our criteria for early gastric cancer.

CASE HISTORIES

The Course of the Elevated Type

Case 1, H. A., 52-year-old man.
Chief complaint: Hematemesis.

The first gastrocamera finding (Plate 54) was an almost healed ulcer at the angulus and general atrophic gastritis. After six years the patient returned with slight epigastric pain. GTF-A examination revealed a small crater on the posterior wall of the antrum (Plate 49) (IIa+IIc). This lesion resembled a small erosion but somewhat like the gastrocamera finding of six years before (Plate 54) the pathology had proved to be cancerous invasion limited within the submucosal layer. This is a typical IIa+IIc of early gastric cancer.

The Course of the Depressed Type

Case 2, T. I., 62-year-old man.
Chief complaint: Discomfort, nausea, heartburn at mealtime.

The first GTF-A examination showed a gastric ulcer at the angulus (Plate 52) (Type III). GTF-A examination after one month showed a markedly healed lesion (Plate 18-7) but the fibroscopic biopsy confirmed the cancerous tissue around its ulceration. Histological section proved the cancerous tissue only at the mucosal layer. This was a phase (IIc+III) of the malignant cycle in the depressed type of early gastric cancer. We had discovered this phenomenon clinically at first in 1965.

Elevated Type (IIa), (Plate 48)

Case 3, O. O., 63-year-old man.
Chief complaint: Anorexia.

A moderately elevated lesion was seen on the lesser curvature at the pyloric antrum. There was an erosion on the tip of the lesion. Only mucosal invasion was proven by histologic section.

The Flat Type (IIb), (Plate 50)

Case 4, Y. H., 52-year-old woman.
Chief complaint: Epigastric pain.

We found a peptic ulcer at the angulus. About 8 months later this lesion had healed completely as shown in the picture. The fiberscopic biopsy proved adenocarcinoma in this lesion. This is a typical case of Type IIb of early gastric cancer.

The Protruded Type (I), (Plate 47)

Case 5, H. K., 65-year-old man.
Chief Complaint: Right side abdominal pain.

For the past two years the patient had noted heavy feeling in the upper abdomen. Because of the right sided abdominal pain he came to the clinic and was diagnosed a gastric cancer. At surgery there was cholelithiasis and early gastric cancer, Type I confirmed.

The Depressed Type (IIc), (Plate 51)

Case 6, M. I., 47-year-old woman.
Chief complaint: Epigastric pain.

For the past two months the patient had noted a heavy sensation and pain in the epigastrium. At surgery early gastric cancer Type IIc was found. Histologic section showed invasion at the mucosal layer.

REFERENCES

1. S. Tasaka, and T. Sakita: Progress of gastrocamera examination. *Proceedings of the first Congress of the International Society of Endoscopy*, Tokyo. 70-77, 1966.
2. T. Sakita: Diagnosis of early gastric cancer with gastrocamera. Recent advances in gastroenterology. *The Proceedings of the Third World Congress of Gastroenterology*, Tokyo. I, 275-281, 1966.
3. S. Tasaka, and Y. Oguro: Fundamental studies on the optimum photographic conditions of the gastrofiberscopic and gastrocamera examinations. *Proceedings of the First Congress of the International Society of Endoscopy*, Tokyo. 320-327, 1966.
4. The Committee of early gastric cancer of the National Hospital of Japan (Chief of the Committee: T. Sakita): Report on Retrospective and follow-up studies of the early carcinoma of the stomach, after surgery, 1971 (written in Japanese).
5. T. Muto et al.: A study of end results of early gastric carcinoma: Stomach and Intestine, 5,541, 1970 (written in Japanese).
6. T. Hayashi: End results of early gastric cancer. *Gastroenterological Endoscopy*, 11, 114, 1969 (written in Japanese).
7. T. Hayashida et al.: End results of early gastric cancer, collected from 22 institutions: *Stomach and Intestine*, 4:1075, 1969 (written in Japanese, but with English abstract and explanations of Tables, etc.).
8. Y. Yoshitoshi: Prognosis of gastric cancer. *Gastroenterological Endoscopy*, 7:126, 1965 (written in Japanese).

CHAPTER 19

GASTRIC LYMPHOMAS, SARCOMAS, GRANULOMATOUS AND RELATED DISORDERS OF THE STOMACH

ROBERT S. NELSON

IN ADDITION TO CARCINOMA, the stomach is the site of other malignant tumors as well as a miscellaneous variety of rare infiltrations, some of which are found so infrequently as to be true curiosities. Of the malignant tumors, by far the most common are lymphoma and sarcoma. The endoscopic investigation of these malignancies is still in an early stage. Their relative rarity and the tendency to subject all radiologically demonstrated gastric abnormalities to early surgery account for the scant gastroscopic experience available in the literature. Those workers who have a large clinical supply of such tumors are few, but it can be demonstrated that preoperative gastroscopy may be very valuable in outlining treatment and in follow-up.

MALIGNANT LYMPHOMA

Malignant lymphomas constitute 0.5 to 8 per cent of all cancerous lesions of the stomach, the incidence varying in individual institutions and averaging about 3 to 5 per cent.[1] The main tumor types, in order of frequency, are lymphosarcoma, reticulum cell sarcoma, and Hodgkin's disease (rare as primary). In generalized lymphomatosis, from 30 to 54 per cent of patients with these three diseases will have stomach lesions,[2, 3] although not all will be symptomatic. The patient with primary gastric lymphoma without other evidence of disease usually presents with upper gastrointestinal symptoms and radiologic evidence of abnormality or tumor. In generalized lymphoma, symptoms may be mild and no roentgenographic studies may be available when the patient is referred, although often these have been performed and show some type of abnormality. The high incidence of gastric involvement in the latter situation should make all symptomatic patients suspect until proven otherwise.

For years, the endoscopist has been intrigued by the possibility of preoperative diagnosis of lymphoma and its differentiation from adenocarcinoma, which it so often resembles grossly. Many patients with primary or secondary gastric lymphoma are poor surgical risks or have massive involvement which renders surgery essentially impossible. Identification of this group without surgery would allow irradiation or chemotherapy without the risk of exploration. Even in the low-risk patient or those with resectable lesions, there would appear to be advantages to a firm gastroscopic diagnosis prior to surgery.

Gross Features

Unfortunately, attempts to make an accurate appraisal of these tumors based on gross characteristics alone have been disappointing. The lesions may often be identified as malignant infiltrations, but a conclusive opinion as to the type of tumor, and in particular the differentiation from carcinoma, has in most cases proved impossible.[4, 5] Gross classifications based on gastroscopic observations of surgically proved lymphomas, such as infiltrative, ulcerative, nodular, polypoid, and combined, are useless in diagnosis since other tumors and in particular carcinoma, present in the same fashion.[6, 7] It has gradually become apparent that only definite histologic proof would be of real value in gastroscopic diagnosis.

This conclusion has been reached only with the passage of time, however. Gastroscopy has not been employed widely enough in lymphoma over the years to allow a definitive conclusion as to its value. In many of the largest series reported, it has apparently not been used at all,[4] and in a group of 270 patients collected over twenty-five years in one large clinic, it is not mentioned.[8] In more recent studies, it has been referred to occasionally.[9, 10] In none has the record as to gross diagnosis been good. The largest published series in which gastroscopy was compared to roentgenography shows that neither has been satisfactory in making a definitive diagnosis.[4, 11]

There appears to be one limited exception to the rule of noncharacteristic features in lymphoma. In approximately one third of all reticulum cell sarcomas, a raised, volcano-like crater ulcer is noted which appears to be diagnostic, permitting an extremely strong suspicion of this tumor. We have, in fact, made the correct diagnosis in several instances on this lesion alone. In thirty-nine patients with primary and secondary gastric lymphoma, twenty with lymphosarcoma, sixteen with reticulum cell sarcoma, and three with Hodgkin's disease, the *crater* ulcer was noted in five patients only, all with reticulum cell sarcoma[12] (Plate 55). In addition, we have had the opportunity of making a correct diagnosis based on this lesion in two other patients seen elsewhere, for a total of seven with this type of ulcer.[13] Although diagnostic when seen, this observation is of relatively small importance when viewed in the perspective of gastric lymphoma as a whole, in which the gross lesions are so varied as to defy diagnostic classification.

Lymphoma arises and spreads through the submucosa, and the gross masses and enlarged folds noted at gastroscopy and roentgenoscopy are frequently only the "tip of the iceberg." When gross abnormalities are noted throughout the stomach, it is easy to determine the extent of visualized tumor, but localized masses are no guarantee that there is not substantial submucosal extension.[11]

Gastroscopic Biopsy

Before the advent of fiberoptic instruments which permit extremely accurate directed biopsy, few histologic diagnoses of lymphoma were made by this means. In 1961, a review noted that seven cases were found in the literature in which biopsies had been obtained up to that time.[11] Of these,

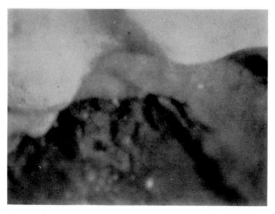

Figure 19-1. Reticulum cell sarcoma with massive infiltration and large folds, grossly indistinguishable from adenocarcinoma. Ulcerating lesion of distal greater curvature was diagnostic on gastroscopic biopsy.

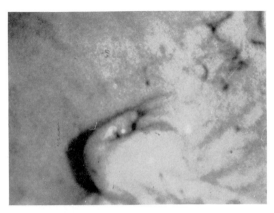

Figure 19-2. Elevated, rolled-edge "crater" lesion on greater curvature of distal stomach in patient with generalized reticulum cell sarcoma. The stomach contained two similar lesions in upper third.

three only were positively identified as lymphoma, the remainder being interpreted as carcinoma or gastritis. Since then, occasional reports of single successful biopsies[14, 15] and one of positive results in four patients[16] have appeared. Recently, more determined efforts have produced slightly improved results,[17, 18] although proportionately they were still poor.[18]

The accuracy of results of guided gastroscopic biopsy at The University of Texas M. D. Anderson Hospital and Tumor Institute has been somewhat better. We obtained a total of twelve positive results in fifteen patients (83.4%) with gastric lymphoma (reticulum cell sarcoma and lymphosarcoma). The technic employed was multiple biopsies (six to nine) taken as deep as possible in the edges of ulcerating lesions, polypoid areas, and

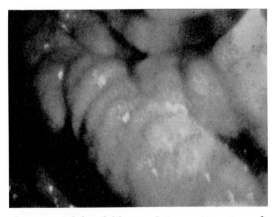

Figure 19-3. Large boggy, nodular folds involving entire stomach in a patient with lymphosarcoma. Biopsies obtained from many areas of these folds all gave positive results.

at the base of the large, meaty folds often found in lymphoma. One excuse given for the failure of biopsy in other series has been the submucosal nature of lymphomatous invasion.[18] This is a definite problem, but we found that by putting considerable pressure on the biopsy tip, the submucosal area can often be penetrated (Figs. 19-1, 2, 3). It may also be true that varying the areas in which specimens are taken is a distinct advantage, since in some cases only one or two specimens will be diagnostic, although six to nine are obtained. Likewise, initial biopsies have on occasion given negative results, with a second attempt successful. Pathologists often have difficulty in distinguishing lymphoma from undifferentiated carcinoma. In patients with disseminated disease, comparison with previously obtained biopsy material (usually from lymph glands) may help to resolve an equivocal reading. Practice in evaluating the small gastric biopsy specimen is also an aid, and review by the gastroenterologist of all gastric biopsies is recommended.

Cytology

Cytologic examination has been essentially unsatisfactory in gastric lymphoma. Scattered reports indicate that gastric washing has been successful in establishing the diagnosis in individual patients,[19, 20] and a recent review[21] listing eleven publications reports positive results in five of twelve cases from the world literature by 1967. Thus far, we have been unable to diagnose lymphoma by brush cytology of individual lesions in any patient, although this procedure is now routine in all tumors seen on our service. The results are in contrast to those obtained with carcinoma, in which brush cytology is strongly supportive.

Gastroscopic Objectives

As stated previously, although gastroscopy has been seldom used in patients with gastric lymphoma, and much more work needs to be done in all centers, sufficient information is available to outline avenues of present and future usefulness in this particular tumor. Endoscopy should prove valuable in: (1) establishing a histologic diagnosis, (2) determining the extent of stomach involvement, and (3) following up treatment.

The gross differentiation of lymphoma from carcinoma is impossible gastroscopically, but proper technics, multiple biopsies and adequate pathologic examination should make the diagnosis histologically possible, in a majority of patients. This will be of great advantage in the future treatment of patients, particularly those who are poor surgical risks.

Lymphoma of the stomach is a submucosal tumor which tends to spread widely, involving large areas. The gross lesions noted at roentgenoscopy and gastroscopy are often indicative of only a small part of gastric infiltration. The determination of gross gastric involvement by both inspection and biopsy will serve to delineate those patients most likely to have non-resectable lesions. These can then be treated by radiation and chemotherapy without the risk of surgery. There is ample evidence to prove that such treatment can be quite as effective as resection in many patients.[22] Tradition and experience with this relatively rare tumor being what they are, it will take a considerable period to determine just how effective nonsurgical therapy is, but the tools are at hand for this purpose.

Partly resected and nonresected stomachs can now be followed grossly and histologically to determine recurrence in primary gastric lymphoma. We are presently following two patients, one for two and another for four years after irradiation alone, who are without evidence of disease. In two others, it was possible to demonstrate that chemotherapy alone was ineffective. This precise information should be invaluable in prescribing treatment.

LYMPHORETICULAR HYPERPLASIA (PSEUDOLYMPHOMA)

This pleomorphic gastric infiltration may be generalized or localized.[23-26] Many of the lesions present as gastric ulceration, but the nature of the surrounding submucosal infiltrate usually raises the question of carcinoma, and most have been so diagnosed grossly both by roentgenoscopy and gastroscopy. The nature of the infiltrate caused by massive collections of lymphoid follicles on section of the resected specimen has resulted in diagnoses of lymphoma in the past, and it has been postulated that the long-term survivals in some cases of lymphoma have been examples of lymphoreticular hyperplasia, since it is invariably nonmalignant.[27] The more extensive lesions can, however, produce considerable morbidity unless resected (Plate 56).

Gastroscopically, the diagnosis is usually gastric ulcer with suspicious local infiltrate or, in the more diffuse lesions, ulcerating carcinoma. Cytology has been unrewarding,[24] and directed gastric biopsy only partly successful. The specimen obtained shows many lymphocytes but is too small as a rule to demonstrate their collection into discrete follicles.[23, 25] Surgical resection is necessary for both diagnosis and treatment, and results in cure in most patients, particularly those with localized lesions.

LEIOMYOSARCOMA

Leiomyosarcoma, the only important malignant smooth muscle tumor of the stomach, comprises 17 to 20 per cent of all smooth muscle tumors of this organ and about 30 per cent of gastric sarcomas. It represents 1 to 3 per cent of all gastric malignant tumors.[8, 28-31] From the clinical standpoint, the lesion is characterized by epigastric pain, bleeding, anemia, and a palpable abdominal mass in 75 to 100 per cent.[8, 28–33] The large mass is frequently a major deterrent to adequate roentgenologic or gastroscopic studies because of pressure and displacement of the stomach. Tumors with more of an intragastric and less extragastric mass are more easily visualized.

Gross Features

With sufficient intragastric mass, submucosal tumor may be recognized roentgenographically and gastroscopically. The tumor is most frequently located in the upper half of the stomach. A central area of necrosis is often present, representing in many cases the source of recent hemorrhage. At gastroscopy, *bridging* mucosal folds are usually noticed. Those tumors with a single submucosal mass are impossible to differentiate from leiomyomas. With two or more masses, a strong suspicion of leiomyosarcoma, rather than leiomyoma, may be entertained. The surrounding areas are as a rule smooth and show no signs of further infiltration, in contradistinction to lymphoma, in which more general distribution is the rule. Unless the tumor is massive, with marked displacement of the stomach, the remainder of the mucosa appears flexible and essentially normal.

In our small series of six patients, all of whom were studied with the older semirigid gastroscope rather than the newer fiberoptic instrument, identification on gross characteristics alone was poor. In five the lesion was identified as tumor, diagnosed as carcinoma in two, lymphoma in two, and leiomyoma in one. In this last patient only, a secondary diagnosis of possible leiomyosarcoma was made. Comparing this experience with that in eight leiomyomas, which may be indistinguishable from leiomyosarcomas grossly, the correct diagnosis was made in three patients, one was not visualized, and the remaining four were identified as benign tumor, carcinoma, inflammatory tissue, and extrinsic mass. In one of those recognized correctly as leiomyoma, leiomyosarcoma was given as a secondary diagnosis.[4] In four subsequent patients, the correct diagnosis was made employing the fiberoptic gastroscope, with adequate photographs to record characteristic features (Fig. 19-4) (Plate 57). When the leiomyoma occurs near the antrum in the area of gastric peristalsis, it can be noted that peristaltic waves go through the tumor area without interruption. We have had no opportunity to determine whether or not this is true with leiomyosarcoma, but presume it would be unlikely if the tumor were extensive.

In summary, single-lobed leiomyosarcomas may be indistinguishable from leiomyomas grossly, which is not surprising in a tumor which may cause the pathologist considerable indecision when it is of a low grade of malignancy. With an identifiable, very large exogastric mass, often cystic, leiomyosarcoma is a more likely diagnosis, and with the single-lobed sub-

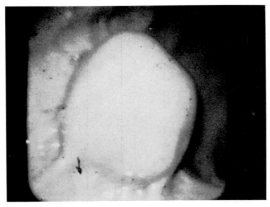

Figure 19-4. Smooth, submucosal tumor on anterior gastric wall was diagnosed as leiomyoma. It consists of a single mass, and there are suggestions of "bridging folds" at the base. The diagnosis was proved on wedge resection of the lesion.

mucosal tumors of medium to small size, leiomyoma can usually be confidently diagnosed.

Gastroscopic Biopsy

Biopsy with the presently available instruments has not been useful in leiomyoma when the surface epithelium is unbroken, but in one patient we were able to obtain a positive specimen from the deep edge of the ulcer crater in an ulcerating lesion. We have had no opportunity to attempt the same maneuver in leiomyosarcoma, but would assume that it would be worthwhile, since the accessibility should be the same. In nonulcerating lesions, however, biopsy has failed.

Gastroscopic Objectives

Gastroscopy in leiomyosarcoma may not differentiate this tumor from leiomyoma, except in ulcerating lesions when material may be available from the ulcer crater (not proven, but probable). In most cases, the tumor can be identified as submucosal, and the extent of involvement delineated. Further study along these lines may prove valuable.

LEIOMYOBLASTOMA

This rare tumor occurs most frequently in the pyloric antrum, with a lesser incidence in the body of the stomach. In 1970, a review listed 112 cases,[34] and two others were reported the same year.[35, 36] The great majority are benign, and the incidence of malignancy, with six of 114 evidencing such change, is extremely low (5.2%). The roentgenographic and gastroscopic appearance is that of any similar intramural tumor, such as leiomyoma or leiomyosarcoma, and there is no report indicating a preoperative histologic diagnosis by biopsy or cytology, all having been confirmed following resection.

LEUKEMIC INFILTRATIONS

Leukemic involvement of the stomach occurs in generalized disease. Review of postmortem material shows an incidence of gastric lesions in 24 per cent, but in those seen clinically the incidence is much smaller. The majority of lesions are microscopic, and the gross lesions represented by massive folds were found in only two of 148 patients.[37] We have never seen such a lesion in an extensive experience at The University of Texas M. D. Anderson Hospital and Tumor Institute. Gastric ulcerations occur frequently in patients with leukemia, especially those subjected to chemotherapy, and unless the diagnosis can be confirmed histologically, it is unrealistic to attribute them to leukemia.[38] Histologic diagnosis has not so far been reported. Lesions recognizable and diagnosable by gastroscopy must therefore be considered extremely rare.

PLASMACYTOMA AND MULTIPLE MYELOMA

Plasmacytomas appear to be unusually rare, and only eighteen have so far been described in the literature.[39, 40] They appear as large, ulcerating tumors and so far as can be determined have not been observed gastroscopically. In generalized myelomatosis, gastroscopic observations have been made of large, nodular folds, indistinguishable from carcinoma or lymphoma. Although this latter form of multiple myeloma is even less commonly seen than the localized plasmacytoma, it should be considered in a patient with multiple myeloma who has roentgenologically demonstrated large folds or infiltrations in the stomach.[13, 41] Biopsy may be valuable (Plate 58).

CARCINOID TUMORS

Primary gastric carcinoids are also rare; they make up 1 to 3 per cent of all gastrointestinal carcinoid tumors. The total so far described in the literature is 102.[19, 42–45] Few roentgenologic and even fewer gastroscopic descriptions exist. Most lesions occur in the distal two thirds of the stomach and may be submucosal and infiltrating or large and polypoid. The tumor has not yet been diagnosed histologically by gastroscopic biopsy, but with the increased use of this method, even this rare lesion probably can be so identified in the future. Histologic verification would appear to be necessary, since there are no characteristic gross findings, and the most common preoperative diagnosis is carcinoma.[19, 42, 44]

TUBERCULOSIS, SYPHILIS, GRANULOMAS, AND VILLOUS TUMORS

The stomach has been shown to be involved by syphilis and tuberculosis in the past, although a close review of some of the cases would indicate that the diagnosis during life was made upon a somewhat tenuous basis when an ulcerating lesion in a patient with one of these diseases healed under treatment without histologic confirmation.[46] We have never had the opportunity to study one of these patients, but it might be suggested for the future that histologic proof be required, now that biopsies can be readily obtained. It is just possible that some of these lesions might be proven to have a different cause.

Granulomas, whether esinophilic or related to regional enteritis, are very rare.[47] The gross gastroscopic picture has seldom been seen, and is not diagnostic. Our single opportunity to view a granuloma related to regional enteritis in a 13-year-old boy appeared gastroscopically as submucosal infiltration, and was correctly diagnosed only on surgical biopsy.

Villous tumors have been found in the stomach in approximately forty-five patients, and again the gross appearance is not diagnostic. They would not appear to be an important differential during endoscopic examination.

REFERENCES

1. Salmela, H.: Lymphosarcoma of the stomach: A clinical study of 39 cases. *Acta chir scandinav, 134*:567, 1968.
2. Bush, R. S., and Ash, C. L.: Primary lymphoma of the gastrointestinal tract. *Radiology, 92*:1349, 1969.
3. Enrlich, A. M., Stalder, G., Geller, W., and Sherlock, P.: Gastrointestinal manifestations of malignant lymphoma. *Gastroenterology, 54*:1115, 1968.
4. Nelson, R. S., and Lanza, F. L.: Endoscopy in the diagnosis of gastric lymphoma and sarcoma. *Am J Gastroenterol, 50*:37, 1968.
5. Kaplan, M. H.: Lymphosarcoma of the stomach (Value of gastroscopy with case report). *Bull Gastrosc & Esophagosc, 6*:15, 1960.
6. Whetsell, J. E.: Primary malignant lymphoma of the stomach: A diagnostic enigma. *Bull Gastrointest Endosc 13*:11, 1966.
7. Dunn, G. D., Moeller, D., and Laing, R. R.: Primary reticulum cell sarcoma of the stomach. *Gastrointest Endosc, 17*:153, 1971.
8. Burgess, J. M., Malcolm, M. D., Dockerty, B., and ReMine, W. H.: Sarcomatous lesions of the stomach. *Ann Surg, 173*:758, 1971.
9. Loehr, W. J., Mujahed, Z., Zahn, F. D., Gray, G. F., and Thorbjarnarson, B.: Primary lymphoma of the gastrointestinal tract: A review of 100 cases. *Ann Surg, 170*:232, 1969.
10. Bilde, T., and Asnaes, S.: Reticulosarcoma of the stomach: Report of 13 cases with follow-up results. *Acta chir scandinav, 136*:617, 1970.
11. Schuman, B. M.: The gastroscopic diagnosis of lymphoma of the stomach. *Bull Gastrointest Endosc, 8*:8, 1961.
12. Nelson, R. S., Lanza, F. L., and Bottiglieri, N. G.: The "crater" ulcer: A possibly exclusive gross characteristic of reticulum cell sarcoma of the stomach. *Gastroenterology, 60*:824, 1971 (abst.).
13. Nelson, Robert S.: *Endoscopy in Gastric Cancer. Recent Results in Cancer Research*, Vol. 32. New York, Springer-Verlag, 1970, p. 39.
14. Heully, F., Gaucher, P., Houplon, M., Penin, F., Bas et Mlle, M., and Macinot,

C.: Lymphosarcome gastrique diagnostique par gastro-biopsie. *Arch franç mal appar dig,* 56:549, 1967.

15. Gadrat, J., Ribet, A., Suduca, P., Pascal, J. P., Duffaut, M., and Prexinos, J.: Le lympho-reticulosarcome gastrique. *Arch franç mal appar dig,* 57:260, 1968.

16. Nelson, R. S., Lanza, F. L., and Somayaji, B. N.: Endoscopic studies in gastric lymphoma. Proceedings XI Pan American Congress of Gastroenterology (In press).

17. Danao, S. C., and Schuman, B. M.: Gastroscopic features of primary gastric lymphoma. *Gastroenterology,* 60:816, 1971.

18. Katz, S., Klein, M., Winawer, S., and Sherlock, P.: Secondary gastric lymphoma: Correlation of endoscopy with directed cytology and biopsy. *Gastroenterology,* 60:818, 1972 (Abstract).

19. Berke, R. A.: Two gastric ulcers adjacent to a mass. *JAMA, 213:2069,* 1970.

20. Bach-Nielsen, P.: The value of gastric cytology in the diagnosis of mesenchymal tumors. *Am J Dig Dis, 11:938,* 1966.

21. Fiol, V. C., Garcia, R. O., Campos, R. O., and Vilardell, F.: Aportacio al cito-diagnostico de las neoplasias malignas gastricas no epiteliales. *Rev expano enf ap dig, 26:1193,* 1967.

22. Cook, J. C., and Corbett, D. P.: Roentgen therapy of primary gastrointestinal lymphoma. *Radiology, 78:562,* 1967.

23. Bahk, Y. W., Ahn, J. S., and Choi, H. J.: Lymphoid hyperplasia of the stomach presenting as umbilicated polypoid lesions. *Diag Radiol, 100:277,* 1971.

24. Kobayashi, R., Prolla, J. C., and Kirsner, J. B.: Reactive lymphoreticular hyperplasia of the stomach. *Arch Intern Med, 125:1030,* 1970.

25. Gagnon, M., and Dreyfuss, J.: Le pseudolymphome gastrique: probleme diagnostique et therapeutique. *Union Med Canada, 96:1079,* 1967.

26. Eras, P., and Winawer, S. J.: Benign lymphoid hyperplasia of the stomach simulating gastric malignancy. *Am J Digest Dis, 14:510,* 1969.

27. Valdes-Dapena, A., Affholter, H., and Vilardell, F.: The gradient of malignancy in lymphoid lesions of the stomach. *Gastroenterology, 50:382,* 1966.

28. Garvie, W. H. H.: Leiomyosarcoma of the stomach. *Brit J Surg, 52:32,* 1965.

29. Stanley, W. M., and Groshong, L. E.: Leiomyosarcoma of the gastrointestinal tract. *Am Surgeon, 35:809,* 1969.

30. Phillips, J. C., Lindsay, J. W., and Kendall, J. A.: Gastric leiomyosarcoma: Roentgenologic and clinical finding. *Am J Dig Dis, 15:230,* 1970.

31. Salmela, H., and Kohler, R.: Roentgenological characteristics of mesenchymal tumours of the stomach. *Ann Clin Res, 1:57,* 1969.

32. Salmela, H.: Smooth muscle tumours of the stomach: A clinical study of 112 cases. *Acta chir scandinav, 134:384,* 1968.

33. Nance, F. C., and Cohn, Jr., I.: The management of leiomyosarcoma of the stomach. *S Clin North America, 50:1129,* 1970.

34. Bose, B., and Candy, J.: Gastric leiomyoblastoma. *Gut, 11:875,* 1970.

35. McBee, J. W., and Aboumrad, M. H.: Leiomyoblastoma of the stomach. *Gastrointest Endosc, 17:17,* 1970.

36. Fagin, R. R., Levinson, J. D., Prolla, J. C., Kobayashi, S., and Singer, H. C.: Myogenic tumors of the stomach (gastroscopic and pathologic observations). *Gastrointest Endosc, 17:30,* 1970.

37. Prolla, J. C., and Kirsner, J. B.: The gastrointestinal lesions and complications of the leukemias. *Ann Intern Med, 61:1084,* 1964.

38. Bynum, T. E.: Gastroscopic appearance of multiple gastric ulcers associated with lymphatic leukemia. *Gastrointest Endosc, 17*:38, 1970.
39. Jocu, M. K.: Plasmocytome gastrique ulcere. *Arch franç mal appar dig, 57*:1033, 1968.
40. Beard, R. J., Lee, E. C. G., Haysom, A. H., and Melcher, D. H.: Noncarcinomatous tumours of the stomach. *Brit J Surg, 55*:535, 1968.
41. Feingold, M. L., Goldstein, M. J., and Lieverman, P. H.: Multiple myeloma involving the stomach. *Gastrointest Endosc, 15*:107, 1969.
42. Brodman, H. R., and Pai, B. N.: Malignant carcinoid of the stomach and distal esophagus. *Am J Digest Dis, 13*:677, 1968.
43. Reiss, R.: Extra-appendicular carcinoid tumors of the gastrointestinal tract. *Arch Surg, 96*:312, 1968.
44. Parks, T. G.: Malignant carcinoid and adenocarcinoma of the stomach. *Brit J Surg, 57*:377, 1970.
45. Okeon, M. M., and Bieber, W. P.: Carcinoid tumor of the stomach resembling carcinoma: Report of a case. *Radiology, 103*:314, 1968.
46. Bockus, H. L.: *Gastroenterology.* Philadelphia, Saunders, 1963, Vol. 1, pp. 836-874.
47. Caffarello, J. R., Gallego, O., and Sabagh, R.: Granuloma eosinofilo ulcerado de estomago: A proposito de un caso. *Arch arg enf ap digest, 136*:1451, 1970.

CHAPTER 20

POSTOPERATIVE DISORDERS OF STOMACH*

BASIL I. HIRSCHOWITZ

SYMPTOMATOLOGY

ALL TYPES OF GASTRIC SURGERY cause fundamental alterations in the anatomy and physiology of the upper digestive tract. While most patients after gastric surgery suffer few or no complaints, it has been reported that 10 to 30 per cent of patients have significant and frequently disabling symptoms or complications after gastric surgery.[1-5]

Most of these patients have two or more symptoms—the commonest are pain, vomiting, bleeding, weight loss, dumping, diarrhea, and anorexia. In general the symptoms are relatively non-specific and physical examination is even less specific, so that investigation of the symptomatic postgastrectomy patient has to be systemic and thorough. Since proper therapy depends on a clear understanding of the causes of symptoms; this chapter presents a guide in the form of a classification of the various possible syndromes which may occur after gastric surgery. It will also emphasize the advan-

* This work was supported by grants AM-4978 and TIAM-05286 from the USPHS, a grant from the State of Alabama Department of Educational Vocational Rehabilitation Service and from the Wappler Foundation.

tages as well as the limitations of fiberoptic endoscopy, not only because this is a book on endoscopy, but also because endoscopy is the single most important technic in the study of the symptomatic postgastrectomy patient.

POSTGASTRECTOMY SYNDROMES

Our classification is largely derived from a ten-year study of 580 symptomatic postgastrectomy patients,[6] each one of whom was gastroscoped in our unit. Most of the detailed data have been presented elsewhere.[6, 7] The problems after gastric surgery may be divided into the *immediate* (before discharge from hospital) and *delayed,* or late symptoms, which may appear after a trouble-free interval of months to years.

Immediate Syndromes

Endoscopy is important in the correct diagnosis of some of the immediate problems after gastric surgery, especially bleeding, vomiting, and dysphagia. The endoscopist should keep in mind the risk of disrupting a suture line by excessive distention by air during endoscopy, and air should be used very sparingly until at least ten days after surgery. However, endoscopy may be performed safely in experienced hands at any time after surgery. The problems may present in some of the following ways. The first three are endoscopic diagnoses, the others are not.

1. *Bleeding* from the suture line, from the original ulcer or from an overlooked second ulcer, or from stress ulceration is generally diagnosable endoscopically. Thus, the gastric or anastomotic suture line often looks worse during the first four to eight days after surgery than it really is. It may appear as an irregular red-purple or purple-black line raised from the surface and with visible sutures in it. Usually there is a little fresh blood at this site, but it seldom is a cause for major bleeding. As for bleeding from an ulcer, if the ulcer were left behind, e.g. proximal gastric or duodenal (in pyloroplasty) the crater may be seen (Plate 59). Acute ulceration (stress ulcer) may be difficult to distinguish from tube (suction) erosions, as is the case in the unoperated stomach. It must be remembered that an ulcer which has bled may not be bleeding at the time of endoscopy.

2. *Obstruction* may be due to several different causes. Stomal edema may completely obliterate the stoma and may last up to four weeks after surgery. Occasionally prolapsed jejunal mucosa (with or without edema) may obstruct the stoma similarly. The efferent loop may be obstructed by a kinked or twisted jejunum. Thus obstruction needs both endoscopic and x-ray study.

3. Varying degrees of *esophagitis* may result from nasogastric intubation especially with recumbent nursing, and may cause dysphagia or bleeding. It is more likely to occur where nasogastric intubation has also been

used for preoperative suction. Secondary moniliasis may complicate matters in those who are debilitated or receiving antibiotics.

4. *Suture-line leak*, especially of the duodenal stump, leading to peritonitis, abscess, or fistula—mostly are not diagnosable by endoscopy.

5. *Infection*, abscess, or inflammation of pancreas, subphrenic space, peritoneum, mesocolon, or abdominal wound.

6. Inadvertent *ligation* of the common bile duct, pancreatic duct, or a major artery.

7. *Miscellaneous* general postsurgical or postanesthetic metabolic, pulmonary, cardiac, renal, hepatic, and electrolyte disorders.

Delayed and Late Syndromes

Despite apparently successful surgery, the patient may have a number of problems to contend with as he returns home to his normal environment, activity, and diet. Though many of these problems can be classified as to probable time of onset of surgery, the majority may start anywhere from a few days to months after leaving the hospital. Thus the remaining classification will be based on mechanism. The major groups of postgastrectomy syndromes are as follows: (1) Mechanical, (2) Anatomical-pathological, (3) Physiological-metabolic-nutritional, (4) Miscellaneous.

Mechanical (Table 20-I)

A. ESOPHAGUS: Hiatal hernia may either preexist or may result from surgery, thus exploration of the paraesophageal tissues for the vagus nerves may disturb the hiatus enough to produce or increase a hiatal hernia. A hernia will allow free reflux, without nausea, especially with a small gastric reservoir. This should be distinguished from vomiting due to other causes. With a hernia, the esophagus is at risk from acid reflux. If the stomach juice has no free acid, it is equally at risk from pancreatic/biliary juices which can produce severe *alkaline* esophagitis and, later, stricture. Esophagitis is diagnosed by endoscopy with or without biopsy.

B. STOMACH: 1. The small stomach syndrome[5]: With 50 per cent or more of the stomach resected, the capacity of the stomach becomes impaired, with post-prandial bloating, fullness, and easy satiety, often with less than an ordinary sized meal. Subconsciously the easy satiety leads to a gradual reduction of food intake, and an intake of 1,500 calories per day or less is not uncommon. This is a frequent cause of significant symptoms following subtotal gastrectomy. These symptoms may be aggravated by coexisting conditions, viz., hiatal hernia, gastritis, obstruction, or ulcer, causing regurgitation, pain, or weight loss. The size of the stomach remnant may be judged by x-ray and by endoscopy, and the diminished intake documented by a good nutritional history.

TABLE 20-I

ANATOMICAL-MECHANICAL POSTGASTRECTOMY SYNDROMES

Type	Symptoms	Complication
Esophageal:		
(i) Hiatal hernia	Regurgitation	Esophagitis
(a) Pre-existing		
(b) Due to surgery (vagotomy)		
(ii) Esophagitis	Dysphagia, pain	Stricture
Stomach:		
(i) Small stomach, proportional to resection	Fullness, vomiting	Dec. food intake, wt. loss
(ii) Poor emptying due to vagotomy	Fullness, vomiting	Dec. food intake, wt. loss
(iii) Retained antral cuff in Billroth II	Ulcer pain, bleeding	Recurrent ulcer
Stoma:		
(i) Obstruction due to:	Vomiting, pain	Dehydration, malnutrition, and anemia
(a) Edema after surgery	Vomiting, pain	
(b) Stricture	Vomiting, pain	
(c) Prolapse of jejunal mucosa	Vomiting, pain	
(d) Bezoar	Vomiting, pain	
(e) Suture extrusion	Pain, bleeding	
(ii) Double-barrel stoma	Vomiting, pain, bleeding	Multiple (see text)
(iii) Too large	Dumping	Dumping, weight loss
Afferent Loop:		
(i) Too long or obstruction of jej.-gastric orifice	Postprandial pain, vomiting	Infection → diarrhea
(ii) A-loop orifice directed into stomach (double barrel)	Bilious vomiting	Gastritis, esophagitis
(iii) Infected A-loop, result of (i) or (ii)	Diarrhea, steatorrhea	Malnut., anemia
Efferent Loop:		
Obstruction due to bezoar, stricture, twist, adhesions, or ulcer	Vomiting	Malnutrition
By-Pass:		
(i) Duodenal-pancreatic-biliary by-pass (B-II anastomosis)	Steatorrhea	Weight loss
(ii) Jejunal by-pass	Severe diarrhea	Malnutrition
(a) Inadvertent gastroileal anastomosis	Severe diarrhea	Malnutrition
(b) Ulcer-induced gastrojejunocolic fistula	Severe diarrhea	Malnutrition

2. Poor emptying due to vagotomy: Denervation of the antrum of the stomach by truncal vagotomy may cause loss of gastric motility. Though this is usually only a problem in the immediate postoperative period, it may persist and cause gastric retention later.

3. Retained antral cuff or the pseudo Zollinger-Ellison syndrome: If a portion of the antrum is left attached to the duodenal stump in a gastrectomized patient (or in the now-abandoned antral exclusion operation), the alkaline medium in this stump will produce a continuous high output of gastrin which is not subject to feedback cutoff by acid secretion. This produces continuous acid secretion from the residual stump and may cause marginal ulcer. Serum gastrin is also increased, and it may thus mimic the Zollinger-Ellison syndrome.

C. STOMA: 1. Obstruction of the stoma may be due to a variety of causes, such as:

a) Edema may cause virtual obstruction of the gastroenterostomy for up to four weeks, and in unusual cases may progress to stricture. If due to late ulcer recurrence, it may require further surgery. Endoscopy is essential in these diagnoses.

b) Prolapse of jejunal mucosa from the afferent loop may cause obstruction of both the stoma and the afferent loop. This condition can be diagnosed with certainty only by endoscopy and requires stomal conversion.

c) A bezoar will occasionally form in the postgastrectomy stomach, act as a ball valve, and cause persistent vomiting. In at least one instance in our series, the patient had symptoms for six months. This may be diagnosed either by x-ray or by endoscopy, and usually resolves in a few days with liquid diet with or without papain. In addition, partial mechanical breaking up of the bezoar can be accomplished by a biopsy forceps through an endoscope.

d) Submucosal or extruding sutures may cause obstruction because of edema or tissue reaction to silk, though more commonly causing ulceration, often with bleeding, and may be seen endoscopically from ten days to four years or more after surgery.[8] When extruding, sutures may sometimes be removed with a biopsy forceps transendoscopically.

2. Double-barrel stoma: The importance of this finding in about 10 per cent of symptomatic patients[1, 2, 7, 9] lies in the fact that it seems to be associated with a very high rate of other complications, including ulcer, bleeding, jejunitis, and it is probably responsible for most of the afferent loop disorders seen after gastric surgery. It is easily recognized by endoscopy, which is the only way of making the diagnosis (Plate 60) (Fig. 2). Once recognized, revision of the stoma is essential, preferably by conversion to Billroth I.

3. Large stoma: If a Billroth II stoma is greater than 2.5cm in diameter,

dumping often occurs. Endoscopy is important in confirming this diagnosis.

D. AFFERENT LOOP: The afferent loop disorders comprise several syndromes. The commonest are 1. Obstruction of the jejunogastric orifice by stricture, ulcer, or by twisting of the afferent loop around the gastro-jejunostomy. If the obstruction is partial, the symptoms will consist of pain, usually in the right upper quadrant, starting about fifteen to twenty minutes after meals and persisting until there is sudden relief with the emptying of the loop contents into the stomach or into the small intestine. If these contents empty into the stomach, this will often cause bilious vomiting after the patient has been relieved. The pain is usually cramping, and occasionally a mass may be felt in this area. It is not uncommon with the double-barrel syndrome and almost invariably requires surgical correction. The cause of the narrowing can usually be determined by endoscopy.

2. Infected afferent loop: Generally occurs as a result of partial obstruction or of double-barrel stoma. Occasionally because of the loop being too long, infection of the stagnant contents of the afferent loop will result in what is known as *blind-loop syndrome* in which the bacterial population exceeds 10 million per ml. Diarrhea and usually steatorrhea will result. This condition is treated on a temporary basis by antibiotics and more definitively by the appropriate drainage of the obstructed or overlong afferent loop by revision or conversion to Billroth I. The condition may be studied endoscopically and the loop contents may thus be aspirated for culture.

Bilious vomiting is a common symptom after gastric surgery, occurring more commonly in women than in men.[1, 10] Bile is vomited because the afferent loop empties into the stomach preferentially or because there is frequent regurgitation from the duodenum through an incompetent pylorus or stoma. Bile reflux to the stomach is frequently seen endoscopically, often in the absence of symptoms. It is difficult to treat medically and may require the conversion from one type of anastomosis to another, or construction of a Roux-en-Y loop.[2] Bile regurgitation may also produce gastritis and esophagitis.

E. EFFERENT LOOP: The efferent loop may be obstructed at the stoma due to bezoar or to stricture, or it may occur as the result of a twist of the gastro-jejunostomy anastomosis, or some distance down the efferent loop due to jejunal ulceration. Vomiting is invariable with higher degrees of obstruction. With lesser degrees of obstruction, the symptoms include easy satiety and frequent vomiting after meals, and may resemble the small stomach syndrome. Often, however, pain and vomiting after eating are significant symptoms. Endoscopically, obstruction of the stoma may be diagnosed easily. Distal obstruction of the efferent loop may produce a dilated afferent loop. X-rays are especially useful in these disorders.

F. By-Pass: Pancreatic-Biliary and Jejunal: These two conditions are not diagnosed by endoscopy.

Anatomical-Pathological Complications (Table 20-II)

All these conditions are recognizable by endoscopy, at which time tissue may be taken for histological confirmation.

A. Postoperative Gastritis: Even without surgery, gastritis of some degree is common. After surgery for duodenal or gastric ulcer, gastritis is very common and in some cases severe with troublesome symptoms.

One possible mechanism of postoperative gastritis may be bile reflux. Gastritis of this sort is also seen in those individuals who drink an excess of alcohol. The diagnosis of this condition is made only by endoscopy, confirmed by biopsy. Its treatment is often unsatisfactory and it may ultimately progress to gastric mucosal atrophy.

B. Gastric Mucosal Atrophy: Marked mucosal atrophy develops only occasionally in the postoperative stomach. It is diagnosed only by endoscopy.

C. Postoperative Stomatitis: Inflammation of the stomal rim is the commonest diagnosis made endoscopically in the symptomatic postgastrectomy patient, occurring in 26 per cent of the patients in our series.[6] It often occurs by itself, not as part of a general gastritis, and consists of localized inflammation often with superficial patchy ulceration and slow bleeding in the 1cm perimeter of the stoma. Ulcer-like pain after eating is a common symptom. The localization of pathology in this area suggests that the blood supply to the junctional area may be partly impaired, e.g. by sutures placed too close together or drawn too tightly, leaving the stoma less able to repair minor damage than either the adjacent jejunum or stomach.

D. Recurrent Peptic Ulcer: This condition after surgery for duodenal ulcer is not an uncommon condition. In the present series approximately 22 per cent of symptomatic patients were found to have marginal ulcer. While most seem to be related to a persistent ulcer diathesis, two occurred in complete absence of any acid secretion with repeated maximal histamine stimulation. On the other hand, only five out of 127 were due to Zollinger-Ellison syndrome with high acid secretion. Approximately 10 per cent of recurrent ulcers were related to suture extrusion at the anastomosis.[6] Of all ulcer recurrences 8 per cent were in the gastric stump away from the stomal margin, i.e. gastric ulcer; 12 per cent were in the jejunum more than 1cm from the stomal margin, i.e. jejunal ulcer (Plate 61); and 80 per cent adjacent to the stoma. While only 35 per cent of these were diagnosed by x-ray, the great majority (more than 90%) were diagnosed by

TABLE 20-II

ANATOMICAL-PATHOLOGICAL COMPLICATIONS

Type	Symptom	Causes	Complication
A. Gastritis	Dyspepsia (some pts.)	Unknown ? bile reflux Alcohol	Bleeding Gastric mucosal atrophy
B. Mucosal atrophy	None	Gastritis ? loss of gastrin	B_{12} deficiency Fe^{++} deficiency
C. Stomatitis	Pain, bleeding	? vascular impairment at stoma	Bleeding
D. Ulcer	Pain, bleeding, vomiting	Persistent ulcer diathesis, suture extrusion, double-barrel stoma, Zollinger-Ellison syndrome, retained antrum	Bleeding, obstr. of stoma or A and E loop, fistula
E. Jejunitis	Pain	Unknown ? acid	Bleeding, jejunal ulcer
F. Bleeding, visible/persistent occult		Ulcer, chronic and acute, gastritis, jejunitis, drugs, various others	Anemia

TABLE 20-III

PHYSIOLOGICAL-NUTRITIONAL-METABOLIC COMPLICATIONS OF GASTRIC SURGERY

Type	Symptoms	Causes	Complication
1. Weight loss, malnutrition	Loss of energy and strength	Various	
2. Anemia			
A. Iron deficient	Weakness, dysphagia		
(i) Secondary to bleeding			
a. Pre-operative blood loss		Suture extrusion	
b. Persistent occult bleeding		Esophagitis,	
c. Recurrent gross bleeding		stomatitis, drugs	
(ii) Decreased Fe intake or uptake			
B. B₁₂ deficient	Weakness, mental depression	Loss of H⁺, bypass	Gastric atrophy
		Loss of I.F.	Subacute combined degen.
		(atrophic gastritis)	
C. Folic acid deficiency	Weakness	Dietary	
D. Malnutrition		Various	
3. Diarrhea		Jejunal by-pass	
a. Watery	Diarrhea, weight loss	Vagotomy, ZE syndrome	
Persistent or	Weakness, paralysis	Biliary-pancreatic	
Episodic	(K⁺ depletion)	insufficiency	
b. Steatorrhea		Blind loop, sprue	Steatorrhea
c. Other	Milk intolerance	Lactase insufficiency	
4. Carbohydrate disorders			
a. Reactive hypoglycemia	Hypoglycemia 2-3 hrs. after meals	Loss of normal insulin and glucagon regulation	
b. Diabetes	Weight loss	Unknown	
c. Low K⁺ (pseudo-dumping)	Weakness 1 hr. after meals	Rapid deposition of glucose	Dehydration
			K⁺ depletion,
			Cachexia
5. Dumping	Early after meals	Loss of gastric reservoir function	Weight loss
6. Calcium depletion	Osteomalacia	Duodenal by-pass,	Muscle weakness,
		steatorrhea	fractures, bone pain

endoscopy. Practically all the patients had pain or bleeding. With the Zollinger-Ellison syndrome the time of recurrence of the ulcer is generally within a few weeks of surgery, whereas most of the recurrences in partial gastrectomized patients occurred between one and five years. In the patients with gastroenterostomy, recurrences did not appear for ten to twenty years after surgery. The double-barrel stoma was frequently associated with marginal ulcer[7, 9] (Plate 62).

E. JEJUNITIS: Jejunitis occurred as an apparently primary condition in a number of patients. This took the form endoscopically of an edematous jejunal mucosa not infrequently with small superficial ulcerations, with friability, and bleeding (Plate 63) (Fig. 3), not necessarily associated with either stomatitis or gastritis. These patients generally had dyspeptic symptoms suggestive of ulcer, including pain, anorexia, and vomiting.

F. RECURRENT BLEEDING: Approximately 36 per cent of the 580 symptomatic patients presented at various times after gastric surgery because of bleeding. The various causes for bleeding could be determined in approximately 80 per cent of the patients by endoscopy and included chronic ulcer, acute ulcer, stomatitis, jejunitis, gastritis, varices, and vascular anomalies and a number of drugs including aspirin, alcohol, anticoagulants, and reserpine. With few exceptions, endoscopy is the only way to find the source of bleeding, though after bleeding has stopped it may be impossible to determine the source of bleeding. In some instances, no specific lesion can be identified with bleeding at the stomal margin.

Physiological-Metabolic-Nutritional (Table 20-III)

A number of such syndromes occur, some very frequently following gastrectomy. For the most part these are not diagnosable by endoscopy or by x-ray, but by special metabolic studies. They are detailed in other reports[6] and summarized in Table 20-III. Their importance or clinical significance to the endoscopist lies in the fact that needless endoscopies may be avoided and failure of endoscopy to reveal explanations of symptoms may be better understood.

Miscellaneous (Table 20-IV)

The above category along with the Miscellaneous group summarized in Table 20-IV are included in this discussion, primarily to indicate that endoscopy, while invaluable in the study and analysis of the multiple syndromes of the postoperative stomach, must not mistakenly be thought of as a single solution to all problems of the postoperative patient. An endoscopist must be first and always a well-trained clinician. In this regard I must mention in some detail the Psychological Postoperative Syndrome.

In approximately 5 per cent of patients undergoing gastric surgery, there

TABLE 20-IV

MISCELLANEOUS COMPLICATIONS

Type	Symptoms	Causes	Complication
1. Psychological	Failure to improve		Invalidism, multiple operations
2. Initial misdiagnosis with persistence of original disorder	Original symptoms		
3. Pulmonary tuberculosis	Weight loss, cough	Malnutrition unknown	
4. Neurological	Mental changes, cerebellar changes peripheral neuritis	? Malnutrition, unknown	Ataxia

is an inexplicable total failure of patient improvement. This group of patients has been found in many series[4, 11, 12] to be incapacitated by psychologic disorders. Review of their preoperative histories often reveals intractability without really specific indications for surgery.[12] Chronic invalidism results and not infrequently such patients undergo repeated surgery without benefit.[2] It should be emphasized, however, that because of the wide variety of possible organic postoperative syndromes, that no patient should be dismissed as psychologically incapacitated without an extremely thorough investigation. This includes a further look for a diagnosis other than the one thought to be the cause of symptoms at the time of surgery, including pancreatic disease, biliary tract disease, hiatal hernia, cardiac, and vascular disease.

Pulmonary tuberculosis has come to be recognized as a late complication of gastric surgery in as many as 7 per cent of patients.[1, 13]

PLAN OF INVESTIGATION
Symptomatic Patient

The general plan of investigation of the symptomatic postgastrectomy patient rests on several well established principles. It is essential to know the exact disease the patient had before surgery, the indications for surgery, and a precise description of the surgical procedures, including the measured extent of the resection, the type of anastomosis, the estimated length of the afferent loop, the arrangement of the afferent and efferent loops, whether or not vagotomy was done, and a complete pathological description of removed tissue. It is important to know also whether the hiatus was repaired as part of the procedure and whether the surgeon explored the abdomen thoroughly for other diseases, including gallstones, pancreatitis, and pancreatic tumor.

The patient should have a careful systematic history, followed by physical examination (noting especially pulse and blood pressure lying and standing at time of symptoms) and a daily weight record. Laboratory studies should include blood count, serum Fe^{++} and TIBC, vitamin B_{12} and folate, glucose tolerance, serum K^+, stools for occult blood, xylose absorption, fat balance, serum carotene and cholesterol, and when indicated x-rays of the bones, with alkaline phosphatase, Ca^{++}, P, and Mg^{++} studies. With recurrent ulceration, histolog gastric analysis, Hollander test, and gastrin determination should be done.

Upper gastrointestinal x-ray may detect 35 to 50 per cent of recurrent ulcers, indicate the length and diameter of the afferent loop, rule out obstruction at the stoma or efferent loop, and hiatal hernia.

Endoscopy, as we have pointed out previously[6, 7, 9, 14] is the single most valuable means of diagnosing both the anatomic-mechanical and the anatomic-pathological lesions. *There are a variety of lesions which are simply not amenable to diagnosis by any other means. Endoscopy includes in summary the source of bleeding, varying degrees of gastritis, esophagitis, stomatitis, jejunitis, extruding sutures, vascular abnormalities, and anatomy, and arrangement of the stoma.* In addition the gastroscope or esophagoscope can be used to remove sutures and to obtain biopsies and specimens for culture.

Asymptomatic Patient

The great majority of patients have few or no symptoms after recovery from good ulcer surgery, though even in this asymptomatic group thorough routine study may reveal weight loss, anemia, carbohydrate disorders, steatorrhea, osteomalacia and vitamin B_{12} deficiency in varying degrees. These findings may occur in gastric resection[1, 4] vagotomy alone or gastroenterostomy.[13] It is, therefore, important for patients after surgery for peptic ulcer to have periodic thorough checkups, including endoscopy, for a number of years.

One should not lose sight of the well documented findings that may be only mildly symptomatic, developing at any time apparently from one to fifteen years. Such is the case with anemia, for example, due to loss of intrinsic factor but mostly due to iron deficiency after gastrectomy.[4]

It may be impractical to do all of the tests described here away from big teaching centers, but endoscopy today should be at the very center of adequate postoperative follow-up after all types of surgery for gastroduodenal disease.

TECHNIC OF ENDOSCOPY*

For the most part the technic is the same as in the intact stomach. Either the forward-viewing esophagoscope or esophago-duodenoscope, or the side-

---

* These technics and findings are all illustrated in a 16mm color movie[7] made in our unit recently.

viewing gastroscope may be used, and each has some advantage.[14] The forward-viewing instruments are well suited to combine esophageal, gastric stump, and jejunal inspection. If the stoma is in the distal or dependent part of the pouch, it may be readily visualized, but if it is on one of the vertical walls (anterior or posterior), the esophagoscope may provide only a tangential view. Lesions on the jejunal wall just beyond stoma may be overlooked in the same way that lesions of the upper gastric walls just beyond the esophagus may be overlooked. The esophagoscope, however, can be more readily directed into each of the two jejunal loops and is more convenient for biopsy, for suture removal, and for aspiration of contents from stomach or jejunum.

The lateral viewing gastroscope is superior for comprehensive inspection of the gastric stump and for those relatively blind areas in the walls just distal to the esophagogastric and gastrointestinal junctions. It is also generally better for viewing stomas on either of the vertical walls of the stomach. Control of the distal end is a distinct advantage with either instrument. In a small stump retroflexion of the instrument may not be possible.

The following points should be noted with each endoscopy in the postoperative stomach:

Esophagus

Inflammation, narrowing or stricture, presence of hiatal hernia.

Gastric Stump

(1) *Size*, which may be judged to nearest 20 per cent.

(2) *Mucosa*, which may vary from that seen in the Zollinger-Ellison syndrome where it is thick, very healthy, pink, and actively secreting, through varying degrees of gastritis and atrophy to total atrophy. Though the gross appearance may not always correspond to the histological, it is reasonable to diagnose varying degrees of atrophy and varying degrees of redness with or without friability and petechiae and to report these as mild, moderate, or severe gastritis, with minimal, moderate, or advanced atrophy of the mucosa, occurring as a localized, patchy, or generalized phenomenon.

(3) *Stoma*

(a) Report on the location, size (estimate in cm at its widest), and whether there is any motility of the stoma.

(b) Stomatitis[6, 7, 9] may occur as an isolated inflammation with or without edema, exudation, superficial ulceration, or friability of the 0.5 to 1cm periphery of the stoma.

(c) In the double-barrel stoma[9] (see Plate 64, Fig. 1), the afferent and efferent loop orifices appear side by side in the gastrojejunostomy, separated by a bridge of jejunum which is at the same level as the gastric mucosa, so that the A and E loops do not communicate except via the cavity of the gastric stump. This is often associated with a number of further complications,[9] and can only be diagnosed endoscopically.

(*d*) An attempt should be made to remove any extruding suture or metal clips.[6, 11]

(*e*) A healed suture line may be seen as a linear white scar or as a series of short white parallel lines due to sutures. It indicates no known pathology.

(*f*) Bleeding should be noted, localized, and characterized.

(*g*) Ulcer location and character should be noted (Plate 63).

Jejunum

Can be seen through the patent gastrojejunostomy. The loop is identified by observing the peristalsis and the flow of bile and bubbles toward the stomach. The E loop is generally empty. The relative size of the two loops and the direction of bile flow and anatomic orientation of the two loops to each other and to the stomach should be noted. Disparity in the size of the two loops will indicate disease or obstruction in one. Jejunitis will appear as abnormal redness, edema, or friability, whereas the normal jejunum is brown-pink with thin Kerckring folds (Plate 65). With the focussing gastroscope the villous nature of the normal jejunal mucosa can be made out in close-up view. Either loop may be intubated and inspected for considerable lengths, and the ampulla of Vater may be seen in the A loop.

The Billroth I Stoma

The duodenal mucosa can be easily differentiated from the gastric by its brown-pink color and thin folds. The Billroth I stoma is generally irregular in shape and with 50 per cent or greater gastric resection, may have no motility. Bile reflux is commonly seen endoscopically but is not necessarily significant and may even reflux more easily because of air distension.

In the Stomach With No Resection

Pyloroplasty will show a deformed pylorus but not necessarily a patulous one. Usually the antral contraction wave does not end in a nice circular wave at the expected pylorus. A gastroenterostomy may be hard to locate, especially a posterior distal antral one. Very often such a stoma can not be intubated, and one may have to be content with only a partial or tangential view.

Miscellaneous Observations

(1) The lack of a pylorus after gastrectomy allows air to enter the intestine very readily, and it is not unusual for the patient to pass excessive flatus within five to ten minutes of beginning endoscopy.

(2) Another problem is that bubbles tend to form much more readily in the postoperative stomach, especially from the air-distended A loop, often obscuring the view. These can be easily eliminated by injecting 3 to 5ml of diluted methyl-polysiloxane liquid (silicone antifoam) through the gastroscope.[7]

(3) The instrument may occasionally be used for other purposes under direct vision, e.g. to dilate a strictured A or E loop orifice; to aspirate contents for culture or chemistry; to biopsy mucosa; or to remove sutures with a biopsy forceps.

REFERENCES

1. Goligher, J. C., Pulvertaft, C. N., deDombal, F. T., Conyers, J. H., Duthie, H. L., Feather, D. B., Latchmore, A. J. C., Shoesmith, J. H., Smiddy, F. G., and Willson-Pepper, J.: Five to eight year results of Lees/York controlled trial of elective surgery for duodenal ulcer. *Br Med J, 2*:781-787, 1968.
2. Herrington, J. L.: Remedial operation for postgastrectomy syndromes. In *Current Problems in Surgery.* Chicago, Year Book, 1969.
3. Postlethwait, R. W.: *Results of Surgery for Peptic Ulcer.* Philadelphia, Saunders, 1963.
4. Stammers, F. A. R., and Williams, J. A.: *Partial Gastrectomy.* London, Butterworth, 1963.
5. Woodward, E. R.: *The Postgastrectomy Syndromes.* Springfield, Thomas, 1963.
6. Hirschowitz, B. I.: Classification of the postgastrectomy syndromes based on observation of 580 patients. *Ala J M Sc, 8*:50-66, 1971.
7. Hirschowitz, B. I.: The symptomatic postgastrectomy patient. 16mm moving picture, color with sound tract, National Medical Audiovisual Center, Atlanta, Ga., Cat. No. M-1714, 1970.
8. Imhof, J. W., Wiebenga, A. H., and Ten Thije, O. J.: Persisting sutures casting off into the stomach after gastric operations. A gastroscopic study. *Gastroenterologia, 96*:291-300, 1961.
9. Demaret, A. N., Luketic, G. C., and Hirschowitz, B. I.: The double-barrel stoma. *Scand J Gastroenterol, 6*:77-86, 1971.
10. Wells, C. A., and McPhee, I. W.: The afferent loop syndrome—bilious regurgitation after subtotal gastrectomy and its relief. *Lancet, 2*:1189-1191, 1952.
11. Morgan, D. B., Hunt, G., and Paterson, C. R.: The osteomalacia syndrome after stomach operations. *Q J Med, 39*:395-410, 1970.
12. Small, W. P., Cay, E. L., Dugard, P., Sircus, W., Falconer, C. W. A., Smith, A. N., McManus, J. P. A., and Bruce, Sir John: Peptic ulcer surgery: Selection for operation by "Earning." *Gut, 10*:996-1003, 1969.
13. Wheldon, E. J., Venables, C. W., and Johnston, D. A.: Late metabolic sequelae of vagotomy and gastroenterostomy. *Lancet, 1*:437-440, 1970.
14. Hirschowitz, B. I.: Progress in esophagoscopy. *Endoscopy, 2*:75-77, 1970.

CHAPTER 21

PART I: ACUTE AND CHRONIC GASTRITIS

Leonidas H. Berry and Jonas Adomavicius

HISTORICAL AND INTRODUCTORY STATEMENT

THERE IS NO SUBJECT in gastroenterology which has been more widely discussed and studied for a longer period in medical history than the subject of "Inflammation of the Stomach" or "Gastritis." There is probably no subject in gastroenterology which remains more controversial in spite of many decades of study and many volumes of discussion than the subject of gastritis. Gastritis is a subject which, in our opinion, must be faced and should not be swept under the rug as some authorities have done because of the lack of absolute proof in fitting the disease pattern into established rigid categories. When one goes into the many ramifications of clinical manifestations, etiology, gross endoscopic and microscopic characteristics, there are yet a set of hard facts which stand out and which would seem to us to justify a minimum of controversy and definite common ground upon which many authorities would agree.

322

Since the era of gastroscopy, the subject of gastritis has had a great boon due to the fact that the mucosal surfaces of the living stomach can now be observed under all types of conditions. As more observers entered the field of gastroscopy, it became generally obvious that one could not always correlate the degree of gastroscopic gastritis with clinical symptoms. Severe gastroscopic changes were seen when the patient had a few symptoms of epigastric distress, and many patients with severe or frequent or prolonged epigastric distress often had mild gross gastroscopic changes. This was true when no disease could be demonstrated in other digestive organs. This experience led many gastroscopists to doubt the clinical significance of chronic gastritis. Others however point to the fact that the inflammatory changes in other organs frequently fail to show a proportional correlation between organic findings and symptoms.

Schindler set forth a simple endoscopic classification[1] of chronic gastritis early in his career. Later he wrote a monograph[2] of considerably more complex classification of chronic gastritis to which he added microscopic concepts. While we are sure that important additional information was added to the general body of facts about this elusive disease, it also added to the complexity of correlated understanding of the disease. When endoscopic gastrobiopsy became possible, it was immediately thought that the whole pathologic question of inflammation of the stomach would be settled. After a few years of these studies, it was evident that one could not consistently correlate in a large percentage of cases the histologic findings with the widely accepted gastroscopic classification of chronic gastritis.[3–5]

It was then argued that since histologic gastritis was not always found with gastroscopic or gross gastritis, gross gastritis therefore does not exist. Extreme positions on this difficult subject are untenable. It should be pointed out that gross pharyngitis, tonsillitis, and rhinitis are diagnosed routinely by ENT specialists and treated appropriately without biopsy or concern for histologic proof. When the dermatologist observes redness, swelling, local fever and pain, this is inflammation of the skin. Biopsy may be used in its differentiation from other lesions or to find a causative organism, but not to prove the existence of inflammation.

GASTROSCOPIC PATHOLOGY

At this point, the gross endoscopic concepts of gastritis will be discussed. The modern anatomic concepts of gastritis based upon direct observations of the living stomach began with Rudolf Schindler and the semiflexible lens gastroscope. His original simple classification has much to justify its continued use, with some modifications. Like all classifications of disease, the Schindler classification of gastritis must not be regarded as absolute.

TABLE 21-I

GASTROSCOPIC CLASSIFICATION OF ACUTE AND CHRONIC GASTRITIS

I. *Acute Gastritis*
Localized or diffuse.
Hyperemia, edema, mucous exudate, whitish or grayish with or without petechiae, mucosal hemorrhages, tiny hemorrhagic or gray erosions.

II. *Chronic Superficial Gastritis*
May be indistinguishable from acute, except in terms of partial healing and repeated recurrences in varying degrees of severity or mildness.

III. *Chronic Atrophic Gastritis*
Localized or diffuse.
Often associated in varying degrees with superficial gastritis, thus II and III may be combined.
Visibility of venules and arterioles, patchy pale to pearly gray areas, effacement of folds, diminution of size and number without regard to amount of inflation, with or without petechiae, tiny hemorrhagic erosions.

IIIa. *Atrophic Gastric Mucosa*
(Primary atrophy not preceded by superficial gastritis.)
May be indistinguishable from atrophic gastritis, except often more extensive and unassociated with superficial gastritis.
Usually associated with pernicious anemia, malnutrition, other chronic debilitating diseases.

IV. *Chronic Hypertrophic Gastritis* (Gastropathy)
(Other Forms: Giant Gastric Fields, Menetrier's Disease, etc.)
Localized or diffuse.
Controversial—may or may not be manifestation of inflammation. Irregular, often flat topped and polygonal nodules presenting cobblestone pattern on anterior and posterior walls, between folds, on the crests of folds ("caterpillar-like" segmentation), uniformly pale pink with diminution of highlights or reflections, may or may not be associated with petechiae or tiny erosions.

V. *Mixed Gastritis*
May be a combination of any of the above in the intact or postoperative stomach.

Primarily it is a mechanism of convenience and a gross guideline for the anatomic study of inflammatory changes of the stomach.

Table 21-I shows the gastroscopic classification of acute and chronic gastritis, with a succinct description of each form. We now continue with further discussion of the endoscopic findings in this disease.

Acute and Chronic Superficial Gastritis

There is very little difference gastroscopically between the acute and chronic superficial forms of inflammatory reaction of the gastric mucosa. The picture consists for the most part of localized or disseminated areas of hyperemia (Plate 66) which are readily recognized by the trained eye when there is a clear concept of the basic, accepted orange-red color of the normal gastric mucosa. It is important to work with standard quality and quantity of light. Fortunately, the major manufacturers of standardized endoscopic equipment have solved this problem for the endoscopist. There is always the advantage of comparing the hyperemic area with surrounding or adjacent areas of normal orange-red mucosa. Seldom is there complete homogeneous hyperemia of the entire stomach. If so, the process is severe and easily recognized. The more intense and extensive the hyperemia, the more there is likely to be also gray or dirty gray flecks or sheets of mucus. Some of this mucus appears to adhere to the mucosal surface, including the crevices between the folds. The highlights or reflections are usually increased in proportion to the intensity of the inflammation. There are often scattered, pinpoint to pinhead sized or larger, petechial hemorrhages into the mucosa (see Chapter 22). One may see tiny, trickling streams of blood from the larger or older petechiae. These may have become very superficially eroded. They should then be called tiny hemorrhagic erosions. The total picture may then be referred to as superficial erosive gastritis. A few scattered petechiae or tiny hemorrhagic erosions often occur without diffuse hyperemia and adherent mucus. Such isolated tiny hemorrhages into the mucosa should not be called gastritis. Superficial gastritis may be complicated by hemorrhage and is then called superficial hemorrhagic gastritis. Occasionally a localized oozing surface is iatrogenic, produced by the instrument, especially in friable areas.

Chronic Atrophic Gastritis

True atrophic gastritis begins as superficial gastritis, probably after repeated injury of the surface epithelium and many recurrent episodes of interstitial infiltration of the lamina propria by inflammatory cells and edema. Many glands are destroyed and the depth of the mucosa is reduced. The submucosa with its loosely arranged connective tissue is seen gastroscopically through the thinned mucosa as pale gray areas mottled by branching blue and red vessels (Plate 67). The atrophic process causes effacement of folds, so that fewer folds are seen gastroscopically. Many are smaller or flatter than normal. The highlights are moderate. In some instances, superficial gastritis is seen in juxtaposition to the atrophic changes. The inflammatory picture may be localized or extensive and should be described as mild, moderate or severe. Atrophic gastritis may be seen commonly at any age. Although partial reepithelization does occur, the residue of atrophic gastritis tends to remain. Berry and Cole[6] reported these observations in an eight-year therapy study of chronic atrophic gastritis with gastroscopic control. Because of the tendency for atrophic changes to remain for reasons in addition to aging, more atrophic changes may be seen in the elderly. Schindler always said that a small degree of atrophy in the region of the cardia is normal. Yamada et al.[7] in Japan claimed to have confirmed the opinion of Ruffin[8] and others that excessive distention of the stomach with air may bring some vessels into gastroscopic view. They devised a method of measuring the amount of air pressure during gastroscopic examination, and they have suggested differential criteria for visualization of normal and abnormal vessels.

Atrophic Gastric Mucosa

In almost 100 per cent of cases, pernicious anemia is associated with atrophic gastric mucosa. It is probably not correct to refer to the gastric changes in pernicious anemia as atrophic gastritis. These changes are more properly regarded as primary atrophy and are not preceded by acute and chronic superficial gastritis. Changes in pernicious anemia are often more severe and extensive than other types of gastric mucosal atrophy. However, reepithelization may occur to some degree with extensive antipernicious-anemia therapy.[9] Studies by Berry[10] have shown that a high incidence of atrophic changes in the stomachs of patients without pernicious anemia but suffering from malnutrition may show mucosal improvement on improved diet and large doses of vitamin B_{12} or B complex.

Hypertrophic Gastropathy

There is a pattern of apparent hypertrophic change seen by the gastroscopist which at present is the subject of considerable controversy. For the serious student of gastritis, review and study of some of the available monographs and literature on this subject is recommended. In this chapter no attempt will be made to discuss all the problems of so-called hypertrophic gastric mucosa. Instead, the principal characteristics of chronic hypertrophic gastropathy will be considered under the headings of Chronic Hypertrophic Gastritis, Hypertrophic-Hypersecretory Gastropathy, Giant Hypertrophic Gastritis of Menetrier and Simple Enlargement of Gastric Folds.

Chronic Hypertrophic Gastritis

The gastroscopic picture of chronic hypertrophic gastritis originally described by Schindler[1,2] consists primarily of the cobblestone pattern of nodularity or pebbling on the crests and in the valleys between folds. The folds are often enlarged. The color of the mucosa is orange-red or slightly pale, with diminished reflections or highlights producing a dull, velvety appearance. The cobblestones are flat-topped, polygonal, closely arranged and separated by tiny slitlike crevices (Plates 68, 69, 70). They are uniform or slightly irregular in size and appear soft to the trained endoscopist's eye. Distribution of these changes may be localized or extensive. Other forms of endoscopic gastritis, namely the superficial or the atrophic forms, may or may not be observed in the same areas or in other parts of the stomach. It is not uncommon to observe tiny hemorrhagic gray or white erosions or petechial hemorrhages associated with so-called hypertrophic gastritis. Sometimes frank hemorrhage occurs. Gastroduodenal ulcer, cancer or other lesions may be present with hypertrophic gastritis. The enlarged folds are not consistently seen on x-ray.[11] Conversely, the enlarged folds seen on x-ray are not always seen at gastroscopy.

These observations by a number of workers raised some doubt that the size of rugal folds alone could be used as a criterion of hypertrophic gastritis. It was also soon pointed out by critics of the Schindler concept that the cobblestone pattern or pebbling was remarkably similar to the état mammelonné or areae gastricae described by postmortem anatomists as normal. Schindler contended that areae gastricae described by anatomists in the cadaver are not seen in the living stomach by the gastroscopist. There is some evidence that the normal areae gastricae and foveolar pits described by anatomists are seen only with magnification (10 to 25×).[12] (See also Chapter 2, Fig. 2-4). Schindler and those who support his point of view feel that the nodularity seen gastroscopically is either hypertrophy of the areae gastricae mosaics or that the areas are exaggerated by submucosal edema or some previous gastritic mechanism.

As more and more gastrobiopsies were done there was an increase in the number of observers who contended that microscopically the hypertrophic gastritis described gastroscopically is not an inflammatory disease (see Chapter 21-II). By this is meant that infiltration of lymphocytes or inflammatory cells, cyst formations, lymphocytic nodules, edema and degenerative changes in surface epithelium do not occur. Stempien et al.[13, 14] state that histologic inflammatory changes are seen in some cases of this disease and inferred that more positive signs of inflammation may have occurred and disappeared. Benedict[15] stated that the chronic hypertrophic gastritis commonly seen gastroscopically is a normal variant. A number of other workers in various parts of the world accept this point of view. Consequently, the net result at this time is that chronic hypertrophic gastritis is a questionable and unresolved entity. More sophisticated methods, such as studies of function, histochemistry and electron microscopy, may resolve the issue in the future. Until that time it is our opinion that gastroscopists may just as well continue to use the term "hypertrophic gastritis" (as long as it is in quotation marks), rather than continuing to becloud the issue with new and insufficiently supported terms.

Stempien and associates[13] reported on a group of 15 patients in 1964. In 1971 they added 50 more with the hypertrophic pattern and found them hypersecretory as well. They proposed the term "hypertrophic hypersecretory gastropathy." These workers state that their findings are comparable to the Schindler concept of chronic hypertrophic glandular gastritis.

Hypertrophic Hypersecretory Gastropathy

Gastroscopically this lesion may be indistinguishable from that described as chronic hypertrophic gastritis. The gross nodularity produced by numerous polygonal nodules may be localized or diffuse. More often the process is extensive. The gastroscopist will observe that the nodular areas appear soft and that the nodules may be slightly irregular in size. The color is the normal orange-red or may be slightly redder or paler than normal, depending on the presence or absence of superimposed superficial gastritic changes. As the mosaic of *cobblestone* nodularity becomes more extensive, the pattern is seen not only in the *valleys* between folds but on the crests of many folds. This produces the so-called caterpillar segmentation of folds. Usually there is a striking absence or diminution of highlights, resulting in a dull, velvety appearance. If, on the other hand, there has been a recent marked secretion of mucus, the highlights may not be strikingly reduced. Other pathologic changes which may be regarded as complications are frequently seen. These changes or lesions may be petechiae, tiny erosions, gastroduodenal ulcer or other forms of gastritis.

Histologically, hypertrophic hypersecretory gastropathy is said to be frequently similar to Schindler's chronic hypertrophic glandular gastritis. That includes marked hypertrophy of the glandular elements in the lamina propria, with increase of the total parietal, chief and mucus-producing cell mass. There may or may not be marked infiltration by inflammatory cells. It is contended by Stempien et al.[13, 14] and a number of other observers that only sections taken from surgically resected specimens show the true picture. These observers believe that gastrobiopsies seldom bite through the total mucosa and muscularis in hypertrophic cases, and that therein lies the error of workers who base their concepts entirely on blind or directed gastrobiopsy.

Gastric secretory studies reveal an increase in hydrochloric acid, pepsin and mucus. There is no hypoproteinemia due to loss of serum protein in the gastric juice.

The hypertrophic picture seen gastroscopically in the Zollinger-Ellison syndrome belongs to the group of hypertrophic hypersecretory gastropathy. This syndrome is associated with gastrin-producing pancreatic islet cell tumors. As is well known, there is also a high incidence of gastroduodenal ulcer in this disease. Symptoms may be very severe, requiring total gastrectomy. In hypertrophic hypersecretory gastropathy without gastrin-producing pancreatic tumors, the disease responds to vagotomy and pyloroplasty or to x-radiation.

Giant Hypertrophic Gastritis of Menetrier

In the year 1888, Menetrier[16] reported the classic description of thickening of the gastric wall due to marked proliferation of the gastric mucosa. Despite the rarity of this disease, it is remarkable how popular and well entrenched it has become in the literature of gastroenterology. Gastroscopically, the disorder is characterized by enlarged gastric folds, which may be localized but more often are diffuse. The classic *pebbling* or nodularity produced by polygonal, irregular nodules is seen and appears perhaps indistinguishable from the classic characteristics described in other forms of hypertrophic gastropathy.

This disease is associated with excessive secretion of mucus and loss of serum albumin in the gastric juice. This can be demonstrated by electrophoresis or by serum albumin tagged with I^{131}, according to Citrin et al.,[17] or by the method of Waldman et al.[18] It should be obvious that whenever significantly enlarged folds are suspected, special as well as ordinary secretory studies should be performed.

Excess mucus has been observed gastroscopically on or between the hypertrophied fold; this may be in contrast to the hypertrophy associated with the Zollinger-Ellison syndrome where there is excessive acid secretion. Tortuosity of folds, especially on the greater curvature or fundic area has been likened to a bag of worms or to cerebral convolutions. Superficial changes may overlay the classic hypertrophic findings in Menetrier's disease, but apparently the association of peptic ulcer is rare. There is always the problem, however, of distinguishing malignant infiltration and even polypoid malignancy from so-called "tumor-simulating gastritis."

Histologically the causes of the hypertrophic changes are seen, namely, marked hyperplasia of the surface epithelium and degenerative changes in glandular elements of the lamina propria. Mucus cysts and inflammatory cellular infiltrations have frequently been reported.[19-22] Interestingly, several observers found normal mucosa with suction and gastrobiopsy but classic hypertrophic findings on deep sections of surgical specimens.

Secretory studies have shown histalog refractory achlorhydria or hypoacidity and marked increase of serum albumin in the gastric juice. Blood serum albumin levels are usually low, and the patient shows corresponding peripheral edema and epigastric pain, often severe.

Simple Enlargement of Gastric Folds

Giant gastric folds with secretory disturbances are relatively uncommon. Chronic hypertrophic gastritis as described gastroscopically is often seen. There remains a group of cases not infrequently seen by the gastroscopist which are referred to in terms such as "the folds are somewhat enlarged." These folds which appear slightly enlarged are most commonly seen on the greater curvature or fundic area. They may also be somewhat tortuous. In this category are those folds which are not associated with the cobblestone mosaic or *pebbling*. They may or may not appear enlarged on x-ray. When such folds are seen on gastroscopic examination, increased inflation has been used to test whether they can be reduced in size. This maneuver is meant to determine whether the enlargement is real or an artefact.

Sometimes the apparent enlargement of folds can be traced to the closeness of the gastroscope objective to the mucosa. It should be remembered that increased inflation to attempt reduction in rugal size also pushes the folds farther away from the objective, and this also reduces apparent size. When enlargement is thought to be significant, experience is needed in estimating the distance of the gastric wall from the gastroscope objective. The stomach may purposely be deflated through the suction channel or by inducing belching to solve this problem. We use the "multiple positions" technic (see Chapter 6) in some of these patients or manual pressure against the abdominal wall. It should be reiterated that variation in size of rugal folds in the same individual from time to time may occur on a physiologic basis. The works of Forssell[23] and Berg[24] have shown these changes to be due to the contractile activity of the muscularis mucosa.

RADIOLOGIC CONCEPTS

Since the very beginning of x-ray study of digestive diseases, attempts have been made to diagnose chronic gastritis radiographically. When gastroscopy came into wide use, it was generally conceded that x-ray played a minor role in diagnosis of chronic gastritis. In more recent years, especially with advanced technics of mucosal relief studies, air contrast and cine radiology, older concepts have changed. Particularly in Japan, where roentgenologists and gastroscopists work very closely together, the importance of roentgenography has come to light.

Indirect role: Routine roentgenography serves the important role of general screening of the gastric silhouette to help rule out more significant lesions in the entire stomach. X-ray shows the forest while forward-viewing endoscopy, which is the present trend, demonstrates the trees. Only the experienced expert in gastroscopy understands the forest completely. Gastroscopists often take x-ray contributions for granted, without being cognizant of the part x-ray plays in screening out filling defects. This role prevents the gastroscopist from concentrating on an intriguing and questionable area of chronic gastritis, for example in one part of the stomach, when there may be a more significant small tumor elsewhere. Endoscopy time is saved when, for example, x-ray screening shows apparent hypertrophic folds high in the fundus, thus directing the endoscopist immediately to this area.

Direct Role: There is a definite, important, continuing need for closer collaboration of roentgenologist and endoscopist in the study of diffuse lesions of the stomach. Mucosal relief, spot filming and ciné radiography help in differentiating chronic gastritis from early gastric cancer, especially the small, flat, slightly elevated or depressed forms (see Chapter 18). When tiny translucencies and thickened rugae can be confirmed in the same area by endoscopy, physiologic effects are better ruled out. Certain forms of gastritis and gastropathies extend into the submucosal and deeper layers of the gastric wall. The hypertrophic nodular forms, subacute phlegmonous[25] and emphysematous gastritis,[26] are examples of gastritic lesions in which x-ray diagnosis is of major importance. It must not be forgotten that in some cases gastroscopy will be unsuccessful or contraindicated.

CLINICAL CONCEPTS

Every disease has its clinical aspects. By this we mean the correlation between the symptoms on the one hand and the organic and physiologic findings on the other. Without this co-relationship, the pathologic and physiologic studies are mere exercises in futility; they become scientific games with no benefits toward improving the quality of life.

In order to emphasize this correlation, some aspects of the etiologic and symptomatic relationships of gastritis will be reviewed.

Etiology and Incidence

The causes of acute and chronic gastritis may be divided into exogenous and endogenous categories. Table 21-II summarizes those exogenous substances which have been associated with inflammation of the stomach in the opinion of physician and patient over the years. Listed also are those endogenous conditions for which there is evidence of a causal relationship to gastritis. The subject will not be greatly elaborated in this discussion. Some of the exogenous substances with which the gastroscopist will be concerned will be referred to and references cited for further study.

Aspirin ingestion has been widely demonstrated as causative in many cases of mild or massive upper gastrointestinal hemorrhage.[27-30] In these cases the gastroscopist often finds scattered petechial hemorrhages in the mucosa of varying ages—bright red, reddish brown to purplish. In some cases hemorrhagic erosions will also be seen, some oozing of a trickle of blood. Usually the erosions are tiny or conglomerate with a reddish base. Others may have a gray or white base. It is uncommon to find more than petechiae and tiny erosions and hemorrhage. Therefore, the term "aspirin gastritis" is seldom warranted. Aspirin ingestion is sometimes followed by

TABLE 21-II

ETIOLOGY OF ACUTE AND CHRONIC GASTRITIS

| | | Exogenous | |
Chemicals	*Infections*	*Foods*	*Miscellaneous*
Alcohol	Pyogenic organism	Highly seasonal	Irradiation
Aspirin	Streptococcal	condiments	Foreign bodies
Steroids	Other organisms	Gastric over-	Other rare causes
Antiarthritic		loading, etc.	
Corrosive			
Others			

| | | Endogenous | |
| *Other Digestive* | | *Psychosomatic* | |
Diseases	*Systemic Diseases*	*Disorders*	*Miscellaneous*
Peptic ulcers	Cardiovascular	Primary G.I.	Post-op stomach
Carcinoma	Renal diseases	disorders of	Primary, rare
Other neoplasms	Malignancies	function	gastric diseases
Gallbladder	Pernicious anemia	Secondary	e.g. syphilis
Liver	Other blood dyscrasias	disorders of	Hodgkins, etc.
Pancreatic	Respiratory disorders	function	
	Endocrine factors		
	Others		

hematemesis when the patient has gastric or duodenal ulcer. The presumption is, and sometimes the evidence indicates, hemorrhage from the peptic ulcer.

Alcohol ingestion since the earliest times has been suspected and often incriminated as an important cause of acute and chronic gastritis. There is little question that alcoholic beverages can cause acute inflammation of the stomach. The effectiveness of alcohol in producing chronic gastritis is another matter. Berry[31] was first to show that gastroscopic evidence of chronic gastritis was not found in more than one third of a large group of severe chronic alcoholic addicts. These individuals, so-called vagabonds from Chicago's Skid Row, were induced to undergo gastroscopy. Although average consumption per individual was three pints of liquor per day, none had complaints of sufficient significance to seek medical care. Gray and Schindler[32] examined a similar number of alcoholics from the same neighborhood, confirming the findings of Berry. The gastritis found was mostly of the superficial type; in one third to one half of the cases. Normal gastric mucosa or a few scattered petechiae were found in the remainder. Biopsies were not available at that time, but since have shown variable evidences of histologic gastritis.

We have continued the gastroscopic study of chronic gastritis associated with chronic alcoholism for many years at the Cook County Hospital.[33-34] Comparing the hospitalized group with the asymptomatic addicts, we found the incidence of chronic gastritis to be higher in the hospitalized group.

Many drugs and chemicals have been incriminated as causal in gastritis. In Caracas, Venezuela, the commonest cause of gastritis in a large series was caustic substances (see Chapter 21-II). Other substances, as indicated in Table 21-III, include steroids, antihypertensive and antiarthritis drugs.

TABLE 21-III

COMPARATIVE CLASSIFICATION OF GASTRITIS BASED UPON GASTROSCOPY, BIOPSY AND HISTOPATHOLOGY

Schindler *Gastroscopy*	*Magnus Surgery* *and Histopathology*	*Benedict et al.* *Gastroscopy and* *Histopathology*
(1) Chr. superficial gastritis	(1) Acute erosive gastritis	(1) Acute gastritis
(2) Chr. atrophic gastritis	(2) Chr. gastritis (atrophic)	(2) Chr. atrophic gastritis
(3) Chr. hypertrophic gastritis	(3) Gastric atrophy of P.A. ETAT Mamalone (normal)	(Normal variant)

Certain forms of chronic gastritis might better be discussed in a special category. They are well described in the gastroenterology literature and will only be mentioned here.

Phlegmonous gastritis[25] is of bacterial origin and involves mostly the submucosa. It may occur in the acute, subacute and chronic forms.

Granulomatous gastritis[36] has been reported as a form of Crohn's disease, affecting the small intestines and colon more often than the stomach. The gastroscopic picture may show granulomatous changes but has no specific gastroscopic pattern.

Emphysematous gastritis[26] is a rare disorder characterized by formation of gas within the gastric wall, most commonly by bacteria or injury due to ingestion of caustics. Other causes have been cited. X-ray provides a spectacular method of diagnosis. Symptoms are often too acute for gastroscopy.

Postoperative alkaline reflux gastritis[37] is being reported increasingly in the literature of recent years. The gastroscopic classification of postoperative gastritis has been made since the early years of gastroscopy. The causative role of failure of physiological adaptation and regurgitation has long been postulated. Postoperative syndromes are discussed in Chapter 20.

The incidence of chronic gastritis has been as controversial a problem as any other aspect of the disease. From the time of Broussais, when everyone had gastritis, to periods when nobody had it, there have been several cycles of incidence reported. From the early days of gastroscopy, the incidence of chronic gastritis among patients gastroscoped was about 35 per cent.[38, 39] An incidence evaluation by Schindler at Billings Hospital among mostly middle-class patients showed a relatively high rate of hypertrophic gastritis. During the same period a large group of economically disadvantaged patients in Berry's Clinic at Provident Hospital, a few city blocks away, showed a relatively high incidence of chronic atrophic gastritis. Recently an interesting gastritis study of gastrobiopsies in a randomized rural Scandinavian population was made by Siurala et al.[40] This was a screening approach in a nonpatient population. This kind of study correlated with x-ray and endoscopy in mass screening may help in the solution of the problem of incidence in the future.

Symptomatology

Long before there were x-ray or gastroscopic concepts of gastritis, epigastric distress was associated with inflammation of the stomach. Other symptoms attributed to gastritis are nausea, sometimes vomiting and occasionally hematemesis. Because of the compact interrelations of digestive organs in the upper abdomen, there are many overlapping syndromes[41] referable to this area. There is no symptom complex specific for any type of gastritis. Usually, the distress of chronic gastritis comes on during or immediately after a meal, especially one of heavy or highly seasoned foods. In the presence of hypertrophic gastropathies with hyperacidity or of many erosions, the distress may resemble the peptic ulcer syndrome.

One of the most controversial aspects of chronic gastritis is the failure, in the opinion of many workers, to find a consistent correlation between gastroscopic or histologic gastritis and chronic epigastric distress. They point out that there may be much distress and very little gastritis, and vice versa. Therefore, chronic gastritis has no clinical significance. Yet it has been shown repeatedly that the organic signs of gastritis may heal and recur again and again. Thus, the problem of timing must be considered in correlating organic changes with symptoms. There is no disease in which the severity of symptoms can always be correlated with the extent of organic changes.

Because of overlapping syndromes in diseases of the liver, gallbladder, pancreas, duodenum and stomach and because gastritis is frequently associated with other diseases in the gastrointestinal canal, such as peptic ulcer and cancer, the problem of assessment of gastritic symptoms remains a difficult one.

Psychoneurotic Aspects

Every gastroenterologist sees patients with digestive distress in whom he can find no physical, biochemical or x-ray evidence of disease in the digestive system. Such disorders are frequently regarded as of functional or psychogenic origin. In a certain number of these patients there will be gastroscopic evidence of chronic gastritis in varying degrees of severity. Sometimes the epigastric symptoms are long-standing and persistent. If the physician has the time, he will often observe anxieties and other emotional manifestations in the patient. Some observers are therefore of the opinion that much chronic gastritis is of psychosomatic origin and that much of the symptomatic complaint is entirely a functional manifestation. Masuda[42] studied two groups consisting of 1,021 patients with chronic gastritis diagnosed gastroscopically and radiologically. He used the Cornell Medical Index to classify the patients by neuropsychiatric standards. It was found that 25 per cent of clinic patients belonged to the psychologically normal group and 75 per cent to the neurasthenic group in varying degrees. Of a second group of gastritis patients obtained by gastric mass survey, 91 per cent belonged to the psychologically normal group and 9 per cent to the neurasthenic group. Masuda concluded that many of these patients had symptoms of psychoneurotic origin, regardless of the clinical significance of the gastritis itself.

CORRELATION AND COMMON GROUND

Controversy has been the lifeblood and the secret of progress in medicine. Occasionally great controversy is brought to an end by dramatic discovery. When Von Mering and Minkowski observed swarming flies around the urine of pancreatectomized dogs, the problem of the cause of diabetes was dramatically solved. While we await this dramatic moment in the history of gastritis, there is much that can be counted as progress. If 60 per cent of gastroscopic gastritis does not have corresponding histologic findings of gastritis, the 40 per cent that does should not be discounted. If the symptoms of chronic epigastric distress appear not to be consonant with organic findings, perhaps the recuperative powers of the stomach should be credited rather than discrediting the disease concept. Closing the communications gap should shrink the area of controversy.

If the histologist never looks through the endoscope and the endoscopist never looks through the microscope, neither may recognize their common ground. If the gastroscopist never sits with the fluoroscopist and the gastroenterologist refers his problems to the psychiatrist, the patient and science may be denied the benefits of correlated understanding.

Table 21-III illustrates the kind of correlation which should be recognized by students of the problems of gastritis. The table shows the relationship of concepts of clinical endoscopist, surgeon and histopathologist.

As we strive toward the moment of truth in gastritis, let us accept gross gastroscopy by the standards of the gross pathology of inflammation, and endoscopy-directed gastrobiopsy by the standards of the histopathology of inflammation. We should accept both on the basis of their individual strengths and leave the clinical significance to the clinician without the confusion that the findings of one must completely negate the value of the other.

REFERENCES

1. Schindler, R.: *Gastroscopy: Endoscopic Study of Gastric Pathology.* Chicago, Chicago Pr., 1937.
2. Schindler, R.: *Gastritis.* New York, Grune, 1947
3. Shallenberger, Paul L., DeWan, C. H., Weed, C. B., and Reganis, J. C.: Biopsy through the flexible operating gastroscope. *Gastroenterology, 16*:327-340, 1950.
4. Atkins, L., and Benedict, E. B.: Correlation of gross gastroscopic findings with gastroscopic biopsy in gastritis. *Engl J Med, 254*:641, 1956.
5. Debray, C., Laumonier, R., and Houssét, P.: Confrontation des donnees gastroscopiques et des biopsies muqueuses gas triques dans les gastrites. *Arch mal app digest, 41*:922, 1952.
6. Berry, Leonidas H., and Cole, T. Jonathan: Therapy of chronic atrophic gastritis with eight years' gastroscopic control. *JAMA, 138*:485, 1948.
7. Yamada, K., Suzukis and Takemoto, T.: Re-evaluation of various forms of gastritis by controlled intragastric pressure simultaneously visualized by gastroscopy. *Gastrointest Endosc, 18*:111-113, Feb., 1972.
8. Ruffin, J. M., and Brown, I. W.: The effect of inflation of the stomach upon the gastroscopic picture. *Am J Dig Dis Nutrition, 7*:418, 1940.
9. Ardeman, S., and Chanarin, I.: Steroids and Addisonian pernicious anemia, *N Engl J Med, 273*:1352, 1965a.
10. Berry, Leonidas H.: Chronic atrophic gastritis and malnutrition. Proceedings of the central society of clinic research. *J Lab & Clin Med, 32*:1521-1522, 1947.
11. Kelly, Charles H., Lawlah, John, and Berry, Leonidas H.: Mucosal relief technic correlated with gastroscopy in 150 cases. *Radiology, 36*:77, 1941.
12. Cunningham, D. J.: *Textbook of Anatomy.* 8th ed. New York, Oxford, 1943.
13. Stempien, S. J., Dagradi, A. E., Reingold, I. M., Heiskell, C. L., Goodman, J. R., Bloom, A., and Weaver, D. S.: Hypertrophic hypersecretory gastropathy. *Am J Dig Dis, 9*:471, 1964.
14. Deogracias, T. D., Stempien, S. J., and Dagradi, A. E.: The clinical spectrum of hypertrophic hypersecretory gastropathy. *Gastrointest Endosc, 18*:2, 1971.
15. Benedict, E. B.: Gastroscopic biopsy. *Gastroenterology, 37*:445, 1959.
16. Menetrier, P.: Les polyadenomés gastriques et des leurs rapports avec le cancer de l'esto mac. *Arch physiol norm path, 20*:32, 1888.
17. Citrin, U., Sterling, K., and Halsted, J. A.: The mechanism of hypoproteinemia associated with giant hypertrophy of the gastric mucosa. *N Engl J Med, 257*:906, 1957.
18. Waldman, A., Steinfeld, J. L., Dutcher, T. F., Davidson, J. D., and Gordon, R. S.: The role of the gastrointestinal system in idiopathic hypoproteinemia. *Gastroenterology, 41*:197, 1961.
19. Baker, W. G., Jr., Kolodny, M., and Colker, Goldin H.: Gastroscopy in Menetrier's disease. *Gastrointest Endosc, 15*:209, 1968.
20. Schindler, R.: *Gastroscopy, the Endoscopic Study of Gastric Pathology,* 2nd ed. Chicago, University of Chicago Press, p. 235, 1950.
21. Palmer, E. D.: What Menetrier really said. *Gastrointest Endosc, 15*:83-109, 1968.
22. Moutier, F.: *Traite de Gastroscopie.* Paris, Masson, 1935.

23. Forssell, G.: Studies of the mechanism of the movement of the mucous membrane of the digestive tract. *Am J Roentgenol, 10*:87, 1923.

24. Berg, H. H.: Röntgenuntersuchungen innenrelief des verdauungskanals. Leipzig, G *Thieme Verlag,* 1930.

25. Bandler, M.: Phlegmonous gastritis mimicking gastric neoplasm. *Gastrointest Endosc, 17*: August, 1970.

26. Clearfield, H.: Emphysematous gastritis, secondary to lye ingestion. Report of a case. *Am J Dig Dis, 14*:195-196, March, 1969.

27. Cooke, A. R.: Aspirin, ethanol and the stomach. *Aust Ann Med, 3*:269, 1970.

28. Hoon, J. R.: Aspirin gastritis examined with intragastric photography. *Ind Med,* 38:52-61, 1969.

29. Croft, D. N., and Wood, P. H. V.: Gastric mucosa and susceptibility to gastrointestinal bleeding caused by aspirins. *Br Med J,* 1:137, 1967.

30. Menguy, R.: Gastric mucosal injury by aspirin. *Gastroenterology, 51*:430-432, September, 1966.

31. Berry, Leonidas H.: Chronic alcoholic gastritis: Evaluation of the concept with gastroscopic studies in 100 cases. *JAMA, 117*:2233-2236, 1941.

32. Gray, S., and Schindler, R.: Gastric mucosa of chronic alcoholic addicts: a gastroscopic study. *JAMA, 117*:1005, 1941.

33. Berry, Leonidas H.: Nouvelle conceptions sur la gastrite alcolique études gastroscopique: Proc IVe Congress de l'association des Societes Nationales Europeannes et Mediterraneennes de Gastro-Enterologie. Paris, Masson et Editeurs, 1954.

34. Berry, Leonidas H., Alavi, S., Mitaniyama, A., and Adomavicius, J.: Analysis of 6,000 consecutive fiberoptic and lens gastroscopies. Proceedings of the 2nd World Congress of Gastrointestinal Endoscopy, Padova, Italy, Piccin Medical Books, 1972.

35. Gonzalez-Crussi, F., and Hackett, R. L.: Phlegmonous gastritis. *Arch Surg, 93*:990, 1966.

36. Comfort, M. W., Weber, H. M., Baggenstoss, A. H., and Kiely, W. F.: Nonspecific granulomatous inflammation of the stomach and duodenum: its relation to regional enteritis. *Am J Med Sci, 220*:616-632, 1950.

37. VanHeerden, J. A., Priestley, J. T., Farrow, G. M., Phillips, S. F.: Postoperative alkaline reflux gastritis—surgical implications. *Am J Surg, 118*:427-429, Sept. 1969.

38. Schindler, R.: The incidence of various types of gastric disease as revealed by gastroscopic study. *Am J Med Sci, 197*:509, 1939.

39. Berry, Leonidas H.: Analysis of 1400 consecutive gastroscopic examinations. *Proc Inst Med Chicago, 16*:237, 1946.

40. Siurala, M., Isokoshi, M., Varis, K., Kekki, M.: Prevalence of gastritis in a rural population, bioptic study of subjects selected at random. *Scand J Gastroent,* 3:1968.

41. Berry, Leonidas H.: Differential diagnosis of the multiple syndromes of the upper gastrointestinal tract. *Rev Gastroenterol, 19*:715, 1952.

CHAPTER 21

PART II: HISTOPATHOLOGY OF GASTRITIS

Joel Valencia-Parparcén and Blas Bruni-Celli

Introduction
Acute Gastritis
Chronic Gastritis
   Chronic Superficial
   Chronic Atrophic
Atrophic Gastric Mucosa
Incidence
Hypertrophic Hypersecretory Gastropathy and Malignant Neoplasia

INTRODUCTION

Chronic gastritis as a clinical entity goes back for many, many years. Only in more recent years has it been possible to diagnose the disease anatomically. In the earlier years there was the problem of postmortem autolysis and the distinction between this and antimortem changes. It is our opinion that while gastroscopy and x-ray have made some supportive contributions to the concept of gastritis, only the blind biopsy method is of primary importance in this diagnosis. Our experience tends to confirm the simple classification of chronic gastritis as described by Wood and Taft[1] and Palmer.[2]

The most common symptoms of gastritis are epigastric pain, post-prandial fullness, belching and flatulence. In our series, almost two thirds of the cases presented epigastric pain and more than one-half showed free acidity. Very often true gastritis is present without discomfort and with good appetite.

Gastritis as we find it, is classified in the following forms: Acute gastritis, chronic gastritis, which may be chronic superficial or chronic atrophic and atrophic gastric mucosa, which is not of inflammatory origin but because of its close similarity to chronic atrophic gastritis, it is included in this discussion.

338

ACUTE GASTRITIS

The essential histological findings in acute gastritis are as follows: Infiltration of the lining epithelium by polymorphonuclear cells, vacuolation and pyknosis of the lining cells, severe vasodilatation of capillaries. There is also polymorphonuclear and plasmocytic infiltration just under the surface epithelial cells. There is also pyknosis of the chief and parietal cells of the neck glands and plasmocytic and polymorphonuclear infiltration of the deep lamina propria.

CHRONIC GASTRITIS

In most instances our biopsies have been obtained from patients who have chronic gastritis. If there is acute gastritis present, biopsy procedures are frequently contraindicated.

Chronic Superficial Gastritis

The histologic picture in superficial gastritis is characterized by changes which take place in the superficial one third of the mucosa. There are inflammatory cells in the superficial lamina propria. Some of these cells are polymorphonuclear. However, many of them are lymphocytes and plasma cells. There is flattening and irregularity of the lining epithelium and infiltration of the glandular epithelium by inflammatory cells[1] (Figs. 21-1a, b, c, d).

Chronic Atrophic Gastritis

There is evidence that chronic atrophic gastritis is an extension of the chronic superficial form of gastritis in most instances. The most frequent changes are as follows[3] (Figs. 21-2a, b, c, d): There is partial loss of the lining epithelium, edema develops in the mucosa causing distortion of the gastric crypts. There is infiltration by lymphocytes and plasma cells and to some extent polymorphonuclear cells. These infiltrations affect the upper two-thirds of the mucosa and spread through the entire lamina propria. There is a decrease in the number of fundic glands and a decrease or absence of parietal and chief cells. Usually, there is an increase in fibrous tissue and of the formation of lymph follicles. A very frequent characteristic is the development of intestinal metaplasia. This is characterized by the presence of goblet cells. Because these cells are more characteristic of the intestines, it is called intestinal metaplasia when such cells are seen in the gastric mucosa (Figs. 21-2a, b, c).

ATROPHIC GASTRIC MUCOSA

It is now well known that the gastric mucosa is found to be atrophic in nearly 100 per cent of cases of untreated pernicious anemia. Histological-

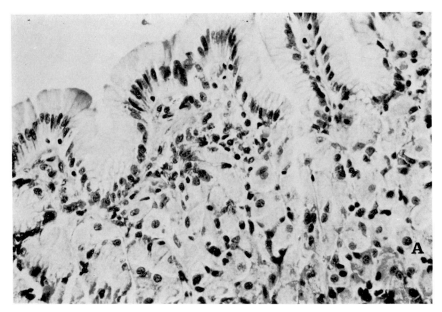

Fig. 21-1a

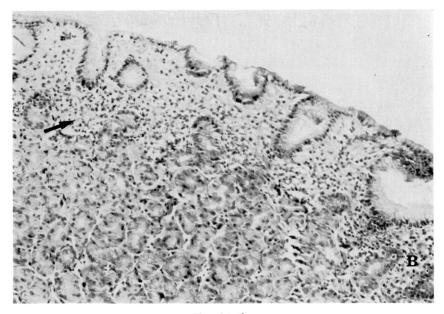

Fig. 21-1b

Figure 21-1a, b. (1a) Normal gastric mucosa (H.E. 200×). (1b) Light superficial gastritis (H.E. 160×). The arrow marks the lymphocytic infiltration area in the superficial corium.

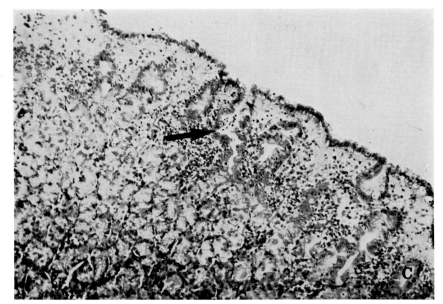

Fig. 21-1c

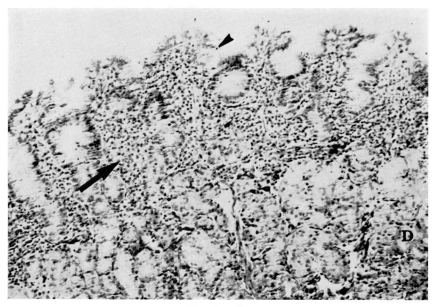

Fig. 21-1d

Figure 21-1c, d. (1c) Mild superficial gastritis (H.E. 160×). The inflammatory infiltration is great and gastric fossae contain many polymorphonuclear cells (arrow). (1d) Severe superficial gastritis (H.E. 160×). The large arrow marks intense inflammatory infiltration. The small arrow indicates focal necrotic areas.

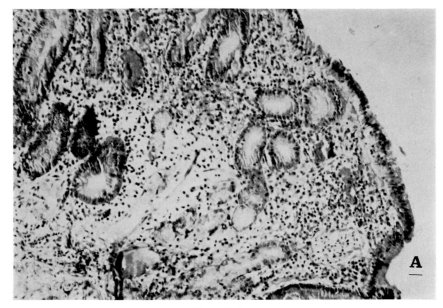

Fig. 21-2a

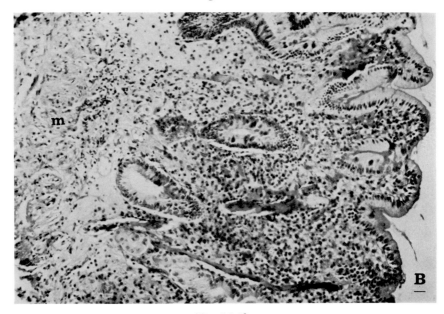

Fig. 21-2b

Figure 21-2a, b. (2a) Light atrophic gastritis (H.E. 160×). There is diffuse infiltration of inflammatory cells, edema in the corium and numerous calciform cells in the superficial epithelium. (2b) Mild atrophic gastritis (H.E. 160×). Inflammatory infiltration is intense, the glands are scant and the mucosal thickness reduced.

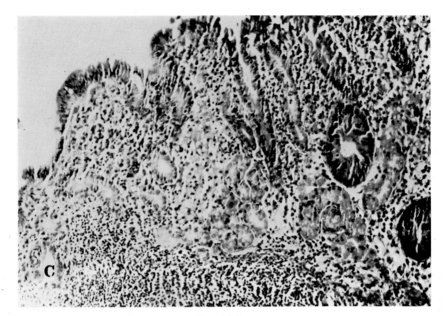

Fig. 21-2c

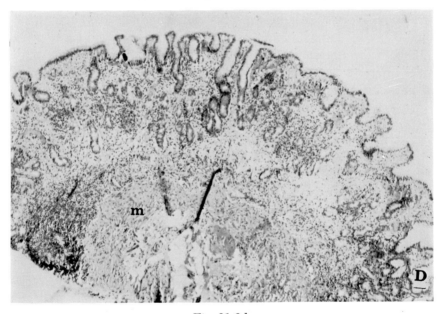

Fig. 21-2d

Figure 21-2c, d. (2c) Severe atrophic gastritis (H.E. 160×). Inflammatory infiltration is very severe, with almost complete glandular atrophy. Calciform cells and a portion of a lymph follicle in the lower right area can be seen. (2d) Gastric atrophy (H.E. 160×). Irregular small gastric fossae, glandular atrophy and inflammatory infiltrations are present.

ly, there is a close resemblance between the atrophic changes in chronic atrophic gastritis and those of atrophic gastric mucosa. There is considerable evidence that the atrophic gastric mucosa of pernicious anemia did not begin as chronic superficial gastritis. Williams and Coghill[4] have studied the mucosa of pernicious anemia patients with the use of biopsies. They made two biopsies in 90 per cent of their studies. In our studies we found it more appropriate to make three biopsies in the classification and accurate description of gastritis.[5] In our histologic studies of chronic gastritis, we have found the use of the flexible tube of Wood to be an excellent instrument, and the preferred method of the collection of biopsies.

It is important to carefully select patients for this procedure to be sure that there are no contraindications and to follow them appropriately after the collection of the biopsy. Our patients are checked with reference to their blood pressure, their hematocrit and general clinical condition before they are allowed to leave the clinic. Joske[6] emphasized the need of the collection of adequate tissue in the biopsy of prompt preparation and the assurance that the sections are cut perpendicularly. We[7] have confirmed the opinions of Joske and other observers with reference to the importance of the manner of collection and of processing of biopsies. We have found a correlation in our studies between histologic findings and the correct provisional diagnosis is to be 54.54 per cent. Very seldom are there any complications in the use of the blind biopsy tube of Wood in our experience. Vilardell[8] reports hemorrhage as a complication of the blind gastrobiopsy as 0.7 per cent in 12,381 such biopsies.

INCIDENCE

We have found that gastritis is a very frequent disease. In our study of 2,000 consecutive biopsies with the blind Wood tube, performed from 1958 to 1961, we obtained a positive finding of gastritis in 26.1 per cent of biopsies taken. Of these cases of positive gastritis, 77.1 per cent was superficial gastritis and 19.5 per cent was atrophic gastritis, with 3.4 per cent unclassified. At the present time, we have sat at 5,000 gastric biopsies and found percentages are relatively the same.[9] The incidence of gastritis associated with various diseases of the digestive tract in 1,478 patients in our clinic was found to have the following distribution: Caustic esophagogastritis 71.6 per cent, gastrectomized patients 63.7 per cent, gastric carcinoma 54 per cent, gastric ulcer 38.5 per cent, duodenal ulcer 17 per cent, clinical gastritis 29 per cent, radiological duodenitis 29.5 per cent, hiatal hernia 24.9 per cent, biliary lithiasis 31.6 per cent, portal hypertension 32.1 per cent, portal cirrhosis 12.6 per cent, intestinal malabsorption 41.6 per cent, viral hepatitis 5.5 per cent, neuroses 20 per cent, and ulcerous recto-colitis 9.4 per cent.

It is obvious that caustic esophageal gastritis has a disproportionately high incidence in our population sample. We admit that in this report there is some selectivity in the cases coming under our observation.

HYPERTROPHIC HYPERSECRETORY GASTROPATHY AND MALIGNANT NEOPLASIA

Menetrier in 1888 described diffuse hypertrophy of the gastric wall caused by excessive proliferation of the mucosa associated with achlorhydria and protein loss.[10] In 1937 Schindler[11] described hypertrophic gastritis and stated that it could only be confirmed by surgical specimens. He differentiated from Menetrier's disease primarily by the fact that there is increased acidity and no protein loss in the hypertrophic gastritis. Histologically, Schindler described an increased glandular mass with thickening of the mucosa and formation of superficial nodules. In 1962, Stempien, et al.[12] described "hypertrophic, hypersecretory gastropathy," which they state is very similar to Schindler's "glandular hypertrophic gastritis." In 1969 Valencia-Parparcen and Bruni-Celli[13] described the first published cases of "hypertrophic, hypersecretory gastropathy" (Figs. 21-3a, b, c, d) in Venezuela, and furnished the necessary data to differentiate it from Menetrier's disease.

During the last two years at "Centro Medico of Caracas," we have studied 20 patients with upper gastrointestinal symptomatology and radiologic and endoscopic findings of thick gastric folds. Three groups of patients were reviewed. The first group consisted of five patients, where extensive gastric resection was done. On gross appearance the surgeons were unable to differentiate the lesion from cancer. The second group consisted of three patients, who also had surgery and a biopsy and frozen section was obtained, thus differentiating the hypertrophic gastritis from cancer, and eliminating the need for gastrectomy.

A third group of cases consisted of twelve patients, where in addition to routine radiography and endoscopy, two other investigative procedures were employed. (1) Double contrast Barium meal with air insufflation and (2) multiple gastric biopsies by means of the blind Wood's tube from various regions of the stomach (Figs. 21-4a, b, c, d). In all of these patients a definitive diagnosis of hypertrophic, hypersecretory gastropathy was made without resorting to surgical intervention.

We agree with Stempien et al., that "hypertrophic, hypersecretory gastropathy" is more frequent than has previously been suspected, during the last decade. We agree that this condition should be suspected in the presence of hypertrophic folds by x-ray and gastroscopy, associated with low gastric pH. Our observations indicate that gastric biopsy and surgical biopsy are necessary for confirmation. However, in our experience it is unneces-

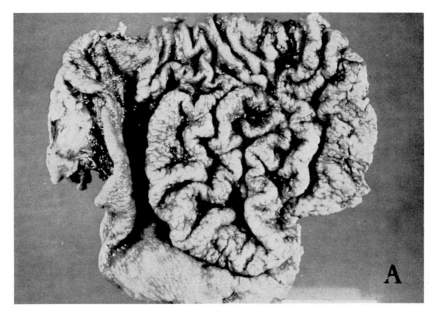

Fig. 21-3a

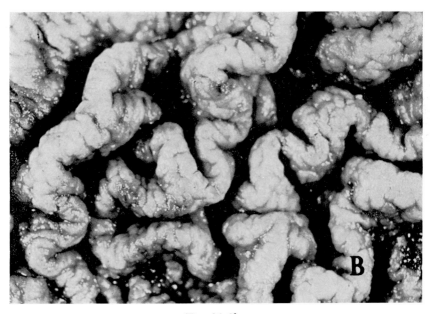

Fig. 21-3b

Figure 21-3a, b. (3a) Surgical specimen of a case of hypertrophic-hypersecretory gastropathy. Note the tortuous folds and nodularity. (3b) A high power view of the same specimen shows "encephaloid" appearance, deep crevices and nodules on the crests of folds.

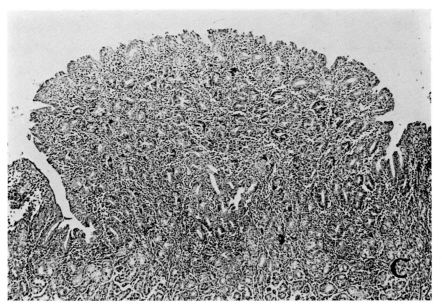

Fig. 21-3c

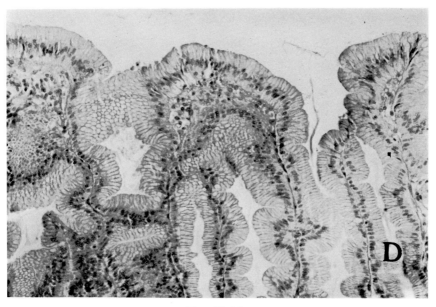

Fig. 21-3d

Figure 21-3c, d. (3c) Microphotograph from surgical specimens with prominent folds. The mucosal thickness appears increased. There is marked lymphocytic infiltration. (3d) A high power view in a similar case of hypertrophic mucosa shows deformity of small gastric fossae and prominent folds (H.E. 200×).

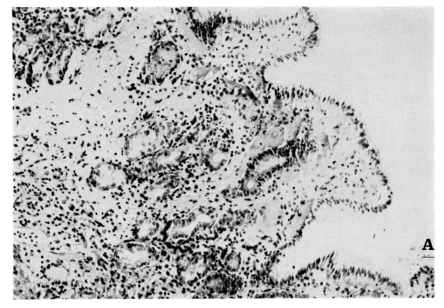

Fig. 21-4a

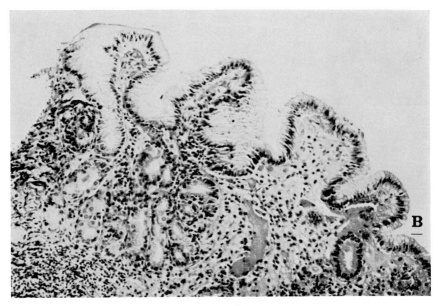

Fig. 21-4b

Figure 21-4a, b. (4a) Section from blind suction biopsy. The gross specimen showed markedly enlarged gastric folds. (4b) In this section prominent folds are seen with moderate cellular infiltration.

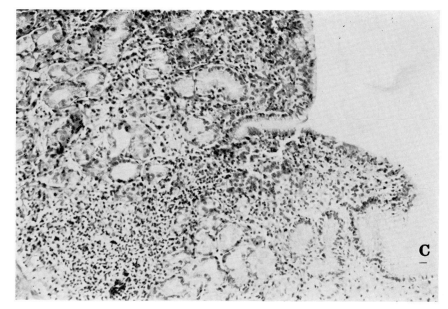

Fig. 21-4c

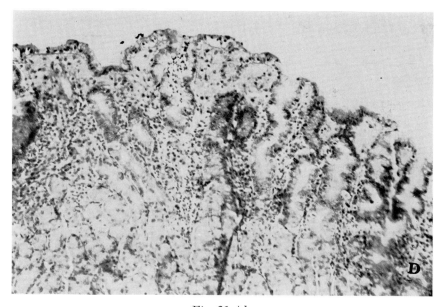

Fig. 21-4d

Figure 21-4c, d. These microphotographs show hypertrophic-hypersecretory gastropathy. (4c) shows irregular distribution of marked cellular infiltration. (4d) shows hypertrophy of folds. Sections are from blind suction biopsy.

sary to have surgical specimens for the diagnosis. We find that blind gastrobiopsy with the Wood's tube is adequate, when combined with the finding of hyperchlorhydria, double contrast x-ray and gastroscopy. With this method we have been able to differentiate diffuse gastric malignancy and save the patient a high gastric resection.

REFERENCES

1. Wood, I. J., and Taft, L. I.: *Diffuse Lesions of the Stomach.* London, Edward Arnold Publications Ltd. 1958.
2. Palmer, E. D.: Gastritis: a revaluation. *Medicine, 33*:199, 1954.
3. Valencia-Parparcén, J., Romer, H., and Salomón, R.: Gastritis: clinic and diagnosis. *GEN, XVII*:258, 1963.
4. Williams, A. W., Coghill, N. F., and Edwards, F.: The gastric mucosa in pernicious anemia: biopsy-studies. *Brit Haemat, 4*:457, 1958.
5. Valencia-Parparcén, J., Bruni-Celli, B., Salomón, R., and Romer, H.: La biopsia gástrica múltiple en la clasificación de las gastritis. *GEN, XX*:281, 1965.
6. Joske, R. A., Finckh, E. S., and Wood, I. J.: Gastric biopsy, a study of 1000 consecutive successful gastric biopsies. *Quart J Med* (N.S.), *24*:269, 1955.
7. Valenca-Parparcén, J., Carbonell, L., Bruni-Celli, B., and Madureri, V.: Diagnosis of gastritis: a review and a report of the use of blind biopsy. *Am J Dig Dis,* (N.S.), *6*:813, 1961.
8. Vilardell, F.: Enfermedades difusas del estómago. Editorial *Científico-Médica,* Barcelona, 1962.
9. Valencia-Parparcén, J.: Diagnóstico y concepto actual de las gastritis. En *Controversias en gastroenterología* de Valencia-Parparcén, J., p. 135. Grafos Impresores Asociados C.A., Caracas, 1967.
10. Vilardell, F.: Gastritis crónica. Tipos especiales. Su relación con otras enfermedades. *Gastroenterologia,* por H. L. Bockus. Tomo I, Cap. 23:428. Salvat Editores S.A., 1965.
11. Schindler, R.: Gastroscopy. The endoscopic study of gastric pathology. Chicago, University of Chicago Press. 1937.
12. Stempien, S. J., Dagradi, A. E., Reingold, I. M., Heiskell, Ch.L., Bloom, A., and Weaver, D. S.: Benign hypertrophic hyperchlorhydric gastropathy. Analysis of 13 cases. Proceedings of the II World Congress of Gastroenterology. Munich, 1962, Tomo II: 243, S. Karger, Basel, 1963.
13. Valencia-Parparcén, J., Bruni-Celli, B., Baquero González, R., and Márquez Reverón, A.: Enfermedad de Menetrier vs. gastritis hipertrófica hipersecretoria. *GEN, XXIV*:281, 1970.

CHAPTER 22

SUPERFICIAL EROSIONS: HEMORRHAGIC, NON-HEMORRHAGIC, PETECHIAL HEMORRHAGES

WOLFGANG ROESCH AND RUDOLF OTTENJANN

INTRODUCTORY STATEMENT

THE HISTORY OF the endoscopic concept of gastric erosions and petechial mucosal hemorrhages probably begins with the early writings of Rudolf Schindler in the late 1920s and especially following his introduction of the first lens-semiflexible gastroscope in 1932. Since the beginning of the era of fiberoptic endoscopy, interest in the clinical significance of superficial erosions and petechial mucosal hemorrhages has increased. The anatomical existence of these defects was well known by pathologists and surgeons long before the observations of the endoscopist. The ultimate clinical significance of these lesions remains as yet an enigma of gastroenterology. There are certain facts, however, which can be documented by the endoscopist and confirmed by gastrobiopsy, surgery and histopathology. The etiology and clinical significance as far as can be substantiated at this stage of our knowledge is of importance to the beginner as well as the ad-

351

vanced student of gastrointestinal endoscopy and will be discussed in this chapter.

DEFINITION AND HISTORY

The term "erosion" is limited to a defect of the mucosal layer which does not penetrate the muscularis mucosa histologically. Morgagni[1] in 1761 was already talking of multiple erosions and hemorrhagic suggillations in describing gastritis. Beaumont[2] in his servant, Alexis St. Martin, found occasional eruptions or deep red pimples arising from the surface of the mucous coat and frequently filled with white purulent matter especially after alcoholic excesses. These findings were later confirmed by Wolf[3] in another gastrostoma patient following stress situations. In 1897 Nauwerck[4] coined the phrase "gastritis ulcerosa chronica" when he had to deal with a stomach showing several ulcers and multiple erosions.

Konjetzny[5] postulated an inflammatory genesis of erosions, Hauser[6] favored circulatory disturbances. This idea was advanced by Virchow[7] in 1856. Buchner[8] preferred the peptic origin of gastric erosion and ulcer. Henning and Schatzki[9] could demonstrate erosions by endoscopy and radiology for the first time intravitally. Schindler[10] described aphtae-like lesions with a gray base surrounded by a red halo and stressed the edematous character of the surrounding mucosa. He also differentiates between petechial hemorrhages and erosions by the conception that the petechiae are subepithelial and that their tiny surfaces may become sloughed by gastric acidity to become erosions. Bleeding may then occur. Otherwise petechiae may fail to erode, become dark red and finally resorb. Their origins in the first place may be due to capillary fragility or changes in the clotting mechanism. Berry[11] calls attention to the fact that non-hemorrhagic superficial erosions are seen by the endoscopist which may reach 1cm or more in diameter. Their bases are shallow and covered with a brilliant white or off-white porcelain-like exudate with irregular shapes and borders. Occasionally a red halo may be seen and they may be single or multiple. Inflammatory changes with localized areas of hyperemia and edema are often associated. These lesions are usually benign but occasionally a spreading superficial carcinomatous lesion may have to be differentiated.

Routine gastroscopy and the vigorous diagnostic approach to acute upper gastrointestinal hemorrhage[12] not only disclosed that gastric erosions were quite common and that about 20 per cent of the patients were bleeding from acute gastric mucosal lesions but also demonstrated the need for endoscopic classification of these lesions.

PATHOLOGY AND CLASSIFICATION

Due to the fact that every loss of surface epithelium and/or mucosa qualifies as an erosive defect, we have devised these categories:

Hemorrhagic-erosive Gastritis

Hemorrhagic-erosive gastritis is characterized by innumerable, pin-point-sized hemorrhages on the mucosal surface with erythro-diapedesis and engorged blood vessels within mucosa and submucosa. This hemorrhagic gastritis with loss or dehiscence of the surface epithelium does not usually show cellular inflammatory reaction and may be diffuse or localized to the fundic or antral region.

Incomplete Erosion

Incomplete erosion is also called flat erosion or hemorrhagic fleck.[13] It is a simple defect of the mucosal layer without reaction of the surroundings, either single or multiple (Fig. 22-1).

Complete Erosion

Complete erosion is characterized in the acute phase by a hematin-covered floor surrounded by an elevated border (Dellengastritis, gastritis varioliformis Moutier) (Fig. 22-2). The black central depression of the erosion is usually followed within 24 to 48 hours by a whitish, gray-yellow coat which is confirmed as fibrinoid necrosis on biopsy. Kawai[13a] divides these complete erosions into two categories (Plate 71):

(a) Mature Type

Mature type, in which the surrounding mucosal elevation is irreversible due to fibrosis. Thus the erosion may persist for years. We could never con-

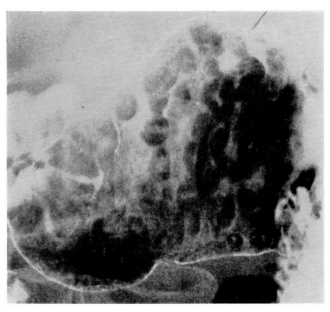

Figure 22-1. Radiological demonstration of multiple antral erosions.

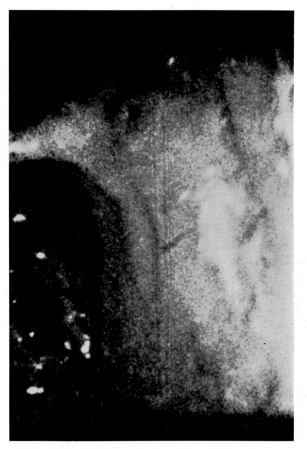

Figure 22-2. Complete erosion with hematin-covered floor near the angle.

firm the existence of intra- or submucosal fibrosis of the lamina propria in chronic complete erosions as suggested by Kawai.[13a] So, we think, the persistence of the bulging border is mainly due to a continuous proliferative stimulus.

(b) Immature Type

Immature type, where the bulging border is due to edema. On histologic examination one may find "foveolar pseudo-hyperplasia" which means elongation of the cristae. These lesions seem to disappear within a few days when re-epithelization takes place. Occasionally, large areas of denuded surface epithelium are covered by a whitish slough. Here, too, re-epithelization takes place within a few days. We never saw and we do not know of any well documented evidence that gastric erosions penetrated the muscularis mucosa and became a true gastric ulcer, substantiated by follow-up examination.

Frequency rate varies from 2 to 80 per cent depending on the different approaches to the problem of gastric erosions. The highest incidence is reported in resected stomachs by Puhl.[14] The pathologist Eder[15] found erosions to be the most common cause (28%) of bleeding in his autopsy material; Waldman[16] found erosions in 2.1 per cent of all autopsy cases, Frik[17] in 2 per cent of routine gastrointestinal series.

For clinical purposes the differentiation between acute erosions, synonymous for bleeding erosions, and chronic (persistent) erosions seems sufficient. Long-term follow-up studies may decide whether there is a direct development toward true polyps or early gastric cancer as suggested by Kawai.[13] We have three patients with multiple chronic erosions in fundic mucosa under observation for up to three years without any change in number and size of the lesions. These patients, by the way, are all asymptomatic and show histamine-refractory achlorhydria.

It was not always possible to classify or group incomplete and complete erosions because both types were sometimes present. Every mucosal protrusion with central depression was qualified as complete erosion. Occasionally, the lesion did not show central necrosis perhaps due to re-epithelialization so that differential diagnosis of a broad based polyp could be raised.

Routine inspection of the duodenal bulb confirmed data from pathologist[18] that duodenal erosions are less common than gastric erosions, the relationship to the latter being 1 to 4. The same types may be found: bleeding, flat and elevated.

GASTROBIOPSY AND HISTOPATHOLOGY

In 60 patients with gastric erosions (no bleeders), a directed biopsy was performed via forceps. In about one-third the erosive defect could be demonstrated directly. Surprisingly inflammatory reaction with cellular infiltration seems not to be the rule, superficial gastritis—a common finding —could also be a pre-existing disease. Whether "Leistenspitzenerosion" (denudation of the superficial epithelium at the neck region) represents the beginning or the healing of the erosive defect has to remain unsettled, the necrotic floor usually reaches down to the chief cell area. Foveolar pseudohyperplasia corresponds to the bulging border of the complete erosions and is characterized by an elongation of the neck area probably due to an intracellular edema[19] (Table 22-I).

TABLE 22-I

RESULTS OF DIRECTED BIOPSY IN GASTRIC EROSIONS

Leistenspitzenerosion or necrotic floor	11
Foveolar pseudohyperplasia	9
Superficial gastritis	23
Chronic atrophic gastritis	5
with acute leucocyte infiltration	1
Normal mucosa	11

TABLE 22-II

AGE AND INCIDENCE OF GASTRIC EROSIONS

Age	11-20	21-30	31-40	41-50	51-60	61-70	71-80	81-90
	2	6	15	19	19	10	4	—

Gastric erosions are most frequently seen between the age of 30 to 60, in our study we had a relative male preponderance (58 males, 21 females) (Table 22-II).

Follow-up examinations in several patients revealed that incomplete and complete erosions heal rapidly within 2 to 8 days but there was one patient in whom multiple complete erosions could be documented endoscopically and histologically at eight examinations within two years. There was no fibrosis or granulation tissue in the elevated border.

Only in a few patients radiological demonstration of erosions was possible prior to gastroscopy. This was possible in the complete type showing a central depot surrounded by halo (Fig. 22-1). Therefore, endoscopy seems to be the diagnostic method of choice in detecting superficial mucosal defects.

ENDOSCOPY AND EXPERIMENTAL EROSIONS

Experimentally one may observe the development of gastric erosions endoscopically after intravenous injection of 2mg per kg body weight Betazoldihydrochloride. Within ten minutes multiple circumscribed hemorrhages in the mucosa arise, predominately in the fundic region, which may change from incomplete type to complete type erosions and may even become demonstrable on x-ray examination (Fig. 22-2). The appearance of these histamine-induced lesions seems to be typical, their demonstration first shown by Katz and Siegel[20a] explains the well known fact of bloody discoloration of the aspirate in gastric analysis (Plate 72).

There is experimental evidence that a prolonged and increased vagal phase of acid production together with enhanced capillary permeability and anoxia of the surface epithelium contribute to the formation of gastric erosions. It seems not to be histamine-specific; we also saw these lesions after pentagastrin-stimulated gastric secretion studies and even lost a patient due to massive upper gastrointestinal hemorrhage from fundic erosions in a case of extreme hyperchlorhydria (PAO 168 mvalHCL/h).

ENDOSCOPIC DATA ANALYSIS

In a total of 1,859 gastroscopies during 1968 and 1969 on patients with upper gastrointestinal tract symptoms, we found 79 cases of gastric ero-

TABLE 22-III

ENDOSCOPY IN ACUTE UPPER G.I. BLEEDING (65 CASES)

Bleeding source
Gastric erosions 14
Gastric ulcer 11
Esophageal varices 8
Stomach ulcer 4
Gastric carcinoma 2
Erosive esophagitis 2
Mallory-Weiss syndrome 2
Fiberoleiomyoma 1
Blood dyscrasia 1
Cause undetermined by endoscopy (including 8 duodenal ulcers) 18
Bleeding from the retronasal space 2

TABLE 22-IV

PEAK ACID OUTPUT IN GASTRIC EROSIONS

10mEq	*10mEq*	*25mEq*	*25mEq*
8	12	27	

sions (4.2%). This figure includes 14 acute bleeding lesions; therefore the incidence was higher than that of Kawai[13] with 3.2 per cent.

Complete erosions	51	(64.6%)
Incomplete erosions	24	(30.4%)
Hemorrhagic gastritis	4	(5%)

In 14 patients diagnosis of erosions was established at an emergency procedure (Table 22-III).

In 47 patients with gastric erosions an augmented histamine test was performed. Most of them showed hyperchlorhydria. This correlates well with the bioptical findings when atrophic gastritis was uncommon (Table 22-IV).

SYMPTOMS AND ASSOCIATED PATHOLOGY

Most patients with gastric erosions except the bleeders with hemorrhage related symptoms complain of vague upper abdominal discomfort, fullness, epigastric pain and heartburn. In our series, 21 patients (27.8%) had a history of gastric or duodenal ulcer, six patients were chronic alcoholics and six had known portal hypertension due to liver cirrhosis. Complete erosions in a stomach bearing an ulcer or a carcinoma were seen eight times. In one patient *Crohn's* disease of the stomach was most probably the underlying cause with granuloma demonstrated in a biopsy specimen from the elevated border[21] (Plate 73).

In another case amyloidosis of mucosal blood vessels seemed to be the primary lesion of multiple bleeding antral erosions (Plate 74). In a case of a young girl, gastroscopy was performed three weeks after a Billroth II operation because of severe hemorrhage from multiple erosions. Endoscopically multiple polypoid lesions could be seen in the stump whereas at operation only erosive defects scattered within the stomach could be demonstrated.

SUMMARY AND DISCUSSION

During 1,859 gastroscopies in patients with upper gastrointestinal tract symptoms, 79 patients with gastric erosions were found. These erosions were classified as hemorrhagic-erosive gastritis, incomplete and complete erosions. In 60 patients a directed forceps biopsy was performed, and in one-third the floor of the erosions showed fibrinoid necrosis or the elevated border with foveolar pseudo-hyperplasia could be demonstrated. Most patients with erosions showed hyperchlorhydria, the middle-age group seemed more often affected. Repeated examinations in several patients revealed a great healing tendency of erosions, usually within two to eight days, but in some patients the lesions persisted for up to two years.

The subject of gastric erosions and petechiae, the pathogenesis of which is still unsettled, is gaining increasing interest. There is some evidence that increased capillary permeability at the neck of the gastric glands may lead to hemorrhage and subsequently to anoxia of the surface epithelium. The desquamation of the superficial layers is followed by peptic necrosis.[20] There are some reports which call for allergic reactions as pathogenetic mechanism,[10] there are also some cases where antigastric antibodies could be demonstrated by indirect immunofluoroscopy.[13] Most incriminated factors involved in the production of acute gastric lesions like drugs, stress, hypovolemia, head injury and burns may act by vagal stimulation or histamine release. The model of histamine or aspirin-induced erosions observed by gastroscopy and documented by biopsy at different intervals may bring some new ideas about the development of petechiae and erosions.

Our figures of the frequency rate of gastric erosions are in agreement with the literature. During the vigorous diagnostic approach in acute upper gastrointestinal hemorrhage, erosions have been found to be one of the most common causes of bleeding (Table 22-V). This corresponds well with the autopsy findings of Eder[15] (28% of all gastrointestinal bleeding in 4,117 autopsies were due to erosions) and Martinoli[18] (6.1% hemorrhagic erosions in a total of 11,353 autopsies). There are several reports showing a male preponderance;[13, 20] the middle age group is the most affected. According to Martinoli,[18] ulcer patients show twice the incidence of erosions as non-ulcer patients.

Further studies may reveal whether chronic erosions exist in reality and

TABLE 22-V

ETIOLOGY OF UPPER GASTROINTESTINAL BLEEDING IN
REPRESENTATIVE SERIES

Author	Endoscopy	Year	No. of Cases	Percentage of Erosive Gastritis
Brown et al.	No	1950	324	—
Marthin et al.	No	1953	246	5
Atik and Simeone	No	1954	293	2
Berkowitz et al.	No	1956	500	1
Zimmermann et al.	No	1956	200	—
Palmer	Yes	1952	121	22
Jones	Yes	1956	1,910	30
Palmer	Yes	1962	650	15
Katz et al.	Yes	1963	150	26
Hirschowitz et al.	Yes	1963	216	22

Table from Katz, D. P. Douvers, H. Weisberg, R. Charm, W. McKinnon: Sources of bleeding in upper gastrointestinal hemorrhage: A re-evaluation *(Amer J Dig Dis 9:447, 1964)*.

if there is connective tissue proliferation in the lamina propria as Kalima and Tomoda[19, 22] suggested based on examination of surgical specimens. We were not able to show fibrosis in our guided biopsies.

Biopsy may prove helpful in defining an underlying cause which may lead to the erosive defect like granulomatous disease, vascular involvement by a systemic disorder or submucous spreading carcinoma.

Routine gastroscopy in every bleeding patient should be performed as soon as possible since in every patient with known varices, ulcer or malignant growth, there is a probability that erosions and not the primary, known lesions are bleeding.

Furthermore gastroscopy should be emphasized in all patients with bizarre upper abdominal complaints and negative x-ray findings.

Gastric erosions are far more common than generally accepted; whether the patient's complaints have to be related with circumscribed, rapidly disappearing lesions like erosions or whether they are due to more diffuse processes like (antral) gastritis has to be investigated.

REFERENCES

1. Morgagni: *De causis et sedibus morborum*, 1761.
2. Beaumont, W.: *Experiments and Observations on the Gastric Juice and the Physiology of Digestion*. Plattsburg, J. P. Allen, 1833.
3. Wolf, S.: *The Stomach*. New York, Oxford University Press, 1965.
4. Nauwerck, G.: Gastritis ulcerosa chronica. Beitrag zur Kenntnis des Magengeschwuers. *Muench Med Wochenschr*, 44:955, 1897.
5. Konjetzny, G. E.: Die Entzuendungen des Magens. In: Henke, F., O. Lubarsch, *Handbuch der speziellen pathologischen Anatomie und Histologie*, Bd. 4, II. Berlin, Springer, 1928.

6. Hauser, G.: Die Haemorrhagische Erosion. In: Henke, F., O. Lubarsch, *Handbuch der speziellen pathologischen Anatomie*, Bd. 1. Berlin, Springer, 1926.

7. Virchow, R.: Historisches, Kritisches und Positives zur Lehre der Unterleibsaffektionen. *Virchows Arch,* 5:5281, 1856.

8. Buchner, F.: *Die Pathogenese der peptischen Veraenderungen.* Jeng, Fischer, 1931.

9. Henning, N., and Schatzki, R.: Gastrophotographisches und roentgenologisches Bild der Gastritis erosiva. *Fortsch Roentgenstr,* 48:177, 1933.

10. Schindler, R.: *Gastroscopy.* New York, Hafner, 1966.

11. Berry, Leonidas H.: Personal communication to the authors.

12. Palmer, E. D.: *Diagnosis of Upper Gastrointestinal Hemorrhage.* Thomas, Springfield, 1961.

13. Kawai, K., Wakabayasci, T., Ida, K., Chikamatsu, S., Kadotani, H., Murakami, K., and Misaki, F.: The process of erosion—so called erosive gastritis. *Stomach and Intestine,* 2:30, 1967.

13a. Kawai, K., Shimamoto, K., Misaki, F., Murakami, K., and Masuda, M.: Erosion of gastric mucosa-pathogenesis, incidence and classification of the erosive gastritis. *Endoscopy,* 3 (in press).

14. Puhl, H.: Ueber die Entstehung and Entwicklung des Magen-Duodenalgeschwuers. *Arch klin Chir,* 158:1, 1930.

15. Eder, M., and Castrup, H. J.: Die gastrointestinale Blutung aus der Sicht des Pathologen. *Chirurg,* 40:97, 1969.

16. Woldman, E. E.: zit. in W. Frik. *JAMA, 149*:984, 1952.

17. Frik, W., and Hesse, R.: Die roentgenologische Darstellung von Magenerosionen. *Dtsch Med Wochenschr, 81*:1119, 1956.

18. Martinoli, E., and Gantner, J.: Die Haemorrhagischen Erosionen von Magen und Duodenum im Vergleich mit den akuten und chronischen Ulcera in einem Sektionsgut von 11 352 Erwachsenen. *Schweiz Med Wochenschr, 100*:37, 1970.

19. Tomoda, M.: Beitrag zur Kenntnis der Geschwuersbildung in Magen und Duodenum. *Arch klin Chir, 190*:254, 1937.

20. Katz, D., and Siegel, I.: Erosive gastritis and acute gastrointestinal mucosal lesions. In: *Progress in Gastroenterology,* Vol. 1. Grune and Stratton, New York, 1968.

20a. Katz, D., Siegel, I., Glass, and G. B. Jerzy: Acute gastric mucosal lesions produced by augmented histamine test. *Am J Dig Dis, 14*:447, 1969.

21. Rosch, W., Elster, K., and Ottenjann, R.: Morbus Crohn des Magens unter dem Bild der kompletten Erosionen. *Endoscopy, 1*:178, 1969.

22. Kalima, T.: Pathologisch anatomische Studien ueber die Gastritis des Ulcusmagens. *Arch klin Chir, 128*:20, 1924.

SECTION IV

ENDOSCOPY OF THE DUODENUM

CHAPTER 23

BULBAR DUODENOSCOPY, TECHNICS AND PATHOLOGY

JOSEPH P. BELBER

INTRODUCTION

THE DUODENAL BULB IS of prime interest to the endoscopist because it commonly is the site of peptic disease, a disease which is responsible for an untold amount of minor human suffering, and may be associated with serious and potentially fatal complications, including massive hemorrhage, perforation and obstruction. Objective diagnosis in the past has depended upon radiology, which is helpful when an ulcer crater can be demonstrated, but is not a reliable indicator of the presence of active disease if a crater cannot be identified. The recent development of suitable instruments and techniques for endoscopic examination of the duodenal bulb now permits an accurate diagnosis of duodenal ulcers, including many not demonstrable by x-ray and provides a reliable diagnosis of duodenitis, both in association with ulcers and as an isolated finding as well. A comparison of x-ray and duodenoscopy gives a clear advantage of endoscopy in the accurate identification of morphologic abnormalities. As an example, in a recent series[1] 70 duodenal ulcers were positively identified.

Endoscopy visualized 66, or 94 per cent using instruments since superceded by improved models, compared to 45 or 65 per cent discovered by x-ray. In addition, radiology diagnosed 10 additional ulcers subsequently found not to exist, compared to zero false positives for endoscopy. The significant advantage of endoscopy is predictable, since the endoscopist can inspect the area thoroughly and obtain biopsies if any doubt remains. Furthermore, his ability to determine the extent and degree of duodenitis adds a dimension to the evaluation of the patient's disease state not obtainable by other means.

HISTORICAL STATEMENT

Duodenoscopy became feasible with the development of the first fiberoptic gastroscope by Hirschowitz[2] in collaboration with the American Cystoscope Makers Inc. (ACMI) in 1958. It met with only limited success. In 1963 the instrument was modified by substituting a fiberoptic light guide system for the incandescent bulb, and placement of the objective lens close to the tip of the instrument, a necessary requirement for better visualization within the duodenum. With this instrument, the author was eventually able to enter the duodenum in approximately 35 per cent of attempts without resorting to complicating auxiliaries such as a previously swallowed guide string, fluoroscopic control, or general anesthesia. In the absence of a guidance system it was frequently necessary to manipulate the instrument through the pylorus by using a hand on the abdominal wall, or by altering the patient's attitude on the table. These basic techniques are still occasionally useful even with more sophisticated instruments. Once in the duodenum the view was often adequate and duodenal ulcer, duodenitis, and deformity were all visualized, photographed, and clearly comprehended. The descending duodenum was occasionally entered and the papilla of Vater seen often enough to appreciate its endoscopic characteristics. In 1969 the author used this basic instrument with a distal deflecting tip to enter the duodenum in 76 of the first 100 attempts,[3] ultimately reaching a rate of 85 per cent. However, by 1969 side-viewing endoscopes specifically designed for duodenal visualization and cannulation of the papilla of Vater had been developed in Japan by the Machida Manufacturing Company and the Olympus Optical Company with the cooperation of a number of endoscopists including Oi, Shindo, Soma, and Niwa. With these instruments, the duodenum could be entered in 95 to 100 per cent of attempts with excellent visualization in the overwhelming majority of cases.[4-7] In the United States, ACMI concentrated its major effort on a forward-viewing all purpose endoscope, which has been found to be effective in the duodenal bulb as well as the esophagus and stomach by the author,[1] and by Cavallaro and McCray[8] in the United States, and Classen and Demling[9] in Germany. Olympus and the Eder Manufacturing Company also produce all purpose endoscopes, Eder combining forward and side viewing in the same instrument.

INDICATIONS AND CONTRAINDICATIONS

The indications for endoscopy of the duodenal bulb include the following:

1. Evaluation of symptoms in patients with a history of peptic disease or alcoholism.
2. Upper gastrointestinal hemorrhage, whether overtly manifested by hematemesis or melena; or merely suggested by occult blood in the stools or unexplained iron deficiency anemia.
3. Equivocal or indeterminate x-ray findings including the radiologically deformed duodenal bulb.
4. Gastric outlet obstruction.
5. Unexplained abdominal distress.
6. Any suggestion of neoplasm.

Contraindications are few. We include the following:

1. The uncooperative or unwilling patient.
2. Probability of perforated viscus.
3. Shock.
4. Serious associated illness such as myocardial infarction or pneumonia unless immediate endoscopic diagnosis is absolutely necessary for the performance of life saving therapy.

CHOICE OF INSTRUMENTS

The choice between a side-viewing or a forward-viewing lens system for examination of the duodenal bulb is influenced primarily by the indication for a given endoscopy. Either system, when provided with a wide angle lens and versatile deflection controls will furnish an excellent view throughout the average duodenal bulb. Both systems may require supplementation by the other system to visualize the occasional blind spot, which is most likely to be directly behind the pylorus, inferiorly for the side-viewer and posteriorly for the forward-viewer. Since peptic disease and alcoholism are responsible for most of the pathology seen in the upper gastrointestinal tract and may involve esophagus, stomach, and duodenum we normally use an all purpose forward-viewer to visualize all three areas in order to fully evaluate the patient's symptoms. We do not hesitate to use a side-viewer for supplementation and find that it improves diagnosis in about 10 per cent of cases. One definite advantage of the forward-viewer is that orientation is simpler especially for the inexperienced. In the presence of outlet obstruction the instrument with the smallest diameter is preferred.

TECHNICS

Although upper gastrointestinal endoscopy can be performed with little or no premedication, I prefer using it in ample amounts unless it is specifically contraindicated. Sodium pentobarbital 100mg and meperidine 100mg are given intramuscularly one half hour prior to the procedure, to allay the anxiety the patient may suffer while awaiting the examination. Atropine 0.6mg is injected at the same time, primarily to reduce salivation. Just before the procedure liquid simethicone is given to prevent bubble formation and the posterior pharynx is swabbed with 2 per cent pontocain. In twenty-five years we have never seen an unfavorable reaction. Next, an average dose of 10mg of diazepam is given intravenously, more in the young adult and considerably less in the elderly. The stomach is always emptied with a large bore tube and irrigated if blood or retained food is recovered. We prefer using a truncated wedge bite block between the right upper and lower molars rather than the oval ring between the incisors currently in vogue.

The endoscope is passed with the patient in the left lateral decubitus position. If a forward-viewer is used the esophagus is examined thoroughly, but biopsy is deferred until later. The stomach is surveyed rapidly, but a detailed examination including retroversion inspection of the cardia is not accomplished until after the duodenal bulb has been completely visualized. The endoscope is advanced in the sagittal plane of the stomach spiralling it clockwise as it is passed into the antrum, being sure to flex the tip upward enough to keep it from impinging on the greater curvature. The pylorus is usually readily visible with a side-viewer, but frequently more than 90 degrees of upward deflection is required to locate the pylorus with a forward-viewer. Once in the antrum the endoscope is maintained in the sagittal plane and advanced directly to the pylorus, often passing through easily. With a side-viewing instrument the inferior margin of the pylorus must lie under the scope during passage, and if visible the tip of the instrument must be momentarily raised to clear it. If difficulty is encountered either in entering the antrum or approaching the pylorus the patient may be rotated onto his back and the head of the table depressed to help straighten the stomach. If this is not sufficient, the instrument may be moved forward by raising it upward and to the right with a hand placed on the lower abdomen. If there is difficulty in passing the pylorus, moving the tip of the instrument by pressure from a hand in the epigastrium may be helpful. It is easier to enter an open pylorus, but even a closed pylorus will often yield to a well centered tip. If the pylorus remains closed and cannot be passed, or if peristalsis is too active to permit satisfactory visualization, propantheline hydrobromide, 30mg, may be administered intravenously or intramuscularly and is usually beneficial.

Once past the pylorus the instrument often comes to rest against the mucosa at the superior flexure of the duodenum and must be withdrawn slightly to obtain a clear view of the flexure, which then serves as an orientation landmark. The duodenal bulb is inspected by slowly withdrawing and advancing, rotating and deflecting the tip up and down or sideways as required to see all quadrants and to see behind folds. Deflecting the tip sharply and advancing tends to flex the scope upon itself, increasing retrovision; in fact, if the Olympus JFB is faced superiorly, flexed sharply upward and advanced it is possible to obtain a retroversion view of the base of the bulb, provided there is not excessive deformity.[4] However, in the presence of significant deformity there may be a potential risk of impaction. Complete inspection should be accomplished prior to biopsy since even a small amount of bleeding may obscure limited portions of the mucosa.

NORMAL DUODENAL BULB

In this chapter, the terms "duodenal bulb," "first portion," "superior portion," or "proximal duodenum" are used interchangeably. The duodenal bulb, as seen with a forward-viewer is a tubular structure of variable length only slightly larger in diameter, if at all, at its proximal end than at its distal end. Within its extent no angle or bend is regularly present. It terminates at the "superior flexure" or "superior angle" of the duodenum, a structure resembling an inverted angulus. The angle is not fixed and may change depending upon the position of the patient or the pressure applied by the endoscope. It may display considerable anatomic variation from person to person. The apex of the duodenal bulb is considered to be located at the superior flexure and the terms are used synonymously.

The walls of the proximal duodenum are smooth, with an occasional low mammilation and although longitudinal, circular or crosshatched folds occur in some individuals, Kerkrings folds or valvulae conniventes are not usually present proximal to the superior flexure. The duodenal mucosa is paler and more beige in color than the salmon pink gastric mucosa. It has a granular or shaggy texture due to the presence of villi, the tips of which can be readily distinguished with closeup focussing.

Duodenal motility is more rapid than that of the stomach and consists of contractions of either long or short length, partially or completely occluding the lumen and moving rapidly for varying distances in either direction. Rapidly repeated rosetting contractions may occur at any one level and then suddenly subside. This is the endoscopists view of rhythmic segmentation, peristaltic rushes, reverse peristalsis, in fact all the activities employed by small bowel in mixing and then propelling the intestinal content. The typical slow, stripping, gastric Type II wave is not seen in the duodenum and may be considered a hallmark of the stomach.

PATHOLOGY

In the succeeding paragraphs duodenal ulcer, duodenal deformity, and duodenitis are classified separately, but the descriptions of each necessarily include all three of these entities, since they frequently coexist and it is important to describe their interrelationships.

Duodenal Ulcer

Duodenal ulcers are the most important pathologic lesions occurring in the first portion of the duodenum. They are polymorphic and manifest great diversity in size, shape, and surrounding inflammatory reaction. Most ulcerations are situated within three centimeters of the pylorus although a small percentage may occur at the superior flexure or beyond. They are fairly uniformly distributed around the circumference of the lumen, although fewer are seen in the inferior quadrant. In a series[10] of 100 consecutive duodenal ulcers 31 were anterior, 27 superior, 27 posterior, and 15 inferior. Lesions in the inferior quadrant may be somewhat more difficult to see in the presence of gross deformity. Circumferential localization may not coincide precisely with the x-ray impression, but the two modalities are usually within 90 degrees of each other, endoscopy tending to be the more counterclockwise.

The typical duodenal ulcer (Plate 75) is small, the majority being under 1cm in diameter. In a series[10] of 100 ulcers with a size range from 3mm to 6cm, only 12 ulcers were over 1cm, 24 were approximately 1cm, 42 were from 5 to 10mm, and 22 were under 5mm. The larger ulcers tend to be round or oval and of considerable depth, and therefore easily identifiable radiologically. The smaller ulcers usually are superficial and frequently are triangular, stellate, or spindle shaped. This is not to imply that the ulcerations necessarily originated in the form first seen by the endoscopist, since they may undergo change in shape as they heal. The oval or round ulcer tends to become stellate or triangular and finally becomes a small white dimple detected primarily by telltale surrounding hyperemia. The elliptic ulcer becomes linear or spindle shaped and resolves as a thin white line surrounding by vascular engorgement and resembles a centipede in configuration. Superficial ulcerations may undergo these metamorphoses within a matter of days and can entirely heal in ten days to two weeks. Even ulcers which have been responsible for gross bleeding may be small and superficial and rapidly disappear.

An interesting characteristic of some duodenal ulcers is their resemblance to ulcerated intramural neoplasms. These ulcers are surrounded by a broad collar of edema and inflammatory infiltrate, and the entire complex including the ulceration appears to project into the lumen as a tumor mass. When the mass is intensely hyperemic and the site of superficial erosions, especially if the ulceration is irregular in shape, the appearance strongly suggests carcinoma. A large inflammatory mass may also complete-ly occlude the lumen particularly if it is in the base of the duodenal bulb or near the superior flexure.

Duodenal Deformity

If distortion of the duodenal bulb is produced largely by edema and in-flammatory infiltrate it may resolve with surprisingly little residue. Many duodenal bulbs, however, are permanently deformed as a result of scar-ring and contracture and the deformity may remain unchanged as ulcers come and go. The deformity itself may conceal an ulcer crater from the radiologist, particularly if the ulcer is small and superficial; but it does not prevent the endoscopist from obtaining a satisfactory view and accurate-ly determining whether ulceration or duodenitis is present or not. Three

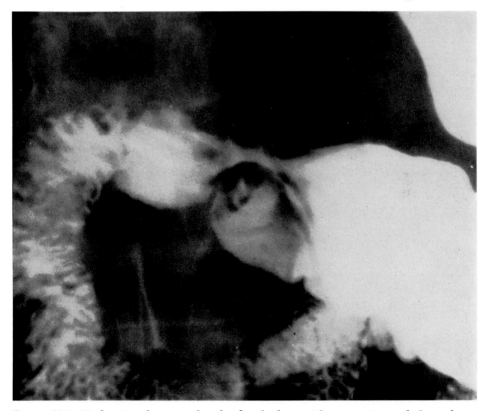

Figure 23-1. Deformity due to pyloroduodenal ulcer with eccentricity of the pylorus, loss of the superior recess of the duodenal bulb and greater curvature filling defect due to large folds. Endoscopically the pylorus was patulous and a small active ulcer was present.

significant persistent deformities are of special interest to the endoscopist. The first is the deformity associated with pyloroduodenal ulcers[11] (Fig. 23-1) most of which lie wholly or in part within the duodenum. These ulcerations (Plate 76), situated superiorly, lead to longitudinal contraction of the distal antrum and the superior recess of the duodenum. The resultant foreshortening tends to flatten the superior recess and cause the pylorus to appear eccentric, and pulls the superior recess proximally so that a duodenal ulcer may radiologically appear to be in the stomach. The lower quadrants of the pyloric area, being unaffected, become redundant and project into the lumen as pseudopolypoid folds. Although pyloric stenosis may occur, in many instances the pylorus is not significantly constricted and may even be patulous once the redundant tissue is pushed out of the way with air inflation. Pyloroduodenal ulcerations may not heal completely, or having healed show a strong tendency to recurrence. It is not unusual for erosions to form in the scar of an old ulceration even in the absence of frank recurrence. Endoscopy is generally more reliable than radiology in differentiating small persistent lesions from retracted scars or in determining the presence of erosions in the bed of the scar.

The second deformity is the contraction ring or incisura which most

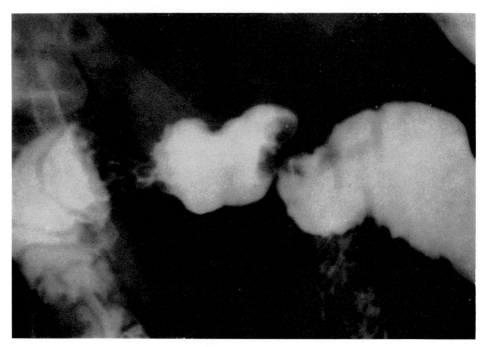

Figure 23-2. Mid bulb contraction ring, unchanging over a 10-year period despite three episodes of gross bleeding. Endoscopy in 1969 visualized two circumferentially oriented superficial ulcers on the proximal face of the ring. Arrows point to ring.

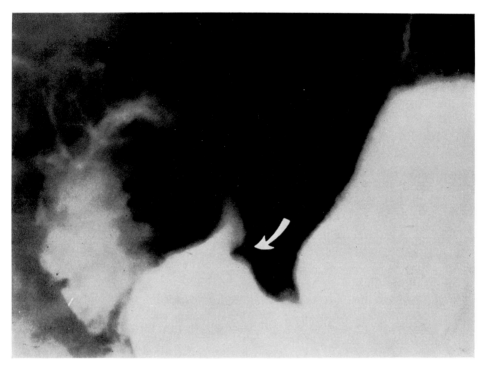

Figure 23-3. Longstanding pseudopolypoid mass almost completely filling the bulb, due to scarring from duodenal ulcer and eventually requiring surgery for post-pyloric obstruction. Endoscopy revealed a widely patulous pylorus and a large pseudopolypoid mass projecting from the inferior aspect of the bulb with erosive duodenitis on its presenting surfaces. The arrow points to the pylorus.

commonly occurs 2 to 3cm distal to the pylorus (Fig. 23-2). Endoscopically a circumferential fold is seen which may partially or completely encircle the lumen. One segment of it may be flattened and secondary folds may occasionally radiate obliquely into that area (Plate 77). It presumably represents the scar of previous ulceration. Large pseudodiverticula may be formed between the ringlike fold and the pylorus usually superiorly or inferiorly. When both diverticula are present the cloverleaf bulb results. Recurrent ulcers tend to occur on the crest or proximal face of the encircling fold rather than in the pseudodiverticula. Occasionally they occur at the intersection of the radiating folds, but frequently they are found elsewhere on the circumference. Although large ulcers may occur, ulcerations in this setting tend to be small, superficial, and may be multiple. Regardless of size they may be responsible for gross hemorrhage. They furnish the bulk of the ulcers detected endoscopically and overlooked radiologically. Elliptic or spindle shaped superficial ulcers oriented circumferentially may be particularly difficult to detect by x-ray. Commonly, in addition to ulceration there is diffuse duodenitis proximal to the contraction ring; but much less commonly is there either ulceration or duodenitis distally, suggesting that the formation of a contraction ring has influenced the subsequent course of the disease, protecting the area beyond the ring from peptic activity. As a rule there is no difficulty in passing the endoscope through the contracted zone, but obstructing stenosis may occur in some cases.

The third deformity presents as a large pseudopolypoid fold usually arising from the inferior aspect of the bulb and often occupying a considerable portion of the lumen (Fig. 23-3). The pseudopolypoid fold may be eroded, but the actual ulceration, frequently sizeable, is adjacent to, but not on the pseudopolyp; distinguishing it from the tumorlike ulcer previously described. Some degree of obstruction may occur with this type of deformity particularly when there is an acute exacerbation of inflammatory disease.

Diverticula

True diverticula of the superior duodenum may occur rarely, and when they are located in the immediate post-pyloric area the appearance may suggest deformity secondary to ulcer disease. The complete absence of any inflammation, the oval orifice similar to those located elsewhere in the gastrointestinal tract suggest their true identity to the endoscopist.

Duodenitis

Duodenitis is diagnosed endoscopically if there is obvious inflammation manifested by hyperemia, intramural hemorrhage, or superficial erosion. It may be diffuse, or patchy in distribution, and can be either localized or generalized. There may be little swelling so that the mucosal contour is not significantly distorted. In other cases folds are enlarged and hyperemic and contain localized beads or nodes. Between folds the node appears as a mammillation 5 to 10mm in diameter showing vascular engorgement and petechia on its surface. Visually it is appropriate to divide duodenitis into two groups: superficial, showing little distortion of the mucosa; and hyperplastic, in which thickened folds, nodes, or prominent mammillations are present (Plate 78). The superficial variety does not significantly distort the x-ray contour, the hyperplastic variety does. Microscopically, duodenitis is characterized by vascular engorgement, intramural hemorrhage, edema, and varying numbers of round cells and eosinophils. If the lesion is particularly acute, polymorphonuclear leukocytes may be present as well. Mucosal erosion may or may not be present. Unfortunately even normal mucosa contains eosinophils and round cells, so that the histologic distinction between mild duodenitis and normal mucosa is blurred and the endoscopic impression must be relied upon. In such circumstance the endoscopist should be circumspect and not make a positive diagnosis on endoscopic findings which are equivocal.

One interesting and uncommon form of duodenitis is manifested by placques of hyperemic mucosa in which there is an intermixture of small petechiae and tiny white erosions (Plate 79). It may be similar to the lesion described by Oi[12] as pepper and salt. However, he refers to ulceration and the lesions depicted herein are not, although ulcerations may be present elsewhere in the same duodenum. Biopsies have revealed an intense, nonspecific acute duodenitis with erosions.

In the presence of acute ulcer (Plate 80) some degree of duodenitis is invariably present, at times confined to the immediate area of the ulcer, but in other cases it may be widespread and intense, giving the impression that the ulceration is only a small part of the whole inflammatory process. Duodenitis, in any form may be encountered in the complete absence of ulceration and can be responsible for peptic symptoms. It may also persist for months after a companion ulcer has healed, indicating that the pathologic process is continuing and may be expected to flare again.

Neoplasms

The superior duodenum may occasionally be the site of neoplasms, both benign and malignant, including most of the varieties found elsewhere in the gastrointestinal tract. Space does not permit a full discussion in this chapter. Those lesions which involve the mucosa may be diagnosed by biopsy, but submucosal tumors may escape histologic diagnosis since the biopsy forceps often avulses normal mucosa from the surface of the tumor.

Primary malignancies include adenocarcinoma, the lymphoblastomas and sarcomas, and carcinoid. Metastatic malignancy usually involves the submucosa but may undergo central ulceration forming the *bullshot* lesion. This is particularly characteristic of melanoma. Malignant invasion from adjacent structures, particularly the pancreas may form ulcerating lesions in the duodenal bulb.

Of the benign tumors adenomas are the most frequently encountered and may be composed of mucosal cells or the cells of Brunner's glands. Lipomas and leiomyomas are the commonest of the wide variety of submucus tumors which may occur.[13] Pancreatic cell rests and gastric mucosal cell rests[14, 15] may also be encountered in the duodenal bulb.

Miscellaneous Disorders

Granulomatous lesions, both specific and nonspecific, including Crohn's disease, may occur in the duodenum and may require biopsy for identification. Unfortunately, the small size and superficial nature of the specimens obtainable may not always yield specific enough information.

Those malabsorptive states with diffuse mucosal involvement such as Whipple's disease, may be diagnosed, but the superior quality of suction biopsy specimens makes them more suitable for diagnosis than the specimens secured transendoscopically.

ALCOHOLIC AND THE DUODENUM

The alcoholic is prone to duodenal involvement, but does not seem to display any special pathology not seen in the nonalcoholic. However, there is an increased incidence of duodenitis in the absence of ulcer, and a higher incidence of the hyperplastic form of duodenitis than in the nonalcoholic. Although all pancreatitis is not the result of alcoholism, much of it is and it is worthy of mention that duodenitis due to spread of inflammation from pancreatitis may occur both in the duodenal bulb and in the descending duodenum. The author has encountered such cases. Pancreatic pseudocysts may produce extrinsic pressure on the duodenum with or without associated duodenitis.

REFERENCES

1. Belber, J. P.: Endoscopic examination of the duodenal bulb; a comparison with x-ray. *Gastroenterology, 61*:55, 1971.
2. Hirschowitz, B. I., Curtiss, L. E., and Peters, C. W.: Demonstration of a new gastroscope, the "fiberscope." *Gastroenterology, 35*:50, 1958.
3. Belber, J. P.: Duodenal bulb visualization with the Hirschowitz gastroduodenal fiberscope and the Hirschowitz gastroduodenal fiberscope with deflecting tip: A comparative study. *Gastroent Endosc, 17*:34, 1970.
4. Ogoshi, K., Tobita, Y., and Hara, Y.: Endoscopic observation of the duodenum and pancreatocholedochography using duodenal fiberscope under direct vision. *Gastroent Endosc* (Tokyo), *12*:83, 1970.
5. Oi, I.: Additional report on study of duodenofiberscope. *Endoscopy, 10*:420, 1968.
6. Shindo, S., and Kankie, Yanagisawa, F.: Duodenofiberoscopy. *Gastroent Endosc* (Tokyo), *12*:70, 1970.
7. Soma, S., Fujita, R., and Kidokoro, T.: Clinical application of duodenofiberscope. *Gastrointest Endosc* (Tokyo), *12*:97, 1970.
8. Cavallaro, J. B., and McCray, R. S.: Duodenoscopy: initial experience with 135 examinations. Presented at the Annual Meeting of the American Society for Gastrointestinal Endoscopy, Miami Beach, Florida, May 12, 1971.
9. Classen, M., and Demling, L.: Duodenal Ulcer: Improved diagnosis through endoscopy. Abstracts of Scientific Reports, IInd World Congress of Gastrointestinal Endoscopy, Copenhagen, Denmark, July 9-11, 1970.
10. Belber, J. P.: Unpublished data.
11. Belber, J. P.: Pyloroduodenal ulcer: Endoscopic aspects. *Gastroent Endosc, 12*:34, 1965.
12. Oi, I.: Endoscopic examination of the duodenum. *Clinical All Around, 19*:307, 1970, as quoted in reference 15.

13. River, L., Silverstein, J., and Tope, J. W.: Benign neoplasms of the small intestine; a critical comprehensive review with reports of 20 new cases. *Internat Abstr Surg, 102*:1, 1956.
14. Belber, J. P., and Musick, R.: Ectopic gastric mucosa in the duodenum. Abstract, annual meeting of the American Society for Gastrointestinal Endoscopy, Boston, Mass., May 20, 1971.
15. James, A. H.: Gastric epithelium in the duodenum. *Gut, 5*:285, 1964.

CHAPTER 24

POSTBULBAR DUODENOSCOPY; TECHNICS AND PATHOLOGY PAPILLA CANNULATION

ITARU OI

INTRODUCTION

IN 1958, A FLEXIBLE FIBEROPTIC INSTRUMENT was successfully introduced in gastrointestinal endoscopy by Hirschowitz[1] and named the "gastro-duodenal fiberscope." Hirschowitz reported that the duodenal bulb was frequently seen with this instrument and that the duodenal papilla was also observed in some cases. Most subsequent papers,[2-4] however, showed this fiberscope to be valuable in gastroscopy but not in duodenoscopy.

Using the Hirschowitz fiberscope, the duodenal papilla was clearly visualized by Watson[5] in five cases in 1966. According to his article, pancreatic juice was demonstrated to pour out from the duodenal papilla.

In 1968 McCune and associates[6] reported cannulation and opacification of the pancreatic duct, using the modified Eder fiberscope, to be successful in 25 per cent of patients. On the other hand, Rider,[7] Oshiba,[8] and others tried to make duodenal fiberscopes but failed.

On the basis of our experiences[9] with the Machida Fiber-Gastroscope, type FGS-CL—which we were able to insert into the duodenal bulb in 75 per cent of cases, with occasional successful visualization of the duodenal papilla—a new duodenal fiberscope, the Machida Fiber-Duodenoscope, type FDS-Lb,[10] was made in February 1969. Successful results with this instrument were reported at the annual meetings of the Japanese Endoscopic Society and the American Society of Gastrointestinal Endoscopy in the same year. This Machida FDS-Lb satisfied the fundamental qualities of a duodenal fiberscope. It made possible visualization of the duodenal papilla in 47 per cent of cases,[11] biopsy from many duodenal lesions, and cannulation and opacification of the pancreatic duct.[11, 12]

The Machida Fiber-Duodenoscope, type FDS-Lb, was the original model of the now improved fiber duodenoscopes, which were mainly intended to see and cannulate the duodenal papilla and to take biopsy specimens from duodenal lesions. The FDS-Lb was 150cm long and was supplied with an external light source. The tip of this lateral-viewing instrument was very short (28mm) and contained the lens and the air and biopsy channels. The biopsy channel was set parallel to the lens in order to shorten the instrument tip. The tip could be flexed, extended, and rotated through a wide range.

Our reports have been verified and extended by Kobayashi, Takagi, Ogoshi, Shindo, Kasugai in Japan, McCray in the United States, Classen in West Germany, Laurent in France, and others using the recently improved instruments.

INSTRUMENTS

The present fiber duodenoscopes used for postbulbar duodenoscopy are made by the Machida and the Olympus companies in Japan[10, 11, 13–15] and by the American Cystoscope Makers, Inc., New York (see also Chapter 5). The qualities of these instruments are almost the same and the fundamental structures are similar to that of the Machida FDS-Lb. These fiberoptic instruments are about 150cm long and about 10mm in diameter, with an external light source. The tip is very short, 20 to 28mm in length, and contains a lateral-viewing lens, light-guide fiber bundle, and air and biopsy channels. The biopsy channel is set parallel to the lens system in order to make the tip short. The tip is flexed and extended through more than 90 degrees by operating the angle knobs. The tip of the Machida FDS is rotated about 60 degrees to the right and left. The Olympus JF has the side-flexion angle instead of the tip rotation mechanism. The A.C.M.I. duodenoscopes are entirely similar, with certain technical differences.

PREMEDICATION

Postbulbar duodenoscopy including cannulation of the duodenal papilla is performed under intramuscular injection of 0.5mg atropine sulfate and 20mg Buscopan, plus local pharyngeal anesthesia with 4 per cent xylocain solution.[10, 12] Tranquilizers are useful in nervous patients. Fluoroscopy is not necessary in duodenoscopy except for opacification of the pancreatic duct. The fiberscopes are carefully kept away from x-ray exposure because radiation damages the fiberoptics, resulting in a gradual decrease in image resolution.

TECHNIC

With the patient lying in the left lateral position, the duodenoscope is inserted into the deep antrum as in gastroscopy. When the pyloric ring is seen in the center of the visual field, the tip of the scope is flexed toward the pyloric ring. The scope is gently advanced along the greater curvature of the antrum, while observing the midline of the lesser curvature, until the elastic resistance of the pyloric ring is felt.[10, 12] The tip then passes readily into the duodenal bulb.

Once within the duodenal bulb, air is insufflated and the tip of the scope is extended and turned to the right. This is done both by twisting the entire instrument and by rotating the tip of the instrument so as to see the superior duodenal angle which is a landmark between the bulb and the superior flexure of the duodenum (Fig. 24-1). The circular folds, which are never flattened by air insufflation, appear on the superior flexure of the duodenum. Then the tip is flexed and gently inserted into the superior flexure, turning the scope about 90 degrees farther to the right. When the

Endoscopic Landmark of the Duodenum

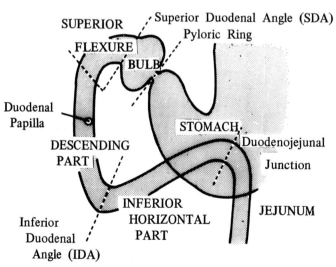

Figure 24-1. Topographic anatomy for duodenoscopy (From Oi, I., et al.[17]).

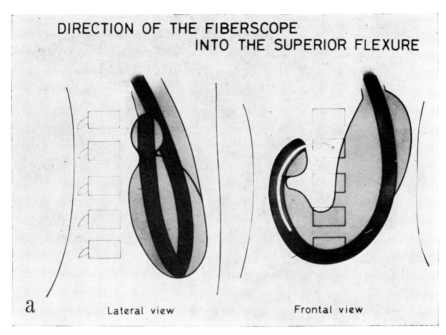

Figure 24-2a. Direction of duodenoscope when passed into superior flexure. Lateral view is 90° to the right (From Oi, I., et al.[10]).

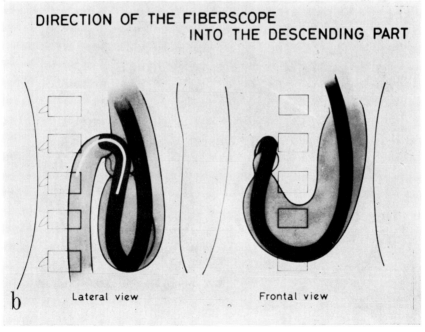

Figure 24-2b. Direction of duodenoscope when passed into descending part of duodenum. Lateral view is 90° to the right (From Oi, I., et al.[10]).

descending part of the duodenum is seen, the scope is turned about 90 degrees to the left and gently advanced through the superior flexure.

This technic of passing the scope through the superior flexure is one of the most difficult procedures in duodenoscopy, because during this procedure the scope should be strongly turned posteriorly (Figs. 24-2a and b), which is also required in order to see the duodenal papilla in the frontal view.

In the descending part of the duodenum, the duodenal papilla is usually observed from the center to the left side of the visual field. The duodenal papilla usually appears as a whitish hemispheric protrusion at the lower end of the longitudinal fold of the duodenum (Pl., Fig. 1). Occasionally, the accessory duodenal papilla is also observed above and to the right of the duodenal papilla.

At the lower end of the descending part is the inferior duodenal angle, a landmark between the second and third portions of the duodenum. Passing through the inferior duodenal angle, the scope is inserted into the

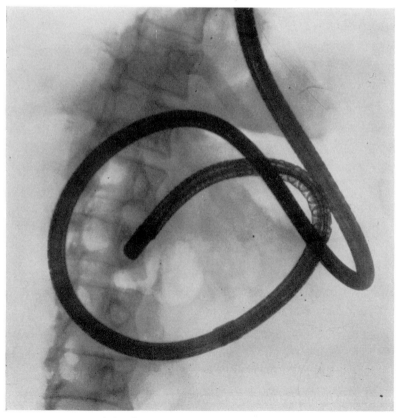

Figure 24-3. X-ray view of duodenoscope with tip in superior portion of jejunum (From Oi, I.).

third portion of the duodenum, if necessary. In some cases, the duodeno-scope may pass the duodenojejunal junction into the upper jejunum, as shown in Figure 24-3. However, the duodenoscope is not long enough to pass this junction commonly, as the intestine is strongly flexed anteriorly similar to the strong posterior flexion of the duodenum from the bulb to the descending part.

Duodenoscopy should be performed gently but as rapidly as possible. If the examination is too prolonged or if gastric stimulation by the scope is excessive, increased duodenal peristalsis and secretion may prevent further effective visualization and interfere with good control of the instrument. In some cases, the injection of additional Buscopan suppresses the strong peristalsis. The duodenal fluid may be aspirated through the cannula or with the suction mechanism of the scope.

Biopsy may be safely taken from any point of the duodenum except the orifice of the duodenal papilla. The duodenal papilla should be biopsied with great care because of its rich blood supply and because of possible in-terference of function secondary to postbiopsy scar formation.

ENDOSCOPIC ANATOMY OF DUODENAL PAPILLA

The main duodenal papilla (papilla Vater), simply called the "duo-denal papilla," and the accessory duodenal papilla (papilla Santorini) are both visualized in most instances. The duodenal papilla is located at the distal end of the longitudinal fold of the descending part of the duode-num. This longitudinal fold is considered to be formed by the intramural common bile duct. The accessory duodenal papilla is seen above and to the right of the duodenal papilla, approximately the border between the su-perior flexure and the descending part of the duodenum.

The duodenal papilla is fundamentally constituted from the base and corona and is accompanied by the covering fold and frenula, as shown in Figure 24-4 (see also Plate 81). The corona shows characteristic features, with or without the circular grooves, and appears whitish in most cases. In the center of the corona, the single or double orifices which are the open-ings of the pancreatic and/or biliary ducts have the appearance of a sea anemone. A close-up view demonstrates that the orifices and the corona are made up of large, whitish villi. Sometimes the sulcus, which has the same structure as the corona, is seen on one of the frenula.

In our recent series of 200 cases,[16] the covering fold is seen in 91 per cent, the corona in 73 per cent, and frenula in 100 per cent, the sulcus in 18 per cent. The circular groove is observed in 23 per cent of the coronas. There are some instances in which the frenula and the longitudinal fold are not clearly visualized.

Although the shape and color of the duodenal papilla vary among indi-

Diagram showing
Structure of the Duodenal Papilla (after Oi)

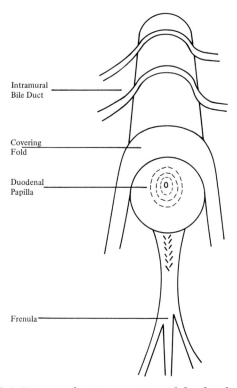

Fig. 24-4. Diagram showing structure of duodenal papilla.

viduals, it may be classified into four types: hemispheric, oval, flat, and special types, including those with double main duodenal papillae (Table 24-I). The features of the orifice of the duodenal papilla are not constant in any individuals, but it is roughly divided into villar type, granular type, lacerated type, slit type, and rigid-hole type.

These numerous features of the duodenal papilla and its orifice will be studied from the clinical and pathologic points of view in the future.

TABLE 24-I

CLASSIFICATION OF DUODENAL PAPILLAE AND ORIFICES

Duodenal Papillae	Incidence (%)	Orifices	Incidence (%)
Hemispheric type	71	Villar type	52
Oval type	19	Granular type	15
Flat type	4	Lacerated type	13
Special types	6	Slit type	11
		Rigid-hole type	3

The accessory duodenal papilla is usually seen as a small mucosal notch. Sometimes it looks like a true duodenal papilla with a hemispheric mucosal protrusion (with or without the corona), but even then it may be distinguished from the main duodenal papilla by its smaller size. The clinical significance of the accessory duodenal papilla is much less than that of the duodenal papilla.

PATHOLOGY OF POSTBULBAR DUODENUM

Ulcer is rare in the postbulbar duodenum[17] and is usually a manifestation of malignant tumor, in our experience.

Duodenitis is occasionally found in the duodenal bulb. Acute duodenitis with mucosal edema and reddening and with scattered mucinous fur involving the entire duodenum is found in some patients with acute gastrointestinal erosions, with or without duodenal ulcer. Localized inflammation of the duodenal mucosa is commonly observed in carcinoma of the pancreatic head and biliary system.

Tumor-like lesions include polyp, submucosal tumor, and polypoid lesion. These are difficult to distinguish even with biopsy, because Brunner's glands are present in the submucosa as well as in the mucosa of the duodenum. Tumor-like lesions in the postbulbar duodenum, however, are mainly polyps and submucosal tumors, in contrast to those found in the bulb, which are mostly polypoid lesions formed by the proliferation of duodenal epithelium. As for diagnosis, these tumor-like lesions are not difficult to find by duodenoscopy, but their nature is revealed only by histologic examination of the operated materials. Plate 82 shows a large submucosal tumor after biopsy at the superior flexure of the duodenum.

Diverticulum is frequently found in the descending part of the duodenum, particularly in the peripapillary region. In most of these cases, the duodenal papilla is visualized adjacent to the edge of the diverticulum. The base of the diverticulum shows normal mucosa without circular folds. No evidence of diverticulitis was found in any of the cases examined.

True tumor of the duodenum is rare. One case of primary duodenal carcinoma,[18] one of duodenal sarcoma, one of benign leiomyoma and few adenomas were found in our series. In the primary duodenal carcinoma, a sizable, eroded tumor with a large crater was seen at the lower end of the descending duodenum and proved to be adenocarcinoma by biopsy. Duodenal sarcoma was seen as a deep ulcer surrounded by normal mucosa without inflammation. In the case of leiomyoma, a large tumor with shallow ulceration on one side was seen and led us to strongly suspect malignant sarcoma. However, a biopsy revealed a benign lesion and this finding was confirmed at operation.

Carcinoma of the papillary region was diagnosed in eight patients.[19]

There were six cases of papillary carcinoma and two of carcinoma of the terminal common bile duct. All showed localized tumor at the papillary region, with a crater or eroded granular orifice on the tumor (Plate 83). Diagnosis of carcinoma at the papillary region is not difficult by duodenoscopy and is frequently confirmed by endoscopic biopsy. Carcinoma of the terminal common bile duct is characteristically seen as a localized tumor just at the proximal side of the duodenal papilla (the part of the intramural bile duct).

In carcinoma of the pancreas and biliary duct, ulceration, bleeding from the duodenal orifice, and compression with or without inflammation of the mucosa are seen, frequently accompanied by the papillary tumor and eroded granular orifice. Bleeding from the normal papilla is characteristic in carcinoma of the biliary system, even though it is seen in only 25 per cent of all biliary carcinomas. Compression and rigidity of the duodenal wall are often present, depending on the location and size of the tumor. Usually, the eroded mucosa covers this compressed and rigid part of the duodenum. Although these findings are not direct evidence of carcinoma, they strongly suggest carcinoma at that location. Biopsy from these eroded mucosa, however, shows only inflammatory changes without evidence of malignancy, except when tumor infiltrates directly through the duodenal mucosa, producing ulceration. Opacification of the pancreatic and biliary ducts, when performed at the same time as duodenoscopy, is valuable in the diagnosis of carcinoma of the pancreas and biliary system.

DUODENOSCOPIC PANCREATOCHOLANGIOGRAPHY

This is a new technic designed to opacify the pancreatic and biliary ducts using the duodenoscope.[20, 21] Premedication is exactly the same as that for routine duodenoscopy. However, fluoroscopy with an image intensifier is essential for this technic, because the injection of the radiocontrast material should be monitored to avoid injecting an excess amount into the pancreatic duct. As the radiocontrast material, 60 per cent Urographin has been used in our clinic.

This procedure requires skillful technic and considerable experience. However, once the technic of cannulation has been mastered, the procedure can be performed within fifteen minutes and without excessive discomfort for the patient.

Technic of Pancreatography

The duodenoscope is inserted into the descending part of the duodenum as quickly as possible. The duodenal papilla is caught in the frontal view in the center of the visual field. Then the cannula, which is passed through the biopsy channel of the scope, is cannulated into the orifice of the duodenal papilla for about 1 to 2cm (Plate 84). During the cannulation, the curved cannula should be passed to the orifice in the same direction as that of the pancreatic duct. It is important that the cannula is completely filled with contrast material before cannulation in order to prevent injection of air or duodenal fluid from the cannula into the pancreatic duct.

Under continuous fluoroscopic control, 2 to 4ml of the contrast material is injected using a 20ml syringe; this amount is sufficient to fill the entire pancreatic duct from head to tail. When the cannula is not correctly inserted into the pancreatic duct, overflow of the contrast material in the duodenum is seen directly with duodenoscopy and also fluoroscopically, while the pancreatic duct is not visualized.

With more recent, improved duodenoscopes, the pancreatic duct was successfully opacified in seventy-eight of one hundred cases. Examinations were unsuccessful in two cases of papillary carcinoma, four of carcinoma of the pancreatic head and two of peripapillary diverticulum. Excluding these, visualization rate of the pancreatic duct is 85 per cent. There are some cases of unknown cause in which the cannula is inserted into the duodenal papilla but the pancreatic duct is not opacified.

Results

Figure 24-5 shows a pancreatogram obtained by this technic. The main pancreatic duct and its branches are clearly demonstrated. Abnormal findings on pancreatograms are obstruction, dilatation, compression, filling de-

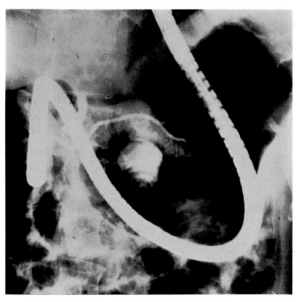

Figure 24-5. Transendoscopic pancreatogram with duodenoscope *in situ*. The main pancreatic duct and its branches are well visualized, demonstrating the shape of the pancreas. The lower part of the common bile duct is also visualized due to overflow of contrast material from the pancreatic duct.

fect, and irregular filling of the main pancreatic duct and its branches. The space-occupying lesions—carcinoma, cyst and pseudocyst, and tumor—are diagnosed by pancreatography without much difficulty. As severe chronic pancreatitis is rare in Japan, chronic pancreatitis was diagnosed only in a few cases in our series that showed irregular caliber of the ducts and terminal small cysts. The visualization of the branches of the pancreatic duct is important to find a small tumor and to diagnose moderate chronic pancreatitis.

There has been no severe complication, such as acute pancreatitis, after pancreatography by this method. Serum amylase levels are elevated to about two to three times normal three to six hours after injection of the contrast material in most patients, but these levels return to normal within two days.[22-25] The volume of contrast material is strictly restricted to the minimum amount required to diagnose the pancreatic diseases—usually less than 4ml.

Technic of Cholangiography

For cholangiography, the technic is the same as in pancreatography. With completion of pancreatography, the cannula is resting approximately 1cm in the pancreatic duct. At that point the cannula is bent upward in the direction of the common bile duct in order to opacify the biliary system. In some instances in which the opening of the common bile duct is separate from that of the pancreatic duct on the same papilla, the cannula is withdrawn and reinserted into the opening of the common bile duct in the same way as described before. The presence of the cannula in the common bile duct is confirmed by injecting a small amount of contrast material under fluoroscopic visualization. The whole biliary system which contains the common bile duct, the gallbladder, and the intrahepatic bile ducts may be opacified by the further injection of 10 to 15ml of the contrast material. During the entire procedure of cholangiography, it is essential to avoid injection of excess contrast material into the pancreatic duct. X-rays should be taken in various positions to visualize all parts of the biliary system (Fig. 24-6).

As it is more difficult to cannulate the common bile duct than the pancreatic duct using a duodenoscope, cholangiograms were taken in fifty-six of the 100 patients examined. Duodenoscopic cholangiography was not performed in twenty patients suspected of having pancreatic disease, so that the net success rate of cholangiography is 70 per cent (fifty-six of eighty cases).

All diseases—including cancer, stone, and stenosis—are demonstrated as

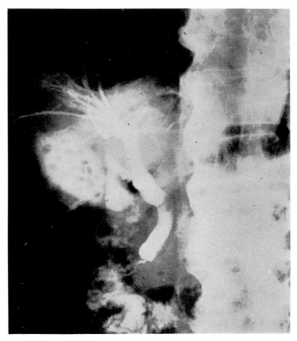

Figure 24-6. Transendoscopic cholangiogram, showing one stone in the common bile duct and many in the gallbladder. Note shaft of scope. The oral and intravenous cholangiograms did not reveal stones in this case (From Oi, I., et al.[22]).

clearly on cholangiograms taken by this method as with percutaneous transhepatic cholangiography.

ANALYSIS OF PANCREATIC AND BILIARY FUNCTION

The technic of cannulation of the pancreatic and biliary ducts makes it possible to collect pure pancreatic juice and bile under various conditions. Analysis of the pure pancreatic juice reveals more precisely the excretory function of the pancreas and its physiology.[25] Cytologic examination of pancreatic juice would be an important diagnostic method in cases of cancer of the pancreas in which results of endoscopic biopsy would be negative.

The excretion of bile is studied over a period of time using the duodenoscope. The thin colored bile is usually excreted intermittently under normal conditions. After stimulation with Pancreozymin (1 unit/kg body weight), thick bile comes out continuously from the opening of the duodenal papilla. The analysis of the bile flow in many conditions and under many stimulations will reveal the functional disorders of the biliary system.

CONCLUSIONS

Duodenoscopes have been accepted throughout the world for the examination of the duodenum and also the pancreas and biliary system, and have proved to be valuable in diagnosis of many related diseases.

Duodenoscopic pancreatography and cholangiography which are applied technics of duodenoscopy, have been found to be most valuable diagnostic methods for the study of the pancreatic and biliary ducts. With these methods, small tumors of the pancreas and biliary duct can be visualized without great difficulty.

Although duodenoscopy and its applied technics are very new, they will have an inevitable major role in diagnosis of diseases of the duodenum, pancreas, and biliary duct.

REFERENCES

1. Hirschowitz, B. I., et al.: Demonstration of a new gastroscope, the "fiberscope." *Gastroenterology, 35*:50, 1958.
2. Fulton, W. F.: The fiberscope in gastroscopy. *Am J Gastroenterol, 38*:290, 1962.
3. Burnett, W.: An evaluation of the gastroduodenal fiberscope. *Gut, 3*:361, 1962.
4. Cohen, N. N., et al.: Experience with 1,000 fibergastroscopic examinations of the stomach. *Am J Digest Dis, 11*:943, new ser., 1966.
5. Watson, W. C.: Direct vision of the ampulla of Vater through the gastroduodenal fiberscope. *Lancet, 1*:902, 1966.
6. McCune, W. S., et al.: Endoscopic cannulation of the ampulla of Vater: Preliminary report. *Ann Surg, 167*:752, 1968.
7. Rider, J. A.: The fiberduodenoscope: A preliminary report. *Am J Gastroenterol, 47*:21, 1967.
8. Oshiba, S.: Experience with duodenal fiberscope. *Gastroenterol Endosc (Jap.), 6*:149, 1965.
9. Oi, I., et al.: Direct visualization of the duodenal mucosa by fibergastroscope. *Shindan to Chiryo (Jap.), 56*:1690, 1968.
10. Oi, I., et al.: Fiberduodenoscope; its quality and usage. *Gastroenterol Endosc (Jap.), 11*:272, 1969.
11. Oi, I., et al.: Fiberduodenoscope: Direct observation of the papilla of Vater. *Endoscopy, 1*:101, 1969.
12. Oi, I.: Fiberduodenoscopy and endoscopic pancreatocholangiography. *Gastrointest Endosc, 17*:59, 1970.
13. Shindo, S., et al.: Duodenal fiberscope. *Gastroenterol Endosc (Jap.), 12*:70, 1970.
14. Ogoshi, K., et al.: Endoscopic observation of the duodenum and pancreatocholangiography using duodenal fiberscope under direct vision. *Gastroenterol Endosc (Jap.), 12*:83, 1970.
15. Fugita, R., et al.: Endoscopic examination of the duodenum. *Gastroenterol Endosc (Jap.), 12*:97, 1970.
16. Oi, I., et al.: Unpublished data, 1971.
17. Oi, I., et al.: Endoscopic examination of the duodenum. *Sogorinsho (Jap.), 19*:307, 1970.
18. Oi, I., et al.: A case of primary duodenal cancer diagnosed by duodenoscopy and scopic biopsy. *Endoscopy, 2*:134, 1970.

19. Oi, I., et al.: Fiberduodenoscopy: Early diagnosis of cancer of the papilla of Vater. *Surgery, 67*:561, 1970.
20. Oi, I.: Endoscopic pancreatography using the fiberduodenoscope, type FDS-Lb. *J Jap Soc Gastroenterol, 66*:880, 1969.
21. Oi, I., et al.: Endoscopic cholangiography. *J Jap Soc Gastroenterol, 67*:165, 1970.
22. Oi, I., et al.: Endoscopic pancreatocholangiography. *Endoscopy, 2*:103, 1970.
23. Takagi, K., et al.: Retrograde pancreatography and cholangiography by fiber duodenoscope. *Gastroenterology, 59*:445, 1970.
24. Oi, I.: Pancreatograms obtained by fiberduodenoscopy. *J Therap (Jap.), 53*:798, 1971.
25. Kozu, T., et al.: Duodenoscopy and its clinical application to diagnosis of pancreatic diseases. *Shindan to Chiryo (Jap.), 57*:2143, 1969.

SECTION V

TRANSENDOSCOPIC TECHNICS IN UPPER GASTROINTESTINAL ENDOSCOPY

CHAPTER 25

EXTRAGASTRIC STILL PHOTOGRAPHY: TECHNICS

Jean Laurent and Pierre Housset[*]

HISTORICAL STATEMENT

Endoscopic photography is an important tool for teaching the subject of endoscopy and as an objective means of recording the endoscopic appearances of various lesions for future comparisons and in the confirmation of the radiological appearances. Conscious of these advantages endoscopists have tried to devise simple means of photographing what is seen through the endoscope. Let us first survey briefly the history of endoscopy. This may be seen as having developed through three eras, beginning with the use of the rigid scopes (1868-1932) which was followed by the era of semiflexible scopes (1932-1958) and finally by the fiberscopes of the present since 1958 (see further discussion in Chapter 1).

Lange and Meltzing[1] were probably the first to attempt intragastric photography by using a very small camera mounted at the tip of a thin rubber tube which was introduced into the stomach for taking blind photographs of the interior of the stomach. No satisfactory pictures were obtained. The same principle was used by Heilpern and Back who used a small arc lamp as the light source which would burn out after each exposure. Hen-

---

[*] The authors acknowledge the valuable assistance of Drs. M. Merle, F. Vicari and B. Watrin.

ning, realizing that blind photography was unsatisfactory constructed a photographic attachment to the rigid gastroscope of Schindler and the first photographs with visual control were made by Henning and Keilhack in 1938.[2] Their results were not satisfactory due to the lack of sensitivity of the film and insufficient light.

The problem grew more difficult with the introduction of the semiflexible scopes in 1932 by Wolf and Schindler. The large number of lenses used here caused a significant absorption of light. Hull[3] was the first in 1940 to obtain black and white photographs with the Wolf-Schindler scope. During this time intragastric photography was largely unsatisfactory due to the poor light sources and limited by the available films which were of low sensitivity.

In 1948 Segal and Watson[4] made the first satisfactory pictures in color, thanks to the better light source and the flash which reduced the exposure time. These workers used a tungsten lamp which could be stepped up from 25 to 80 volts during the exposure. Nelson[5] modified the instrument making it simpler to use and published his results in 1956.

In France Debray and Housset[6, 7] resolved the problem of insufficient light by using an electronic flash lamp which permitted the use of slow speed film such as the Kodachrome II resulting in good color saturation, better detail and clearer enlargements.

Colcher et al.[8] using a large tungsten lamp and fast color film, obtained excellent movies through the fiberscope. Hirschowitz[9] obtained good results with color movie photographs through the fiberscope using the Camex camera. In the following years the quality of fiberscopes was greatly improved particularly in the sphere of glass fiberoptics and light transmission. These developments with the availability of high speed color films have made it possible to take excellent photographs during endoscopy.

GENERAL PRINCIPLES

Generally speaking, the taking of endoscopic pictures is similar to routine photography. However, local factors, including reflections from the mucosal surfaces and the secretions sometimes obscuring an important area, may cause problems. Local movement, such as pulsations of underlying great vessels, peristalsis, and the motion due to respiration, tends to give a loss of sharpness. These movements are usually overcome by the short-exposure times made possible by better illumination and faster films. The reflection of light from mucosal surfaces is variable, and what can be well appreciated by the endoscopist may not be reproduced on the photograph. For instance, in gastric atrophy light is poorly reflected and there may result dark pictures with poor detail. Shadows cast by a large lesion may make the surrounding areas come out poorly on the photograph, whereas the lesion itself may stand out very well. The depth of field is also a factor that sometimes limits the reproduction of everything that is seen by the endoscopist.

Good cooperation from the patient and proper positioning are also equally important for best results.

PHOTOGRAPHIC OPTICS

The aim of photographic optics is to obtain an image of the picture precisely as seen through the ocular and transmitted to the film, keeping the maximum brightness, contrast and sharpness. The choice of photographic optics requires a knowledge of the nature of the scopes, the light sources, and the sensitivity of the film.

In endoscopy we use small tele-lenses whose focusing distance, 24-36 camera, varies within a moderate range. While using the special lens objectives of various manufacturers, it may be mentioned that the aperture for the lens is not very important, but that the number of the lens components is very important. The larger the number, the greater will be the loss of light. The choice of the focusing distance is also critical, since it determines the field of vision and hence the area photographed.

In practice, with a doubling of the field of vision and thereby the area photographed, one must increase the light by a factor of four. This is because the intensity of illumination at a surface is inversely proportional to the square of the distance from the light source. It is better to get a picture of a small area perfectly exposed than to have an underexposed one of a larger area. On the other hand, the good light transmission of the rigid scopes and the use of flashes permit good photographs of large areas. The lenses used by the better manufacturers are of good quality, small in size, without any diaphragm, and are very well adapted to the ocular. Focusing must be very precise because the tele-lenses have little depth of field.

Optical fibers are silica conduits with small sections transmitting light. They are made of two materials.[1] The central fibers having a high refractive index N_1 1.62. Its role is to transmit light.[2] The revetement with a lens of higher refractive index of N_2 2.52. It prevents the light from going out of the conduit, permitting the propagation of light. The two materials in each case are made of glass of excellent clarity and durability.

The best fiberscopes have very precise focus (from a few millimeters to a few centimeters). To preserve their optical qualities, fiberscopes must be handled with great care when they have been left at low temperature. One should also avoid too strong *beguillages* and long exposure under x-rays that yellow the fibers.

We have tested many rigid scopes and we think that Lumina and Hopkins optics give the best results. Most firms have adopted the exoflash light for the taking of photographs.

LIGHT SOURCES

The light sources of an endoscope need reflection to obtain good pictures. It is impossible to classify all the light sources used in photography. We have selected a few for their qualities.

Light Sources for Rigid and Semirigid Endoscopes

We can use four types of light sources with these.
a. The survoltage of the usual blister
b. The exoflash
c. The endoflash
d. The very powerful sources chiefly used for cinema.

The use of the Fourestier-Gladu-Vulmiere universal endoscope allows both still photography and cinematographic sequences by using a double-quartz conduit for transmitting the proximal flash. This gives good results, but the low color temperature requires films that are balanced for artificial light.

Light Sources for Fiberscopes

The usual lighting comes from a distal spark, and a survolted spark makes photography possible. This is true for old Olympus scopes, type GFB, which use a "hot lighting." Their light source is produced by a current generator for the usual lighting and by a condensor for the survoltage of the flash (color temperature, 3200K). Presently the Olympus firm uses cold light. With the cold-light generator the same light is used for the examination and the photography. This is true for all Olympus scopes that are provided with supple-lighting conductors.

Following are the most used:

1. The Olympus CLE. This is equipped with a hologen lamp whose color temperature requires the use of film balanced for artificial light. An electromagnetic Obturator set in front of the spark opens completely for the taking of views. The time of exposure is automatically set by a photoelectric cell put in the fiberscope camera. The time of exposure varies from 10 to 200 milliseconds.

2. The Olympus CLS is provided with a xenon arc lamp, and its color temperature is like that of daylight. It possesses a photoelectric cell regulating the time of exposure and the fibers used are a function of the sensitivity of the color emulsion.

3. The Olympus CLX we think is a most improved one. It permits the selection of films as well as pictures. It uses an xenon arc also and lasts 500

hours. The taking of photographs is completely automatic. The fiberscope camera contains a photoelectric cell and an electronic integrator. The time of exposure varies from 10 to 250 milliseconds.

4. The Machida RX500. The Machida firm produces the most powerful light sources. The RX500 is equipped with an xenon arc lamp. Its intensity can be regulated, although it has nonincorporated electric cell for integrator.

5. The AEMFCB 1000 light sources requires the use of photoelectric-celled cameras to determine the time of exposure.

CHOICE OF THE FILM

The improvements in endoscopic photography are due to the availability of emulsions of high sensitivity and the improvements in the light sources. Photographic emulsions are based on the trichromatic principle of Young which states that it is possible to reform any color with the combination of three primary colors, blue, green and red in varying proportions. The color film has three layers of coatings, each of which is sensitive to one of the primary colors. Depending on the light composition of the object photographed, the three layers are reduced in varying proportions and the final result is the development of the original color.

The color film has to be balanced for the type of the light used. The spectral composition of the light used depends on the temperature to which the element of the light source is heated. The greater the color temperature, the greater is the proportion of white light. The color temperature of daylight is 5500 K and it has almost equal proportions of the three primary colors. Hence, when using light source which approach the composition of daylight, the film used must be balanced for the light, meaning that the layers of the three emulsions are also in the same proportions.

With the use of high speed films, which are of high sensitivity, it is possible to use far shorter exposure times but with high speed films, the rendition of reds suffers and the blue predominates. Generally the reds are ren-

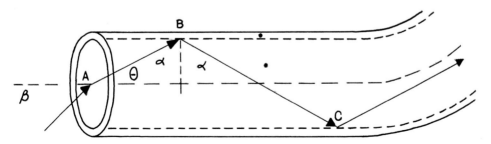

Figure 25-1. Transmission of light through bundle of optical gloss fibers.

dered best with slower speed films. The graininess and the resolving power also suffer with the use of films of high speeds. Generally speaking, good results are obtained with the use of High Speed Ektachrome (Kodak) with an ASA rating of 160 and balanced for daylight with the light sources used today.

THE CHOICE OF CAMERA

It is quite easy when you know the qualities required. It must be a reflex camera, mono-objective, with an interchangeable objective.

It must be provided with bright view and have an automatic advancement of the film following each exposure. It must be light, compact and easily transported.

Many 35mm cameras answer these conditions. The Olympus Pen-F and Pen FT T are widely used now. The American Cystoscope Makers, Inc., of New York (ACMI) have recently introduced a good 35mm camera for endoscopes called ALPA. In rigid endoscopy, many 35mm cameras give very good results (see Figs. 25-1 and 2).

PRACTICAL PHOTOGRAPHIC HINTS

A large variety of good 35mm cameras can be adapted for good photography by fiberscope manufacturers. In photography, the difficulties range

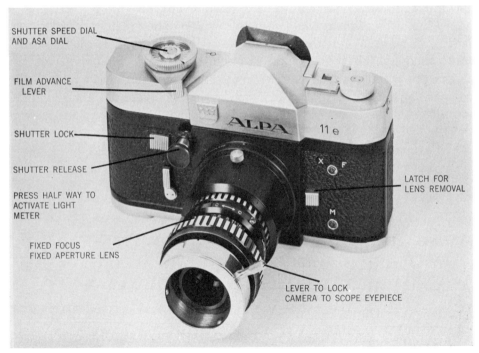

Figure 25-2. ALPA reflex camera introduced by the American Cystoscopy Makers, Inc., of New York.

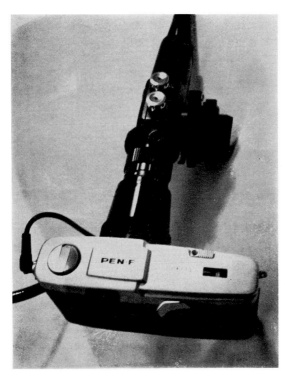

Figure 25-3. Pen-F Olympus Camera attached to GIF Olympus endoscope.

from those due to the small depth of field to those due to dirt on the optics. So that all firms equip their instruments with a very good washing-suction system, some endoscopists recommend putting a few drops of silicone on the objective, before the introduction, to reduce dirt. In fact, silicone is quickly eliminated by the different washings. Moreover, it may alter the quality of the optic when drying. Some fiberscopes have a constant depth of field, so that one must photograph the lesion within that space, to improve these conditions. Other scopes have focuses with adjustment varying from a few millimeters to several centimeters without changing the depth of field. One can thus photograph the lesions from a certain distance. This very sensitive focus requires both a great deal of skill and extensive experience.

Esophagogastroduodenoscopes are often used. They offer a great depth of field, but the pictures obtained are often imprecise.

We must always be sure of the cleanliness of the optic before making an exposure. To photograph the lesion, it must be approached in the clear field, avoiding the necessity of multiple exposures. In general a lesion must be photographed several times so that its size, form and position may be estimated. As fiberscopes give pictures of very small areas, the area and distance estimations take a great deal of experience.

With lateral-viewing duodenoscopes and jejunoscopes, there are some photographic difficulties stemming from the small diameters of the pictures. The number of the fibers is reduced and the field of observation is reduced. Moveover biliary pancreatic secretions constantly dirty the optic, even though there is a washing-suction system. Cold light sources equipped with arc lamps should be used for better lighting.

REFERENCES

1. Lange, F., and Meltzing, D.: Photographie d. Mageninneren. *Munchen med Wchnschr*, 50:1585, 1898.
2. Henning, N., and Keilhack, H.: Die gezielte Farbenphotographie in der magenhohle. *Deutsche med Wchnschr*, 64:1329, 1938.
3. Hull, W. M.: Inside the body. *Pop Sc*, May, 1940.
4. Segal, H. L., and Watson, J. S., Jr.: Color photography through the flexible gastroscope. *Gastroenterology*, 10:575, 1948.
5. Nelson, R. S.: Routine gastroscopic photography. *Gastroenterology*, 30:661, 1956.
6. Debray, C., and Housset, P.: La Gastrophotographie au flash electronique et la gastrocinematographie a l'aide du gastroscope flexible: Premiers documents en couleurs, *Ann otolaryng*, 4:209, 1957.
7. Debray, C., and Housset, P.: Color gastro-photography with an electronic flash. *Am Gastroscop Soc Bull*, 5:9, 1958.
8. Colcher, H., and Katz, G. M.: Apparatus for intragastric color cinematography. *Bull gastrointest endosc*, 1:5, 1961.
9. Hirschowitz, B. I.: Fiberduodenoscopy and cinefiberduodenoscopy; presented at meeting of the American Gastroscopic Society, May 24, 1961, Chicago.

CHAPTER 26

ENDOSCOPIC CINEPHOTOGRAPHY

Henry Colcher

HISTORY

CINEPHOTOGRAPHY THROUGH ENDOSCOPES developed gradually during the past fifty years. Progress depended on the technical advances of each component of this technique. Adequate cinematography requires a good source of light and the correct transmission of a well illuminated image to the camera film. With intraluminal electric bulbs, the limiting factor has been the danger of burns by an overheated filament. External sources of light require a good system for transmission into the organ to be photographed. At first, only simple telescopic systems were used to reduce the loss of brightness of the image. Similarly, the less complicated the camera lens, the less illumination is required. Initially, black and white film was used because of its higher sensitivity (ASA ratings of 100 to 1,000). Color film was made with ASA ratings of 10 to 25. Then faster film was introduced with ratings as high as 800 ASA. But, as the light sources became brighter and transmission through the endoscopes improved, slow color films could again be used. They are now preferred because of their excellent quality. Filming at slow speeds (eight frames per second) requires less illumination. Filming can now be done at 16, 24 and even 32 frames per second. Originally, simple camera lens systems were used to avoid loss of brightness, whereas now illumination is available even for complex zoom lens systems.

The system developed by Brubaker in the 1940s,[1] provides excellent photography through rigid endoscopes, such as bronchoscopes, esophagoscopes and sigmoidoscopes. It consists of an external light transmitted through a system of mirrors via air; the image is transmitted to the motion picture camera through straight telescopes. Debray and Segal[2] adapted the system of external illumination with transmission through quartz rods, which had been used for bronchoscopes, to straight scopes, such as esophagoscopes, proctoscopes, sigmoidoscopes and peritoneoscopes. They produced excellent films with a 16mm reflex camera (Beaulieu). The quartz rod system could not be applied to gastroscopes with lens systems, such as the Wolf-Schindler scope, since this instrument assumes a variety of curves during the examination.

The author and Doctor George Katz,[3] an engineer, obtained the first color motion pictures through a Benedict Operating gastroscope by using a bundle of fiberglass to carry light from an external source. A Truflector projection bulb was used. A system of mirrors was placed at the distal end of the Benedict gastroscope to illuminate the gastric mucosa. Since the lens system of the Benedict operating gastroscope absorbs a large amount of light, we used high speed film (So270 by Kodak), through a lens reflex camera, Camex 8mm, filming at eight frames per second. Debray and Housset[4] obtained color motion pictures through their gastroscope which has a smaller number of lenses, by increasing the voltage to the internal bulb. They could photograph only for brief periods, ten seconds at most, to avoid overheating the bulb and gastric burns. Doctor Katz developed a special power supply unit for intermittent internal illumination.[5] The lens gastroscopes of all makes were then adapted for this system, which supplied a burst of illumination when the film was advanced to the back of the shutter. Color cinematography became simplified when fiberscopes were developed in the late 1950s.[6] The internal bulb supplied sufficient illumination without intermittency because the loss through the image carrying bundle is much less than through the lens system. We adapted the system of intermittent illumination to the American and Japanese fiberscopes,[7] which supply more light during the burst and allow the bulb to cool off while the film is advanced in the camera. This technique is therefore safe for prolonged periods.

In the 1960s, the system of external illumination with a bundle of fiberglass to carry light from an external source was applied to practically all new models of fiberscopes. Good cinematography could therefore be achieved through esophagoscopes, gastroscopes, duodenoscopes and colonoscopes.[8] Simple projection bulbs were replaced by Halogen bulbs and Xenon lamps. With improvement in the quality of fibers of the light conducting bundle and image transmission, as well as the quality of color film emulsions, cinematography became easy. In 1967, we started to use simple cameras, namely the Instamatic Super-8 camera by Kodak, making cinematography inexpensive and convenient. Though excellent systems for automatic exposures are available, they are still extremely costly.

VALUE OF CINEMATOGRAPHY IN ENDOSCOPY

Color cinematography is the best method to document endoscopic findings. The endoscopist needs no longer depend on visual impression and memory, nor regret his inability to visualize once again a lesion he saw briefly. No longer must the endoscopist reach a decision regarding some unusual aspect of the findings on the basis of a fleeting image. With objective documents he can review, analyze these images, and discuss them with colleagues. If the entire examination was filmed, he may notice details which escaped his attention during the examination or which he considered insignificant, for he must concentrate on observation as well as on the patient's comfort. These minute changes may assume greater importance as the disease process evolves. A tiny elevation of the mucosa, a slight change in color of the mucosa, a minimal irregularity at the edge of an ulcer, may be more consequential a few months later as these changes continue or spread. By comparing motion pictures of different periods, one can improve the ability to interpret each minimal change and therefore be of greater use to his patients in the future. This self-teaching or self-improvement has been one of the greatest benefits of cinematography.

With still photography, one tends to visualize a lesion and photograph it repeatedly, but minute changes cannot be evaluated in relation to distance of lesion to the objective lens, changes in intensity of color and changes during peristalsis. Therefore they cannot be compared adequately during subsequent examinations. Even with still photography, one could insist on photographing the entire examination and the entire stomach, then go back and evaluate discrete changes and learn from them. Yet, this is done much better with cinematography. By reviewing motion and changes in appearance of a lesion during various phases of the peristaltic contraction, one obtains almost a three-dimensional impression of the examination. This is much closer to the impressions gained during viewing, whereas still photography gives only a two-dimensional document. Stereoscopic still examination could improve this aspect of photography but this technique is cumbersome. The endoscopist has learned to use one eye to obtain three-dimensional information as given by motion, rather than use both eyes. This point is even more pertinent when filming a procedure carried out through fiberscopes, such as a biopsy, cannulation of the papilla of Vater, when taking electrical measurements with electrodes, or doing electro-surgery. For all these procedures, the third dimensional aspect is important and this can be recorded only by movies. Changes in electrical potential, while an electrode is moved from the duodenum into the stomach, touching a lesion, or being suspended in mid-air, cannot be properly documented with still photography. They must be correlated with movements of the stomach. The effect of a peristaltic wave on a disease process, the demonstration of movement involving rigid portions, can best be evaluated by cinematography. The sliding of an esophageal mucosa over an extrinsic lesion in the mediastinum or of the gastric mucosa over an extrinsic lesion in the abdomen, can be recorded only by cinematography and thus masses outside the organs and those which involve the organ itself can be distinguished. Pulsations of vessels, filling and emptying of varices, changes of a hiatus hernia with respiration can be evaluated only with motion pictures.

Color cinematography has another great advantage. It is the only method for training endoscopists since it reproduces exactly the living phenomena observed during the examination. Certainly, television systems with tape recording could do as much, but at present this is extremely costly and requires sophisticated equipment.

When a permanent record is required to demonstrate the total examination, either for self-review or to reach a diagnosis by group opinion, cinematography is the best system available. Motion pictures can be used to exhibit the problem to other physicians, radiologists, surgeons, pathologists, and others interested in the care of a particular patient, and, at times to explain to the patient the importance of certain decisions. These films are also extremely useful in the training of residents and endoscopists since they can be added to clinical findings and subsequent pathological findings and follow-up examinations, to prove or disprove the initial interpretation.

TECHNICS OF ENDOSCOPIC CINEMATOGRAPHY

Equipment has been developed all over the world which permits selection from a variety of cameras, film emulsions and light sources. Fairly automatic systems have been devised; others are semiautomatic, and still others offer a certain latitude to the experienced photographer who may vary his exposure factors, speed of filming and size of image on the frame.

The quality of cinematography depends on correct illumination, which in turn depends on the source of light, the filtering system before reaching the light transmission bundle, the interconnecting systems between the light source and the fiberbundle, the length of the bundle and its composition. Most modern fiberscopes use an integral bundle without the extra connection at the head of the instrument which causes loss of light. The longer the bundle, the more light is lost. By compensating for this loss with changes of filters, one can use any length desired. Within the organ, for instance the stomach, illumination depends on the distance between the fiberscope and the lesion. In the automatic system of exposure, this is corrected by a light sensing device, either in the fiberscope or the camera. In the semiautomatic systems, the light meter in the camera corrects for distance. With experience, the endoscopist develops a sense of distance and degree of illumination and can vary the opening of the camera lens or speed of filming to correct for changes in distance. The latter method is somewhat confusing when the film is projected. The antrum may be photographed at 24 frames per second, whereas the fundus, photographed from a distance, may be filmed at only eight frames per second, and the film will probably be projected at a constant speed. The endoscopist may use his own judgment with the semiautomatic or automatic controls to improve his results. Automatic settings must be adjusted manually, for different endoscopes and types of film, and for the conditions of the examination. Light reflections from the organs vary with the state of health. A gastric mucosa which is somewhat congested and hypersecreting will appear brighter and reflect more light than a markedly atrophic mucosa. A mucosa covered with mucus will appear brighter than one covered with residual blood. The automatic adjustments of filters, or opening of the diaphragm or other systems, is not as reliable as the photographer's judgment. A lesion may be in the shadow or dark portion of the stomach and therefore requires adjustments other than what the light sensing device will do in response to the entire amount of illumination. At times one must *bracket* the exposure, as with still photography. Thus, the lesion will be photographed at different speeds or with different lens openings to allow for some overexposure and underexposure. Then one can select the best portions of film obtained with this technique. With the automatic systems this can be done by changing the filter which reduces or increases the total amount of light supplied. The amount of light that reaches the film in motion depends on the illumination of the lesion being photographed, the loss of transmission through the fiberscope which is related to the quality of glass and its length. Loss also occurs through the lens system of the ocular and of the camera lens. The more complicated the camera lens, namely the Zoom systems, the greater the loss.

Film emulsion should be selected according to the quality of external light source. At present, we have great latitude, ranging from Kodachrome-II, daylight or artificial light, to Kodachrome-X and a variety of Ektachromes. The endoscopist can obtain guidance from the instrument makers as to the proper film for the specific fiberscope and light source. This is a matter of personal choice. The film emulsion that renders the most satisfactory visual impression to the individual endoscopist is not an absolute value of color but a synthesis of personal training and memory of colors. A gastric lesion that was viewed with a Schindler lens gastroscope and artificial illumination by the electric bulb in a specific setting and a certain distance, does not give the same impression of color values as when examined with different fiberscopes and different sources of light, internal bulb or external illumination. The same lesion, filmed with the same light but at different distances, gives different color values with the same film emulsion.

Cameras

During the first decade of cinegastroscopy, the author used regular 8mm and 16mm film in Camex and Arriflex cameras. The Camex was an excellent through-the-lens camera, adapted for medical photography. It is no longer available. The Arriflex 16mm camera is an excellent and versatile professional instrument. It permits total transmission of the image to film through the lens viewing system and the rotating mirror. With the motor at varying speeds, one can obtain professional quality motion pictures. In recent years, the 8mm camera was replaced by Super-8, at first the Beaulieu and then the Kodak Instamatic (M20, M30, M9). The Arriflex was replaced by the Beaulieu 16 and 16R. These cameras are lighter, extremely versatile, and their optical systems are of high quality. At present the author prefers the Super-8 Instamatic Kodak cameras which are inexpensive and convenient because of the instant loading of cartridges. This is also available in other Super-8 cameras.

Attachments for Camera to Fiberscope

To obtain clear motion pictures, one must have a simple attachment system which will permit automatic alignment without disturbing the controls of the ocular of the camera lens. Initially, the author had a variety of systems which were custom-made but this is no longer necessary. The instrument manufacturers provide simple attachment devices that are satisfactory. The ocular of the fiberscope is kept at the infinity setting as is the camera lens. Since the new fiberscopes are made with fixed focus systems, the film is usually perfect. There are still a few fiberscopes with focusing devices. It is easy to learn to keep the image in perfect focus, both for the eye and the camera film. Future motion picture cameras will probably include systems for self-focusing in the manner of modern still cameras.

Additional Technical Details

Processing of film is best done by commercial processors. Since the author uses only film made by Kodak, processing is done by the Kodak Company. However, equipment is available for Ektachrome processing in institutions that may be far away from commerical laboratories.

Film Identification

Many systems of identification have been used. At the beginning or end of the examination, one can film a serial number of a filing system or the patient's name, his hospital or social security number. At times it is of interest to film the patient or parts that would illustrate distinct pathology—jaundice, spiders, exostoses, ascites, abdominal varices, or other skin manifestations that would be useful in the interpretation of the endoscopic finding. It may be worthwhile to photograph a wall clock with its movement to document time of injection of drugs or speed of changes within the stomach when speed of filming is variable.

Editing of Film

Some editing is required to eliminate poor quality portions which may be of little import and waste time during projection. Editing should not be done to document only the important pictures of an examination. What appears as insignificant at that time may be very important for subsequent comparison. What appears important to one observer, or less so to him, may be of significance when viewed by a group. Therefore, one should have a motion picture of the total examination.

Filing of Film

The cost of photographing a patient on a full roll of file is approximately $5.00. After editing, one is left with 40 to 45 feet of film which should be kept on the standard spool. Square plastic boxes, 82 x 82 x 14mm in depth fit the standard spool. An 80 x 80mm file card should include the patient's name, serial number, date of examination, instrument used and diagnosis. On the back of the card one can add several clinical or other details. The square boxes can be filed numerically in metal filing cabinets or cardboard boxes. Subsequent examinations maintain the same serial number with the suffix B, C, D, and are filed together.

Sixteen millimeter films are more expensive and can be limited to 20 to 30 feet per patient. Special studies may require several hundred feet of film and can be carried out with the Arriflex or Beaulieu cameras equipped with magazines of 100 to 400 feet of film. Filing is again done individually. A spool may therefore contain varying lengths of film. The spools are kept in metal containers and are filed numerically in metal cabinets or special cardboard boxes. Sixteen millimeter films can also be mounted for microfilm viewers. Some equipment permits rapid selection of individual frames.

For interesting cases, a sound tape recording is made of the clinical history and endoscopic findings, as well as subsequent developments. Such data, either on cassettes or magnetic tape, are kept together with the film collection since they are of similar size and shape. This adds to the teaching value of such collections. Teaching motion pictures can then be prepared with optical recordings of sound.

Film Projection

Considerable progress has been made in projection equipment. The 8mm films of interest were transferred to self-winding cartridges which were used for table model projectors. This made it convenient to study such patients in a less expensive manner. Super-8 film is loaded similarly in the automatic cartridge devices supplied by Kodak. They can be projected on screens or on special viewers available for partially dimmed rooms. Teaching movies on 8, super-8 or 16mm can also be prepared with a variety of audio systems for individual or group projection.

SUMMARY

Equipment is available for convenient cinematography in color of all endoscopic procedures. Simple equipment is available to permit filming with instamatic motion picture cameras and automatic settings to make cinematography available to all endoscopists. Filing and studying of such films may seem somewhat awkward at the beginning but once this is organized, one reaps the benefits of excellent documentation of the endoscopic studies. These result in better care of patients, better self-training and teaching of other endoscopists.

REFERENCES

1. Brubaker, J. D., and Holinger, P. H.: An endoscopic motion picture camera for otolaryngology and bronchoesophagology. *J. Biol Phat Assoc*, 15:171-192, 1947.
2. Segal, S.: Oesophagoscope derive de L'appareil de F.G.V. In Traite Pratique de Photographie et de Cinematographie Medicales. Paris, Pub. Photo-cinema Paul Montel, 1960, p. 200.
3. Colcher, H., and Katz, G. M.: Cinegastroscopy II. External source of light for color cinematography through the gastroscope. *Amer J Gastroent*, 35:5, May, 1961.
4. Debray, C., and Housset, P.: Personal Communication to author.
5. Colcher, H., and Katz, G. M.: Cinegastroscopy: Intermittent illumination with standard bulbs for color cinematography through the gastroscope. In McHardy, G. G. (Ed.): *Current Gastroenterology*, New York, Hoeber, 1962, p. 51.
6. Hirschowitz, B. I., Curtiss, L. E., Peters, C. W., and Pollard, H. M.: Demonstration of a new gastroscope, the "Fiberscope." *Gastroent*, 35:50, 1958.
7. Colcher, H.: Cinegastroscopy with two new gastroscopes. *Amer J Gastroent*, 47:16, 1967.
8. Colcher, H.: Gastrophotography and Cinegastroscopy. In, *Progress in Gastroenterology*, George B. Jerzy Glass, (Ed.). New York, Grune and Stratton, 1968, p. 97.

CHAPTER 27

DIRECT VISION CYTOLOGY, WASHING AND BRUSHING TECHNICS

TATSUZO KASUGAI AND SEIBI KOBAYASHI

WASHING TECHNIC

FOR THE REASON THAT routine washing or lavage for cytology did not yield a satisfactory result in early (superficial) gastric carcinoma confined to the mucosa and submucosa, direct vision washing technic under fibergastroscopy was developed by Kasugai et al. in 1964[1] and the results have further been reported.[2, 3]

Several types of gastroscopes are used for this purpose. The latest model of the instrument used is shown in Figure 27-1. Washing solution is jetted

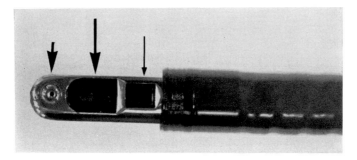

Figure 27-1. Gastroscope for direct vision washing (Machida FGS-CL). Short arrow: Jet opening; Long arrow: Lens for visualization; Fine arrow: Light system.

409

through a small opening near the tip of the gastroscope, and the direction of the stream can be controlled under direct vision with a flexible tip, with which it is easy to direct the jet of washing solution so that it will cover the entire lesion. Hanks' tissue culture solution is utilized as washing solution with which preservation of exfoliated cells proved to be better than with saline or other solutions.[4, 5]

The patient is fasted overnight. Thirty minutes prior to the examination, 0.5mg of atropine sulfate is given subcutaneously. The throat is anesthesized with viscous xylocaine and the patient is sedated with 35mg of intravenous pethidine hydrochloride (Meperidine Hydrochloride).

A preliminary washing of the stomach is carried out by introducing a Levin type gastric tube and aspirating residual gastric juice, which is discarded. The stomach then is washed with Hanks' tissue culture solution until the aspirate is clear. The fibergastroscope then is inserted into the stomach and visualization of the entire stomach is performed. All suspicious areas are thoroughly washed and the force of the jetting stream is regulated, depending upon the location and the features of the lesion. Bleeding and exfoliation of necrotic tissue are seen in most cases. Following washing of the entire lesion, the fibergastroscope is withdrawn and a Levin type gastric tube is again introduced into the stomach to retrieve the washing solution. The solution is then centrifuged at 3000 RPM for five minutes and the sediment is smeared on glass slides which are stained with Papanicolaou stain. The slides are then screened and the results are reported either positive or negative.

Results

A total of 512 patients with proven gastric cancer were examined and of these, 494 (96.0%) were positive. One hundred twenty-eight cases were of early gastric carcinoma which did not extend into the muscularis propria, and of these 122 (93.5%) were positive and six were negative (Table 27-I).

This technic was compared with the routine blind washing method in 84 cases. Sixty-nine of these cases had advanced gastric carcinoma; 61 (88.4%) by blind method and 66 (95.7%) by direct vision washing were positive. In

TABLE 27-I

DIAGNOSTIC ACCURACY OF WASHING CYTOLOGY
UNDER DIRECT VISION IN STOMACH CANCER

	Total	Positive	Accuracy (%)
Early cancer	128	122	93.5
Advanced cancer	384	372	96.9
Total	512	494	96.0

TABLE 27-II
COMPARISON OF DIRECT WASHING WITH ROUTINE
WASHING IN 84 CASES OF STOMACH CANCER

	Method	Positive	Accuracy (%)
Early cancer	Routine	6	40.0
15 cases	Direct	13	86.7
Advanced cancer	Routine	61	88.4
69 cases	Direct	66	95.7
Total	Routine	67	79.8
84 cases	Direct	79	94.0

15 cases of early gastric carcinoma, 6 (40%) by blind method and 13 (86.7%) by direct vision washing were positive. When these two groups are totaled, 79.8% by blind method and 94.0% by direct vision washing were positive (Table 27-II).

BRUSHING TECHNIC

Because of the complexity of the washing method, brushing cytology method was established at the Gastrointestinal Endoscopy and Cytology Laboratories, University of Chicago in August, 1968.[2] Likewise, the technic has been in use at the Aichi Cancer Center Hospital since June, 1970[6] for the main reason of easiness in processing nd screening.

Fiberscopes for biopsy (see Fig. 27-2a and b) can be used for this purpose in the esophagus, stomach and duodenum. Preparation of the patient is the same as that of direct vision washing as mentioned above. After the lesion has been brought into the center of the visual field with a fiberoptic instrument, a nylon brush is introduced through the channel for biopsy forceps, and advanced to the lesion as shown in Figure 27-3. At least two brushings are performed. Bleeding is usually seen at the site or in the

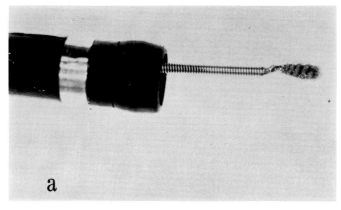

Figure 27-2a. Instrument for brushing cytology. Tip of esophagoscope (Olympus EF).

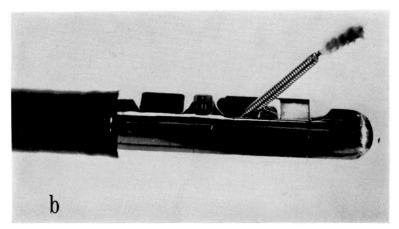

Figure 27-2b. Instrument for brushing cytology. Tip of gastroscope for biopsy (Machida FGS-BL).

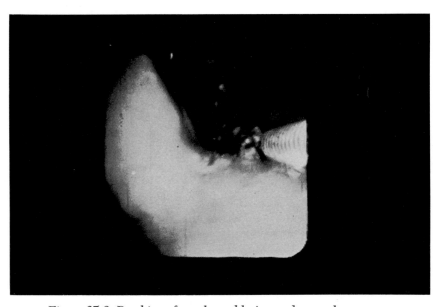

Figure 27-3. Brushing of esophageal lesion under esophagoscope.

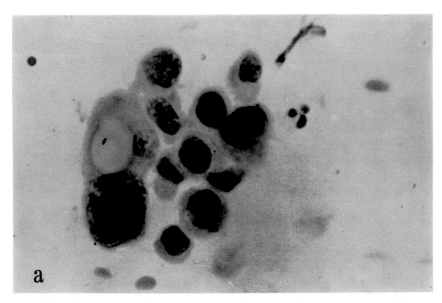

Figure 27-4a. Specimen of direct vision washing containing other materials in the background.

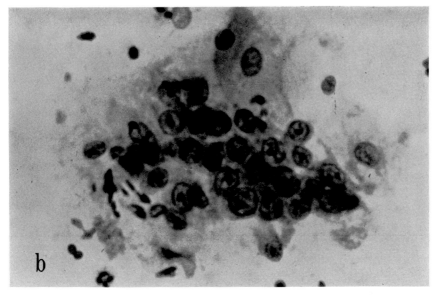

Figure 27-4b. Specimen of direct vision brushing demonstrated a clean background making screening much easier.

TABLE 27-III

COMPARATIVE DIAGNOSTIC ACCURACY OF VARIOUS METHODS
(UNIVERSITY OF CHICAGO)

| | No. Cases | No. of Cases Positive by Each Method | | | |
		X-ray Film	Endoscopy	Cytology	Biopsy
Carcinoma of esophagus	4	4	4	4	4
Carcinoma of cardia	4	3	4	4[†]	3
Carcinoma of stomach	19	13	15	18[†]	16[*]
Total carcinomas (%)	27	20	23	26	23
		(74.1)	(83.2)	(96.3)	(88.5)
Lymphoma	2	1	1	2	2
Leiomyosarcoma	1	1	1	1[†]	0
Total nonepithelial malignancies	3	2	2	3	2
Total malignancies (%)	30	22	25	29	25
		(73.3)	(83.3)	(96.7)	(86.2)

[*] Biopsy not performed in one case of gastric carcinoma due to severe thrombocytopenia.
[†] Includes three cases where brushing cytology was not performed because washing cytology was already positive.

TABLE 27-IV

DIAGNOSTIC ACCURACY OF BRUSHING CYTOLOGY UNDER
DIRECT VISION IN UPPER GI MALIGNANCY
(Aichi Cancer Center Series)

	Total	Positive	Accuracy (%)
Carcinoma of the esophagus	17	16	94.1
Carcinoma of the cardia	12	11	91.7
Carcinoma of the stomach	24	17	70.8
Total	53	44	83.0

TABLE 27-V

RESULTS OF COMBINED USE OF CYTOLOGY AND
BIOPSY UNDER DIRECT VISION

| | Cytology (+) | | Cytology (−) | | Total |
	Biopsy (+)	Biopsy (−)	Biopsy (+)	Biopsy (−)	
University of Chicago[7] Simultaneous use of brushing in gastro-esophageal cancer	23	2	1	0	26
Aichi Cancer Center Separate use of washing in early gastric cancer	119	4	8	0	131

TABLE 27-VI

COMPARISON OF DIRECT VISION METHODS WITH ROUTINE WASHING OR
BLIND LAVAGE

		Direct Vision Method		
	Routine Washing	Washing	Brushing	Biopsy
Technique	Simple	Complicated	Complicated	Complicated
Burden on patient	Less	More	More	More
Screening	Time-consuming	Time-consuming	Rapid Easy	
Cell Preservation	Poor	Moderate	Good	
Exfoliation	Poor	Excellent	Excellent	
Background	Contaminated	Contaminated (Figure 4A)	Clean (Figure 4B)	
Against a stenotic lesion	Ineffective	Ineffective	Effective	Ineffective
Accuracy	Less	High	High	High
Diagnosis	Cytological	Cytological	Cytological	Histological

shape / size	without stalk	intermediate	with stalk	total
less than 5mm	000000000 ●●●●●	0000		18
5-10mm	00000000000 ●●●●	000000000000 00 ●●●●●●	000000 ●●●●●●	46
11-20 mm			00000000 ●●●●●●	15
larger than 20 mm			000 ●	4
total	29	24	30	83

0=positive recovery
from stomach after
amputation

●=negative recovery
from stomach
amputation

vicinity of the lesion after successful brushing. The material is smeared on glass slides immediately after withdrawing the brush. Fixation, staining and reading are subsequently made as stated in the washing technic (Fig. 27-4a and b).

Results

University of Chicago Series[7]

During the period from August 1968 through December 1969, 30 cases of esophageal and gastric cancer were investigated.

Table 27-III shows the diagnostic accuracy of brushing method in comparison with other diagnostic procedures, i.e. roentgenographic examination, endoscopy and biopsy in all 30 cases. This table includes three cases in which brushing cytology was not performed because blind washing cytology had already been done with positive results. Of 26 cases of upper gastrointestinal tract malignancies, 25 (96.3%) were positive by the brushing cytology method. Only one negative case was noted in a lesion with adenocarcinoma of linitis plastica type in the distal antrum of the stomach.

Aichi Cancer Center Series

During the period from June, 1970 to August, 1971, 53 cases of upper gastrointestinal malignancy were examined.

Table 27-IV tabulates the diagnostic accuracy of brushing cytology. At present the technic is utilized mainly for the cases in which biopsy failed to obtain malignant tissues or was not applicable for the reason that the presence of a marked stricture did not allow a biopsy forceps to advance to the site of the lesion.

COMBINED USE OF DIRECT VISION BRUSHING CYTOLOGY AND BIOPSY

When direct vision biopsy was performed simultaneously or at different times with brushing cytology, the diagnostic results went up to 100 per cent in both series at the University of Chicago and Aichi Cancer Center Hospital as shown in Table 27-V.

Table 27-VI shows comparison of direct vision methods with routine washing or blind lavage.

REFERENCES

1. Kasugai, T., Yamaoka, Y., and Kobayashi, S.: The cytodiagnosis by chymotrypsin lavage under fibergastroscopy. *Japanese Society of Clinical Cytology*, 3:141, 1964.
2. Kasugai, T.: Gastric lavage cytology and biopsy for early gastric cancer under direct vision by the fibergastroscope. *Gastrointest Endosc, 14*:205, 1968.
3. Kobayashi, S., Kasugai, T., Yamaoka, Y., Yoshii, Y. and Naito, Y.: Improved tech-

nique for gastric cytology utilizing simultaneous lavage and fibergastroscopy. *Gastrointest Endosc, 15*:198, 1969.

4. Kasugai, T.: Evaluation of gastric lavage cytology under direct vision by the fibergastroscope employing Hanks' solution as washing solution. *Acta Cytologica, 12*:345, 1968.

5. Yoshii, Y.: Experimental and clinical studies on washing solution used in lavage cytology under direct vision by fibergastroscope. *Japanese Society of Clinical Cytology, 9*:1, 1970.

6. Kobayashi, S., Prolla, J. C., and Kirsner, J. B.: Brushing cytology of the esophagus and stomach under direct vision by fiberscopes. *Acta Cytologica, 14*:219, 1970.

7. Kobayashi, S., Prolla, J. C., Winans, C. S., and Kirsner, J. B.: Improved endoscopic diagnosis of gastroesophageal malignancy: Combined use of direct vision brushing cytology and biopsy. *JAMA, 212*:2086, 1970.

CHAPTER 28

PART I: BIOPSY; HISTORY, USES, TECHNICS

DAVID KATZ

INTRODUCTION

EARLY IN THE HISTORY of gastroscopy, visualization of any given lesion was of surpassing importance since histological diagnosis was impossible to obtain preoperatively. Biopsy instruments were subsequently developed, which allowed the examiner to obtain adequate specimens where diffuse lesions of the stomach existed, but guided biopsies were usually not feasible. As attempts at guided biopsies went floundering, cytologic diagnosis became far more precise. In recent years, newer biopsy instruments have been devised and precise biopsies can now be obtained by the gastroscopist.

The crucial problem in attempting to delineate the nature of any lesion is obviously visualization of the lesion. Consequently, as we talk of the capabilities of any biopsy instrument, the feasibility of any given instrument to visualize various areas of the stomach must be evaluated. I would, at the outset, suggest that in the opinion of many of us, there is no one instrument which can best visualize all areas of the upper gastrointestinal tract. The choice of instrument must thus depend upon the location of the lesion, and observer prejudice.

FORCEPS BIOPSY WITH LENS SCOPES

Bruce Kenamore introduced a forceps biopsy attachment for the Schindler lens gastroscope in 1940.[1] It had an element of real danger and could be used only in the upper portion of the stomach. It was not widely used. The first widely known gastroscopic instrument devised in the United States was the ACMI Benedict[2] operating gastroscope (Fig. 28-1). This instrument was the "Big Bertha" of gastroscopes. It had an excellent lens system but was somewhat less flexible and slightly larger in diameter than the Wolf-Schindler and the Cameron-Schindler lens scopes of that era. As with all semiflexible lens gastroscopes scrutiny of the dome of the stomach, portions of the posterior wall, and often the important prepyloric lesser curvature were incomplete. However, the instrument was quite effective for most local and diffuse lesions of the stomach. Much of the correlative work in comparing gastroscopic observations of gastritis and pathologic diagnosis of gastritis was done with the Benedict gastroscope. In areas where gastroscopic observation was good, direct extension of the biopsy forceps to a lesion allowed for a positive biopsy at the time of gastroscopy. Because of its inconveniences, however, the instrument never attained general use and today it is rarely used. The principle of the instrument, however, has remained and the same type of biopsy forceps is now used in many of the fibergastroscopes we will discuss.

SUCTION BIOPSY INSTRUMENTS

In terms of chronology the next type of biopsy instrument devised was one which utilized a suction principle. Suction would be applied so that the contents of the stomach were withdrawn and a negative pressure obtained. Tissue was thus drawn into the biopsy port. By means of a guillotine device activated by the examiner a biopsy was then obtained. This principle was incorporated in the Wood's[3] intragastric biopsy tube.

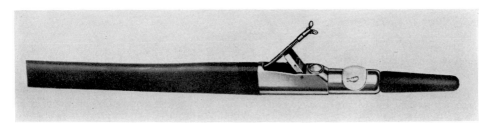

Figure 28-1. The Benedict ACMI operating gastroscope with extended biopsy forceps.

The Wood's tube, a blind biopsy instrument, is relatively effective and has been used widely in the investigation of the natural history of chronic gastritis. A modification of the Wood's tube now used in this country is the Quinton (Rubin) tube which allows for multiple biopsies of stomach or small intestine and immediate delivery of the biopsy specimen. Because of the patchy nature of gastritis, multiple biopsies which can be performed with the Quinton instrument reduce the possibility of error in investigating populations with chronic gastritis. Obviously, no effective accuracy can be obtained with this type of biopsy device even under fluoroscopic control.

The principle was also incorporated into a gastroscopic assembly built as a permanent attachment for the Schindler gastroscope by Tomenius[4] but accurate biopsy of isolated lesions was very difficult with this instrument. Berry[5] utilized the suction principle in the development of a direct vision, detachable, biopsy instrument designed to fit as a sheath over the small calibre (9mm), Eder-Palmer gastroscope. The complete gastrobiopsy assembly was passed only when a biopsy was to be taken. Otherwise the instrument could be readily disassembled in a quick maneuver for simple viewing. See (Fig. 28-2a) and (Fig. 28-2b).

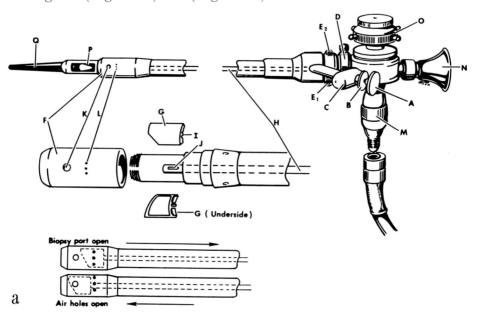

Figure 28-2a. Berry biopsy instrument, schematic drawing. A, Cutting plunger; B, flanged bushing; C, slotted bushing; D, locknut; E_1, inflation connector; E_2; suction connector; F, cutting head; G, biopsy knife; H, cutting wire; I, knife key; J, cutting wire key slot; K, biopsy port; L, air holes. Eder-Palmer gastroscope parts also shown include: M, light switch; N, eyepiece; O, remote control handle; P, objective window; Q, tip.

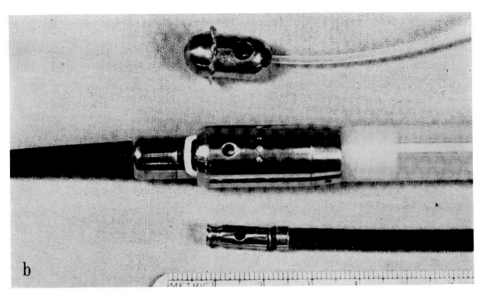

Figure 28-2b. Comparison of biopsy ports of Crosby capsule (top), Berry flexible tube instrument (center), and Rubin multipurpose instrument (bottom).

The suction principle biopsy instruments were difficult to use with predictable accuracy for small localized lesions. When the gastroscope could be abutted against a lesion effective suction biopsy could be obtained. However, a hard lesion might not be successfully biopsied because suction pressures utilized were not capable of pulling all lesions into biopsy port.

The suction type of biopsy instrument, whether blind tube or incorporated in a gastroscope, still may be quite effective in the investigation of diffuse gastric lesions such as gastritis. Our group's work on the biopsy of patients with acute gastrointestinal bleeding was performed with the Berry instrument. Successful biopsy was invariably performed and multiple specimens could be trapped in the storage compartment making it unnecessary to withdraw the scope after each bite. In addition in the past, we have been successful in diagnosing diffuse lesions such as Menetrier's disease and lymphoma by means of the Berry assembly. To my knowledge, no one has ever devised a suction type instrument which can be extended from the gastroscope and reach for a lesion in order to effect a biopsy.

FORCEPS BIOPSY WITH FIBERSCOPES

In recent years various biopsy instruments have been adapted to fibergastroscopes. These instruments are variations of the Benedict-principle (Fig. 28-3). Forceps are introduced through biopsy channels and biopsies can be obtained under direct vision. Great accuracy can be obtained with these instruments and multiple biopsies can be performed. Biopsy forceps are

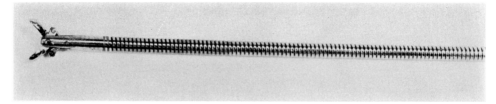

Figure 28-3. Olympus fiberscopic biopsy forceps. The greatest diameter of the open jaws is slightly over 2mm.

withdrawn between attempts and after removal of the specimen, the forceps can be reintroduced and subsequent biopsies then performed.

The first fiberscopic gastric biopsies were those obtained through the American Cystoscope Makers Inc. Lo Presti[6] fiberesophagoscope. Similar biopsies were obtained somewhat later through the Olympus EF fiberesophagoscope (Fig. 28-4). It was noted that when the fiberesophagoscope was passed full length it became a relatively effective instrument with which to examine the proximal stomach. The view was forward, and the distal tip could be deflected. In the post-subtotal gastrectomy stomach the fiberesophagoscope was quite effective in the investigation of stoma and anastamotic jejunum. The biopsy forceps provided with the Lo Presti fiberesophagoscope were initially relatively fragile and effective biopsy was, on

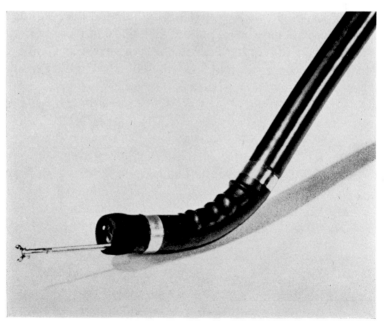

Figure 28-4. The Olympus EF fiberesophagoscope with biopsy forceps extended through the deflected distal portion.

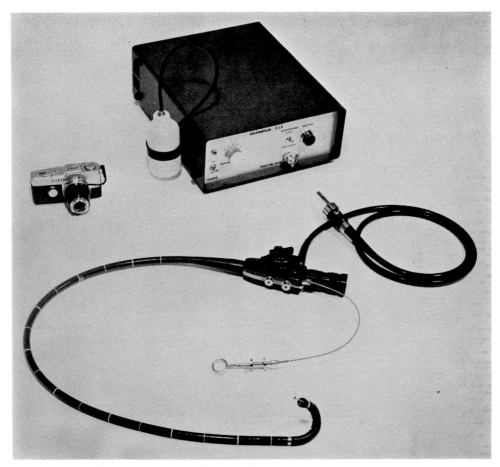

Figure 28-5. Olympus GIF. The fiberesophagoscope principle is incorporated into a lengthened instrument which allows for forward vision in esophagus, stomach and duodenum. Biopsy may be obtained in each area.

occasion, not obtained because of failure of the forceps. The Olympus biopsy forceps were, however, quite effective from the inception of their use. We have also had the opportunity to use the Machida forceps and of late the latter type forceps, which are quite effective, have been incorporated into ACMI instruments and are now widely used. The area about the cardia is effectively visualized with fiberesophagoscopes and the forward view allows for easy approach to any given lesion. Unfortunately the area of the dome of the stomach was not well seen with the early fiberesophagoscopes and with these instruments it was quite difficult to perform a U-turn. Hence, one should consider the dome of the stomach a relatively blind area with the early fiberesophagoscope. The earlier failing of shortness which precluded the use of the fiberesophagoscope as a total gastroscope has been corrected by ACMI and their newer 7087 and 7089 instruments have been lengthened so that one now can easily reach the area of the pylorus. Similarly Olympus has now fabricated a lengthened GIF (Fig. 28-5). With the newer long forward-viewing endoscopes one has a good view of the entire stomach. Both ACMI and Olympus have recently incorporated deflecting tips which in our experience obviate the necessity for performing wide U-turns (Fig. 28-6). When the instrument lies beneath the angulus, deflecting the tip 135° allows the examiner to visualize the cardia and dome of the stomach. The longest of the forward-viewing fiberscopes (ACMI 7089, Olympus GIF) can now be used as effective panendoscopes visualizing esophagus, stomach and duodenum. All areas visualized can be effectively biopsied through the forward-viewing scopes. Biopsy when the tip is completely deflected is slightly more difficult since one is reaching for a distant lesion.

The earliest lateral viewing fibergastroscope with an internal biopsy port was the ACMI 5004 which was basically an external light Hirschowitz fibergastroscope with an internal biopsy channel. The instrument failed since it did not have a tip which could be deflected and the biopsy forceps could not be well directed. In addition the biopsy forceps were initially similar to those provided with the Lo Presti instruments and they were technically poor. The next generation of fibergastroscopes with lateral viewing which

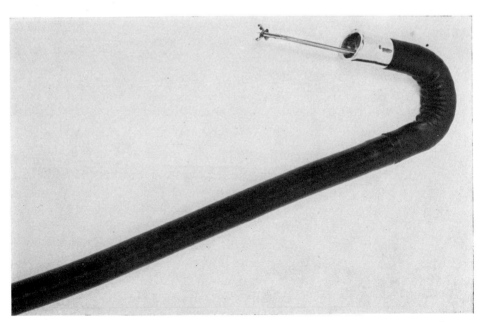

Figure 28-6. ACMI 7098 Polydirectional Panendoscope: This instrument is analogous to the Olympus GIF. Retroflexion obviates necessity for U-turn. As the instrument lies beneath the angulus, retroflexion brings the cardia into view.

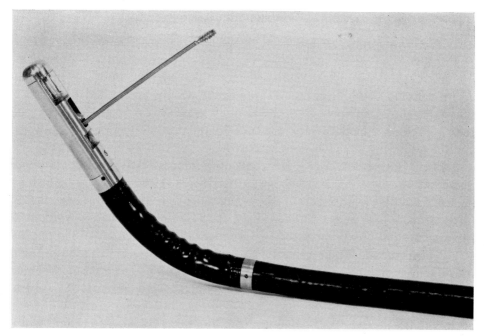

Figure 28-7. Olympus GFB: A lateral viewing fibergastroscope with deflecting tip and biopsy port shown.

could biopsy were the ACMI 5007 and the Olympus GFB (Fig. 28-7). In addition Machida manufactured an instrument similar to the Olympus GFB.

Surprisingly, the side-viewing fibergastroscopes are quite effective in all areas of the stomach in spite of the fact that one is quite frequently biopsying from a distance, in contrast to the forward-viewing fibergastroscopes which usually allow one to approach the area of the lesion and biopsy from relatively close. However, effective biopsy is still quite feasible and the term target biopsy was coined using this type of instrument.

TECHNICS
Preparation of the Patient

A prothrombin time above 50 per cent is required as are normal bleeding and clotting times and platelet counts. The patient is fasted for at least four hours. We do *not* routinely aspirate the stomach, reserving aspiration for cases of gastric outlet obstruction. Premedication is given as valium 10mg intramuscularly 30 minutes prior to the procedure with meperidine and atropine administered in standard doses when the patient is called for gastroscopy. In the usual course of events we rarely perform gastric biopsy as an outpatient procedure. Topical anesthesia is obtained by gargle. Our choice of a topical anesthetic is Dyclone.

Instrumentation

Blind Suction Biopsies are used today only for mass correlative studies or the investigation of potential cases of pernicious anemia and for gastric secretory arrest. These instruments are passed transorally, in the manner of a Levin tube. Fluoroscopic positioning is recommended but not essential. Passage between 45 and 55cms is suggested if gastric fundal mucosa is desired. Negative pressure of 7 to 10 inches of mercury is applied and the guillotine device is then actuated.

BERRY DIRECT INSTRUMENT. This ingenious biopsy instrument devised and manufactured by Eder Instrument Co. and Berry[5] was designed to fit over an Eder-Palmer flexirigid gastroscope. A schematic drawing of the instrument (Fig. 28-2a and b) taken from Dr. Francis Owens'[5, 7] chapter in Brown's *Diagnostic Procedures in Gastroenterology*, demonstrates the instrument in detail. When a lesion is seen, the gastroscope must be brought into the area of the lesion with the objective and biopsy port in apposition to the lesion. The sheath is then rotated on the gastroscope in order to open the distal biopsy port. Suction is applied so that a negative pressure of 10 to 15 inches of mercury is reached and the guillotine device activated. Multiple biopsies are possible. The reader is referred to Dr. Ownens' chapter for fuller details.

FORWARD-VIEWING FIBERSCOPE (LO PRESTI TYPE). We consider this type of instrument to be our standard biopsy instrument at present (Fig. 28-6). There is the advantage of frontal viewing with lesions always centered in direct view. Positioning the lesion in forward view brings the biopsy forceps directly to the lesion in the observer's plane of vision. A similar view of the Olympus EF (Fig. 28-4) in 75° flexion demonstrates the same principle.

When the biopsy forceps are introduced into the proximal channel of the fiberscope, care must be taken to keep the cups closed. The cups must remain closed while passage is accomplished through the biopsy channel. When the forceps emerge and are in view, they are extended directly to the lesion as the cups are opened. The forceps are then pressed firmly into the lesion and the cups closed. The forceps are then pulled away from the lesion. Bleeding is common but invariably self-limited. The forceps must be pulled to the outside through the channel in order to deliver the specimen. Accurate target biopsy is quite feasible. One can, for instance, biopsy the Z line separating esophagus from stomach and histologically demonstrate squamous epithelium joining glandular mucosa.

SIDE-VIEWING FIBERSCOPES. The objective is located immediately proximal to the biopsy port in the Olympus GFB (Fig. 28.7). The angle of extension of the forceps can be controlled by a forceps control device ac-

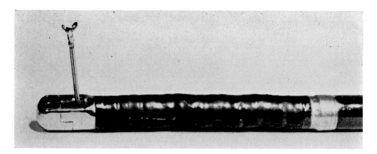

Figure 28-8. Olympus JFB fiberduodenoscope.

tuated from the proximal end of the fibergastroscope and mediated by a deflecting bar in the distal end of the biopsy channel at the port. The forceps can be directed over 100° from its axis.

Biopsy with the side-viewing instruments is more accurate (and invariably more successful) when the instrument lies closer to the lesion. It is thus far easier to biopsy in antrum than attempting to biopsy in cardia after making a U-turn.

An effort must be made to center the lesion in the objective. It is easier to biopsy with the forceps extended at 90° from the instrument in the direct plane of view of the observer. The biopsy is obtained in a similar manner to that described with Lo Presti type instruments. The biopsy forceps utilized in each type instrument and in the Olympus JFB duodenoscope (Fig. 28-8) are similar.

Selection of Sites

Elevated lesions are biopsied directly from the surface. Ulcerated lesions and ulcers are biopsied from the margins. Kobayashi, et al.[3] correctly point out that areas covered by normal mucosa should be avoided since the chance of positive pick up is remote. Areas of nodularity or discoloration should be searched for in elevated lesions. In ulcers, the base should be avoided since necrotic material alone will frequently be obtained. The inner edge of the ulcer margin should be biopsied. Submucosal tumor will be biopsied in this manner which might be missed if the outer edge of an ulcer margin is biopsied. The biopsy cups measure only approximately 2mm at their greatest depth so that submucosal lesions can easily be missed.

Number of Biopsies

We would suggest a minimum of three biopsies in any sitting. We usually biopsy five to seven times. The value of greater numbers of biopsies has been shown in the diagnosis of carcinoma (vide infra). A similar philosophy dictates that we perform cytology in all cases where biopsy is negative since positive findings have occurred even with multiple negative biopsies.

Accuracy Rate

What of the accuracy of biopsy attempts in carcinoma of the stomach? At the meeting of the American Society for Gastrointestinal Endoscopy which was held in Boston in 1970, Dr. T. Yamakawa[7] stated that approximately 55 per cent of individual biopsies taken in proven carcinomas of the stomach were positive. However, if, as Dr. Yamakawa did, up to six biopsies are taken at the same sitting the incidence of positivity rises to 92.7 per cent per examination. Dr. Yamakawa ringed the lesion attempting to get representative biopsies from all sides of the lesion. He did his work with the lateral-viewing Olympus and Machida instruments. At the same meeting Dr. Y. Yoshii[8] reported her experience utilizing the fiberesophagoscopes of the Machida and Olympus companies. Her experience with proximal gastric and distal esophageal carcinomas revealed a 72 per cent rate of accuracy utilizing one or two biopsies in each case. Her most difficult cases were those where submucosal extension of a high gastric carcinoma into the esophagus precluded passage of the instrument into the stomach. Consequently no effective biopsy could be obtained. Her greatest number of successes occurred when gastric carcinoma extended upwards into the esophageal lumen allowing for biopsy in distal esophagus. These biopsies were invariably positive.

In our own group, the forward-viewing fibergastroscopes such as the ACMI 7089 have become our biopsy instruments of choice. We have learned to take multiple biopsies in all carcinomas of the stomach and our success rate lies intermediate to that of Dr. Yamakawa and Dr. Yoshii. We have been relatively disappointed in attempting to biopsy submucosal lesions. We have obtained negative biopsies on multiple bites of leiomyomata when the biopsy forceps could not penetrate deeper than the lamina propria. The late Dr. Rudolf Schindler has on many occasions pointed out that failure to obtain a deep biopsy is a feature of gastroscopic biopsy instrumentation.

COMPLICATIONS

Blind biopsies carry with them a morbidity of 1 per cent due to bleeding. We have never had a bleeding complication in several hundred biopsies with the Berry biopsy instrument but simply consider ourselves fortunate. Bleeding is almost invariable with fibergastroscopic biopsy instruments, but rarely of clinical importance. We would recommend following the patient's vital signs for 4 hours post-biopsy. Perforation should not occur since the biopsy cups are relatively shallow and cannot reach submucosa in the normal gastric mucosa. The careless examiner with excessive pressure could conceivably pass a biopsy forceps through an ulcer, malignancy, or atrophic stomach.

SUMMARY

In summary, we have reviewed the history and techniques of gastric biopsy which have attained popularity in our country. The newer fibergastroscopes have provided us with effective instrumentation with which to visualize all areas of the stomach. Effective target biopsy is now quite feasible. Multiple gastric biopsies should allow for false negative results of 8 per cent or less in gastric carcinoma, while false positive findings are unknown.

REFERENCES

1. Kenamore, B.: A biopsy forceps for the flexible gastroscope. *Am J Dig Dis Nutrition, 7*:539, 1940.
2. Benedict, E. B.: An operating gastroscope. *Gastroenterology, 11*:281, 1948.
3. Wood, I. J., Doig, R. K., Motteram, R., and Hughes, A.: Gastric biopsy, report of fifty-five biopsies using the new flexible biopsy tube. *Lancet, 1*:18, 1949.
4. Tomenius, J.: An instrument for gastrobiopsies. *Gastroenterology, 15*:498, 1950.
5. Berry, L. H.: A new suction, direct vision biopsy instrument presented and demonstrated on a patient before annual session of the American Gastroscopic Society, (May) 1956.
6. Lo Presti, P. A., and Hilmi, A. M.: Clinical experience with a new forobilique fiber optic esophagoscope. *Am J. Dig Dis, 9*:690, 1964.
7. Owens, F.: Gastric biopsy. Use of the Berry suction biopsy instrument, p. 106-111, in Brown, C. H. ed.: *Diagnostic Procedures in Gastroenterology*. St. Louis, Mosby, 1967.
8. Kobayashi, S., Yoshii, Y., Winans, C. S., Prolla, J. C., and Kirsner, J. B.: Use of direct vision biopsy in the diagnosis of gastroesophageal malignancy. *Gastrointest Endoscopy, 18*:23, 1971.
9. Yamakawa, T., Panish, J., Berci, G., Morganstern, L., Sohma, S., Kidokoro, T., and Hayashida, T.: The correlation of target biopsy.
10. Yoshii, Y., Kuno, N., Yagi, M., and Kasugai, T.: Endoscopy biopsy and cytology in esophageal and esophageal and gastric carcinoma with the fiberesophagoscope, *Gastrointest Endoscopy, 17*:150, 1971.

CHAPTER 28

PART II: GASTRIC POLYPECTOMY

Kenji Tsuneoka and Noboru Watanabe*

INTRODUCTION

IN RECENT YEARS, the development and improvement of the fibergastroscope made it possible to conduct observation and biopsy by direct vision for lesions at every site in the stomach. At the same time, pathological studies, particularly those on the specimens obtained in biopsy by direct vision, have led to rather reasonable opinions on the diagnosis of polypoid lesions of the stomach, especially the problem of atypical epithelium and malignant changes in the gastric polyp.

In gastric polyps with a histologically benign picture, operation should be deferred with the indication for operation to be decided after following up the clinical course.

On the other hand, biopsy procedures for polyps being employed at present are still unsatisfactory in some respects so that overlooking of lesions and possible erroneous diagnosis must be taken fully into consideration in arriving at an accurate diagnosis. In view of the problem of follow-up in non-operated cases as well as the patient's anxiety, the possibility of resecting the gastric polyp with a less invasive method has been looked for.

Fortunately, the development and improvement of the fibergastroscope have made it possible to perform transendoscopic polypectomy by direct

* We acknowledge the cooperation and assistance of Dr. T. Uchida and Staff of the Third Department of Internal Medicine, Nippon Medical School, Tokyo, Japan.

430

vision. We observed during a preliminary experience with this technic that the use of biopsy forceps was unsatisfactory. Repeated bites were necessary for removal of even very small polyps. Small portions of the polyps were often left and disturbing hemorrhage sometimes occurred. After this experience, the snare method using a wire loop was devised. With this technic we have monitored the site of polyp removal and developed a satisfactory method of transendoscopic gastric polypectomy for the first time.[1-4]

THE METHOD OF TRANSENDOSCOPIC POLYPECTOMY
Polyps Selected for Amputation

Regardless of the site, any gastric polyp can be treated by this method. It is important, however, to establish the benign nature of the polyp

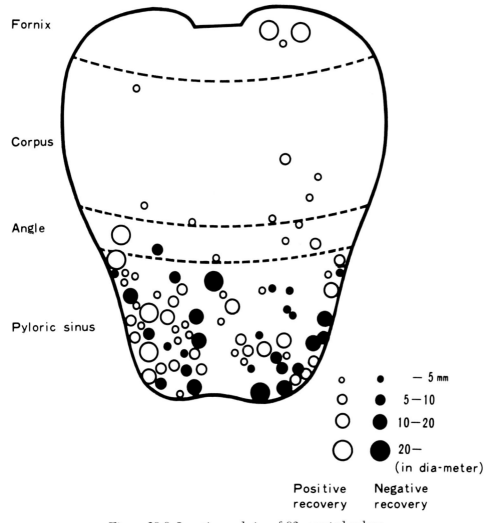

Figure 28-9. Location and size of 83 resected polyps.

through endoscopy and biopsy preoperatively. (In our experience, the result of the preoperative diagnosis by biopsy there were no significant changes of diagnosis from that of chronic gastritis except for 20 polyps which were diagnosed as adenomatous polyp.)

We have already resected 83 polyps with distribution as shown in Figure 28-9. The size and shape of the polyps selected for polypectomy exceeded 20mm in diameter, but in most of the other cases, it was less than 15mm. The shapes of polyps were classified into a type with a stalk, a type without a stalk and an intermediate type. In our experience, the latter two types were slightly more predominant.

Preoperative Preparation

Since this method is carried out by direct vision through a fibergastroscope, preoperative preparation is conducted as in the general observation and biopsy method. Taking hemorrhage into consideration since it is anticipated to occur during or after resection, presence or absence of a hemorrhagic tendency should be tested beforehand.

Administering of hemostatic agent and using sedatives are necessarily combined in order to alleviate the patient's anxieties and fears.

Instruments and Procedure

This snaring or chopping-off method utilizes a stainless steel wire of 0.18mm in diameter. Figure 28-10a illustrates the procedure. The steel loop is folded in two and inserted into the conveying tube and cut slightly longer than the fibergastroscope. Enough of the two ends of the wire should re-

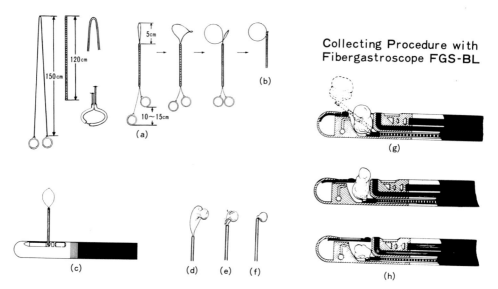

Figure 28-10, a-h. Method I and procedure for resection of polyp.

main so they can easily be grasped outside the conveying tube when the tip of wire protrudes from the tip of the tube by 5cm, as shown in Figure 28-10a.

The difference in distance between the ring and the tube end is adjusted to 10 to 15cm, due to the difference in the length of the two folded wires. The proximal end of the steel wire is then placed through the ring and fixed. This ring for gripping is necessary so that the polyp can be amputated in a direction toward the operator.

When the steel wire protruding toward the operator is pushed into the conveying tube, the doubled-up wire protruding from the tip by 5cm changes into a shape of the loop (Fig. 28-10b). Furthermore, by pushing the grip ring deeper so that two rings are placed together, the folded part at the tip does not change but the wire is spread transversally to form a larger loop. The two grip rings are then pulled together toward the operator. The folded section of the wire is thus trapped at the tip of the conveying tube and the wire forms a loop toward the transverse direction.

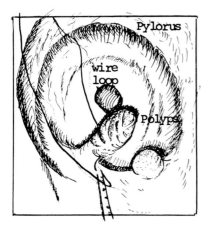

a.

Figure 28-11a. Two polyps at the greater curvature of the pyloric sinus, with opened wire loop and conveying tube.

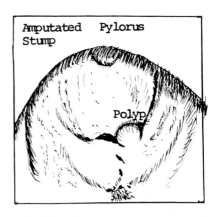

b.

Figure 28-11b. A laceration wound and drained blood after amputation.

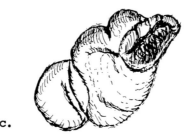

c.

Figure 28-11c. The polyp amputated and removed with method I.

When the ring is pulled further toward the operator slowly but firmly, the folded part is pulled into the conveying tube, forming an open ring due to the tension of the wire (Fig. 28-10c).

These procedures are performed within the stomach through the forceps channel equipped in the fibergastroscope. The size of a wire loop can be adjusted by utilizing the intragastric space and according to the size of polyp to be resected. The loop is placed around the polyp, with the tip of the conveying tube fixed at the base of the polyp. When the grip ring is pulled, the base of the polyp is chopped and amputation is completed (Figs. 28-10d, e, f). The polyp thus resected is gripped with a biopsy forceps inserted anew (Fig. 28-10g), placed immediately in the forceps gutter (Fig. 28-10h) and removed from the body along with the fibergastroscope.

Case one illustrates two polyps on the greater curvature in the pyloric antrum. These polyps were proven to be benign by endoscopic observation and biopsy. Larger polyps are amputated by this method. Figure 28-11a shows a polyp with the opened wire loop hanging around its base. The conveying tube is also shown. Figure 28-11b shows the condition of the amputation site immediately after resection. The hemorrhage was only minimal and it stopped promptly. Figure 28-11c shows the polyp amputated and removed by our method. The cut surface is placed upward. Our histological examination revealed that it was a benign adenomatous polyp.

RESULTS

The results obtained with this resection method are illustrated in Figure 28-9. The site and size of the resected polyps and success or failure of the removal of the amputated polyp from the body of the stomach are also summarized. The summary of the results are as follows:

1. Amputation of the gastric polyp is not very difficult for those who are skillful in gastroscopic observation with gastrobiopsy technic. The sites of the resected polyps were widely distributed to all parts of the stomach (Fig. 28-9). The sizes varied from 3mm to 25mm in diameter and the type with a stalk or intermediate type are slightly more predominant. There were no marked differences seen in the amputation results.

2. When the polyps were located close to the pyloric ring, chances for amputating and retrieval were rather poor. This was due to the amputated polyp falling into the duodenum with the aid of peristalsis in the pyloric antrum. Recently, through the improvement of the instruments and the procedure, we have succeeded in recovering about 75 per cent of the amputated polyps.

3. The histological diagnosis of any recovered polyps should be made with extreme care, especially with regard to the presence or absence of cancer. Up to the present time however, four cases with atypical epithelium

were encounted among 39 cases of adenomatous polyps, but no cancer was found. Moreover, one case of aberrant pancreas and one intramucosal cyst were also found.

ACCIDENTS

Proper consideration should be given against possible accidents, especially hemorrhage. Hemorrhage should be only minimal with proper resection. Such a mild hemorrhage immediately after resection may be favorable compared with that of biopsy, i.e. the former stopped more readily than the latter. After resection, the state of hemorrhage is carefully observed and the procedure brought to an end when hemostasis is confirmed. At least we have never experienced cases that presented any difficult hemostasis or perforations.

MANAGEMENT AFTER POLYPECTOMY

After amputation of the polyp, the patient is made to lie flat for several hours without having any food. For the next two weeks, treatment is given according to general procedures of medical management for gastric ulcer. An endoscopic follow-up is performed after one week, two weeks and one month to confirm the postoperative course and to conduct resection again in cases where some of the polyp remains. One week following polypectomy a shallow ulcer was found in 80 per cent and only reddening was observed in 20 per cent. After another week, ulcer was not found in almost all cases and mucosal elevation was seen in 30 per cent. Except for two cases ulcers completely healed without leaving a trace after one month. The remainder of the polyp recognized as mucosal elevation was easily and completely removed by sampling of several mucosal specimens with the biopsy forceps.

Case two is that of a polyp on the anterior wall at the gastric angulus. The size was 8mm in diameter and 15mm in length. The gross appearance suggested malignancy but biopsy proved it benign (Plate 85). This polyp was amputated and removed with the snare method. A histological examination of removed polyp confirmed it was benign adenomatous polyp. Plate 86 shows the condition of the amputation site one week later, represented by a shallow ulcer with slight gray-white coating. Plate 87 is the picture one month later, the same site shows complete healing.

SUMMARY AND CONCLUSIONS

Excision of gastric polyps has been performed under direct vision by means of a wire snare through the fibergastroscope into the gastric lumen.

1. The method of transendoscopic-gastric polypectomy has been found to be much less difficult and safer in our hands than anticipated.

2. With this method we have found it technically feasible and possible to cut and remove gastric polyps without causing any serious damage to the

surrounding tissues. Fiberoptic gastroscopy is a reliable and effective means for examining the whole area around the gastric polyp tissues. The method described here is also very effective for diagnosing protruding polyps of tumors which may be more difficult to diagnose by conventional biopsy methods. We are, therefore, convinced that our method constitutes an effective diagnostic method for all gastric polypoid lesions.

3. Furthermore, in some of the polyps, especially cancer, exceeding the range of biopsy diagnosis, total polypectomy is very effective for diagnosis.

REFERENCES

1. Tsuneoka, K., and Uchida, T.: Fibergastroscopic polypectomy with snare method. *Gastroenterological Endosc, 11*:174, 1967.
2. Tsuneoka, K., Watanabe, N., Uchida, T., and Kusachi, S.: Fibergostroscopic polypectomy. *Proceedings of the Third Asian Pacific Congress of Gastroenterology,* 356, 1968.
3. Tsuneoka, K., Watanabe, N., and Sato, H.: The present aspect of polypectomy under direct vision. *Today's Therapies and Diagnosis of Gastroenterogical Diseases,* (Igakutosyoshuppan Tokyo), 559, 1972.
4. Tsuneoka, K., Watanabe, N., and Uchida, T.: Endoscopic amputation of gastric polyp. *Naika, 25*:255, 1968.

ENDOSCOPY OF RECTUM
AND COLON

CHAPTER 29

RIGID TUBE PROCTOSIGMOIDOSCOPY: HISTORY, ANATOMY, INDICATIONS, TECHNIC

RAYMOND JOSEPH JACKMAN

439

DEFINITION

As a result of common usage, the word "proctoscopy" has to a large extent supplanted "proctosigmoidoscopy." Throughout this chapter when the word "proctoscopy" is used we imply visual inspection of anal and perianal areas; palpation of the perianal area, anus, and rectum; and visual examination of the anus, rectum, rectosigmoid, and variable amounts of the sigmoid colon. Therefore, synonymous words and phrases for proctoscopy, as the word will be used herein, are "proctosigmoidoscopy," "sigmoidoscopy," and "endoscopy" of the lower bowel. "Rigid tube proctosigmoidoscopy" is in fact what the term implies and is used to distinguish it from "flexible tube endoscopy" to be discussed elsewhere in this treatise (Chapter 30).

Proctoscopy does not require a specialist's skill but should be a part of the diagnostic armamentarium of every clinician, be he general practitioner, internist, or surgeon.

INDICATIONS FOR PROCTOSCOPY

In general, proctoscopy is indicated (1) when there is a history of symptoms relative to the lower part of the large bowel, such as bleeding, pain, constipation, or diarrhea, (2) when any abnormal pathologic process is palpated at digital examination of the anus and rectum, or (3) as part of the annual routine physical examination of older persons, for the detection of cancer. About 70 per cent of all lesions of the entire large intestine, both malignant and inflammatory, can be diagnosed with the ordinary 25cm proctoscope. In general, x-ray studies of the colon should be contingent on the proctoscopic findings.[1]

THE EXAMINING ROOM

The detailed arrangements of the proctoscopic examining room are an individualistic matter, contingent somewhat on the nature of the physician's practice and the number of examinations carried out per day. Figure 29-1 shows the outline of a single examining suite that I found to be satisfactory.

However, there are certain fundamental requirements for any proctoscopic examination room, regardless of how the examination is conducted

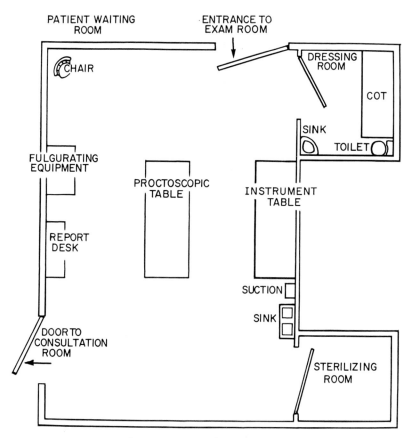

Figure 29-1. General arrangement of a proctoscopic examining room.

or in what position the patient is placed while being examined. (1) A nurse or assistant should be present for numerous reasons, such as properly positioning the patient on the examining table and handing the various instruments to the physician. (2) Immediately adjacent to the examining room there should be a recovery room with a cot, lavatory, and toilet. Reasons for this are obvious. Usually air is left in the lower bowel following the proctoscopic examination and the patient will feel a desire to expel this, thus the necessity of a toilet. (3) Anyone who does proctoscopic examinations should have readily available electrothermia or fulgurating equipment. (Most small polyps—less than 0.5cm in diameter—should be fulgurated when they are first visualized for reasons to be mentioned subsequently.) Equipment for taking of specimens for biopsy and suction apparatus should always be available to the examiner. Certain other ancillary diagnostic equipment to be discussed subsequently should also be at hand.

PROCTOLOGIC HISTORY

It is assumed that for most patients a recorded general history and results of physical examination are available. A more detailed history relative to the anus, rectum, and colon is taken before the proctoscopic examination and is kept as part of the patient's permanent record. This serves as a guide in conducting the examination.

Often, before he is able to arrive at a diagnosis, the physician may have to refer to the more detailed history and physical examination recorded by the internist. If a patient gives a history of transanal bleeding, it is obviously necessary to qualify the character of the bleeding. Bright red blood noticed on the toilet tissue or blood which drips into the bowl after defecation is most likely anal in origin, meaning internal hemorrhoids or an anal abrasion. However, it may be dangerous to assume that such is the case, and the presence of a pathologic process higher in the bowel must be ruled out. Blood from a polyp or neoplasm usually is mixed with the stool and also is bright red. Patients with ulcerative colitis or with most other types of inflammatory processes usually will have variable degrees of diarrhea associated with the bloody discharges. In early ulcerative colitis, a good history may be invaluable because many patients in whom the inflammatory process involves only the distal part of the rectum will give a history of constipation but, on closer questioning, will also tell of an occasional bloody discharge without the passage of stool. It is this type of patient who is sometimes unwittingly operated on for some supposed anal pathologic process, with the result that the wound may heal slowly, if at all, and the colitis may become more active.

Pain made worse by defecation generally is anal in origin as distinguished from high rectal pain that is aggravated by sitting or that extends down the legs.

It is important to know whether rectal treatment has been administered previously, because certain types of medium used in the injection treatment of hemorrhoids may produce intramural tumors (oleomas) which may be confused with other types of tumors.

PREPARATION OF PATIENT

Some physicians prefer to examine the patient without any cleansing of the lower portion of the bowel. They contend that they can learn something about the patient's problem by the character of the stool and by the factor of whether or not the bowel has been completely emptied at defecation. They contend that a soapsuds enema might set up hyperemia which would be difficult to distinguish from an organic inflammatory process. Nonetheless, even though it may be possible on occasions to carry out a satisfactory proctoscopic examination within a few hours after defecation, enough stool often remains in the lower part of the bowel to prevent satisfactory visualization. This is particularly true when one is searching for small polyps.

Patients With Anal Continence

One or more enemas of plain warm water or soapsuds, or enemas continued until the water returns reasonably clear, should be taken within two

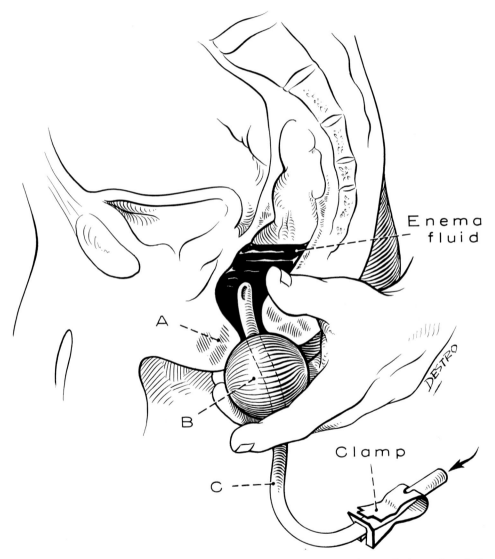

Figure 29-2. For patient with anal incontinence, a 24-F catheter (C) is threaded through hole in soft rubber ball (B) which is pressed against the anus (A) and acts as a plug to retain enema fluid.[4] (By permission.)

hours preceding the examination. Fasting is unnecessary. Catharsis or purgation should be avoided for at least 12 hours before examination because it causes increased irritation of the bowel and usually causes liquid or soft stool to remain in the lower part of the bowel. If a patient comes to the office without preparation or if preparation is unsatisfactory, one of the commercially made enemas of sodium biphosphate or sodium phosphate may be used; this generally gives satisfactory results.

Patients With Anal Incontinence

Cleansing of the lower part of the bowel of a patient who has difficulty retaining liquid creates a different problem and calls for some mechanism such as depicted in Figure 29-2. The enema is prepared in the usual manner, and the patient or nurse is instructed to press the retaining plug firmly against the perineum to keep the fluid in the rectum.

VARIETIES OF PROCTOSCOPES

In 1902, Tuttle produced a proctoscope in which the light-carrier became a part of the instrument itself. A small glass window at the distal end of the light-carrying tube protected the bulb from being soiled by bowel contents. This arrangement is still the basis of most modern proctoscopes. Modifications are available commercially to accommodate the preferences of various physicians; most such variants are entirely satisfactory but some have the disadvantage of being too complicated and are, therefore, difficult to clean and to sterilize.

Regular Anoscopes and Proctoscopes

For active examinations, I prefer the Buie proctoscope which is 25cm long with an outside diameter of 1.8cm. Until recently this scope, which had a tube in its wall to carry the light-stick, used miniature light bulbs that proved to be fragile and expensive. This tube has now been replaced by a fiber-optic that fits into the same channel. Since the light source is several feet from the patient, it has the advantage of being free from the dangers of heat and short circuits. In addition, the transmitted light is of better quality and more uniform intensity, and a single light bulb may last for many years with ordinary use. These scopes are manufactured in various lengths from 25 to 50cm (Fig. 29-3). A small-caliber scope (1.2cm) is advantageous in examining patients with anal or rectal stricture or when a tight stoma exists.

For more detailed examination of the anus or lower rectum, we prefer the Hirschman anoscope which is available in three calibers (Fig. 29-3). When using the anoscope, the fiber-optic light-stick bundle from the Buie proctoscope may be used, or one may use an anoscope with a channel in its wall for the light-stick.

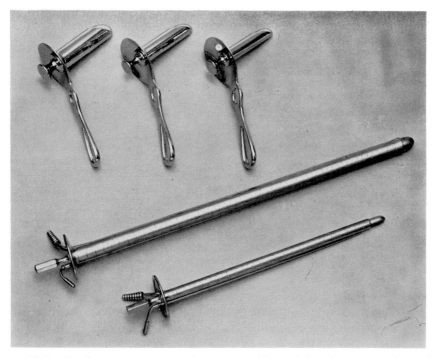

Figure 29-3. Hirschman anoscopes of various calibers (above) and regular caliber (40cm) proctoscope and smaller caliber (25cm) scope (below).[5] (By permission.)

Fiber-Optic Scopes

One recent modification consists of transmission of illumination through bundles of disoriented optic fibers; this is used in two types of instruments. In one type, with integral fiber-optic fibers, a light source external to the instrument is used. The light is transmitted to the fiber-optic bundle built into the wall of the instrument, and these fibers transmit the light to the distal end of the instrument, generally encircling the instrument approximately 2cm from its termination. A second type of instrument utilizes a single, removable fiber-optic bundle which is placed in the channel similar to that used for an incandescent bulb.

Disposable Sigmoidoscopes

Most disposable sigmoidoscopes are constructed of plastic material. Essentially, there are two types: one that readily transmits light and one that does not transmit light. The light-transmitting type is relatively simple because there is no need to have a special part for illumination. The nonlight-transmitting variety requires that a light source be placed in its wall for illumination. Both types are completely adequate for examination. The advantages of disposable instruments include the labor-saving feature plus the constant ready availability of equipment. Disposable instruments generally are less expensive and are economically reasonable for office and hospital use if few proctoscopic examinations are done.

Flexible Scopes

A relatively recent innovation in endoscopy is the use of coated glass fibers of extremely small diameter oriented so that images are transmitted longitudinally within the optical bundle. A parallel bundle of unoriented fibers transmits the light to illuminate the image, and extremely small chromatic lenses are placed at both the distal and proximal ends of the oriented fiber so that the viewer can see the image. Since the glass fibers are pliable, a flexible instrument is achieved which can be threaded through any number of contortions. Further discussion of the technical aspects involved in the use of this instrument will be presented in Chapter 30.

ANCILLARY EQUIPMENT

Suction and Fulguration Apparatus

Some type of suction apparatus should always be available during proctoscopic examination for aspiration of retained enema water, liquid stool, or mucus which might interfere with visualization. The tip of the aspirator should be rounded so that it will not traumatize the mucosa.

Small polyps (up to 0.5cm in diameter) usually should be fulgurated when they are first visualized as suggested previously. These small lesions are usually asymptomatic and are found in about 10 per cent of routine proctoscopies in patients 40 years of age or older. Unless there are some extenuating circumstances, such as firmness, biopsy usually is unnecessary, and to find the polyp again at subsequent proctoscopy might be difficult.

When larger polyps are fulgurated, a Y-type connection in the suction tube facilitates the procedure. One arm of the Y is connected to the smoke aspirator on the fulgurating proctoscope, while the other arm is connected to the liquid aspirator. Each arm of the Y can be closed as desired. During fulguration procedures, liquid and mucus tend to be drawn from the lesion or surrounding bowel as a result of the heat generated, so that from time to time it is necessary to stop the fulguration, close the clamp on the smoke aspirator, and open the clamp on the liquid aspirator to get rid of the accumulated fluid.

Cotton Swabs

Long cotton swabs also should be available during the proctoscopic examination. These are used for two purposes: (1) to push aside a piece of stool or to remove stool which has gotten into the lumen of the proctoscope and is obstructing direct vision, and (2) to ascertain how readily the mucosa of the bowel is traumatized or is made to bleed. Normal intestinal mucosa can be rubbed rather vigorously with a cotton swab without causing any bleeding, whereas the first indication that certain inflammatory processes exist is mucosal bleeding after only slight trauma.

Biopsy Forceps and Removal of Biopsy Specimens

Another instrument that should be available during any proctoscopic examination is the biopsy forceps. Two types of modifications are necessary. The Buie biopsy forceps is used for removal of specimens of tissue from various lesions of the bowel. Bleeding of any consequence is rarely a complication, which means that the practice of fulgurating the site from which a specimen of tissue is removed from an adenocarcinoma or a polyp is largely superfluous. On only one occasion have we seen serious bleeding after removal of a specimen of tissue from a lesion of the bowel. This bleeding occurred in a patient with portal cirrhosis and large rectal varices which extended as far up as the rectosigmoid. The mucosa overlying one varix and the anterior wall was reddened and ulcerated, probably as a result of erosion. Grossly, the possibility of neoplasm had to be ruled out and, when a specimen of tissue was removed from the ulcerated region, blood welled out and filled the rectum within a short time. Hospitalization, the administration of blood, and several days of rectal packing were necessary. Radium packs subsequently were used over the area to produce scar tissue and to help prevent hemorrhage in the future.

To take biopsy specimens from the anus, either local infiltration or nerve-block anesthesia may be necessary. A cutting type of instrument, such as the Myles nasal forceps, is used. Significant bleeding after removal of a biopsy specimen is more likely to occur when tissue is taken from anal lesions, but this bleeding usually can be controlled with a piece of oxidized gauze or with superficial cauterization.

In removing a biopsy specimen when amyloid disease is suspected, it is necessary to obtain a specimen sufficiently deep to demonstrate submucosal blood vessels. This can be done simply by removing the specimen from the edge of a valve of Houston. While not as accurate as a liver biopsy, it is much less formidable. In 25 cases of amyloid disease proved by liver biopsies, 21 rectal biopsies were positive and four were negative. Since it is necessary to obtain a specimen from fairly deep in the tissue and since the arterioles are somewhat rigid and inelastic, fulguration of the biopsied site is sometimes necessary to control the bleeding.

Metal Clips to Delineate Polyps

Sometimes the proctoscopist and the radiologist each identifies a polyp in the sigmoid flexure. Is it the same polyp or two separate polyps? The

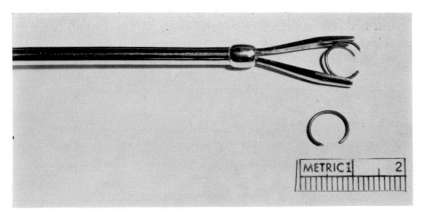

Figure 29-4. Metal ring and application forceps used to delineate lesions.[6] (Printed by permission.)

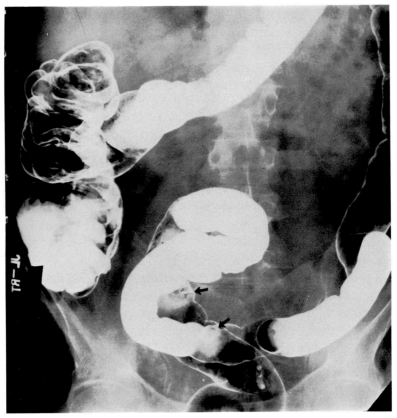

Figure 29-5. Evacuation film. *Upper Arrow,* Metal ring on polyp seen on proctoscopy. *Lower Arrow,* Another polyp located higher in the sigmoid.

question cannot be resolved until the polyp seen via the proctoscope has been removed and the colon has been reexamined roentgenologically. How, then, can the proctoscopist call the attention of the radiologist to the fact that a particular polyp located in the sigmoid has been visualized through the proctoscope? There is a simple way to do this. The proctoscopist applies a partial ring, about 5mm in diameter and made of 23-gauge stainless steel, to the pedicle or near the base of the polyp with a modified Buie biopsy forceps (Fig. 29-4). The ring is more likely to come loose if it is placed in the body of soft adenomatous or neoplastic tissue. This is a safe, simple, and effective method[3] of delineating certain polyps in the sigmoid and spares the patient the ordeal of a second x-ray examination of the colon. It has been our practice to use the metal clip to identify only those lesions situated in the sigmoid, the location in which confusion is likely to occur (Fig. 29-5).

POSITIONS OF PATIENT FOR PROCTOSCOPY

For proctoscopic examination, the patient may be placed in any one of three positions: the left Sims position, the knee-chest position, and the inverted position. In any of these positions, it is desirable that the patient be suitably draped and that a nurse be in attendance.

Left Sims' Position

Use of this position is advantageous if a patient is so ill that the knee-chest position or the inverted position cannot be used. Some physicians prefer to do all their proctoscopic examinations with the patient in this position because patients regard it as less humiliating than the other two positions. However, in our opinion, satisfactory visualization is more difficult when the left Sims position is used. Moreover, this position may cause more discomfort to the patient because the bowel frequently has to be inflated with air in order to pass the proctoscope. If the left Sims position is used, as it sometimes is for patients who are very ill, the examination will be greatly facilitated if the patient is properly placed (Fig. 29-6). The hips of the patient should be at the edge of the bed or examining table. The left leg is extended. The right knee is flexed and the right thigh is drawn well up. The left arm is brought back of the patient, thus permitting the patient's chest to touch the examining table. The hips are in a vertical line. The patient is instructed to sway the back and to allow the abdominal muscles to relax. If the patient is placed thus, the bowel tends to fall away from the pelvis, as in the knee-chest or inverted position, and thus the examination is facilitated.

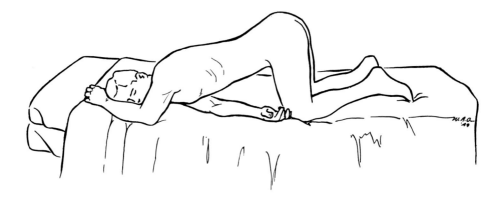

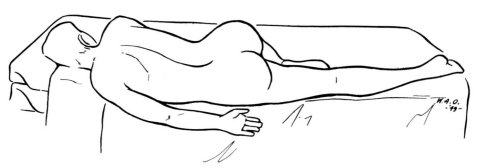

Figure 29-6. *Upper,* Knee-chest position. *Lower,* Left Sims' position.[7] (By permission.)

Knee-Chest Position

This position can be used as a substitute for the inverted position if a satisfactory proctoscopic table is not available. Here again the procedure will be less difficult if the patient is properly placed (Fig. 29-6). When the patient is in the proper position, the thighs are almost vertical and the left arm is placed beneath the patient to bring the chest closer to the examining table. The back is swayed and the abdominal muscles are relaxed; thus, the bowel drops away from the pelvis and the resistance of the abdominal muscles is overcome as the proctoscope is inserted.

Inverted Position

When this position is used, the patient lies on a standard proctoscopic examining table, of which there are many modifications. However, the basic principle is the same. The ideal feature of any proctoscopic table is the

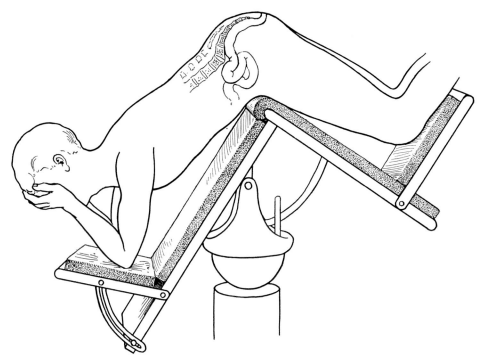

Figure 29-7. Inverted position.[8] (By permission.)

ease with which it can be adjusted to fit the needs of both the patient and the examining physician: the arm and head rest can be removed, the knee rest can be raised or lowered, and the height of the table can be changed as desired. When the patient is inverted, it is important that the abdomen hang free without pressure and that muscle resistance be eliminated (Fig. 29-7).

When a special table is not available, the inverted position also can be used if the patient is placed over the side of a bed or an examining table.

CONDUCT OF EXAMINATION

Vocal Anesthesia

A proctoscopic examination is an office procedure in practically all instances, and the success or failure of the examination depends on the tact and finesse of the physician in obtaining the patient's cooperation. This aspect of the preparation and examination is *vocal anesthesia,* which means simply the practical application of basic psychologic principles, such as anticipating the patient's anxieties and discomforts and advising him of the reasons for these in advance. Buie has made the statement that no one should be permitted to do a proctoscopic examination until he himself has undergone the procedure. We concur in this opinion, because there is no better method of teaching than that based on personal experience.

A short explanation of why the examination is necessary will do much to allay the embarrassments and apprehensions which most persons experience during this procedure. When the patient is properly placed on the examining table and suitably draped, the examining physician might well say something to this effect: "Now I am going to tilt the table forward slowly; you cannot fall. Do not change your position." After the patient is inverted, the examiner proceeds as in any other type of physical examination—that is, inspection and then palpation. After the perianal area has been inspected and palpated the physician remarks: "Now I am going to insert a finger into the anus; if you will try not to resist it, there will be less discomfort."

Digital Examination

In performing the digital examination, it has been our practice to use the left index finger protected by a rubber finger cot. The reason for use of the left index finger is that it leaves the right hand free to receive instruments as needed from the nurse. With the patient in the inverted position and the examiner standing at the patient's left side, the procedure described makes it mechanically feasible to palpate the entire rectal circumference.

First, the anal region should be palpated for abnormalities; then the ischioanal fossae and perineum between the thumb and index finger should be palpated. Then the finger should be brought around the rectal circumference. The examiner should school himself in the same sequence on each rectal digital examination. Personally, after palpating the anal circumference, I insert the finger higher, first examining the anterior wall, then sweeping around to the right side, then the left and posteriorly. For the most part this is actually a bidigital maneuver with the index finger inside the anus and rectum and the thumb outside palpating the intervening tissue of the perineum, ischioanal fossae, and coccyx for areas of tenderness, induration, or tumefaction. Occasionally, it may be advisable to have the assisting nurse bring the table back up to the starting position so that lesions or extrinsic masses situated higher up can be palpated by having the patient strain downward.

An instrument never should be inserted into the anal canal until digital examination has been done or attempted. The reason for this is obvious: Only by digital examination can the examiner learn whether or not it is feasible to use a proctoscope of standard caliber, which is about the size of the average index finger or ⅝ inch in diameter. If a painful anal lesion is causing anal muscle spasm, use of a proctoscope of smaller caliber might be indicated, with some form of topical anesthetic agent. The technique of examination of the patient who has an anal stricture or painful anal lesions will be presented subsequently.

Introduction of Proctoscope

After the digital examination, the assisting nurse hands the proctoscope to the physician, who grasps it firmly in his right hand and makes sure that the obturator is held firmly in position by the thumb. Lubricant is placed

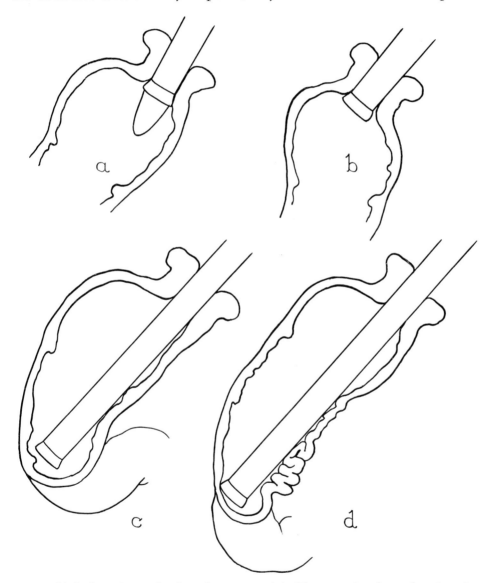

Figure 29-8. Inserting and advancing scope. (a) Obturator in place after inserting through anus. (b) Obturator withdrawn. (c) Scope advanced visually to upper rectum. (d) Bowel usually turns anteriorly as rectosigmoid is entered.

on the anus and, here again, before the proctoscope is introduced, the physician explains to the patient what is to follow: "Now I am going to insert an instrument into the rectum; this instrument is the same size as my finger. If you will try not to resist it by tightening the muscles, it will cause you very little discomfort. Let your back sag down and the abdominal muscles loosen, and continue to breathe slowly through the mouth."

The examining physician must keep in mind the angle between the direction of the anal canal and the direction of the rectum. The proctoscope, still held firmly in the right hand, is aimed in about the direction of the umbilicus and is introduced through the anus (Fig. 29-8). After the resistance presented by the anus is passed, the examining physician transfers the proctoscope to the left hand and removes the obturator with the right hand and puts it aside. The physician maneuvers and passes the proctoscope by continuing to hold the flange in his left hand; this leaves his right hand free to use the suction apparatus, biopsy forceps, fulguration applicator, or other instruments.

Advancing the Proctoscope

From now on, the proctoscope is advanced by direct visualization, meaning that the lumen ahead actually is seen or that a clue to the lumen is seen. As soon as the obturator has been withdrawn, the rectal lumen usually will balloon open as a result of atmospheric pressure if the examining physician has his patient well under control and cooperating. Generally, there is no difficulty in advancing the proctoscope into the upper part of the rectum or into the rectosigmoidal region, where the bowel tends to narrow and to turn anteriorly or to the right or left.

When the proctoscope has been advanced to this point, the physician anticipates what his patient is experiencing or about to experience by saying, "Now, I realize that you have a sensation of fullness which seems like the impulse to defecate, but it is only because the instrument is in the rectum. Your bowel is well prepared. Even though you may have a desire to tighten your muscles, try not to do so, and you will have less discomfort. Continue to breathe slowly in and out through the mouth."

Blind Alley

In my experience, *the proctoscope always can be reinserted as far as it once has been advanced,* and it usually is necessary to withdraw it to determine from what direction a fold of bowel appears. This is a most difficult fact to teach graduate students who are learning to conduct a proctoscopic examination. When the proctoscope seems to be in a so-called blind alley, withdrawal for as much as 5 or 6cm may be necessary. After the fold of

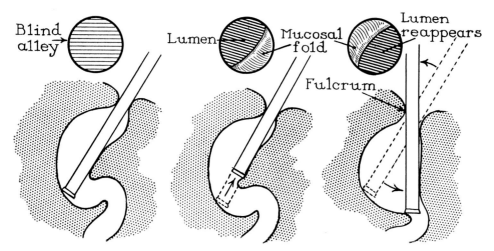

Figure 29-9. Maneuver to overcome "blind alley."[9] (By permission.)

bowel appears in the lumen of the scope, the instrument is advanced again just beyond the fold which is then pushed out of the way. With the anus as a semifixed fulcrum, the proctoscope is angled in the same direction as that from which the fold appeared, until the lumen of the bowel is seen ahead again (Fig. 29-9).

As the proctoscope is advanced into the lower part of the sigmoid, the patient experiences variable degrees of cramp or distress which probably can best be described in the words: "It feels as if I'm going to burst." Hence, the examiner reassures the patient as follows: "Yes, I realize you are having some distress in the lower part of your abdomen, but the examination will soon be over, and it is important that you do not try to protect yourself by tightening your muscles."

Use of Bellows

Most of the detailed examination is carried out as the proctoscope is withdrawn. Use of bellows to inflate the bowel is now permissible, but inflation should be used cautiously because it will only add to the patient's distress. Actually, inflation of the bowel with air to aid in passing the proctoscope is of little value; it causes the patient more distress and can convert a cooperative patient into a tense, apprehensive one who fears that he is going to have a bowel movement.

After the instrument has been inserted the full distance, the patient is reassured in some such manner as this: "Now, I am going to take the instrument out. This might make you feel as if your bowels are moving, but this will not happen; it is only the sensation you have."

When the instrument has been removed, the physician may wish to examine the anus and lower part of the rectum in more detail with an anoscope. This procedure will be described subsequently.

Gentleness and consideration for the patient's anxieties are of utmost importance to successful completion of the proctoscopic examination. Complete cooperation of the patient is absolutely necessary for effective proctoscopy.

If one of the main rectal complaints is protrusion at the time of defecation, it probably is advisable to have the patient strain down while seated on the toilet, and to examine him while he is in the squatting position. Frequently, the degree of protrusion found will be out of proportion to the patient's statement.

Anoscopic Examination

More careful inspection of the anus can be carried out with the Hirschman type of anoscope, of which there are three sizes: large (2.3cm in caliber), medium (1.8cm in caliber), and small (1.5cm in caliber) (Fig. 29-3). The size of the anoscope selected for the examination depends on anal contraction, anal muscle spasm (as caused by a painful anal lesion), and ability of the patient to cooperate. The purpose of the anoscopic examination is to obtain better inspection of the anal canal, such as a search for the primary source of a fistula or for anal ulceration which may have been difficult or impossible to visualize with the standard proctoscope. Moreover, the anoscope affords better visualization of lesions low in the rectum. Before the anoscope is removed, the obturator should be replaced in the instrument. When this is done, the discomfort of the patient is less as the anoscope is withdrawn.

Examination of Patient Who Has Painful Anus

If there is a break in the continuity of the anal skin, such as occurs in anal fissures, anal abrasions, or various types of malignant or inflammatory ulcers, the associated anal muscle spasm may render any examination most unsatisfactory and may cause the patient much discomfort. To relieve such a situation, we use a topical anesthetic agent. A small wisp of cotton is moistened with the anesthetic solution and is inserted into the anal canal with a wooden applicator. The wisp of cotton saturated with the anesthetic agent should be left in place for a few minutes before an attempt is made to insert a finger or an instrument.

Examination Under Anesthesia

Proctoscopic examination with the patient under anesthesia is rarely necessary. In the course of 19,294 proctoscopic examinations at the Mayo Clinic in 1955, only 38 patients (approximately 0.2%) were hospitalized for examination under anesthesia.

Two reasons necessitated the use of an anesthetic agent during these 38 proctoscopic examinations. In 25 cases, although the patient had cooperated well when the examination was attempted clinically, it was the impression of the examining physician that he might have overlooked some pathologic process, such as a deep-lying abscess of the ischioanal fossa, which might possibly be revealed after more satisfactory muscular relaxation was obtained by anesthesia. In 13 cases, the patients were fearful of the examination, some justifiably so because of past experience and some because of an actual painful lesion, but all refused to have the procedure carried out unless it was done while they were under anesthesia.

The type of anesthesia used in all instances was caudal and sacral block, with the patient in the inverted position. Yet, even though preoperative sedation and caudal and sacral block anesthesia are used, the patient usually will experience some degree of abdominal discomfort as the proctoscope is advanced into the sigmoid, because the sympathetic nerve supply to the bowel is not affected by block anesthesia. Since the examining physician is guided to a great extent by the patient's reactions to this procedure, it is necessary to exercise more caution and judgment in passing the proctoscope when the patient's senses are dulled by sedation and block anesthesia.

Use of Analgesics and Sedatives in the Office

I rarely resort to the use of orally or hypodermically administered analgesics, sedatives, or narcotics in either adults or children for the following reasons: If the drug is administered orally, it will take 20 minutes to an hour for it to reach its full effect. While the effect is more rapid if administered hypodermically, in either case it has been my experience that the dulling impact of the drug makes for a less cooperative patient. Proctoscopy, as in many other diagnostic procedures, is a cooperative effort between examiner and patient. This should be explained to the patient and he should be assured that the examination will be stopped if he so requests. I have done this many times to get the patient's confidence, asking him to return a day or two later when he is less apprehensive. More times than not the examination can be successfully completed at the subsequent visit.

I think my main objection to the use of drugs in carrying out a diagnostic office procedure is the hazard that a patient might encounter when released from the office and before the effect of the drug has worn off.

In the case of infants and children who are not old enough to cooperate, it has been my experience that it is far better to have an assistant gently but forcibly restrain them during the examination.

Incomplete Proctoscopic Examination

The usual proctoscope is 25cm long and ⅝ inch in caliber. If the patient is cooperative—and much of this desideratum is contingent on the physician's ability to inspire confidence in the patient—the proctoscope can be passed the full distance, unless some pathologic process in or around the lower part of the bowel prevents it.

In the 19,294 proctoscopic examinations referred to previously, the proctoscope could not be passed the complete distance in 2,864 (14.8%). However, most of these 2,864 patients had some type of pathologic condition that interfered with complete passage of the instrument. Normal anatomic variations such as a short mesosigmoid, inability of the patient to cooperate, and low threshold for pain are other reasons for incomplete passage of the proctoscope.[2]

PERFORATIONS AND INJURIES FROM PROCTOSCOPIC EXAMINATIONS

Over a 20-year period, during which some 350,000 proctoscopic examinations have been performed in the Section of Proctology of the Mayo Clinic, there have been only four severe injuries to the lower portion of the bowel.

Three of these injuries were tears, rather than perforations, at the site of anastomosis in patients who had undergone low anterior resection for carcinoma of the upper part of the rectum. The caliber of the lumen of the bowel through the scarred site of anastomosis was ample for passage of a proctoscope of standard caliber. As the instrument was passed into the rectosigmoid and the sigmoid above, anterior angulation of it was required. This maneuver exerted a pull on the scarred site of anastomosis, and the relatively nonresilient scar tissue gave way. None of the patients complained of discomfort, and the examiner was greatly surprised to see a rent in the scarred anastomosis as the instrument was being withdrawn. Bleeding at the site of the rent was minimal because of the scarring, and, in all three patients, suspicion was first aroused when peritoneal fat was visualized at the site of the tear. Laparotomy was performed in all three patients, and closure was effected within two hours. Recovery of the three patients was uneventful.

The lesson to be learned from these three unfortunate incidents is that any examination of the bowel above the site of an anastomosis may be dangerous when considerable manipulation or levering of the proctoscope is required. Since the scar is relatively insensitive, the examining physician cannot be guided by the patient's reactions.

The fourth patient, a woman in her 80's who sustained a perforation during examination, had what might be considered to be an inevitable predisposition toward this accident. The proctoscopic examination was uneventful except that the patient complained considerably when a specimen of tissue was removed with the biopsy forceps from what seemed grossly to be proliferative tissue that appeared to be invading the bowel from an extrinsic process. During that day, the patient complained of progressively increasing abdominal distress, with fever and rigidity of the lower part of the abdomen. Laparotomy and exploration performed approximately 10 hours after the proctoscopic examination revealed abdominal carcinomatosis and also early pelvic peritonitis. A perforation was noted at the site from which the specimen of tissue had been taken for biopsy. Carcinoma was seen to be invading the bowel in this region, so that perforation probably would have occurred spontaneously within a matter of days.

PROCTOSCOPIC EXAMINATION OF INFANTS AND CHILDREN

In general, infants and children are prepared in the same manner as adults, and proctoscopic examination of them is the same as in adults. Despite the advertising by certain commercial firms to promote the sales of so-called infant-type proctoscopes, we examine children with an instrument of the same length and caliber as that used for adults, unless some anomaly or pathologic process exists. When proctoscopy is done on infants and younger children who are not old enough to cooperate, it usually is necessary to have a nurse hold them in position on the examining table while the procedure is carried out. In some instances, when the child is frightened or difficult to manage or when fulguration of a polyp is required, some sedation may be necessary. Actually, from a technical standpoint, insertion and passage of the proctoscope generally are easier in a child than in most adults because the lower part of the bowel of children has not been subjected to the aging processes and as a rule has not been affected by various surgical procedures or inflammatory conditions that may make the bowel less mobile. Older children tolerate well the examination by the same procedure and vocal anesthesia as used for adults.

REFERENCES

1. Jackman, R. J.: The importance and technic of proctoscopy. *Dis Colon Rectum,* 2:139-148, 1959.
2. Salazar, M., and Jackman, R. J.: Reasons for incomplete proctoscopy. *Dis Colon Rectum, 12*:19-21, 1969.

3. Spencer, R. J., Jackman, R. J., and Witten, D. M.: New device for delineating polyps of lower bowel. *Proc Staff Meet Mayo Clin,* 37:451-453, 1962.
4. Jackman, R. J.: Technique of proctoscopy. *JAMA, 166*:1510-1513, 1958.
5. Jackman, R. J.: Technique of proctoscopy. *JAMA, 166*:1510-1513, 1958.
6. Spencer, R. J., Jackman, R. J., and Witten, D. M.: New device for delineating polyps of lower bowel. *Proc Staff Meet Mayo Clin,* 37:451-453, 1962.
7. Jackman, R. J.: Technique of proctoscopy. *JAMA, 166*:1510-1513, 1958.
8. Jackman, R. J.: Technique of proctoscopy. *JAMA, 166*:1510-1513, 1958.
9. Jackman, R. J.: Technique of proctoscopy. *JAMA, 166*:1510-1513, 1958.

CHAPTER 30

FIBEROPTIC COLONOSCOPY HISTORY, ANATOMY, INDICATIONS, TECHNICS AND PATHOLOGY

Hiromi Shinya, Howard J. Eddy, Jr. and Bergein Overholt

HISTORICAL DEVELOPMENT

I N THIS CHAPTER, THE TERM "colonoscopy" is used interchangeably with "coloscopy," a term preferred by some authorities.

In 1957, flexible fiberoptics were first utilized in a medical instrument in the form of a gastroscope reported by Hirschowitz, Peters and Curtis.[1] Six years later[2] successful fiberoptic colonoscopic examinations were being performed with fiber-sigmoidoscopes ranging from 50 to 60cm in length. Subsequent refinements by American Cystoscope Makers, Olympus Corporation of Japan and other manufacturers have allowed production of instruments to view not only the sigmoid and descending colons (Fig. 30-1), but the entire colon even to the cecum (Fig. 30-2).

Instruments commonly used today incorporate the following features: (A) Fiberoptics for visualization and for light transmission from an external illuminating source. (B) Control of distal tip movement 180 degrees in any direction. (C) A flexible instrument throughout its effective length. (D) Channels for water irrigation and air insufflation. (E) An accessory channel for aspiration of luminal contents or for the passage of a biopsy forceps, a probe, or a cautery-snare device for polypectomy and (F) A proximal end incorporating the various control levers, channels and attachment areas for cameras. The length of these instruments varies

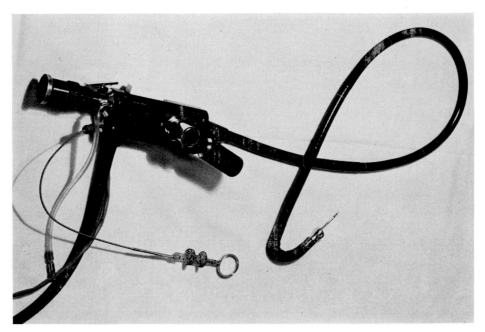

Figure 30-1. One hundred and five cm poly-directional colonoscope with biopsy forceps (ACMI).

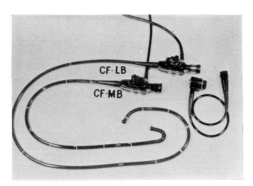

Figure 30-2. Colonofiberscopes. Models: CF-LB (long bundle), CF-MB (medium bundle) and Teaching Attachment (Olympus).

up to 105cm for visualization to the proximal transverse colon to 185cm for visualization of the right side of the colon and terminal ileum.

A.C.M.I. recently produced an operating colonoscope with an extra channel for securing the polyp with a forceps while polypectomy is being performed.

APPLIED ANATOMY

The entire colon can usually be visualized with a colonoscope 150cm or longer. Colonoscopes of 105cm length usually allow visualization of the sigmoid, descending, splenic flexure and right transverse colon.

The sigmoid colon begins at the rectosigmoid junction. It continues to the pelvic brim, often forming a looped or sigma configuration. Thus, this portion of the colon can be expanded tremendously permitting the full introduction of a 105cm of colonoscope unless the technics of sigmoid straightening are applied. In the sigmoid colon, the lumen is of greater diameter and has prominent semilunar configurations. Once the descending colon is reached, one encounters a long straight tube indented along its margin by shallow colonic folds, although an occasional redundant sigmoid can demonstrate a similar configuration. In the proximal portion of the descending colon, one encounters the splenic flexure, a curve occasionally difficult to traverse. The transverse colon typically appears with prominent triangular folds.

The normal mucosa of the colon demonstrates the same soft glistening appearance as does the rectal mucosa. The prominent veins seen often in the distal rectum are not seen above the rectosigmoid junction but a fine capillary network of vessels is readily apparent. Haustral markings are seen throughout the colon.

The hepatic flexure is not as prominent nor does it have the dome-like appearance of the splenic flexure. Because of anatomical variations and less maneuverability of the instrument, the passage of the hepatic flexure and ascending colon is more difficult. The ascending colon is similar to the transverse colon with less prominent folds, less redundancy and a wider lumen.

The cecum is quite large and subdivided into pouch-like recesses by prominent folds and taenial compressions. The ileocecal valve is located in the side wall of the proximal ascending colon, approximately 10 to 15cm from the inferior-most extent of the cecum. The shape and orifice of the ileocecal valve are variable in position, size and configuration.

INDICATIONS AND CONTRAINDICATIONS

The flexible fiberoptic colonoscope, by direct visualization of intracolonic pathology, affords a near-perfect diagnostic tool. It gives the earliest possible means of diagnosing colonic disease.

This is an excellent method of evaluation, and all patients being considered for x-ray should be scheduled for a colonoscopy. However, because of the limitations of time and personnel, this is not yet practicable. Therefore, the specific indications for colonoscopy are:

Table A: Diagnostic Applications

1. Evaluation of the etiology of symptoms referable to the colon in the face of negative x-rays (i.e. bloody mucus, etc.).
2. Evaluation of questionable x-ray findings.
3. Diagnosis of intracolonic neoplasms.
4. Repeated polyp development previously demonstrated by proctosigmoidoscopy, x-ray or laparotomy.
5. Patient with a family history of rectal or colon carcinoma.
6. Regular follow-up for patients with previously-treated colon or rectal carcinoma.
7. Evaluation of the colon prior to all cases of colon surgery, including colostomy closure.
8. Patient with diverticular or inflammatory ileocolic disease, to locate possible pathology masked by the disease process.
9. Evaluation of the "irritable-bowel syndrome."
10. Diagnostic biopsy for parasitic disease.
11. Color-slide and cinephotography for teaching purposes.

Table B: Therapeutic Applications

1. Colonoscopic polypectomy—Shinya Technique.
2. Injection of chemotherapeutic agents directly into malignant neoplasms of the colon.
3. Intraluminal, electrosurgical removal of obstructing neoplasms.

The following conditions should be considered as contraindications for its use:

1. Acute fulminating ulcerative colitis.
2. Acute diverticulitis with systemic reaction.
3. Suspected perforation of the bowel.
4. Abdominal and iliac aneurysm.
5. Paralytic ileus with peritonitis.
6. Partial or complete small intestinal obstruction.
7. Acute inflammatory disease of the anus.
8. Pregnancy.

PREPARATION AND PREMEDICATION
Examining Room Facilities

Complete x-ray facilities, including a tilting table and an image intensifier, are a necessity. A television fluoroscopy viewer is extremely helpful. As the experience of the operator increases, fluoroscopy is used less frequently, and the more skillful endoscopist will seldom have need of these facilities.

Emergency Supplies

An intravenous solution is running when the patient reaches the x-ray suite. The usual emergency medications and oxygen are readily available. Additional analgesics and tranquilizers are also available for use during the procedure, because the patient's comfort is essential to the success of the procedure.

TABLE 30-I

PREOPERATIVE PREPARATION AND MEDICATION FOR COLONOSCOPY

Two days prior to procedure
  Clear liquid diet and Vivonex 100 diet, if desired
Morning of admission
  9:00 AM
    Magnesium Citrate, oz 10 (one bottle) by mouth
Hospital orders if in-patient (or out-patient laboratory studies)
  On admission (approximately 1:00 PM):
    Usual laboratory tests and chest x-ray
    EKG
    SMA$_{12}$ and electrolytes
    Continue clear liquid diet
    Other medications as needed
Day of procedure (procedure usually performed at 1:00 PM):
  6:00 AM
    Fleet Phospho-Soda oz 1-2, by mouth
  1½ hours prior to procedure
    Enemas, half-normal saline, 1 qt., 1 to 2, or until clear
    Prior to procedure start intravenous infusion. Administer meperidine hydrochloride and diazepam intravenously, as needed, in the radiology suite.

The regimen followed in preparing the patient for colonoscopy is explained in Table 30-I.

TECHNIQUE OF COLONOSCOPY

Complete preparation and proper premedication are essential. It is wise to explain to the patient why the examination is being performed and what to expect. As stated above, the procedure is performed in an x-ray room. All equipment, including the light source, instrument, air, water, suction, and biopsy forceps must be checked before each use, and extra light bulbs should be available.

The colonoscope is well lubricated and inserted into the rectum with the patient in the left-lateral position. As with all endoscopic procedures, extreme care and gentleness cannot be overemphasized. The least possible amount of air should be used and excess air aspirated when possible. It is helpful, occasionally, to have an assistant advance and retract the instrument, using a teaching attachment for simultaneous visualization.

Immediately upon insertion of the colonoscope, the entire rectal mucosa should be visualized carefully. Minute mucosal lesions and enema-tip mucosal lacerations can be detected easily with this instrument.

An inexperienced operator may find it difficult to pass through the rectosigmoid junction. However, unless an obstruction is present, with the use of the following techniques, this segment should be negotiated. Changing the patient's position is advisable when a difficult segment of the colon has been reached. The knee-chest position is tried first. If the lumen cannot be observed, "persuasive pressure" may be employed. The result of using this technique is that the steady pressure slides the instrument along the curve of the colon. It is essential that the mucosa be observed to slide by the tip of the colonoscope easily and with a minimum of pressure. If this "slide-by" cannot be seen, the instrument is withdrawn until the lumen can be observed again. The above procedures are repeated as many times as necessary.

If these maneuvers are unsuccessful, Gastrografin is injected through the biopsy channel with the assistance of the radiologist, and the direction to proceed is determined by fluoroscopy and/or spot films.

When the instrument has reached the sigmoid colon, a number of anatomical variations may be present. The most frequent is a long loop of sigmoid colon which may be in the form of a figure eight, an "S" curve, a "J" loop, or a combination of all three. With a long, redundant loop, passage of the instrument through the rectum serves only to increase the size of the loop as the sigmoid is stretched; and the tip, rather than advancing, may be actually retracting, since the force applied is being exerted against the outer periphery of the curve, rather than at the tip. Therefore, it must be kept in mind that the number of centimeters of instrument passing through the rectum is in no way related to the distance the tip is advancing in the colon. For this reason, if for no other, fluoroscopy is essential, as it is possible to insert the entire instrument into a redundant sigmoid while the tip remains at the sigmoid-descending junction.

At this point, with the instrument at the sigmoid-descending junction, the physician is usually looking up the lumen of the descending colon. Another technique is now employed to proceed further. This technique consists of hooking, gentle withdrawal, and straightening with counter-rotation. That is, by maintaining a hook of extreme flexion the instrument is gently withdrawn and rotated in the direction indicated by fluoroscopy, and the sigmoid is thus straightened, leaving the position of the tip of the instrument unchanged (Figs. 30-3a, b, c; 4a, b; and 5). The instrument may then be advanced with the driving force transmitted once again to the tip. In other words, when intervening curves or loops occur, advancing the instrument through the rectum merely serves to enlarge the loop of instrument and stretch the colon. This causes the colon to slip forward off the tip of the instrument and results in the actual retraction of the instrument.

Once the descending colon has been reached and the sigmoid straightened, it is a simple matter to ascend the descending colon to the splenic flexure. Occasionally, the above procedures may have to be repeated one or more times if the sigmoid loop forms again. If only a small loop forms in the sigmoid and the splenic flexure is reached easily, the loop may be reduced by hooking into the splenix flexure. Again, gentleness is essential to avoid damaging the spleen.

In a few instances, it is extremely difficult to advance the instrument beyond the junction of sigmoid and descending colon. Under fluoroscopic guidance, from a left-sided inverted "J" (see Fig. 30-4a) the instrument shaft is gently rotated counterclockwise in such a manner that the colon forms a right-sided, inverted "J." As the instrument is advanced, the "J" forms a configuration resembling the Greek letter alpha, called the "alpha loop" maneuver (see Fig. 30-4b). This loop allows the instrument to be advanced smoothly into the descending colon and the splenix flexure. Some colonoscopists form an alpha loop almost routinely as an aid to negotiating the sigmoid colon with its tendency toward loop formation.

Eddy has recently modified the procedure by placing the patient in a right lateral position at the beginning of the examination and immediately forming an alpha loop.

Recently, three other adjuncts have been employed:

1. A flexible steel wire enclosed in a tightly-wound spiral wire is introduced into the biopsy channel after the sigmoid colon has been straight-

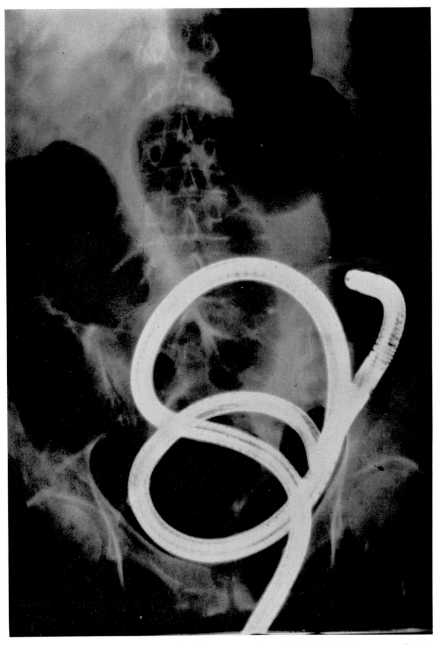

Figure 30-3a. Colonoscope in a redundant sigmoid with a "hook" of extreme flexion.

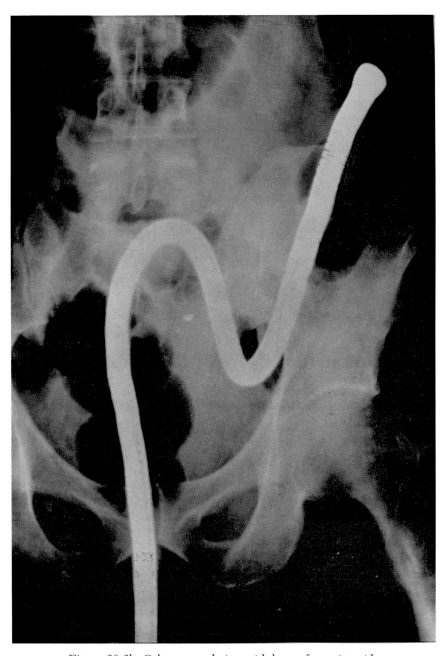

Figure 30-3b. Colonoscope being withdrawn from sigmoid.

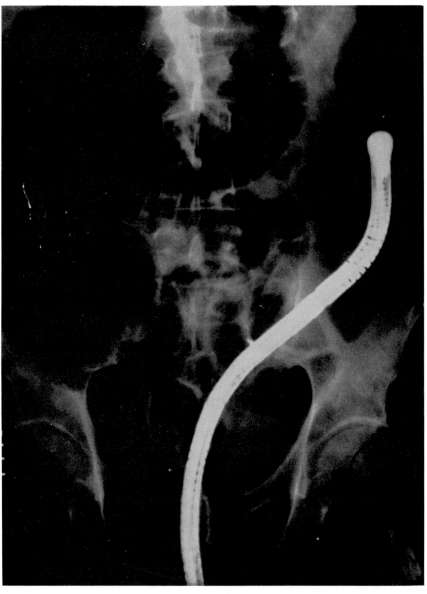

Figure 30-3c. Sigmoid completely straightened with tip in the same position as figure 30-4a.

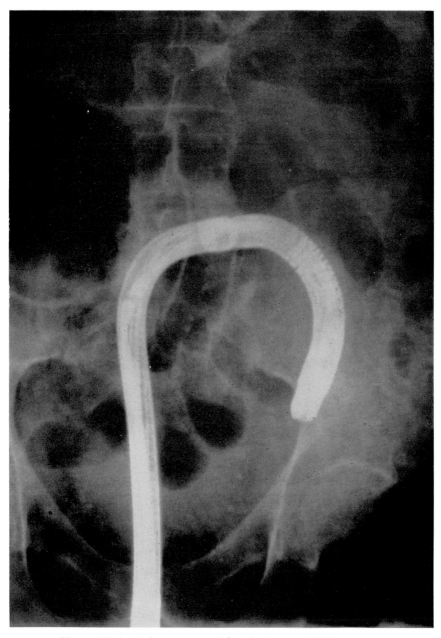

Figure 30-4a. Colonoscope in left-sided inverted "J" position.

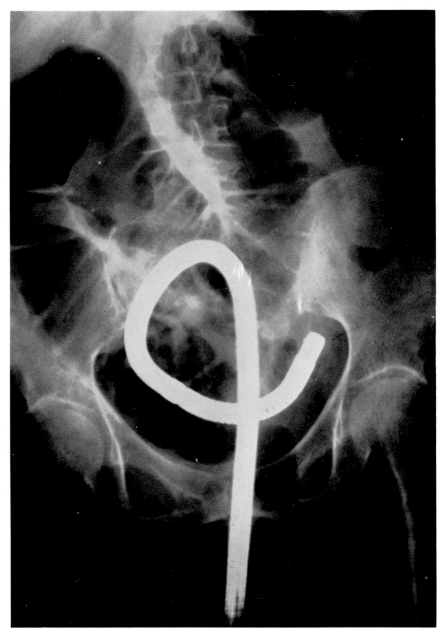

Figure 30-4b. Colonoscope in "Alpha-loop" position.

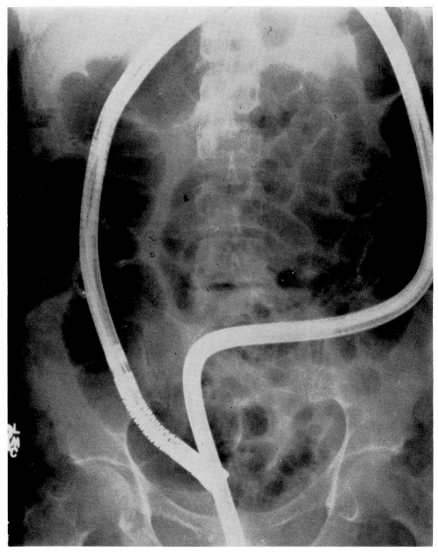

Figure 30-5. Position of colonoscope in the entire colon. Note tip in cecum.

ened. This prevents reformation of the sigmoid loops during later stages of the examination. The wire is usually introduced as far as the mid-descending colon, and thus the instrument can be advanced again. This aid was developed by Peter Dehyle of Zurich, Switzerland.[3]

2. An external "splint" of the colonoscope by use of a splinting tube reaching well into the descending colon, can be applied onto the colonoscope to achieve the same purpose. This method was developed by one of us (Hiromi Shinya).

3. A modification of the Shinya splint has been developed by Eddy, using a number of splints of varying length and stiffness for the purpose of keeping the sigmoid straight.

Once the tip of the colonoscope has rounded the splenic flexure into the distal transverse colon, the redundant sigmoid loop may form again. By repeating the withdrawal-rotation maneuver, the sigmoid loop is again straightened under fluoroscopy. The patient is rotated into the right lateral position and the x-ray table is placed in as much Trendelenburg position as is required for the instrument to reach and round the hepatic flexure. In a number of cases, it is not possible to reach the hepatic flexure by advancing the instrument, due to the presence of a long, redundant, and dependent transverse colon, which is frequently combined with a redundant sigmoid colon. In these cases, attempts at advancing the instrument through the rectum result in withdrawal and retraction of the tip. Therefore, the tip of the instrument can be advanced, by direct vision alone or in combination with fluoroscopy, by the simple expedient of flexing the tip in the direction of the hepatic flexure and actually withdrawing the instrument out through the rectum, thus lifting, straightening, and reducing the angle between the ascending colon and the proximal colon and the proximal transverse colon to as near 90 degrees as possible. At this point the tip of the instrument may be advanced around into the ascending colon or if this can not be done, a further maneuver may be performed, called the "hepatic flip." This involves flexing the tip of the instrument back toward the mid-line in an upward direction as the instrument is withdrawn through the rectum. This results in maximum straightening of the distal-ascending, proximal-transverse angle. Pressure of the hand applied to the abdomen under the transverse colon also facilitates passage of the instrument around the hepatic flexure. Thus, under direct fluoroscopic control, the tip of the instrument is flipped around into the ascending colon. With a colonoscope of 165cm or more this maneuver is not usually necessary. At this point, usually, the instrument may be advanced directly into the cecum (Fig. 30-5), which is about 90cm from the anorectal line when the colon is telescoped onto the instrument and the intervening loops completely straightened. The terminal ileum has been examined to a distance of 50cm in the non-resected bowel.

COLONOSCOPIC POLYPECTOMY

Only well-trained colonoscopists should attempt this procedure. When a polypoid lesion is found by barium enema or endoscopy, histologic verification should be performed. Removal of the polypoid lesion should be done to be certain invasive carcinoma is not present. If evidence of malignancy is absent, treatment is automatically complete.

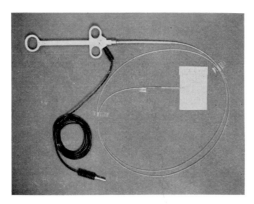

Figure 30-6. Shinya snare-cautery device used through biopsy channel of colonoscope.

Endoscopic excision of benign polyps has many obvious advantages as compared to transabdominal resection of such lesions.[4-6] Polyps beyond the reach of the conventional proctosigmoidoscope can be excised through the colonoscope by Shinya snare-cautery technique.

The Shinya snare-cautery device (Fig. 30-6) consists of a braided, flexible wire of 0.5mm in diameter, doubled over and threaded through a teflon catheter with an outer diameter of 2.7mm. The device is introduced through the biopsy channel of the colonoscope. The snare wire is made to form a loop about 4cm in diameter beyond the tip of the catheter. The wire loop is manipulated around the polyp and tightened about the stalk or the base of the polyp (Fig. 30-6).[5]

Technic, Results

Polypectomy through the colonoscope may be performed both on ambulatory and hospitalized patients, depending on the size and nature of the polyp and general condition of the patient and the skill of the operator. A brief period of hospitalization is preferred for adequate colonic preparation and 24 hours observation after polypectomy.

A complete history is obtained and a thorough physical examination is done before the endoscopic procedure. When the patient is hospitalized, complete blood count, urinalysis, chest x-ray, ECG, blood coagulation studies, relevant blood chemistry determinations and blood typing etc., are performed as routine studies. At the time of the procedure, the patient is given mild sedatives (e.g. diazepam, 5-10mg, meperidine, 25-50mg). The patient is placed comfortably in the left lateral recumbent position. The anal canal and perianal area are well lubricated and the colonoscope is directly introduced. The colonoscope is then advanced as far as feasible and a complete diagnostic examination is performed, if this has not been done previously.

TECHNIQUE OF COLONOSCOPIC POLYPECTOMY

PEDUNCULATED POLYP

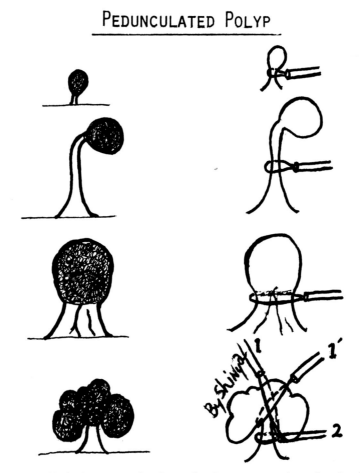

Figure 30-7a. Diagram of technic of polypectomy pedunculated polyp.

Diminutive polyps less than 4mm in size or mucosal excrescences are easily removed simply by taking multiple biopsies. Electrical coagulation or fulguration may also be used for small lesions of this size.

Small sessile polyps measuring in the range of 0.5cm to 1.0cm in size are removed by snare excision or coagulation using the tip of the snare-cautery device. Multiple biopsies of such lesions are taken before destroying them by coagulation.

Larger sessile polyps measuring 1cm to 4cm in diameter can also be excised if they have a narrow base. Broad-based and large sessile polyps may be removed in piecemeal fashion with the snare-cautery technique. The technique of the procedure on both pedunculated and sessile polyps is illustrated (Figs. 30-7a and b). Extreme precaution, skill and experience are mandatory for the performance of this procedure.

After colonoscopic polypectomy, the patient is advised to have a low residue diet, to avoid strenuous physical activity and alcohol intake for about 10 days.

TECHNIQUE OF COLONOSCOPIC POLYPECTOMY

SESSILE POLYP

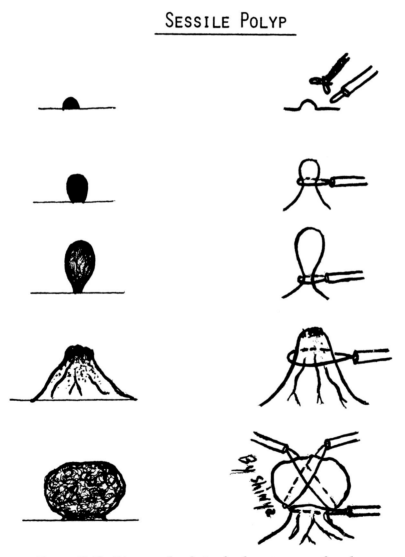

Figure 30-7b. Diagram of technic of polypectomy sessile polyp.

ENDOSCOPIC PATHOLOGY

Malignancies

CARCINOMA: The endoscopic appearance of a malignant lesion is fungoid, crater-like, or ulcerated with puckering or distortion of the neighboring mucosa (Plate 88). Early cancers are often wide-based, polypoid lesions with an irregular, granular surface of reddish-pink color. As the cancer grows, it appears to be a crater-like or elevated plaque-like lesion. A more advanced malignant tumor in the left colon, extends around the colon in an annular fashion, narrowing the lumen. The annular constricting lesion shows heaped up, eroded margins with central ulceration.

In the right colon, cancers are more frequently polypoid and fungating in appearance. The malignant ulcer is usually covered by a whitish, necrotic material.

Infrequently, invasive adenocarcinoma masquerades as a benign sessile polyp under 1cm in size.

CARCINOID TUMORS: These are usually slow-growing tumors occurring in any segment of the colon. Typically, they are light yellow with a *chicken wire* appearance. They may be single or multiple, involve the regional lymph nodes, and may grow to be quite large. They are usually malignant except for the very small lesions found in the rectum.[7, 8]

LYMPHOSARCOMA: Lymphosarcoma is an extremely rare lesion of the colon found almost anywhere in the colon.[9] From an endoscopic point of view it may be suspected but diagnosis will have to rely upon the biopsy.

Polyps and Non-Malignant Neoplasms

POLYPS: The pedunculated polyps are usually adenomatous and are commonly sized from 1 to 2cm in diameter. They are soft, red, raspberry-like tumors, with a long slender stalk of colonic musoca. The tip of the pedunculated polyp (Plate 89) is occasionally congested, necrotic, with fresh blood or blood on the mucosa of the adjacent colon.

A larger, broad-based sessile polyp is usually the villous (papillary) adenoma. It has a soft, pink-red, cauliflower appearance.

Recently, Shinya and Eddy have encountered a number of polyps demonstrating both villous and adenomatous properties in the same polyp.

FAMILIAL POLYPOSIS: These lesions may start out as benign adenomatous polyps, but almost always become malignant.[10] Usually the malignant changes begin to occur in the twenties or early thirties. Endoscopy reveals a complete spectrum of sizes from superficial mamillations to actual pedunculated polyps. Frequently, the bowel has a rug-like appearance due to the tremendous numbers of these lesions.

JUVENILE POLYPS: Classically these are found in children.[11] Most frequently they are single but may be multiple. Grossly, the juvenile (retention) polyps appear to be inflammatory, but are difficult to distinguish from other types of polyps seen after adolescence.

MALIGNANT POTENTIAL OF POLYPS: At present, this is a seemingly impossible task to answer accurately, but after extensive review of the literature, the majority of the material indicates that at least a moderate number of polyps are pre-malignant. Even more important is the fact that a malignant potential appears to exist in that particular patient's mucosa. Furthermore, the true significance of finding a polyp is not so much in the polyp itself, but in the necessity for a complete examination of that patient's colon for further polyps or adenocarcinoma, both at the time of initial discovery and in the future.

Perhaps the best answer to those who claim to have found a specific answer to this problem was stated by Culp,[12] "Ideal proof—or disproof—of the adenoma-carcinoma sequence would require that an adenomatous polyp be removed from the bowel, sectioned for intimate study, reassembled, returned to its original site, and allowed to progress to its ultimate fate." The work of Spratt, Ackerman, and Moyer[13] on the relationship of polyps of the colon to colonic cancer, in 1958, stated that adenocarcinoma of the colon arises de novo and does not develop from pre-existing adenomatous polyps. In 1962, Castleman and Krickstein[14] agreed with this premise.

Since that time, a number of excellent and well-documented articles have been published which would appear to prove, by means of the scientific follow-up and statistical analysis of the results obtained, that varying percentages of polyps are definitely pre-malignant.

At this writing, this author has found several polyps in the four to six millimeter range with varying amounts of atypia present. In one polyp, complete replacement of the adenomatous elements had occurred but without invasion of the basement membrane. In addition, there were four, fully-invasive adenocarcinomas in the six to eight millimeter range. All of these lesions were sessile.

On the other hand, in pedunculated lesions, a complete progression of pathology has been found from atypia to fully-invasive adenocarcinoma involving the stalk.

Most authors agree on the pre-malignant potential of the villous or papillary adenoma.

The preponderance of opinion in the literature of the world today is as follows: that polyps are pre-malignant but that no one can prove that all polyps will become cancer eventually; and that the polyp indicates a potential malignant predisposition of that particular patient's colonic mucosa.

LIPOMAS: The lipoma is usually submucosal and is easily recognized by direct vision. It is a simple matter to palpate it with a biopsy forceps and feel its inherent softness. It may be removed with the electro snare if it is creating symptoms.

LYMPHOID POLYPS (BENIGN LYMPHOMAS): These are usually found in the colon, although they may be found in the rectal area.[15] They may be either single or multiple, and are typically submucosal. They are rare and found more in children. They are smooth, pale, or yellow in appearance.

ANGIOMA: This lesion is extremely rare. Most of these lesions disappear at birth or shortly thereafter. Females are affected more often than males. The lesions originate in the submucosa, and are composed of blood vessels or lymphatics. They may be single or multiple.

FIBROMA: This rare lesion occurs primarily in adults and is found encapsulated in the submucosa. It is usually a single lesion which grows slowly.

MYOMA: This rare lesion is similar to the fibroma but it may be either sessile or pedunculated.

Inflammatory Lesions

Non-Specific Ulcerative Colitis

In the earliest stages, the mucosa shows scattered hemorrhages and marked hyperemia. Later, the mucosa is irregularly ulcerated leaving strips and islands of intact mucosa. If the ulceration is deep, the patches of mucosa between the ulcers stand out prominently.

Crypt abscesses are also noted as pinpoint to 1 to 2mm submucosal blisters. In the chronic active phase, the normal mucosa is completely destroyed and covered with multi-colored, necrotic mucus with multiple pseudopolyps which are usually covered with a whitish mucus (Plates 90 and 91).

In the long-standing inactive cases, the mucosa is markedly scarred and appears markedly atrophic. There are scattered pseudopolyps in various sizes. The length of the colon is markedly reduced and normal configuration of the colonic folds is lost. The lumen of the colon is narrowed and tubular.

There are the specific colitides—amebiasis, bacillary dysentery and tuberculous colitis which vary in incidence throughout the world. With amebiasis, where isolated ulcers are found, moniliasis, bacillary dysentery and tuberculous colitis, all of which can resemble ulcerative colitis, the colonoscope is invaluable for diagnosis.

Colitis of Obscure and Unusual Origin

Monilial colitis, which is on the increase recently, due to the widespread use of broad-spectrum antibiotics, occurs from several days to several weeks following the oral ingestion of antibiotics.

Granulomatous Colitis

This disease usually involves the colon from the cecum to the sigmoid colon and frequently skip-areas of involvement are present. The terminal ileum is involved in a high percentage of cases.

The mucosal appearance may be difficult to distinguish from that of chronic ulcerative colitis in certain stages, especially in the diffuse involvement of the disease from cecum to rectum.[16]

The typical colonoscopic appearance is characterized by skip areas of edematous and erythematous granular mucosa with nodularity accentuated by scattered linear ulceration.

The histologic examination on colonoscopic biopsy is not usually diagnostic. The differentiation between granulomatous colitis and chronic ulcerative colitis in the endoscopic appearance, should be correlated with the radiologic and clinical features.

Diverticular Disease

Diverticular disease classically has been divided into diverticulosis and diverticulitis.[17, 18] Endoscopically the appearance of diverticular disease without inflammation shows marked prominence and thickening of the folds which stand out almost so much as to obscure the view of the lumen. In between these folds are the diverticula of varying sizes. Occasionally the lumen is noted to be actually narrowed. Frequently, inspissated feces are noted within the diverticular orifices. In acute diverticulitis the mucosa may be markedly edematous and erythematous with submucosal petechiae. Much more spasm is noted along with more frequent narrowing of the lumen. In these cases, it is wise to proceed with caution.

Functional Disorders

IRRITABLE COLON: This is often thought of as a functional disease usually occurring in neurotic females and has been variously called spastic colitis, mucous colitis or myxorrhea coli. Colonoscopy reveals moderate to extreme sigmoid colon redundancy with frequent associated transverse colon redundancy. In addition, endoscopy occasionally reveals previously undiagnosed diverticular disease as there can be an overlapping of these two conditions.

Further, it is felt that with the redundancy present, many of these individuals may suffer from intermittent volvulus of the sigmoid and/or transverse colon and again, this discomfort has been reproducible with the colonoscope. The colonoscope is the single best instrument which can be used to evaluate these patients, because the use of it allows the clinician to evaluate the following pathology: the true extent of the redundancy of the sigmoid and transverse colon, the location of previously undiagnosed diverticular or other intra-colonic pathology, the tendency to volvulus, the presence of fixed adhesions, or the existence of actual motor abnormalities.

Miscellaneous Disorders

ENDOMETRIOSIS: This condition occurs during the child-bearing years. It is usually found in the anterior rectal wall, ranging from a few millimeters to approximately 1cm. It is exquisitely tender to palpation. On some occasions, it may even cause a deformity with thickening and/or stricture of the sigmoid colon. It may give rectal bleeding related to the menses.[19]

COLITIS CYSTICA PROFUNDA: Colitis cystica profunda[20, 21] (Plate 92) is a benign condition in which a flattened circumscribed mass which appears to be submucosal or intramural, is found approximately 5 to 12cm above the anal verge but may be found higher up in the colon. Endoscopic appearance can be very similar to that of adenocarcinoma and for this reason extreme care must be exercised in diagnosis and treatment of this condition.

MELANOSIS COLI: In this condition, endoscopically (Plate 93), there is seen a reticulated discoloration of the mucosa which can be almost black depending on how much ingestion has taken place of the anthracene cathartics of which cascara is the most common. This will be noted from the anal rectal line all the way to the cecum. Upon discontinuation of the particular cathartic, the pigmentation will gradually disappear.

PNEUMATOSIS CYSTOIDES INTESTINORUM: This is an uncommon disease in which gas cysts (Plate 94) develop in the walls of the colon which may be located in the subcirrhous or submucosal layers. They may occur in large numbers and vary in size from 1mm to several cm. Endoscopically one notes these clear colored *blebs* which upon biopsy, explode with a *loud pop*.[22]

ISCHEMIC COLITIS: This condition has been described as a transitional phenomenon between a syndrome of abdominal angina and mesentery infarction.[23] A constantly changing picture by radiology and/or endoscopy is pathognomonic of this. The splenic flexure is one of the most common locations although any segment, including the rectum, may be involved. Early endoscopy may show a picture which can be mistaken for ulcerative colitis with ulcerations, edema and friability. This condition can be found in a continuous segment of rectum or colon, or may be seen in skip areas. Later on, the endoscopic appearance shows areas of large superficial ulceration covered with necrotic material. Adjacent mucosa is usually erythema-tous and may actually be hemorrhagic. Still later, stricture formation is present. L. F. Williams, Jr.[24] reports, "The problem of ischemic colitis proximal to carcinoma of the colon, deserves special mention. Since there is often a segment of a normal colon between the neoplasm and the proximal ischemic segment, the carcinoma can be overlooked even on barium enema. At least 40 cases of this problem have been reported, and associated colonic car-cinoma has been found in 10 per cent of the patients with ischemic colitis. So it may be much more common than currently expected."

RADIATION COLITIS: This condition is found in the patient who has received radiation to the uterus or cervix. Usually the lesions are confined to the anterior rectal wall appearing 8 to 10cm proximally in the rectal line. However, occasionally they will occur more proximally with telangiectasia, friability, easy bleeding, stricture, ulceration, or even fistulization.

POST-OPERATIVE LESIONS: Anastomoses may result in narrowing, granula-tion tissue, or even sutures being present. Granulation tissue which may cause sufficient bleeding to give the patient and clinician concern, may be fulgerated easily. Any sutures which are present can be removed with a biopsy forceps reducing the amount of tissue reaction and resulting granu-lation tissue formation.

ACCIDENTS AND COMPLICATIONS:
PREVENTION AND MANAGEMENT
Perforation

The most serious accident which can occur during colonoscopy is per-foration of the bowel. This may occur by pushing the instrument directly through the bowel wall usually in an area of sharp angulation and fixation or through a large diverticulum which has been mistaken for bowel lumen. Conceivably, perforation can be partly caused by excess air insufflation through a diverticulum or a distant blow out of a thin walled cecum. Par-ticular care, therefore, must be exercised in colonoscoping the patient with inflammatory conditions, ulcerated carcinoma, radiation injuries, strictures or atrophic bowel wall.

Polypectomy through the colonoscope with the use of surgical dia-thermy, requires practice, experience and dexterity. The degree or depth of electrical coagulation required for transection of the stalk or of coagu-lation of small polyps is gained only by experience. Colonoscopic removal of polyps should not be attempted until considerable training and skill in the use of the colonoscope is achieved.

We have never encountered any perforation during polypectomy, al-though the snare-cautery technic has been carefully employed as far as the colonoscope can reach even to the cecum. Perforations may occur during the snare-cautery procedure especially when the lesion cannot be visualized well enough for the safe looping of the stalk of a polyp or during faulty sessile polypectomy. Perforations have occurred in a few hospitals following colonoscopic polypectomy. Subcutaneous emphysema of neck and face, pneumoperitoneum with air under the diaphragm and abdominal pain have been noted in these cases.

Bleeding

Insignificant bleeding may occur during the first few days following excision of the pedunculated polyp. In our experience of several hundred electrical excisions of polyps ranging in size from 0.5cm to 5.0cm, we have encountered a 1 per cent incidence of inconsequential bleeding within the first ten days following polypectomy. In no instance did the bleeding require surgical treatment. No complications have occurred following coagulation of the tiny polyps, in our hands.

When larger polyps are incompletely excised or coagulated, bleeding may persist. In instances of persistant bleeding, additional polyps not excised or hemorrhoids can also contribute to the bleeding episode.

Explosions

Hazardous gas explosions during polypectomy are very unlikely because the adequately cleansed colon is free of explosive gases and the gas content of the colon is continuously exchanged by inflation and expulsion of air during introduction of the instrument and colonoscopic polypectomy. However, a flow of inert gases, such as carbon dioxide or nitrogen, can easily be introduced into the colon and to the area of polypectomy through the colonoscope.

Indirect Injury and Medical Complications

Damage to adjacent organs can occur if an excess amount of pulling is exerted during the withdrawal and straightening maneuvers of the various intestinal loops. Caution in the area of the spleen is especially important as the spleen is easily torn.

Careful consideration of indications and contraindications will usually eliminate medical complications. However, the patient must not be subjected to undue physical stress and his general condition must be observed throughout the procedure to avoid possible medical complications. The avoidance of medical complications requires the skills and experience of a doctor who is first and foremost a clinician and only secondarily an endoscopist. Adequate consideration must be given for example to elderly patients who may have no overt or apparent heart or lung lesion but who have chronic disease with low cardiac or pulmonary functional reserve. Patients with chronic congestive heart failure or healed post-myocardial infarction, chronic obstructive lung disease or marked senile emphysemia may be potential candidates for medical complications due to required inflationary and instrumental pressures in the upper abdomen during colonoscopy.

Management

An obvious gross perforation would demand an immediate laparotomy. However, even a gross perforation may be missed and a minimal perforation due to leakage of air through a small diverticulum is even more difficult to determine. Should a question of perforation exist, the usual surgical and medical precautions for a perforated abdominal viscus should be taken. Upright, reclining, decubitus x-ray views of the abdomen along with chest PA and lateral x-rays should be at once performed. Intravenous infusion and appropriate antibiotics should be started. The patient is allowed nothing by mouth. Vital signs are monitored every 15, 30, and 60 minutes or as indicated by patient's condition. Immediate surgical consultation is called and the patient is continuously observed.

If a gross perforation is seen, the instrument is left in place, while immediate x-rays of the chest and abdomen are taken. Appropriate antibiotics are administered not only intravenously but also through the biopsy channel intraperitoneally. While the preparations for surgery are being completed, any further studies can be performed, but the colonoscope should be left in place to facilitate the location of the perforation during laparotomy. Again, immediate surgery is a necessity.

In a case of pneumoperitoneum during gastroscopy, a simple effective procedure is reported in Chapter 32. The patient was having marked cardio-respiratory distress associated with abdominal distension. A spinal puncture needle with obturator was introduced through the abdominal wall and the abdomen deflated while preparation was being made for laparotomy. The patient immediately became comfortable. This procedure would probably be important in a similar situation occurring during colonoscopy.

The management of bleeding can usually be handled conservatively. The same preoperative examinations, arrangements, and preparations which are made before major colon surgery are required before polypectomy. Minor bleeding at the site of biopsy or snare-cautery has not required transfusion. We have known of at least one case of bleeding without perforation which required transfusion and no major intervention.

Drug reactions are managed in the same manner for any gastrointestinal endoscopic procedure and are discussed in detail in Chapter 4.

REFERENCES

1. Hirschowitz, B. I., Peters, C. W., and Curtiss, L. E.: Preliminary report on a long fiberscope for examination of stomach and duodenum. *Univ Michigan M Bull,* 23:178, 1957.

2. Overholt, B. F.: Description and experiences with flexible fibersigmoidoscopes. *Proceedings Sixth National Cancer Conference,* Philadelphia, Lippincott, 1970.

3. Deyhle, P.: Flexible steel wire for the maintenance of the straightening of sigmoid and transverse colon during coloscopy. *Endoscopy,* 4:36-38, 1972.

4. Wolff, W. I., and Shinya, H.: Colonfiberoscopy. *JAMA, 217*:1509, 1971.

5. Wolff, W. I., Shinya, H., and Geffen, A.: Colonofiberoscopy. *Am J Surg, 123*:180, 1972.

6. Wolff, W. I., and Shinya, H.: Colonofiberoscopy: Diagnostic modality and therapeutic application. *Bull Soc Int Chir,* 5:525, 1971.

7. Jackman, R. J.: Submucosal rectal nodules with particular reference to carcinoids. *Am J Surg,* 88:909, 1954.

8. MacDonald, R. A.: A study of 356 carcinoids of the G.I. tract. *Am J Med, 21*:867, 1956.

9. Helwig, E. B., and Hanson, J.: Lymphoid polyp (benign lymphoma) and malignant lymphoma of the rectum and anus. *SG and O, 92*:233, 1951.

10. Morson, B. C.: Some leads to the etiology of cancer of the large bowel. *Proc R Soc Med, 64*:959, 1971.

11. Horrilleno, E. G., Eckert, C., and Ackerman, L. V.: Polyps of the rectum and colon in children. *Cancer, 10*:1210-1220, 1957.

12. Culp, C. E.: New studies of the colonic polyp and cancer. *Surg Clin North Am,* 47:955, 1967.

13. Spratt, J. S., Jr., Ackerman, L. V., and Moyer, C. A.: The relationship of polyps of the colon to colonic cancer. *Ann Surg, 148*:682, 1958.

14. Castleman, B., and Krickstein, H. I.: Do adenomatous polyps of the colon become malignant? *N Engl J Med, 267*:469, 1962.

15. Cornes, J. S., Wallace, M. H., and Morson, B. C.: Benign lymphomas of the rectum and anal canal: a study of 100 cases. *J Path Bact, 82*:371-382, 1961.

16. Edward, F. C., and Truelove, S. C.: The course and prognosis of ulcerative colitis, III. Complications. *Gut,* 5:1-22, 1964. [Excellent review.]

17. Mailer, R.: Diverticula of the colon: a pathological and clinical study. *Lancet,* 2:51-58, 1928.

18. Morson, B. C.: The muscle abnormality in diverticular disease of the colon. *Proc R Soc Med, 56*:798-800, 1963.

19. Spjut, H. J., and Perkins, D. E.: Endometriosis of the sigmoid colon and rectum. *Am J Roentgen, 83*:1070-1075, 1959.

20. Epstein, S. E., Ascari, W. Q., Ablow, R. C., Seaman, W. B., and Lattes, R.: Colitis cystica profunda. *Am J Clin Path, 45*:186-201, 1966.

21. Wayte, D. M., and Helwig, E. B.: Colitis cystica profunda. *Am J Clin Path, 48*:159-169, 1967.

22. Ramos, A. J., and Powers, W. E.: Pneumatosis cystoides intestinalis: report of a case. *Am J Roentgen, 77*:678-683, 1957.

23. Friedman, G., and Sloan, W. C.: Ischemic enteropathy. *Surg Clin North Am,* 52, No. 4, Aug., 1972.

24. Williams, L. F., Jr.: Vascular insufficiency of the intestines. *Gastroenterology, 61*, No. 5:757, 1971.

MISCELLANEOUS SUBJECTS OF IMPORTANCE IN UPPER GASTROINTESTINAL ENDOSCOPY

CHAPTER 31

PART I: AGGRESSIVE ENDOSCOPY IN UPPER GASTROINTESTINAL HEMORRHAGE

Eddy D. Palmer

INTRODUCTORY STATEMENT

THE DESPERATE EMERGENCY created by massive upper gastrointestinal hemorrhage loses some of its sting as soon as the bleeding lesion has been identified. A quick accurate diagnosis is important because when the hemorrhage makes the demand for some radical control measure, the surgical or other manipulative effort can immediately be directed at the responsible lesion. As surgical capabilities improve, the need for specific diagnosis upon the patient's arrival in medical hands becomes more urgent.

It perhaps is no longer necessary to emphasize that an important responsibility of the gastroenterologic endoscopist these days is to make himself quickly available for emergency help with the bleeder. Experience from many quarters during the past several years indicates that, when carried

out in a thoughtful manner by an experienced clinician-endoscopist, endoscopic study is able to furnish information that is essential for optimal
management of the bleeder.[1-7]

POINTS OF TECHNIC

There is no patient who requires more careful individualization than
the patient with severe upper gastrointestinal bleeding. Nevertheless, the
past several years have witnessed the cautious unification of many previously divergent ideas about diagnostic management, so that today certain
steps can be considered *routine*. All can agree that the effort must be a
team project from the moment that hemorrhage is recognized. Many people from many services will share responsibility for management—gastroenterologist, radiologist, surgeon, nurse, laboratory technician, blood bank
technician, electrocardiographer, chaplain, and many others. At the start
there will be a lot going on all at once, emphasizing the need for some degree of team routine.

In addition to assessment of the effects to the moment of the current
bleed, there is need for quick evaluation of the patient's medical background, with special attention to possible cardiopulmonary problems, kidney disease, diabetes, and chronic liver disease. Resuscitation is begun immediately, with emphasis on quick blood replacement.

Ice-water lavage of the stomach immediately follows the history and
physical examination as the most effective emergent move short of surgery
to stop the bleeding, whatever its source, and as the best way to clear the
tract of blood prior to endoscopic and radiologic study. The lavage must
be competently carried out with a large-bore Ewald tube, until the returns
are clear or almost so. The average bleeder requires about two quarts of
ice water instilled and withdrawn successively by 50ml Toomey syringe, for
effective lavage. This takes about twenty minutes. Esophagogastroscopy immediately follows.

Identification of the bleeding lesion[8] and discovery of other abnormalities of the upper tract require, in order, pharyngoesophagoscopy, gastroscopy, hopefully duodenoscopy and upper gastrointestinal contrast roentgenography. All procedures must be carried out with the patient horizontal because of the shock problem, a handicap primarily to the radiologic part of
the investigation.

At what point in the resuscitative effort it is proper to go ahead with the
diagnostic study is not difficult to decide. Restoration of the circulating
volume is the most pressing need. The ice-water lavage has important therapeutic potential and should not be delayed once the patient has com-
menced to come up out of shock. The endoscopic procedures ordinarily
should be carried out as soon as the lavage is complete but only after a

good start has been made at controlling hypotension. A quick diagnosis is essential and the peroral manipulations do not add to the shock; however, continued deep shock clearly demands activities aimed wholly at its treatment.

INDICATIONS FOR IMMEDIATE PANDIAGNOSTIC EFFORT

In the usual general hospital patient population, about half of upper gastrointestinal bleeders are admitted with bleeding that is obviously active, with observed hematemesis or evidence of recent hematemesis on the clothing. The other half raise doubt at first either over whether the bleeding has recently stopped or whether there has been any bleeding at all. In the latter group aspiration of gastric contents by Levin tube at the very start gives information that is invaluable for planning both the diagnostic effort and the therapy.

The usual rule is that, if there is any active bleeding at all, advantage should be taken of it by looking for its source endoscopically. This is so even when the current bleed is of small amount. Although initially the emergency pandiagnostic technic was intended to assist management of the massive bleeder only, it has become adopted for diagnostic management also of the small bleeder as its practicability has proven itself. Taking advantage of the period of active bleeding has been found important, in order to preclude the diagnostic vacuum that so often follows cessation of a small bleed. The technic has worked well in this situation.

The main prerequisite for the endoscopic study, then, is simply active bleeding at the moment, so the endoscopist may find the lesion that is doing the bleeding and hopefully identify it.

PREPARATION OF THE PATIENT

The bleeder is ordinarily a frightened patient. Once explanations have been given regarding the medical problem and the necessary diagnostic and therapeutic manipulations, he almost always becomes a cooperative patient. Even though a great deal of activity is required for early assessment and resuscitative effort, causing everyone concerned to be extraordinarily busy, all must understand that the patient requires explanations and answers to his questions as much as he requires blood. When his fears are attended to, it is unusual for him to employ tactics designed to delay the examination. He wants attention. He wants the study and treatment to go well and without delay. Because of this and because the fresh bleeding directs the endoscopist to the diseased area, endoscopy carried out for the care of the bleeder is likely to be especially easy and productive.

The patient is often unknown to the personnel suddenly charged with his care and is in or close to shock, with unknown drug sensitivities and a poorly understood medical background; therefore, it is usually a mistake to use any sedation or other depressing drug prior to endoscopy. Pharyngeal anesthesia is not used either, because it greatly increases the danger of transadital aspiration when there is incipient shock and because the ice-water gastric lavage has already serendipitously produced excellent cryo-anesthesia down the path to be followed by the instruments.

ENDOSCOPIC TECHNIC

It is rather pointless to argue the advantages of the various endoscopic instruments that are suitable for use in this situation. One will use whatever instrument is available to him and has generated confidence in him. Endoscopists who have used and liked the classical open tube esophagoscope, such as the Eder-Hufford, find it ideal for examining the bleeder, and exactly the same is true for the fiberoptic instruments. Similarly, both the classical glass gastroscope and the fiberoptic gastroscope have enthusiastic supporters.

Whatever the instrument, the examination must begin at the lips. This means that if the Eder-Hufford esophagoscope is used, the obturator must be discarded and the instrument passed under direct vision. Not only is there the need to scrutinize the tract from its very start down as far as the endoscopes will reach, but also the endoscopist must proceed without roentgen assurance that there are no dangerous lesions, such as Zenker's diverticulum, in the way.

The examination must be quick but thorough. The endoscopist travels down the tract rapidly, noting all abnormalities but being especially alert to traces or smears of blood that have appeared since the lavage. The whole point of the examination, quite naturally, is to recognize fresh bleeding—hopefully well controlled by the lavage—and then to trace it back to the bleeding lesion, localize the lesion, and identify it.

Ordinarily thorough esophagogastroscopy under these circumstances should require no more than five minutes, if the Eder-Hufford esophagoscope and classical glass gastroscope are used. The fiberendoscopes usually require a little longer, but experiences differ. If the instrument has duodenoscopic capabilities, permitting a most valuable extension of the visualized area, there will necessarily be some prolongation of the examination period.

ERRORS AND FAILURES

As with any endoscopic effort, the important source of error is simple misinterpretation of the satisfactorily visualized lesion. Only expert instruction, plus extensive experience, can make for endoscopic competence, and even the experts (if there really be such a category) must expect an interpretational error of about 5 per cent in this situation.

A surprisingly small error is contributed by obscuration of the bleeding lesion by blood or clots. Insufficient gastric lavage is the usual explanation, although torrential arterial bleeding can be wholly uncontrollable by any amount of lavage. In any case, even with the patient continuously in the horizontal position, almost never does blood collect in and obscure either the esophagus or duodenum. It is solely gastric diagnosis that is affected.

Failure of the lavage to clean the stomach can sometimes best be explained by compartmentalization of the lavage fluid within the stomach. Subsequent gastroscopic examination leaves no doubt that the instilled water has not reached a large section of the stomach, that now is found to be filled with old blood and clots that spill through the organ as it is inflated with air.

Utter failure of efforts to empty the stomach must be expected if anything less than a large-bore Ewald tube is used. The patient should lie in the left lateral position throughout the lavage. It is not necessary to roll him about, nor is it helpful to massage his abdomen. On the other hand, it is important to lavage the stomach at all levels, withdrawing the tube a few inches or inserting it farther from time to time, whenever the bloody stain begins to clear from the returns.

Clots ordinarily come back freely from the stomach in small pieces or strings. Sometimes, however, a single large conglomerated clot several centimeters in diameter remains. Later at gastroscopy the intense illumination, plus the trapped foreign material, gives such a clot a multicolored appearance with grays, whites and reds, causing confusing similarity to malignant tumor.

When a small amount of clot remains overlying an actively bleeding spot in the stomach, the lesion most often is a small benign ulcer, either acute or chronic. There is no sure means during gastroscopy of moving such a clot out of the way, although sometimes the trick is accomplished by rapid insufflation of air. Clots do not cause this sort of trouble in the esophagus. Experience within the duodenal bulb is as yet too limited to permit assessment of the matter.

The ice-water lavage does not change the appearance of normal esophagogastric mucosa, nor does it alter the features usually relied on for endoscopic diagnosis. Intolerance to insufflated air is not produced.

The amount of mucosa that has remained unscrutinized by the time an endoscopic study has been completed is never known to the endoscopist, and it seems unlikely that there will ever be a way to assess the matter exactly. Whatever the instrument or combination of instruments, it is probably fair to guess that more mucosa remains hidden than suspected.

Once a bleeding lesion has been found and identified, the main error results from assuming that the diagnosis is now complete. The fact is that more than one bleeding site is not unusual, meaning that in every case the diagnostic effort must be pushed to its completion. When there are multiple ulcers within the stomach, especially acute ulcers, or ulcers in both the stomach and the duodenum, all are likely to begin to bleed simultaneously. Unless the location of every bleeding crater is known, bad mistakes may be made at emergency surgery.

Simultaneous bleeding from dissimilar lesions is not as common but the possibility must always be kept in mind. In personal experience, duodenal ulcer and esophageal varices, erosive esophagitis and erosive gastritis, and erosive esophagitis and varices are the combinations most often encountered when there are multiple dissimilar bleeding sites. In most such cases it is not difficult to decide which one of the lesions is contributing mainly to the blood loss, at least at the moment of the diagnostic search. Short of emergency surgery, this knowledge is important only for putting together simplified statistics on the matter, as for Table 31-I. When operation is required to stop the bleeding, information about the patient's total bleeding problem is, of course, essential.

INJURIES AND ACCIDENTS

In regard to aggravation or reinitiation of bleeding, the peroral manipulative procedures and the positioning and pressures required for thorough contrast radiologic study are remarkably safe. There can be little question that long sojourn of a simple Levin tube will produce in some patients bleeding esophageal erosions, and probably it can encourage bleeding from previously intact varices. On the other hand, proper passage of esophagoscopes, gastroscopes and gastroduodenoscopes does not cause significant bleeding from normal tissues nor does it initiate variceal bleeding.

The risk of perforation exists, of course, as during regularly scheduled endoscopy. Perhaps it is somewhat increased under these emergency circumstances, not so much by the need for haste as by the little problems that result because the patient and doctor are often strangers to each other. The need to carry out the endoscopic part of the study prior to roentgen examination should not introduce additional mechanical hazards, provided the esophagoscope is not passed blindly, but it does add to the chance of overlooking nonbleeding lesions.

BLEEDING LESIONS

Experience with endoscopic investigation of the active bleeder has abruptly changed ideas about the frequencies of the common bleeding lesions. Duodenal ulcer has been found to be far less important to the overall picture than formerly thought. The cardia, too often considered in the past a pathologic desert by roentgen opinion, is now known to be the

TABLE 31-I

DATA ON 1,630 PATIENTS WITH SEVERE UPPER GASTROINTESTINAL
HEMORRHAGE, MANAGED BY THE VIGOROUS DIAGNOSTIC APPROACH

Bleeding Lesion*	Incidence No. of Cases	%	Blood Replacement Requirements, Average Per Bleed, ml	Emergency Surgery No.	% of Patients With This Diagnosis	Death Due to This Bleed No.	% of Patients With This Diagnosis
Duodenal ulcer	430	26	2,150	79	18	8	2
Varices	341	21	3,510	41	12	90	26
Gastric ulcer	215	13	3,140	68	32	11	5
Erosive gastritis	204	13	3,540	17	8	19	9
Erosive esophagitis	113	7	2,910	6	5	3	3
Mallory-Weiss	80	5	2,140	13	16	5	6
Stomal ulcer	48	3	3,200	14	29	4	8
30 other diagnoses	90	6	—	24	27	16	18
Undetermined or wrong	109	7	—	—	—	—	—

* When more than one lesion was bleeding, case was listed according to the lesion that seemed to be bleeding hardest.

bleeding segment in at least half of city-hospital bleeders. Experiences with incidence and severity of bleeding lesions, their demand for emergent surgical intervention, and mortality are shown for one series in Table 31-I.

The pandiagnostic effort turns up a great many potential bleeding lesions that are playing no part in the current bleed. If radiologic study were not supplemented by endoscopic investigation, no doubt many would erroneously be blamed for the bleed. Among the 1,630 bleeders shown in Table 31-I, for instance, no bleeding lesion could be found in 93, but in the other 1,537 patients 2,430 actual or potential bleeding lesions were found. As many as 162 patients had esophageal varices that were not bleeding, and 175 had nonbleeding duodenal ulcer.

SURGICAL HELP

The chief reason for all this diagnostic effort is to assist the surgeon, when his help is required, to accomplish a quick, accurate and complete hemorrhage-arresting operation, or, when the diagnosis is bleeding varices, to signal the need for esophageal tamponade. Even though the surgeon must carry out his own exploration anyway, there can be no doubt that the preoperative diagnostic effort makes his work much quicker and hopefully it precludes any error of omission that he might otherwise fall into.

DIAGNOSIS OF BLEEDING DUODENAL ULCER

It was hoped that the advent of effective duodenoscopes would make diagnosis of bleeding duodenal ulcer certain and easy. Current disappointment is explained simply by the fact that the duodenoscope's objective is so close to the bleeding lesion that the endoscopist can seldom tell where all the blood is coming from. Short of duodenoscopy, the diagnosis must be made indirectly, by gastroscopic discovery that fresh blood is refluxing back into the stomach through the pylorus, plus later roentgen identification of a duodenal crater.

ESOPHAGOGASTRIC VARICES

In locating the bleeding point along the course of a tangled complex of huge esophageal varices, the endoscopist finds himself thwarted unless his aspirating channel is clear and working well. Even though the blood flow is usually significantly retarded by the ice-water lavage and even though only small amounts of blood ordinarily collect in the esophagus before and during esophagoscopy, the instrument's tip or objective is so close to the action that even a small amount of free blood can obscure its point of origin. With continuous aspiration and constant movement of the instrument up and down the length of the affected esophagus, the endoscopist usually is able to conclude with some confidence that he has located all of the bleeding points.

The main interpretational problem created by bleeding varices on the gastric side of the cardia concerns confusion with a Mallory-Weiss tear, but only when the conditions of visualization are less than good. The latter lesion, when well visualized, is really quite characteristic. It is distinguished from other bleeding lesions by its linear disposition paralleling the axis of the esophagus, and the prominent linear black clot that fills it.

GASTRIC ULCER

Bleeding gastric ulcer is sometimes obscured by overlying clot, but otherwise there is not often a difficult problem in visualization or interpretation. A reliable rule states that a benign gastric ulcer bleeds from its edges, while a malignant crater bleeds from its center. The main diagnostic pitfall, again, is failure to detect a second or third bleeding crater in the stomach.

The bleeding acute or *stress* gastric ulcer is an especially dangerous lesion. Its bleeding is likely to be continuous as well as severe for a long period. If the bleeding is arrested by ice-water lavage, it is likely to recommence quickly. Furthermore, multiplicity is the rule. Quite naturally, the gastroscopist, upon discovering a bleeding gastric ulcer, must do his best to designate it either acute or chronic. In order to do so with assurance he must be able to see all or most of the crater well. The acute ulcer is shallow, no more than a centimeter in diameter, and is surrounded by a rim of hyperemic mucosa. Most important, the acute ulcer is not accompanied by scarring, configurational deformity of the neighboring gastric wall, or radiating folds, all features that may be evaluated with some assurance even when the crater itself cannot be well visualized.

EROSIVE GASTRITIS

This proves to be a straight-forward diagnosis, made with confidence by the gastroscopist. It is true, of course, that underlying the gastritic process there may rarely be some unsuspected specific mucosal disease, such as sarcoidosis or lymphoma. Although the bleeding from erosive gastritis may be torrential when the patient first seeks help, this is capillary bleeding and it is satisfactorily controlled by ice-water lavage.

The gastroscopic picture is that of innumerable bleeding points, slowly bleeding, scattered over various parts of the gastric mucosa or all of it, diffusely or in clusters. Determination of the exact distribution of the erosions requires an empty stomach and careful attention to complete scrutiny of the mucosa. There should be no problem distinguishing erosions from petechiae, but when there are not many erosions the gastroscopist may be unable at first to exclude the diagnosis of multiple small acute gastric ulcers.

EROSIVE ESOPHAGITIS

Bleeding esophagitis is easily recognized, the main feature being simply multiple tiny bleeding points scattered over the distal portions of the mucosa. The hyperemia and surface exudate of esophagitis cannot be recognized under these conditions. It is unusual to find that all of the esophageal mucosa is involved, from cricopharyngeus down. Whatever the extent of the process, the bleeding is always hardest distally, just above the esophagogastric junction. There appears to be no good correlation between this process and erosive gastritis, and as one descends into the stomach, most often the angry bleeding esophageal mucosa gives way suddenly to normal gastric mucosa as the junction is passed. Occasionally universal esophagogastritis is encountered, with bleeding from all surfaces, from cricopharyngeus to pylorus.

The esophagoscopist's main interpretational problem is likely to be uncertainty over whether there are small varices beneath the eroded mucosa, contributing to the bleeding. This may be a more difficult decision than one might think on first consideration. The matter must be decided solely on the basis of the mucosa's surface configuration.

COMMENT

Endoscopic interpretation is often difficult under ideal conditions but, paradoxically, when there is massive hemorrhage endoscopic diagnostic efforts are likely to become remarkably easy, as well as reliable. An accurate endoscopic opinion is vital to selection of optimal treatment. The art of emergency pandiagnostic management of the bleeder requires intense concentration at the time of each study. Diagnostic competence comes only with experience.

REFERENCES

1. Brick, I. B.: Early diagnosis in massive upper gastrointestinal bleeding. *JAMA*, *163*:1217-1219, 1957.
2. Dagradi, A. E., and Stempien, S. J.: Esophagogastroscopy during active upper gastrointestinal bleeding: Technic and experiences. *Am J Gastroenterol, 51*:498-502, 1969.
3. Katz, D., Douvres, P., Weisberg, H., Charm, R., and McKinnon, W.: Sources of bleeding in upper gastrointestinal hemorrhage: A re-evaluation. *Am J Dig Dis, 9* (n.s.): 447-458, 1964.
4. Miniconi, P., Perrin, D., and Delumeau, G., et al.: Le diagnostic étiologique précoce des hémorragies digestives. Justification de la fiberscopie oesophagienne et gastrique fait en urgence. *Presse méd, 78*:2011-2013, 1970.
5. Morse, W. H.: Gastroscopy as a diagnostic aid in upper gastrointestinal bleeding. *Am J Gastroenterol, 53*:323-329, 1970.
6. Moyson, F., and DeScoville, A.: Diagnostic et traitement des hémorragies digestives aiguës. *Acta Chir Belg, [Suppl] 1*: 1-143, 1955.
7. Ortiz Vázquez, J.: *Hemorragias Digestivas Altas.* Barcelona, Sandoz, 1969, pp. 1-221.
8. Palmer, E. D.: *Upper Gastrointestinal Hemorrhage.* Springfield, Thomas, 1970, pp. 1-410.

CHAPTER 31

*PART II: NONAGGRESSIVE ENDOSCOPY IN UPPER GASTROINTESTINAL HEMORRHAGE**

MITCHELL A. SPELLBERG, LESLIE J. SANDLOW AND LEONIDAS H. BERRY

INTRODUCTORY STATEMENT

SCHINDLER'S INTRODUCTION and popularization of the semiflexible, optical gastroscope revolutionized the diagnostic approach to gastric lesions. The advent of the more sophisticated fiberoptic instruments for esophaagoscopy, gastroscopy, and duodenoscopy has furthered the endoscopist's capabilities of accurate diagnosis of lesions in the area of the gastrointestinal tract. Some twenty years ago Palmer[1] demonstrated that immediate gastroscopy and upper gastrointestinal roentgenograms vastly improved the accuracy in diagnosing the source of bleeding in the upper gastrointestinal tract. These observations were extended by other observers,[2-5] and the usefulness of gastroscopy as a diagnostic tool is well established.[6]

During at least the last ten or fifteen years, there has been a popular trend toward early or so-called aggressive endoscopy in gross upper gastrointestinal hemorrhage. A large body of evidence has accumulated to support the advantages of this approach. In the long history of medical science, there always comes a time when innovative trends or practices have

* Supported in part by a grant from General Research Fund, Michael Reese Hospital, Chicago.

499

rightfully been re-evaluated. This is not for the purpose of rejecting good points of established and proved procedures and technics. Rather, reevaluations are for the prime purpose of rejecting that which has not stood the test of time and experience.

UPPER GASTROINTESTINAL HEMORRHAGE

A few years ago a group of us at Michael Reese Hospital entered on a prospective randomized evaluation of aggressive and nonaggressive (conservative) endoscopy in upper gastrointestinal hemorrhage. Our studies soon led us to consider whether the period of morbidity and the mortality rate actually decreased in the group subjected to the aggressive endoscopy approach. To answer this question, our group set up a study for 150 randomized cases of upper gastrointestinal hemorrhage. Numbers in sealed envelopes were randomly assigned to the 150 patients for either the aggressive or the conservative diagnostic approach.

Eighty patients were randomly assigned to the aggressive and seventy to the conservative approach. Those in the aggressive protocol underwent gastroscopy and esophagoscopy with a fiberoptic instrument immediately or within four hours after admission if there was evidence of active bleeding, as demonstrated by hematemesis or nasogastric suction containing blood. In the conservative group of patients x-rays and gastroscopy with similar instruments were done within one week after admission to the hospital. Immediately following the endoscopic examination in the aggressive group, upper gastrointestinal x-ray studies were performed. Both groups were maintained on a strict ulcer regimen, consisting of a bland diet with

TABLE 31-II

CLINICAL DATA IN TWO GROUPS RANDOMIZED FOR AGGRESSIVE
AND CONSERVATIVE ENDOSCOPY

	Incidence in Aggressive Group (%)	Incidence in Conservative Group (%)
No prior history of bleeding	64	68
One previous bleeding	20	22
Multiple bleeding episodes	16	10
Incidence of previous duodenal or gastric ulcer	same	same
Presented with melena	80	73
Presented with hematemesis	72	67
Shock	5	7
Stable vital signs	60	57
Hb 8 Gm%	35	33
Hb 8-11 Gm%	39	51
Hb 11 Gm% or above	26	16

milk and antacids hourly, anticholinergics as indicated, and ascorbic acid orally to substitute for the fruit juices absent from the strict ulcer diet.

Table 31-II shows comparative data for both the aggressive and conservative groups. It is apparent from these data that, for the most part, the two groups were equally ill and had approximately the same degree of hemorrhage of blood loss prior to the institution of the diagnostic procedures and treatment.

Mortality

The mortality rate in Palmer's aggressive endoscopy series of 1,400 patients reported in 1969 was 8 per cent.[7] This result is similar to that found in the 400 cases retrospectively studied by one of us in 1968.[8] The mortality rate in this group was also 8 per cent. Our study[9] likewise confirms the observations of others that when patients with upper gastrointestinal hemorrhage were studied immediately upon entrance to the hospital the frequency of diagnosis of the site of bleeding was much higher than in those studied thoroughly after a period of a week. The diagnostic accuracy in the aggressively studied group was 85 per cent, very similar to another reported series,[7] whereas in patients who were studied at the end of the week an accurate diagnosis was made in only 65 per cent, a significant difference.

Morbidity

It was assumed by many of those involved in this study that the morbidity and hospital stay will be shortened in those patients in whom the diagnosis was established shortly after entrance into the hospital. When the data were analyzed we were surprised that the reverse was true (Table 31-III). Sixty-six per cent of the aggressive group had an uneventful course compared with 87 per cent in the conservative group. Continuous and recurrent bleeding was three times as high in the aggressive group (23.5% vs. 7%). The period of hospitalization was likewise longer in the patients who were diagnosed aggressively. Hospitalization of twenty days or less occurred in 65 per cent in the aggressive group compared with 74 per cent in the conservative group. Hospitalization lasted twenty days or over in 27.5 per cent in the aggressive and in 17 per cent in the conservative group. Emergency surgery was required in 19 per cent of the aggressive group, apparently related to the greater continuous and recurrent bleeding. Only 7 per cent of those in the conservative group required emergency surgery although the two groups were randomly selected. The requirement for blood transfusions was significantly higher in the aggressive than in the conservative group. In summary, then, although the diagnosis was established significantly more often in the aggressively diagnosed

TABLE 31-III

RESULTS IN RANDOMIZED GROUPS

	In Aggressive Group (%)	In Conservative Group (%)
Accurate diagnosis	85	65
Uneventful course	66	87
Continuous and recurrent bleeding	23.5	7
Hospitalized 20 days or less	65	74
Hospitalized 21 days and over	27.5	17
Emergency surgery	19	7
No transfusion	32	40
Transfusion of 1-3 units	30	34
Transfusion of over 3 units	38	26

group, the mortality was the same in the two groups, and the morbidity was significantly higher in those who were studied aggressively.

DISCUSSION

It has been assumed by some who had only a superficial familiarity with the implications of our study that our conclusions would relegate gastroscopy to a secondary position. This is entirely untrue. We are more convinced than ever that gastroscopy, esophagoscopy and duodenoscopy have become very important and integral parts of diagnosis in lesions of the upper gastrointestinal tract. Our study merely places a question mark on the timing of endoscopy and questions whether immediate, posthaste, emergency gastroscopy or endoscopy is of vital importance to the physician and the patient in all cases. Indeed, in the structure of our study all patients who continued to bleed in spite of the conservative regimen were to have endoscopy immediately and prior to emergency surgery to determine the site of bleeding. The policy of the senior author for over twenty years has been that all patients who did not stop bleeding with conservative management should undergo endoscopy before exploratory laporotomy.

It has been the policy in treatment of upper gastrointestinal hemorrhage in former years and indeed also in the classical studies of Muellengracht[10] that patients with gastrointestinal hemorrhage must be made comfortable and placed at ease both physically and emotionally. This was one of the reasons the patient was not to be disturbed even for upper gastrointestinal x-rays. It has been our experience that most patients with upper gastrointestinal hemorrhage want to be *let alone*. They are not eager and some are quite resistant to the rush, urgency, and confusion of an immediate, post-midnight endoscopic examination. Emergency examinations are not done under ideal conditions for the patient or the endoscopist. A rested, alert endoscopist is more astute than one who has worked twelve hours and really desires rest rather than another endoscopy. Another problem is that the emergency gastroscopy may not be done by the most experienced and efficient endoscopist and therefore the conclusions drawn from the examination may not be as valid as those made by a more mature observer. This would probably be the case in most hospitals.

Direct observation of the bleeding lesion is proof of one source of hemorrhage at the time of endoscopy. Many aggressive examinations showed no active bleeding lesions. If only one lesion is found it may be safely assumed that the lesion indeed is the cause of the hemorrhage. However, in some instances, especially those of multiple lesions, the source may be in the esophagus, stomach, and duodenum. We advise endoscopy after the gastrointestinal x-ray series is done at the appropriate time. However, invariably, if no apparent lesion is revealed by roentgenographic examination, endoscopy is carried out. While seeing the blood at the site of the lesion is helpful, it may occasionally also be confusing. When adherent small blood clots are seen but no active bleeding, one may readily conclude that the diagnosis is erosive gastritis, when indeed the clots may have been regurgitated from the duodenum or elsewhere. In one of our patients, not in this series, emergency endoscopy revealed severe esophagitis and gastritis. However, another bleeding lesion in the second portion of the duodenum was not seen because duodenoscopy was not done, the assumption being that all the bleeding was coming from the lesions seen. Our studies emphasize that, while emergency endoscopy improves diagnostic accuracy,[11] it does not decrease mortality, and there is a definite increase of morbidity.

Why do the patients who are studied aggressively have a higher morbidity and a higher incidence of emergency surgery? It is within the realm of possibility that the physical and emotional trauma in acutely ill, bleeding patients during the early critical period does disturb the reparative process enough so that the healing of the bleeding area does not proceed as smoothly as in the group of patients treated conservatively throughout the early period. Another possibility is that the ice-water lavage invariably used before emergency endoscopy, while stopping the bleeding temporarily, may have resulted in rebleeding after lavage is discontinued. Therefore, it would be appropriate to do another study using a third group in which only ice-water lavage is used as the variable.

Emergency gastroscopy is always indicated in an upper gastrointestinal hemorrhage which does not stop after a reasonable period of controlled evaluation and for which emergency surgery is required. Emergency esophagogastroscopy may also be necessary in patients with known liver disease to determine whether the bleeding is occurring from esophageal varices. In such instances, Sengstaken-Blakemore compression, a portacaval shunt, or other method of therapy may be necessary. When there is reasonable probability that esophageal varices are present and are the only source of bleeding, use of a diagnostic Sengstaken tube may be appropriate as a preliminary therapeutic test. A Mallory-Weiss tear may also indicate emergency endoscopy, if the bleeding from this possible source does not stop within a reasonable period, based on good clinical judgment, with ulcer therapy. However, we have seen a patient who on endoscopic examination did have a Mallory-Weiss tear as a source of bleeding; the surgeons elected not to do emergency surgery on him, the bleeding stopped, and subsequently a duodenal ulcer was demonstrated and was a possible source of bleeding. Patients with upper gastrointestinal hemorrhage in whom no source of bleeding is found at the time of a delayed endoscopic and roentgen examination should have emergency endoscopy when a rebleeding incident occurs.

CONCLUSIONS

Emergency endoscopy and roentgenography increase diagnostic accuracy in upper gastrointestinal hemorrhage. Mortality is not decreased by this aggressive diagnostic approach, and morbidity was noted to increase in the *aggressive* group in a randomized prospective study. The aggressively studied patients required longer hospital stay and more blood transfusions than those on the conservative regimen. Emergency endoscopy may be a burden to the physician and to the patient but is always indicated prior to surgery for intractable bleeding. Diagnostic error may be inherent in the emergency endoscopic procedure.

Our experience indicates that not all patients with gross upper gastrointestinal hemorrhage need have aggressive endoscopy. It is also probable that many hospitals will not be equipped for effective and justifiable aggressive endoscopy.

REFERENCES

1. Palmer, E. D.: Observations in the vigorous diagnostic approach to severe upper gastrointestinal hemorrhage. *Ann Intern Med, 36*:1484-1491, 1952.
2. Chandler, G. N., Cameron, A. D., Nunn, A. H., and Street, D. F.: Early investigations of haematemesis. *Gut, 1*:6-13, 1960.
3. Hirschowitz, B. I., Luketic, G. C., Balint, J. A., and Fulton, W. F.: Early fiberscope endoscopy for upper gastrointestinal bleeding. *Am J Dig Dis, 8*:816-825, 1963.
4. Katz, D., Douvres, P., Weisberg, H., McKinnon, W., and Glass, G. B. J.: Early endoscopic diagnosis of acute upper gastrointestinal hemorrhage: Demonstration of relatively high incidence of erosions as a source of bleeding. *JAMA, 188*:405-408, 1964.
5. Katz, D., Douvres, P., Weisberg, H., Charm, R., and McKinnon, W. M. P.: Esophagogastroscopy: An advantage in the diagnosis of acute upper gastrointestinal hemorrhage. *Bull Gastrointest Endosc, 11*:25-29, 1965.
6. Baker, L., Gorvett, E. A., and Spellberg, M. A.: Diagnostic accuracy of gastroscopy in neoplasms of the stomach. *Cancer, 5*:1116-1127, 1952.

7. Palmer, E.: Vigorous diagnostic approach to upper gastrointestinal tract hemorrhage. *JAMA, 207/8*:1477-1480, 1969.

8. Sandlow, L. J.: The enigma of upper gastrointestinal hemorrhage. *Am J Gastroenterol, 50*:366-371, 1968.

9. Sandlow, L. J., Becker, G. H., Spellberg, M. A., Allen, H., Berg, M., Berry, L. H., and Newman, E.: A prospective randomized study of the management of upper gastrointestinal hemorrhage. In Press.

10. Muellengracht, E.: Fifteen years' experience with free-feeding patients with bleeding peptic ulcers. *Arch Int Med, 80*:697, 1947.

11. Katz, D., Douvres, P., Weisberg, H., Charm, R., and McKinnon, W.: Sources of bleeding in upper gastrointestinal hemorrhage: A re-evaluation. *Am J Dig Dis, 9*:447, 1964.

CHAPTER 32

UPPER GASTROINTESTINAL ENDOSCOPIC ACCIDENTS, DIAGNOSIS, MANAGEMENT AND PREVENTION

Leonidas H. Berry

INTRODUCTION

WITH THE INTRODUCTION of the Wolf-Schindler gastroscope in 1932 gastroscopy became accepted as an important method in the investigation of upper gastrointestinal disease. The procedure has become considerably safer and less discomforting to the patient since the introduction of the fiberscope. Like any other investigative procedure, complications will occur. Minor complications are frequently not reported so that the reported accident rate may be lower than the actual rate.

TYPES OF ACCIDENTS

Complications during upper gastrointestinal endoscopy include drug reactions related to premedication, and instrumental injuries. Included also

506

are those reactions or crises occurring during endoscopy, but not directly due to the administered drugs or the instruments used. Several excellent surveys have appeared analyzing the morbidity and mortality in upper gastrointestinal endoscopy.[1-4]

DRUG REACTIONS

Palmer and Wirts[3] in a world-wide survey in 1955 collected data on 307,-715 gastroscopies. There were 42 accidents related to the use of premedication and 10 deaths. Jones et al.[1] found six cases with reactions to local anesthetic medication and five of these were fatal. However, the corresponding number of gastroscopies were not known. Many of the reactions are preventable by avoiding overdosage. The reactions to local anesthetics include cardiovascular collapse and convulsions due to hypersensitivity or overdosage. Reactions to the other drugs used in premedication for endoscopy are covered in the literature. For further discussion of this subject, see Chapter 4.

ESOPHAGEAL ACCIDENTS

Incidence

Esophageal injuries of various degrees followed by esophageal and periesophageal infection are the most common and the most serious complications of upper gastrointestinal endoscopy. These may range from mild bruises to frank perforation.

Esophageal injury following lens gastroscopy is reported by Schindler,[5] Fletcher and Jones[6] and Paul and Lage[7] among others.

Jones et al.[1] found the incidence of esophageal perforation to be 50 in 49,000 gastroscopies with 21 deaths. Nearly all the perforations occurred with the Hermon Taylor lens instrument. Injuries to the upper esophagus were eight times more frequent than those to the lower esophagus.

Smith and Tanner[2] in 1956, during the pre-fiberoptic era, reviewing 7,200 gastroscopies and 605 esophagoscopies reported 29 cases of upper esophageal injuries and five cases of lower esophageal perforations. However, a number of doubtful cases were excluded. All the gastroscopies were done with the Hermon Taylor instrument.

In a study sponsored by the American Gastroscopic Society and reported by Palmer and Wirts[3] there were 267,175 gastroscopies with 84 pharyngoesophageal perforations with 13 deaths. Of 40,540 esophagoscopies, there were 95 perforations resulting in 22 deaths.

In a 1969 survey[4] of the mortality and morbidity in gastrointestinal endoscopy, experience with both fiberoptic and standard instruments was analyzed. Of 32,237 fibergastroscopies there were 24 perforations (0.074%) with 6 deaths. Out of 3,211 cases of fiberesophagoscopies there were three perforations (0.093%) with no deaths. In this study, the rate of perforation was seen to be slightly higher with fibergastroscopy than with standard lens gastroscopy.

Cohen et al.[8] in 1956 reported three perforations (0.19%) in a total of 1,514 examinations with the Hirschowitz gastroduodenal fiberscope. One perforation occurred at the gastroesophageal junction and the other two immediately distal to it. All three patients had hiatal hernia.

Maruyama et al.[9] reported their experience with 45,250 fiberscopic examinations during the period 1962 to 1970 at the Institute of Gastroenterology, Tokyo Womens Medical College and the Toranomon Hospital, Tokyo, Japan. Twenty accidents were encountered, an incidence of 0.44 per cent. These included three anesthetic accidents and nine cases of hemorrhage following gastroscopy. There were only two instances of esophageal perforation in this series.

In this study there were also 2,115 examinations with the Schindler type instrument with eight accidents. These included 1,704 examinations with the Schindler flexible lens scope with an accident rate of 0.23 per cent and 411 rigid (all metal) gastroscopies with an accident rate of 0.97 per cent. the overall accident rate was 0.38 per cent which is higher than the accident rate with the fiberscope.

Diagnosis and Management

Injuries of the esophagus may be crush injuries or perforations. Crush injury may occur in the hypopharynx where the pharyngeal wall may be compressed between the shaft of the instrument and the convexity of the cervical spine. The retropharyngeal fascia usually remains intact limiting infection. The injury becomes obvious several hours after an otherwise uneventful procedure. Fever, progressive dysphagia, pain referred to the base of the neck and difficulty and pain on neck movements develop. If prompt treatment is not given, abscess formation and fistula may result.

The signs and symptoms of perforation of the esophagus and hypopharynx vary depending on the location of the perforation. The pyriform sinuses of the hypopharynx are quite vulnerable to perforation. With perforation of the upper esophagus, the instrument may become arrested in the mediastinum and there may be blood at the tip of the instrument on withdrawal. Extension of the process into the mediastinum gives rise to chest pain, cough, tachycardia, dyspnea and cyanosis. Progressive dyspnea and shock may occur due to pneumothorax and collapse of a portion of the lung. Hemoptysis may also result. Subcutaneous emphysema with crepitation may occur in the neck and submental region. Symptoms of mediastinitis are prominent with lower esophageal perforations, empyema and pericarditis may be a late result. Generally, the course is stormy and the mortality is high. However, the symptoms may be delayed up to 48 hours with only soreness on swallowing and fever initially.[10]

Cohen and Katz[11] stress the statistical importance of esophagograms and chest x-rays in the diagnosis of esophageal perforation. The radiological findings include the presence of air or fluid in the cervical area, mediastinum, the pleural cavity and sometimes the pericordial sac. Special x-ray contrast material may be noted extraluminally in the above areas.

The endoscopist should be aware of the hazards of the procedure. All patients should be watched carefully and observed with reference to vital signs and other evidence of complications all during the procedure and for several hours thereafter. Prompt diagnosis is essential for effective treatment.

Crush injury of the hypopharynx may not become manifest for several hours afterward since the retropharyngeal fascia delays the spread of infection. There is no place for surgery in this situation as there is no actual perforation to suture. Prompt and vigorous treatment with antibiotics and intravenous alimentation with avoidance of swallowing will usually suffice. Taylor[12] advocates splinting the head, neck and the shoulders in a posterior cast to immobilize the area and limit the spread of infection.

If an early diagnosis is not made, an abscess may develop which needs drainage through the neck. If a fistula develops, the patient will need a feeding gastrostomy until the fistula heals. The insertion of a nasogastric tube may be ill advised as it can further traumatize the area.[11] If the instrument has perforated the pharyngeal wall, surgical closure of the tear should be undertaken at once and with antibiotics the complications may be avoided.

In the case of esophageal perforations associated with anaplastic necrotic carcinoma, in the cardio-esophageal area the injury may go unnoticed on x-ray examination. The best course in these cases would appear to be immediate wide thoracotomy with a view to primary suture in case the esophagus is healthy or for radical surgery in case an operable lesion is found. When actual perforation is not suspected during the procedure and the patient is seen some time later with symptoms of lower esophageal injury, the management will depend on the particular case. Aggressive treatment of infection and shock should be started. A wide thoracotomy should be done as soon as possible to drain the area of infection and an approximation of the esophageal tear with loose sutures may be done. A feeding gastrostomy is also done. Other complications which require energetic management include pneumothorax and empyema.

GASTRIC ACCIDENTS

These include gastric perforation, *scrape* injury, post-gastroscopy bleeding and thermal burns of the gastric mucosa. Pneumoperitoneum following gastroscopy in many instances may not be associated with any demonstrable perforation even after a careful examination at laparotomy. These are due to *scrape* injury and inflation forcing air through the wall at the thinned site of injury.

Incidence

Gastric perforation in present day fiberoptic endoscopy is a rare event. However, it did occur occasionally in the era of semiflexible lens gastroscopy.

Schindler[5] collected data on 22,351 gastroscopies involving 50 observers. Eight perforations of the gastric wall were noted. Jones et al.[1] surveying the British experience found nine instances of gastric perforations out of 49,000 gastroscopies. Smith and Tanner[2] reporting their experience at a single institution found no case of gastric perforation in a series of over 10,000 gastroscopies. Palmer and Wirts[3] in the world-wide survey found 75 gastric perforations with 12 deaths out of a total of 267,175 gastroscopies. Most of these cases had pathological lesions which would be expected to weaken the stomach wall. In about half the cases of pneumoperitoneum following gastroscopy, no perforation can be demonstrated at laparotomy in spite of a careful examination.[13] Early reports of pneumoperitoneum without gastric perforation have included those of Schiff,[14] Schindler,[15] Chamberlain[16] and Nelson[17] among others.

Little attention has been paid to the incidence of hemorrhage following gastroscopy.[1] This is no doubt due to the fact that in most situations, it may be difficult to differentiate hemorrhage induced by gastroscopy from that occurring incidentally. Moreover, instances of mild hemorrhage may go unreported. It may be stated that significant hemorrhage as a complication of gastroscopy is remarkable for its rarity.[1]

A few thermal burns of the stomach due to prolonged contact between the tip of the gastroscope and the stomach wall with the Schindler-type instrument, were reported in the past. Belber[18] has reported thermal burns of the stomach with thermal ulcer during the use of Hirschowitz gastroduodenal fiberscope for cinegastroscopy. However, with the development of *cold light* sources, the problem may be said to have been eliminated.

CASE HISTORY

A 60-year-old housewife had symptoms of epigastric distress and weight loss of 20 lbs. over a period of five months. The physical examination was essentially negative. Laboratory findings revealed Hgb of 10gms, occult blood in stools. Barium meal x-ray revealed a niche of approximately 2cm in diameter on the lesser curvature, lower body of the stomach. There was some irregularity at the lower and upper border which raised the probability of malignancy. Gastroscopy was requested. The GFBK Olympus fiberscope with biopsy facility was introduced without difficulty. The gastric mucosa was uniformly pale in the upper portions. A large ulcer defect with dirty-gray base and raised portions of the circumference was seen in a fleeting view on the lesser curvature and posterior wall of the upper antrum. Before the lesion could be further examined, difficulty in keeping the stomach sufficiently inflated for thorough inspection was noted. As more air was introduced, it was observed that the patient was not belching and the abdomen was becoming distended.

The patient appeared quite comfortable but the possibility of pneumoperitoneum was recognized and the examination was interrupted. X-ray of the abdomen in the upright position revealed air under the diaphragm. During transportation and manipulation on the x-ray table, the abdomen remained considerably distended and there was no belching. It was then noted that the pulse rate was 120, blood pressure was normal and there was some difficulty in breathing and the patient complained of the tight feeling in the abdomen but no pain. The elderly surgeon who had referred the patient and was observing had previously treated many tuberculosis patients with pneumothorax and pneumoperitoneum. The question of relieving the patient by deflation was raised. A spinal puncture needle with obturator was introduced through the distended abdominal wall and the air was slowly removed. The respiratory embarrassment was immediately relieved. The pulse rate dropped to 90 and the patient remained comfortable. Laparotomy was performed nearly three hours later. A perforation of 3mm was found in the thinned wall base of a large carcinomatous ulcer. Gastric resection was performed and there was normal recovery. Because the tip of the gastroscope had not reached the ulcer, the perforation was unquestionably caused by the inflation of air against the thinned crater floor of the carcinomatous ulcer.

Diagnosis and Management

In almost all cases, the perforation has occurred in the posterior wall of the stomach at or just below the gastroesophageal junction. Schindler states that this is due to the anatomical peculiarities of the region, the stomach being anchored firmly superiorly and the posterior wall angulating anteriorly due to the retroperitoneally situated pancreas and the upper pole of the left kidney. In all these cases gastroscopy has been unsatisfactory from the beginning. With frank perforation, it may be noted that the most frequent finding is the inability to keep the stomach inflated.

An upright film of the abdomen reveals air under the diaphragm. Subjective symptoms are remarkably few and the patient may only complain of discomfort due to the abdominal distension by escaped air. Objective signs of peritoneal irritation are remarkably absent in most cases.

Relevant to the diagnosis of gastric perforations following gastroscopy is the condition reported as "pseudoacute abdomen."[19, 20] The authors state that this condition should be suspected if not otherwise noted when the patient complains of severe abdominal pain and distension following gastroscopy. The symptoms usually appear during or immediately following the procedure, lasts a few hours and are relieved by nasogastric suction and the passage of flatus. No pneumoperitoneum is seen on x-ray. All of these patients seemed to the authors to have either gastric outlet obstruction or a nonfunctioning gastroenterostomy stoma.

Most patients with gastric perforation go on to uneventful recovery with conservative therapy with continuous nasogastric suction and intravenous fluids, and operation is quite unnecessary.[12]

DUODENAL AND JEJUNAL ACCIDENTS

Rumball[21] reported a jejunal perforation in a patient who had a gastroenterostomy stoma. McBroom[22] reported a single case of jejunal perforation in a patient who had undergone a Billroth II partial gastrectomy for duodenal ulcer 16 years previously. Palmer's[3] survey includes two cases of jejunal perforation and both of their patients survived. In contrast to gastric perforations, jejunal perforations should be treated by surgical repair.

The potential risk of impaction of the fiberscope in a deformed duodenal bulb if retroversion examination of the duodenal bulb is attempted has been referred to by Belber (see Chapter 23).

Transendoscopic pancreatography duodenoscopy is associated with the potential risk of pancreatitis but in practice only mild elevation of serum amylase are noted which return to normal in two to three days. However more serious complications have begun to occur.

IMPACTION INJURY

Impaction of the fiberscope in the esophagus has to be recognized as a real possibility. With the more recent fiberscopes capable of tip deflection of 135 degrees or more it would seem to increase the possibility of this accident in the future. At least seven instances of impaction injury have been recorded in the literature.[22-25] Most of these have involved patients with a short gastric remnant following surgery or in patients with hiatus hernia. In the case of Braucher and Kirsner[23] the fiberscope was impacted in the small gastric remnant of a patient who had undergone a previous gastric resection and surgery was necessary to relieve the impaction. Bralow[24] reported the impaction of a fiberscope tip in a hiatal hernia. Retroflexion of the instrument seemed to have occurred inadvertently. The retroflexed instrument was acutely angulated and removed in this position without any injury to the patient. The instrument, however, suffered considerable damage.

In the case reported by Kavin et al.,[25] the instrument had flexed on itself in the esophagus following retroflexion and the tip was noted at the fauces on a cursory examination of the throat. The instrument was withdrawn by pulling on the tip and the proximal end simultaneously. Barrett[26] reports three instances of impaction of the fiberscope and all were related to the use of the Olympus GTF-A gastroscope after it had been retroflexed. Two of these had hiatus hernia and the other had a rather transverse stomach. One of these who had suffered a rupture of the hiatus hernia due probably to the impaction was treated by surgical closure of the perforation and recovered (Cohen[27]).

In the light of the experience described above, special care must be taken with patients having short gastric remnants and those with hiatus hernia if the retroflexion maneuver is to be carried out in order to avoid accidential impaction.

OTHER COMPLICATIONS

Severe cardiac decompensation or angina should be considered relative contraindications to endoscopy. Endoscopy may be justified in mild cases, with extra care if a shortened procedure is deemed very vital to the immediate health of the individual. Myocardial infarctions have been reported during upper gastrointestinal endoscopy[3] but in view of the large number of the examinations it is not surprising that a few myocardial infarctions have occurred coincidental to endoscopy.

Excessive insufflation of the stomach during gastroscopy may result in cardiorespiratory embarrassment and may diminish the venous return to the heart. Reflex coronary flow changes have also been attributed to endoscopy. Serious cardiorespiratory embarrassment may occur with overdistension of the stomach especially in emphysematous elderly patients with low pulmonary reserve.

PREVENTION

Most of the complications of esophagogastroduodenoscopy are preventable. Attention to premedication with avoidance of undue depression of consciousness and assuring proper patient cooperation by establishing a rapport with the patient are important. The importance of a well trained nurse assistant to continuously attend the patient cannot be overemphasized. Upper gastrointestinal roentgenography should precede all elective endoscopies.

Endoscopy should be performed only by experienced endoscopists or under their close supervision. Anesthetic accidents are avoided by proper attention to premedication (see Chapter 4). Prompt treatment of any of the complications discussed above should generally diminish morbidity and mortality from upper gastrointestinal endoscopy.

REFERENCES

1. Jones, A. F., Doll, R., Fletcher, C., and Rodgers, H. W.: The risks of gastroscopy: A survey of 49,000 examinations. *Lancet,* 1:647, 1951.
2. Smith, C. C. K., and Tanner, N. C.: The complications of gastroscopy and esophagoscopy. *Br J Surg,* 43:396, 1956.
3. Palmer, E. D., and Wirts, C. W.: Survey of gastroscopic and esophagoscopic ac-

cidents. Report of committee on accidents of the American gastroscopic society. *JAMA, 164*:2012, 1957.

4. Katz, D.: Morbidity and mortality in standard and flexible gastrointestinal endoscopy. *Gastrointes. Endosc, 15*:134, 1969.

5. Schindler, R.: Results of the questionnaire on fatalities in gastroscopy. *Am J Dig Dis Nutrition, 7*:293, 1940.

6. Fletcher, C. M., and Jones, F. A.: Risks of gastroscopy with flexible gastroscope. *Br Med J, 2*:421, 1945.

7. Paul, W. D., and Lage, R. H.: Perforation of esophagus caused by flexible gastroscope: Report of case with autopsy. *JAMA, 122*:596, 1943.

8. Cohen, N. N., Huges, R. W., and Manfredo, H. E.: Experience with 1000 fibergastroscopic examinations of the stomach. *Am J Dig Dis, 11*:943, 1966.

9. Maruyama, M., Takemoto, T., Kondo, T., Yokoyama, I., Tanaka, S., Tamiya, M., Kimura, K., and Hirazuka, K.: The retrospective study on the accidents associated with the fiberoptic gastroscopy. *Rinsho to Kenkyu, 48*:878, 1971.

10. Goldstein, M. J., and Sherlock, P.: Silent esophageal performation following esophagoscopy. *Gastrointest Endosc, 13*:22, 1966.

11. Cohen, G., and Katz, J.: The importance of radiographic examination of the esophagus and routine chest radiography after esophagoscopy. *S Afr Med J, 34*:2731, 1960.

12. Taylor, H.: Difficulties and dangers in gastroscopy. *Gastroenterology, 35*:79, 1958.

13. Calem, W. S.: Perforation of the stomach during gastroscopy. *Am J Surg, 103*:640, 1962.

14. Schiff, L., Stevens, R. J., and Goodman, S.: Pneumoperitoneum following use of gastroscope. *Ann Intern Med, 14*:1283, 1941.

15. Schindler, R.: Passage of air through the gastric wall during gastroscopy with no wound demonstrable three hours later. *Gastroenterology, 5*:34, 1945.

16. Chamberlain, D. T.: Pneumoperitoneum following gastroscopy apparently without perforation. *New Eng J Med, 237*:843, 19 7.

17. Nelson, R. S.: Pneumoperitoneum following gastroscopy with spontaneous recovery on conservative therapy. *Gastroenterology, 24*:267, 1953.

18. Belber, J. P.: Thermal burn: a complication of cinegastroscopy with the fiberoptic gastroscope. *Bull Gastrointest Endosc, 11*:23, 1965.

19. Moldow, R. M., Waye, J. D., Cohen, N., and Wolf, J.: Pseudoacute abdomen following gastroscopy. *Gastrointest Endosc, 17*:117, 1971.

20. Rastogi, H., and Brown, C. H.: Pseudoacute abdomen following gastroscopy. *Gastrointest Endosc, 14*:16, 1967.

21. Rumball, J. M.: Perforation of the jejunum during a gastroscopic examination of a resected stomach. *JAMA, 113*:2053, 1939.

22. McBroom, G. L.: Experience with conventional upper gastrointestinal endoscopy, a 13-year study. *Gastrointest Endosc, 16*:213, 1970.

23. Braucher, R. E., and Kirsner, J.B.: Case report: Impacted fiberscope. *Gastrointest Endosc, 12*:20, 1965.

24. Bralow, S. P.: Fibergastroscopic technic for examination of the gastric fundus. *Am J Dig Dis New Ser, 12*:653, 1967.

25. Kavin, H., and Schneider, J.: Impaction of a fiberoptic gastroscope in the esophagus: an unusual complication of gastroscopy. *S Afr Med J, 44*:478, 1970.

26. Barrett, B.: New instruments, new horizons, new hazards. The impaction injury. *Gastrointest Endosc, 16*:142, 1970.

27. Cohen, N. N.: An unusual complication of fiberscope. *Bull Gastrointest Endosc, 11*:19, 1964.

CHAPTER 33

UPPER GASTROINTESTINAL ENDOSCOPY IN DISEASES OUTSIDE THE UPPER GASTROINTESTINAL CANAL

Leonidas H. Berry and Koduri R. Prasadrao

INTRODUCTORY STATEMENT

THERE ARE ENDOSCOPIC FINDINGS which occur in association with diseases of the solid digestive organs or the hepatobiliary system and the pancreas. Some of these relationships are definitively causative. Others are coincidental. It is conceivable that there are common causes as yet poorly understood for coexisting disorders in different parts of the digestive system.

With reference to endoscopy of the upper gastrointestinal canal, one must always justify indications and contraindications. There are many digestive disorder syndromes. They may or may not be specific for a specific disease and there is much overlapping of syndromes in the upper abdomen.[1] Besides this, digestive symptoms are not infrequently associated with systemic diseases in the absence of demonstrable digestive lesions. Finally, digestive symptoms frequently occur in the absence of demonstrable diseases in any of the organ systems of the body. These are the so-called functional dyspepsias or gastrointestinal neuroses. In this chapter, we will discuss justifications for upper gastrointestinal endoscopy or the lack of them in diseases outside the upper gastrointestinal canal.

DISEASES OF THE LIVER AND GALLBLADDER

The question of when upper gastrointestinal endoscopy is indicated in the presence of demonstrated disease of the liver, gallbladder and pancreas is a matter for decision in each individual case. It should largely be determined by whether the demonstrated disorders of the solid digestive organs sufficiently explain the clinical symptoms. Obviously a patient with hepatic cirrhosis and hematemesis should have esophagoscopy, barring contraindications whether or not the esophagograms fail to demonstrate varices. But such a patient may have associated gastric erosions or peptic ulcer disease which may better explain or complicate the possible cause of the hematemesis and require a different course of therapeutic management. The question arises as to whether known viral hepatitis should be a relative contraindication to endoscopy until better sterilization procedures for endoscopies are developed.

Any chronic disease of the liver, benign or malignant may cause esophageal or upper gastric varices and justify esophagogastroscopy.

Upper gastrointestinal bleeding in patients with cirrhosis of liver is due most commonly to multiple superficial gastric erosions, esophageal or gastric varices or to peptic ulcer. Radiological demonstration of varices does not mean that the patient is bleeding from the varices. Erosions as the source of bleeding are usually missed by roentgenology.[2] Endoscopy is therefore essential to demonstrate the source of bleeding. The high incidence of erosions as the source of massive upper gastrointestinal bleeding in cirrhotics is now being recognized. In a recent study of selected patients of cirrhosis with upper gastrointestinal bleeding erosions as the sole source of bleeding was noted in 61 per cent of our cases. Similar findings were noted in a recent autopsy survey.[3]

The frequency of variceal bleeding in patients with cirrhosis of liver and upper gastrointestinal bleeding has varied from 18.5 per cent to 56.2 per cent.[2, 4–6] This variation is due to several factors including patient selection, and endoscopic skill.

The increased frequency of ulcers in patients with cirrhosis seems firmly established.[7] Palmer[8] noted 195 instances of duodenal ulcer in 1,200 patients with proven cirrhosis of liver. Malnutrition, mucosal congestion, decreased hepatic histamine degradation have all been implicated as factors in the increased susceptibility of the cirrhotic patient to peptic ulcer.[9, 10]

In the experience of the senior author alcoholics who have liver and pancreatic disease have a higher incidence of gastritis.[11] There is a large group of chronic alcoholics who do not have an impressive gastritis gastroscopically but who have disseminated petechial mucosal hemorrhages of the stomach and tiny hemorrhagic erosions. These patients may have epigastric distress either with or in the absence of demonstrated liver disease. Endoscopy may be indicated for the possible finding of these changes. The presence of petechial and hemorrhagic erosions may explain the low hematocrit in the absence of frank hematemesis or melena.

Gallbladder diseases, especially cholecystitis manifest themselves by symptoms related to digestive organ functions. It has long been a question as to what is the mechanism of pain, nausea and vomiting in these disorders. Since the early years of gastroscopy an answer has been sought as to whether gastritis and other gastric disorders occur in a causative relationship with acute and chronic gallbladder disease. The senior author has not been impressed with the presence of significant gastritis above average incidence. However, he has observed hypermotility and pyloric hyperspasticity with biliary regurgitation in these cases. These are motor phenomena which may help to explain the mechanism of symptoms in gallbladder disease but do not justify routine gastroscopy for their observation. Because the gallbladder disease may be chronic, long standing and relatively quiescent, the probability of coexisting gastric lesions is a proper indication for gastroscopy.

Lawson[12] reported gastric mucosal changes secondary to duodenal and biliary reflux in experimental animals. Reports are being made of endoscopic and other evidence of so-called alkaline reflux gastritis in postoperative stomachs.

It is well known that chronic pancreatitis may be associated with biliary disease and posterior wall duodenal ulcer may penetrate into the pancreas and produce symptoms of pancreatitis. As more duodenoscopies are performed and more endoscopists develop the expertise of cannulating the papilla of Vater, there will be a better delineation of those gallbladder and pancreatic disorders which are poorly demonstrated by other methods. Reference is made particularly to include such disorders as cystic-duct syndrome or "stasis gallbladder," cholesterosis and biliary dyskinesia. Patients with gallbladder-type symptoms will have more and more indications for panendoscopy of the upper gastrointestinal canal.

PANCREATIC DISEASES

One is often faced with the decision of whether an associated chronic gastritis may not share the cause of digestive distress in the presence of demonstrated recurrent pancreatitis or cancer of the pancreas, especially when epigastric pain immediately after meals is the principal symptom rather than back pain.

CASE HISTORY

An illustrative case of the problem of overlapping syndromes in hollow organ and solid digestive organ disease is that of a middle-aged woman who had nausea and epigastric pain. The preliminary upper gastrointestinal x-ray revealed a questionable gastric ulcer and a negative esophagus and duodenum. Endoscopy revealed a very definite but small healing gastric ulcer of the lesser curvature near the posterior wall of the antrum. It was only when the severity of the pain seemed out of proportion that chemical studies were done and associated pancreatitis was demonstrated. The ulcer was subsequently healed completely with gastroscopic control, while the pancreatic symptoms continued.

Chronic pancreatitis is often associated with chronic alcoholism. Either or both sometimes associated with the endoscopic picture of chronic superficial gastritis or tiny gastric mucosal hemorrhages and erosions. If a patient has negative gastrointestinal x-ray studies but laboratory and clinical evidence of pancreatic disease, endoscopy is indicated. When these combined lesions are demonstrated there is a better understanding of the method of treatment to be employed.

Masses in or about the pancreas may first be recognized endoscopically.[13] Notable among these are the pseudopancreatic cysts and pancreatic carcinoma. Gastric compression by carcinoma of pancreas may be seen as a pyramidal or broadbased tumefaction in the antral area over the posterior wall with smooth overlying mucosa.

DISEASES OF THE COLON AND SMALL INTESTINES

Granulomatous lesions or Crohn's disease have been reported at various sites of the gastrointestinal tract from the esophagus to the rectum. Involvement of the stomach and the duodenum in Crohn's disease is rare. Among recent reports of the endoscopic aspects of Crohn's disease of the stomach and duodenum are those of Elibol and Rankin[14] and Laing et al.[15] These workers reported antral ulceration, nodularity of the mucosa in the antrum and distal body and pallor of the antral mucosa with inflammation and edema of the body and antrum. Polypoid masses in the posterior wall of the body were noted in the patient described by Laing et al.[15] In regional enterocolitis one must be aware of the occasional indication for upper gastrointestinal endoscopy and biopsy.

CARDIOVASCULAR DISEASES

The long association of the diseases of the heart and digestive disorders has its classic example in "acute indigestion" of by-gone days. In acute coronary disease, endoscopy is contraindicated. In chronic congestive heart failure, there is frequently the association of digestive symptoms.

Endoscopy may be indicated after digitalization. Symptoms in these cases are more often due to the generalized congestion which also effects the G.I. tract than to any other demonstrated gastric changes. Bohm and associates[16] found little or no histopathologic gastritis by gastroscopy and gastrobiopsy in patients with congestive heart failure. They stated that the evidence of passive congestion was not studied.

RESPIRATORY DISORDERS

We have long observed that patients with obstructive lesions of the esophagus may present with initial respiratory symptoms due to aspiration pneumonitis. Forty per cent of the patients with cardiospasm reviewed by Breakey[17] and Weens[18] had presented with pulmonary symptoms as the complaint. (In these cases the achalasia comes first and it is presumed that the excessive esophageal mucus associated with achalasia is aspirated during the recumbent position at night.) Unexplained and low grade pulmonary infiltrates should always indicate a study of the esophagus.

Tuberculosis of the esophagus is rare. However, dysphagia in a patient with pulmonary tuberculosis should raise the suspicion of ulcerative or hyperplastic esophageal involvement. Pulmonary tuberculosis patients not uncommonly have epigastric distress. Hardt[19] and others have reported gastroscopic evidence of gastritis and especially the atrophic form in patients with chronic pulmonary tuberculosis. In tuberculous patients, if x-ray screening of the gastrointestinal tract and other tests are negative for gastrointestinal disease, routine endoscopy may not be indicated.

The increased incidence of gastroduodenal ulceration in chronic pulmonary disease, especially emphysema has been well known. About 20 per cent of the patients with chronic obstructive pulmonary disease may have associated peptic ulcer,[20] in contrast to 3 to 4 per cent incidence in the general population.

Bronchogenic carcinoma may occasionally invade the esophagus, sometimes resulting in a bronchoesophageal fistula. Long before this occurs, there may have developed lymphatic invasion of the esophagus. We have observed one case in which esophagogastroscopy and brush cytology revealed class V cells several months before fistula formation. In this same patient, the first symptoms of significance to the patient was dysphagia. Enlarged metastatic bronchial lymph nodes were compressing the esophagus.

ENDOCRINE DISORDERS

Diseases of the endocrine glands associated with digestive symptoms has been observed for many years. The digestive symptoms seen associated with thyrotoxicosis are expressions of excessive metabolic and motor activity and not specific digestive disease states caused by the hyperactive thyroid gland. If endoscopy is done in patients with thyrotoxicosis in fairly acute stages, special caution must be exercised in order not to precipitate a thyrotoxic crisis.

Atypical and recurrent peptic ulcers with massive hypersecretion of acid in Zollinger-Ellison syndrome is well known. Other features that may be observed include multiple superficial erosions in the stomach and the pattern of hypertrophic gastropathy.

A high incidence of peptic ulcer disease in hyperparathyroidism, varying from 10 to 15 per cent has been reported.[21] In a significant number of patients, peptic ulcer may be the presenting feature antedating the symptoms of hyperparathyroidism by several years.[22] A variety of gastrointestinal symptoms are seen in diabetics. Gastric atony with stasis has been noted[23] being called gastroparesis diabeticorum.

HEMATOLOGIC DISORDERS
Anemias

Anemias of undetermined origin constitute a frequent indication for upper gastrointestinal endoscopy. The most common anemia seen by the endoscopist is hypochromic anemia of chronic blood loss. Most of these cases have intrinsic lesions in the upper gastrointestinal tract and are not appropriate for discussion in this chapter. Dysphagia and anemia may occur as part of the Plummer-Vinson syndrome.

Hereditary hemorrhagic telangiectasia may be occasionally localized to the gastrointestinal tract and present with multiple episodes of gastrointestinal bleeding and iron deficiency anemia. Gastroscopic biopsy of the lesions may help in the diagnosis.[24] Among other hemorrhagic disorders of interest to the upper gastrointestinal endoscopist, we should mention aspirin intoxication and other drugs causing upper gastrointestinal hemorrhage. There is evidence to support the involvement of thrombocytes in hemorrhage associated with the ingestion of aspirin and certain other drugs.

Addisonian or pernicious anemia always has the endoscopic picture of atrophic gastric mucosa. These changes should not be referred to as atrophic gastritis because there is no established evidence that an acute or chronic superficial type of gastritis preceded these changes. A roentgen study[25] of 211 patients found gastric carcinoma in 8 per cent and benign polyps in 7.1 per cent. Several reports[26, 27] of high frequency of carcinoma of stomach in pernicious anemia at autopsy suggest the desirability of getting periodic examinations by gastroscopy or x-ray studies at least in suspicious cases.

Leukemias and Lymphoma

Leukemic involvement of the gastrointestinal tract is not uncommon[28] especially in chronic lymphatic leukemia. Plaque-like lesions, nodular infiltrations and diffuse infiltrations with *brainlike* appearance have all been described. Palmer[29] reported visualizing a large actively bleeding ulcer on the posterior wall of the stomach located on a smooth hemispherical mass in a patient with chronic monocytic leukemia. Multiple gastric ulcers have been reported in association with lymphatic leukemia[30] and polycythemia vera.[31] Primary lymphoma of the stomach represents 3 per cent of all primary malignant tumors of the stomach.[32] Despite their rarity, they are important in view of the better prognosis that they carry and the specific modes of therapy available. The radiological methods of diagnosis are not very helpful. Endoscopy and biopsy may be helpful.

The submucosal infiltrating type of lymphoma usually produces prominent folds, deformity of the interior of the lumen and the enlarged folds are not altered by distension. The appearance may simulate Menetrier's disease. Hemorrhagic gastritis has been seen as a source of massive bleeding in patients with lymphoma unrelated to tumor involvement of the gastrointestinal tract. The mechanism is unknown.[33]

COLLAGEN DISEASES

In this group there is a large number of disorders, all of which may have associated upper gastrointestinal manifestations. The principal disorders in this category are scleroderma, dermatomyositis and systemic lupus erythematosis. In the upper gastrointestinal tract, the classic involvement with these diseases occurs in the esophagus. Dysphagia and substernal pain are the principal symptoms of involvement.

Esophageal involvement may be seen early in the disease in scleroderma. Stricture of the mid-esophagus, dilation of the lower esophagus with poor motility, peptic esophagitis with a terminally constricted but open esophagus may be seen. Involvement of the antrum of the stomach with thickened finely nodular mucosa has been seen.[34] The duodenum may be dilated due to the constriction and narrowing of the distal part. The difficulty in getting rid of esophageal secretions may cause aspiration pneumonia and excessive coughing.

In systemic lupus associated gastrointestinal symptoms are common and are usually attributed to serositis and vasculitis. Anatomical lesions have been found in 15 to 20 per cent of cases at autopsy.[35] Esophagogastroscopy in this condition may be indicated.

In dermatomyositis, involvement of the esophagus is common and the striated muscles of the upper esophagus may be affected in over half of these patients. Multiple ulcerations are seen in the stomach which may be a source of gastrointestinal bleeding in some cases.

MISCELLANEOUS DISORDERS

There are many miscellaneous diseases outside the gastrointestinal canal which may be associated with pathological changes in the upper gastrointestinal canal. In their severest forms, they may cause a stress ulcer or mucosal erosions and massive upper gastrointestinal hemorrhage. Genitourinary diseases in the male and the female have a high incidence of gastrointestinal symptoms. Some of these gastrointestinal symptoms have functional bases while others have organic bases. We have seen several cases of acute upper gastrointestinal bleeding following surgery in the genitourinary tract without history of previous gastrointestinal disturbance. One patient had an acute stress type ulceration over an arteriosclerotic vessel which could be seen in the base of the ulcer, in the surgical specimen.

Gastrointestinal complications in patients with intracranial lesions are sufficiently common that they should be quickly recognized.[36, 37] Two such complications are hemorrhage and/or ulceration. French et al. studied 17 cases with various intracranial lesions and gastric lesions. There were five with erosive gastritis and 12 patients with hemorrhagic gastritis. Other systemic disease with upper gastrointestinal manifestations include the so-called gastrointestinal allergies and dermatological diseases. The pioneer gastroscopist François Moutier and his associate Paul Chevelier first called attention to endoscopic changes in severe skin disorders. Pemphigus and epidermolysis bullosa have been known to involve the esophagus with development of strictures. Other rare conditions which may be associated with gastric mucosal changes include those in syphilis, which have been described by several authors.[38, 39]

FUNCTIONAL DIGESTIVE DISORDERS

We now turn to a subject which may be the most important to be encountered by the upper gastrointestinal endoscopist. We refer to the important problem of functional digestive disorders. Their importance to the endoscopist is primarily in terms of the kinds of referrals in which he will be asked to give diagnostic aid. Most of these referrals will involve problems of dyspepsia referable to the upper abdomen which have already been found to be x-ray negative. Many of the patients will have symptoms of such long duration that early, small lesions easily overlooked by x-ray will be unlikely. These patients are often well nourished and have nothing in the physical examination, blood morphology, biochemical or other extensive studies which suggest disease. Their complaints may be any or most of a long list of symptoms and descriptions of distress as they manifest themselves to the patient. These symptoms include such terms as gas, heartburn, bloating, indigestion, belching, gastritis, difficulty in swallowing, nausea, distress after meals, loss of appetite, gas pressure against the heart, palpitation, pain in the upper abdomen, etc. All of these, others and their international equivalents may make up the final list of such complaints.

Even the experienced endoscopist may not dare refuse endoscopy in this group of patients, for fear of missing an occasional early malignancy. Unfortunately, neglect of fair and meaningful endoscopy in such patients will indeed present the embarrassment occasionally of an overlooked early gastroesophageal malignancy. This can happen in a country of low gastric cancer incidence like the United States. It may be even more likely to occur if such patients are not endoscoped in countries of high gastric cancer incidence such as Japan.

When cancer by endoscopy, cytology and biopsy is not found and when peptic ulcer disease is absent, what does the upper gastrointestinal endoscopist find in the repeatedly x-ray negative stomach? First of all, he may find nothing that he can describe as pathological change. If he is very observant, he may identify physiologic states such as hypermotility, hyperspastic areas of activity at the sphincters of the pylorus, the antral incisura, the cricopharyngeus and even the gastroesophageal junction. These findings can most assuredly explain functional complaints.

A third possibility is that the endoscopist may observe what can be psychosomatic effects such as those reported by Wolf and Wolff[40] in *Human Gastric Function* on the fistulous stomach of their subject, Tom. These would be recent and ancient mild manifestations of inflammatory reactions, namely localized, mild superficial gastritic changes and local areas of mild atrophic mucosa.

Finally, and perhaps of most importance, the upper gastrointestinal endoscopist will have helped in ruling out the presence of serious disorders in terms of life-threatening or potentially dangerous organic disease of the upper gastrointestinal canal and more specific dyspepsias.

REFERENCES

1. Berry, Leonidas H.: Differential diagnosis of the multiple syndromes of the upper gastrointestinal tract. *Rev Gastroenterol, 19*:715, 1952.
2. McCray, R. S., Martin, F., Amir-Ahmadi, H., Sheahan, D. G., and Zamcheck, N.: Erroneous diagnosis of haemorrhage from esophageal varices. *Am J Dig Dis, 14*:755, 1969.
3. Sheahan, D. G., and Zamacheck, N.: Multiple superficial gastric erosions (MSGE): An overlooked cause of fatal haemorrhage? *Clin Res, 16*:2, 1968.
4. Merigan, T. C., Hollister, R. M., Gryska, P. F., Starkey, G. W. B., and Davidson,

C. S.: Gastrointestinal bleeding with cirrhosis. *New Engl J Med, 263*:579, 1960.

5. Brick, I. B., and Palmer, E. D.: One thousand cases of portal cirrhosis of liver. Implications of esophageal varices and their management. *Arch Int Med, 113*:501, 1964.

6. Dagradi, A., Saunders, D., and Stemphen, S. J.: Sources of upper gastrointestinal bleeding in liver cirrhosis. *Ann Int Med, 42*:852, 1955.

7. Clark, J. S.: Influence of liver upon gastric secretion. *Am J Med, 29*:740, 1960.

8. Palmer, E. D.: *Upper Gastrointestinal Hemorrhage*. Springfield, Thomas, 1970. p. 186.

9. Bockus, H. L., Ed.: *Gastroenterology*. Vol. 1. Philadelphia, Saunders, 1944.

10. Drapanas, T., Adler, W., Vang, O. J., and McMenamy, R. H.: Primary regulation of histamine metabolism by the liver. *Ann Surg, 161*:447, 1965.

11. Berry, Leonidas H., Villa, F., Adomavicius, J., and Alavi, M.: Unpublished data.

12. Lawson, H. H.: Effect of duodenal contents on the gastric contents on the gastric mucosa under experimental conditions. *Lancet, 1*:469, 1964.

13. Palmer, E. D., and Boyce, H. W.: *Manual of Gastrointestinal Endoscopy*. Baltimore, Williams and Wilkins, 1964, p. 6.

14. Elibol, T. E., and Rankin, G. B.: Crohn's disease of the stomach. *Gastrointest Endosc, 14*:201, 1968.

15. Laing, R. R., Dunn, G. D., and Klotz, A. P.: Crohn's disease of the stomach. *Gastrointest Endosc, 16*:168, 1970.

16. Bohm, R., Gunther, K. H., David, H., Theur, D., and Ginther, H.: Correlation between congestive heart failure (CHF) and stomach: the problem of the so-called congestive gastritis. In: Endoscopy of the digestive system. *Proc 1st Europ Cong Digestive Endoscopy*. Prague, 1968. Karger, Basel/New York. 1969, p. 154. Eds. Marataka, Z. and Setka, J.

17. Breakley, A. S., Dotter, C. T., and Steinberg, I.: Pulmonary complications of cardiospasm. *New Engl J Med, 245*:441, 1951.

18. Weens, H. S.: Pulmonary disease associated with megaesophagus. *Am J Roentgenol, 52*:472, 1944.

19. Hardt, L. L., Wiessman, M., and Coulter, J. S.: Gastric atrophy in far advanced pulmonary tuberculosis. *Am J Dig Dis Nutrition, 9*:404, 1942.

20. Knowles, J. H.: Chronic obstructive pulmonary disease. Bronchitis and emphysema. In Harrison's: *Principles of Internal Medicine*. New York, McGraw-Hill, 1970, p. 1295.

21. Ostrow, J. D., Blanshard, G., and Gray, S. J.: Peptic ulcer in hyperparathyroidism. *Am J Med, 29*:769, 1960.

22. Keating, F. R.: Diagnosis of primary hyperparathyroidism. *JAMA, 178*:547, 1961.

23. Kravetz, R. E.: Gastroparesis diabeticorum. *Gastrointest Endosc, 12*:22, 1965.

24. Sanowski, R. A.: Heriditary hemorrhagic telangiectasia—a clinical and endoscopic study. *Gastrointest Endosc, 16*:224, 1970.

25. Rigler, L. F., Kaplan, H. S., and Fink, D. L.: Pernicious anemia and the early diagnosis of tumors of the stomach.*JAMA, 128*:426, 1945.

26. Kaplan, H. S., and Rigler, L. G.: Pernicious anemia and carcinoma of stomach—Autopsy studies concerning their interrelationship. *Am J Med Sci, 209*:339, 1945.

27. Zamcheck, N., Grable, E., Ley, A. B., and Norman, L.: Occurrence of gastric cancer in patients with pernicious anemia at the Boston city hospital. *New Engl J Med, 252*:1103, 1955.

28. Wintrobe, M.: *Clinical Hematology*. Philadelphia. Lea and Febiger, 1967.

29. Palmer, E. D.: Leukemia, Gastroduodenal ulcer, and the problem of massive gastrointestinal hemorrhage. *Cancer, 8*:132, 1955.

30. Bynum, T. E.: Gastroscopic appearance of multiple gastric ulcers associated with lymphatic leukemia. *Gastrointest Endosc, 17*:38, 1970.

31. Schindler, R.: *Gastroscopy*. New York, Hafner, 1966.

32. Sherlock, P., Winawer, S. J., Goldstein, M. J., and Bragg, D. G.: Malignant lymphoma of the gastrointestinal tract. In: *Progress in Gastroenterology*. Vol. II. New York, Grune and Stratton, 1970. p. 369.

33. Ehrlich, A. N., Stalder, G., Geller, W., and Sherlock, P.: Gastrointestinal manifestations of malignant lymphoma. *Gastroenterology, 54*:1115, 1968.

34. Boleman, A. P., and Rumball, J. M.: Progressive systemic sclerosis (scleroderma) with esophageal and gastric antral involvement. *Gastrointest Endosc, 17*:160, 1971.

35. Harvey, A. M., Shylman, L. E., Tumulty, P. A., Conley, C. L., and Schoenrich, E. H.: Systemic lupus erythematosis. Review of literature and clinical analysis of 138 cases. *Medicine, 35*:291, 1954.

36. French, J. D., Porter, R. W., Von Amerongen, J. K., and Raney, R. B.: Gastrointestinal haemorrhage and ulceration associated with intracranial lesions. *Surgery, 32*:395-407, 1952.

37. Strassman, G. S.: Relation of acute mucosal hemorrhage and ulcer of gastrointestinal tract to intracranial lesions. *Arch Neurol and Psychiat, 57*:145-160, 1947.

38. Palmer, E. D.: *Stomach Disease as Diagnosed by Gastroscopy*. Lea and Febiger, Philadelphia, 1949.

39. Yamaguchi, T.: Clinical observation with biopsy, endoscopic and x-ray examination of gastric lesions in secondary syphilis. In: Endoscopy of the digestive system. *Proc 1st Europ Cong Digestive Endoscopy*. Prague 1968. Karger, Basel/New York, 1969, pp. 82-83. Eds. Marataka, Z. and Setka, J.

40. Wolf, S., and Wolff, H. G.: *Human Gastric Function*. New York, Oxford Univ. Press, 1943.

CHAPTER 34

FRONTIERS AND FUTURE TECHNICS IN GASTROINTESTINAL ENDOSCOPY

Sadataka Tasaka and Sachio Takusu

PRELIMINARY STATEMENT

IN PRECEDING CHAPTERS the "History of Gastrointestinal Endoscopy" has been discussed in considerable detail. Endoscopy is a very important arm in the diagnostic study and in some cases treatment of diseases of the alimentary canal. The procedure had a rugged and disconnected past prior to 1932.[1] It had a fascinating and productive period from 1932 to 1958, and a rapid and dramatic development during the last two decades. Yet, every new and perfected development had its forerunner in crude attempts during previous years of history. There were pioneers who tried to bend a ray of light around a corner before Schindler and the George

Wolf Company. There were pioneers who attempted with only crude success to develop a miniature camera which could be swallowed in relative comfort before Uji and the Olympus Company. There were attempts, not so crude but impractical in its day, to utilize glass fiberoptics in endoscopes before the fiberscope breakthrough of Hirschowitz and Associates and the American Cystoscope Makers. The restless curiosity of scientists in gastroenterology and enteric endoscopy have crossed the frontiers of controllable tip instruments, remote cold light sources, curvi-linear biopsy forceps, pancreato-biliary duct cannulation and colonoscopy in amazingly short periods of time.

We now look forward to newer and increasingly more imaginative horizons in gastrointestinal endoscopy.

VARIOUS ADVANCED DEVICES FOR FIBEROSCOPY

The controllable tip of fiberscopes makes the introduction of an instrument very easy and solves the blind spots completely in competent hands. Four directional control of the tip over 90 degrees is possible in many fiberscopes. Inaba and Sanada reported a gastrofiberscope with two angles. This is made especially for observation en face of the posterior wall of the upper gastric body.[2] On the other hand such a strong angulation damages glass fibers rather considerably. One should move the tip slowly and gently. Further discussion of various instruments currently in use may be found in Chapter 5.

The angle of vision of each endoscope varies between 50 and 70 degrees. For orientation a wide angle of vision is convenient but is unsuitable for detailed observation. A fiberscope equipped with a zoom-lens has been developed to overcome this problem. However, there are still some technical difficulties not yet overcome in developing a miniature practical zoom-lens. In the not too distant future this feature may be constructed in every endoscope.

In the early developmental period of endoscopy, the problem of illumination was very crucial. Kussmaul used a gazogen (a mixture of four parts of alcohol and one part of oil of terebinth) lamp for his first gastroscope. The development of the miniature electric bulb made possible a giant step in endoscopy. Excellent fiberoptics today have now made the miniature electric bulb obsolete, largely because of the heat of the lamp occasionally causing burns of the mucosa. Today light is usually transmitted through a fiber bundle from outside and the danger of burn is completely avoided. As a light source, a halogen lamp or xenon lamp is used and excellent illumination is provided not only for still and cinematography but also for color television. The subject of the remote projection of the endoscopic image on a television screen is further discussed in Chapter 7, Part II.

Among other recent advances are incorporation of automatic mechanisms in endoscopes. For exposure control a small photo-cell is installed inside the fiberscope and light is cut off automatically when enough light for photography is generated. Powered air *feeding* and the device for washing off mucus on the lens by water are already part of the endoscopes by Olympus and other companies. These mechanisms will continue to be improved in the future.

FIBEROSCOPY OF THE JEJUNUM AND ILEUM

The problem of visualization of the mucosa of the jejunum and ileum simply expressed is the problem of introducing a fiberscope along the extensive serpentine course of the small intestines. Hiratsuka et al. have reported their success in the introduction of a 2.5 meter long fiberscope under the guidance of a string which was swallowed previously. The clinical significance of endoscopy in diseases of the jejunum and ileum may be the subject of exploration in the near future. Thus endoscopic observation of the entire alimentary tract from the esophagus to the rectum is now within the range of possibility.

SINGLE INSTRUMENT FIBEROSCOPY OF ESOPHAGUS, STOMACH AND DUODENUM

If endoscopy of the esophagus, stomach and duodenum can be conducted by a single fiberscope, this certainly has important advantages. To meet this purpose, a long forward-viewing fiberscope with four directional movement of its tip has been developed. This is especially useful for location of upper gastrointestinal bleeding, since any of the three upper gastrointestinal organs may be the source of hemorrhage. However, with the forward-viewing endoscopes some difficulties are experienced in adequately visualizing the gastric body, and cannulation of the pancreatic duct is impossible. The side-viewing scopes have definite advantages in viewing the stomach and for the purpose of cannulating the pancreato-biliary duct. However, side-viewing scopes usually cannot be used satisfactorily for viewing the esophagus. The exception being in the case of megaesophagus or in the use of the smaller diameter side-viewing endoscopes.

PROBLEMS WITH FIBERSCOPES AND THEIR FUTURE RESOLUTION

The biggest problem with fiberscopes today concerns their expensiveness and fragility. The resolving power of a fiberscope depends almost entirely on the number of glass fibers incorporated. For better observation the glass fiber should be thinner and the number of fibers should be greater. However, this makes the fiberscope more expensive and more fragile. Even though remarkable technical improvements are made for the assembly of fiber bundles, glass fibers are broken because of the high flexibility of a fiberscope and especially with four directional controllable tips. Insertion of biopsy forceps also damages glass fibers. For the present, endoscopes should be manipulated very carefully in the interest of the instrument as well as the patient.

At the present time the finest fiberscope available is one designed for observation of the ureter, with diameter of 2mm. It is said that with the present manufacturing techniques, production of a finer fiberscope with a minimum diameter of 1.5mm is possible. But, if we must make a finer fiberendoscope, we would have to look for another optical system.

A major shortcoming of the fiberscope is its limited resolving power compared with a scope incorporating an optical lens system only. This is an unavoidable shortcoming of the fiberscope due to the principle of fiber optics, which transmits an image by resolving it into dots of the same number of glass fibers incorporated. There are several ideas to solve this problem. For example synchronized movements of both ends of a fiber bundle make for disappearance of its mosaic pattern and improve the resolving power. However, this theory has not been put into practical use as yet.[3]

Recently a new optical guide called "SELFOC" was developed in Japan.[4] In this optical guide, refractive index decreases quadratically with the distance from its optical axis, and a light beam is transmitted in a sine-curve. With a single rod of this optical material, image transmission is possible. But, before practical application of this principle for the endoscopes can be made, there are many technical difficulties to be solved, such as chromatic aberration. Furthermore, "SELFOC" is now made of glass and not flexible. Recently this has been applied to a very thin rigid arthroscope. But in the future it may be made of plastic materials and be widely used for endoscopes.

FRONTIERS AND FUTURISTIC CONCEPTS OF TRANSENDOSCOPIC PROCEDURES

Biopsy and Cytology

Direct vision biopsy of the stomach was successfully and extensively used with semiflexible lens gastroscopes, but the procedure has been considerably simplified with fibergastroscopes. Today, endoscopic biopsy is performed easily for most any part of the gastrointestinal tract available to endoscopic viewing. Endoscopic forceps biopsy is carried out widely and yields excellent results. Excellently functional biopsy forceps are constructed which are very small in diameter and very flexible. Further discussions of "Biopsy and Cytology" are included in Chapters 27 and 28. In the future suction biopsy, as was applied with the Berry Gastrobiopsy Assembly for Eder-Palmer Scopes (Chapter 28), the Tormenius Attachment for Schindler Scopes and the Debray Gastroscope, may be reconsidered for fiberoptic endoscopic biopsy.

The collection of cells for cyto-diagnosis is performed by brushing, washing the mucosa by water jet and suction through a tube. Biopsy is found superior to cytology by most workers because of its high positive rate in malignant cases and very low frequency of false positives. Furthermore the former is more important even for the diagnosis of benign diseases. Yet in some instances cytology is superior to biopsy.

We cannot agree with the recent tendency to shift the entire responsibility of diagnosis from endoscopic observation to biopsy and cytology. Without an earnest attitude toward gross diagnosis by endoscopic observation, progress in endoscopy cannot be expected. The greatest cause of false negatives in the direct vision biopsy depends on the imperfect observation of a gross lesion.

Vital Staining and Related Technics

To demonstrate minute unevenness of the mucosal surface, dyes such as 0.2% solution of methylene-blue, 0.6% Evans-blue, 0.4% coomasse-blue and other such dyes may be sprayed on the mucosa under endoscopic control.[5] This method is effective for the detection of hyperplasia of the gastric mucosa, a small erosion or a cicatrix of peptic ulcer (Plate 95).

The acid secreting area of the stomach, which decreases with age, can be demonstrated by the method of Okuda et al.[6] as follows: The stomach is lavaged by 5% solution of sodium bicarbonate and 20 to 30ml of 0.3% solution of Congo red is applied on the gastric mucosa by changing the patient's position. Then histalog or gastrin is injected and endoscopy is performed. The acid secreting area changes in color after 20 to 30 minutes following the injection.

After Klinger and Katz of Chile, South America, demonstrated the usefulness of the Tetracycline Test for gastric cancer, Berry with the assistance of the Eder Instrument Company and a miniature electric bulb engineer in 1962 developed a light bulb built into an Eder lens scope, which would emit ultraviolet filtered light. Attempts were made to detect fluorescence in the stomachs of patients with gastric cancer gastroscopically after oral or intravenous administration of Tetracycline. These workers never succeeded in getting enough ultraviolet illumination in the stomach with these instruments for diagnostic purposes. More recently an ordinary fiberscope has been used in Japan for the attempted transmission of ultraviolet fluorescence in gastric cancer diagnosis with limited success.

Special Photography

A gastrocamera with ultraviolet photography already has a history of ten years.[7] An electronic flash lamp is installed at its tip and a filter for ultraviolet ray is placed in front of the lamp. A special film (Kodak, spectroscopic 103-0) is used. Ultraviolet photography exaggerates minute unevenness of the mucosal surface.

Glass fibers cannot conduct ultraviolet ray. With a fiberscope incorporated by a special kind of glass fibers which transmit semiultraviolet ray, a special endoscopic examination of the digestive tract may be possible. Such observation has already been carried out in cystoscopy and its usefulness for detection of carcinoma *in situ* of the urinary bladder has been reported.

In contrast to the rather long history of ultraviolet endoscopy, it is performed apparently only by limited numbers of endoscopists. The clinical significance of this examination in the future is difficult to estimate, but the application of various kinds of illumination for endoscopic observation and photography is a very interesting projection.

Blue-white fluorescence is emitted when the normal gastric mucosa is illuminated by ultraviolet ray, but does not if there are erosions or ulcers on the mucosa.[8] The ordinary gastrocamera can photograph fluorescence almost as well as that of ultraviolet photography if a filter is used which permits only the ultraviolet rays to pass through. With this method in order to get enough of the ultraviolet rays, the electronic lamp must be flashed six times within $\frac{1}{25}$ of a second. Because of the difficulties to get enough of the ultraviolet illumination, this method was never adopted for clinical examination. Intravenous administration of fluorescent drugs such as riboflavin phosphate before photography was reported as not being very effective for the demonstrations of mucosal ulcerations.

Polarization photography has also been tried in endoscopy. The reflex of light on the mucosal surface occasionally disturbs exact observation.[9] The polarization gastrocamera has a filter (polarizer) in front of its lamp and another one (analyzer) before its lens. This instrument is not of practical use because of its failure to photograph small lesions and other difficulties.

With the considerable advances in electronics, color television for endoscopy is now in routine use for floor model and table model sets. Yet to be developed for practical distribution are television facilities for transmission of the endoscopic image to distant and large audiences. Color television for endoscopy is useful especially for teaching direct vision biopsy, measurement of lesions and other manipulations under endoscopic control. A detailed discussion of "Television in Endoscopy" appears in Chapter 7, Part II.

MACRO- AND MICRO-METRIC TECHNICS
Thermometry

Temperature evaluations of gastrointestinal lesions have been studied and found to be of value. This technique may be found to be of considerable importance in the future. A detailed measurement of the temperature of the mucosal surface at the level of 0.01 degree C. has been performed by Tasaka et al. with a thermister.[10] In peptic ulcers, temperature is higher at the margin in its active stage and lower at the center. On the contrary during the healing stage, the temperature is higher at the center than at the margin. Temperature distribution around an ulcer is different in the case of a benign than in the case of a malignant lesion. The studies of Tasaka et al. have been correlated with the distribution of capillaries in microangiographic studies of resected specimens. Temperature studies of gastrointestinal lesions have been performed with the use of endoscopic color television (Plate 96). Intragastric thermometry may be an important development for the future of endoscopy.

Color and pH Measurements

Sakita and Associates are working on the development of a spectrophotometric analysis of the color of the gastric mucosa with a thin fiberbundle inserted through a fiberscope. This may be useful to demonstrate changes of blood flow under various conditions. Berry has experimented with what he calls a "gastroglobinometer" with incomplete results.

The pH at particular areas on the mucosa of the digestive tract can be measured by miniature glass electrodes under endoscopic control.

Radioactive Detection Tests

Distribution of injected radioactive substances such as ^{32}P or ^{67}Ga may be registered with a Geiger Counter or a solid state detector of the catheter type through an endoscope. Accumulation of ^{32}P or ^{67}Ga may be observed in a malignant lesion but its superiority over the visual observations of endoscopy has not yet been confirmed. Nelson, working at the M. D. Anderson Hospital and Tumor Institute in Houston, Texas, summarizes his experiences with radioactive phosphorus (^{32}P) and transendoscopic Geiger Counters in lesions of esophagus, stomach and rectum in a monograph published in 1967.[8] Best results were obtained in the detection of cancer of the esophagus and rectum through rigid endoscopes. The application of these methods with the Eder-Palmer lens scope met with only limited success.

Measurement of Lesions

The American Cystoscope Makers, Incorporated, after the suggestions of Berry, has developed a transendoscopic meter stick for determining apparent and actual size of surface lesions. Japanese manufacturers of endoscopes have also developed flexible rules for measuring the dimensions of lesions. The thickness and stiffness of the gastric wall may conceivably be determined transendoscopically in the not too distant future. When well developed, these studies may contribute to the clarification of gastrointestinal physiology, which will lead us closer to the world of preventive medicine in the gastrointestinal tract.

Microfiberoscopy

Microfiberoscopy will undoubtedly be a technique which will be developed in future years. Suzuki and Associates[11] have developed a microgastrofiberscope. It is 7mm in diameter and is inserted through the channel of a specially build fiberscope. The tip of the microgastrofiberscope is placed against the gastric mucosa. The area of the visual field is 5x5mm and the magnification is thirteen times. The investigators claim usefulness for this instrument in diagnosing the capillary distribution in malignant lesions of the stomach which appear different from benign lesions. A combination of these studies with microangiography will undoubtedly be a development in future years (Plate 97).

TREATMENT TECHNICS

Transendoscopic treatment technics must follow as logical and reasonable goals following the great technical advances in diagnostic fiberscopy. Injection of therapeutic chemicals around an ulcer crater of the stomach was tried by Namiki and Associates in benign ulcers and favorable results have been reported (Table 34-I).[12] As the remedial agents, Beta-methason and Alantoin are chosen and injected once a week. The investigators presume that the steroid hormone injected in the floor of the ulcer crater may depress the formation of fibrosis, which apparently delays healing. The Alantoin injected at the margins of the crater may promote regeneration of epithelium. Complete healing is reported by six to nine injection treatments. Recurrence was experienced in 4.2 per cent. The pathophysiologic basis and indication for this treatment should be investigated. A special needle for this purpose is on the market and its technic apparently is not difficult. These technics in the hands of other workers and with other chemicals apparently have not succeeded.

Endoscopic polypectomy is discussed in Chapter 28, Part II, with reference to the stomach and Chapter 30, with reference to the colon. Namiki

TABLE 34-I

NUMBER OF DIRECT INJECTIONS NECESSARY FOR COMPLETE HEALING
OF REFRACTORY GASTRIC ULCERS

No. of Injections	No. of Cases
2	3
4	10
6	27
8	31
10	21
12	18
14	10
16	9
18	4
20	3
Over 20	3
Total	139

Namiki et al.[12]

et al. have reported a kind of "chemical polypectomy" by injecting the stalk or base of a polyp with Bleomycin, an anticancer agent or with necrotizing substances. It is claimed that the technic is simple and safe.

Removal of a foreign body from the gastrointestinal canal using a fiberscope is rather difficult as compared with the use of rigid endoscopes in the esophagus and rectum. There are some exceptions to the general experience. Among them are the removal of unresolved sutures causing ulceration or inflammation in the postoperative stomach. A special forceps with a cutter is made for this purpose, although this procedure can be performed with ordinary transendoscopic forceps. Transendoscopic electro-coagulation as an emergency treatment for massive upper gastrointestinal bleeding has been tried by some doctors who have reported its usefulness in selected cases. Endoscopic papillotomy by electro-coagulation is also reported for obstructive jaundice by an incarcerated stone. In the future a laser beam may be adapted for transendoscopic manipulations. Direct irradiation of a malignant lesion with a miniature radioactive source inserted through the fiberscope may not be far from reality.

CONCLUSION

It is now more than a century since Kussmaul performed his first gastroscopy. The medical profession can be justly proud of the continuing cooperative achievements of medical science and engineering. Progress has been so rapid in the last decade that it defies the imagination to contemplate the future in gastrointestinal endoscopy. In this chapter some of the more promising of the newer technics which appear on the horizon have been briefly reviewed and discussed.

REFERENCES

1. Killian, G.: Zur Geschichte der Oesophago- und Gastroskopie. *Deutsch Ztsch f Chir,* 58:499-512, 1901.
2. Inaba, E., Sanada, K., and Associates: Swan-type double-bending gastrofiberscope. *Bull of Tokyo Medical and Dental Univ,* 17:307-317, 1970.
3. Kapany, N. S.: *Fiber optics.* New York, Academic Press, 1969.
4. Uchida, T., Furukawa, M., and Associates: Optical characteristics of a light-focusing fiber guide and its application. *IEEE J of Quantum Electronics,* 10:606-612, 1970.
5. Tsuda, Y.: Endoscopic observation of gastric pathologies by the spray of dyes (in Japanese). *Gastrointest Endosc,* 9:189-195, 1967.
6. Okuda, S., Saegusa, T., and Associates: Clinical endoscopic observations of gastric secretion. *Annual Report of Center for Adult Diseases of Osaka,* 7:53-58, 1967.
7. Sakita, T., and Utsumi, H.: Ultraviolet photography of the stomach. *Med Biol Illus,* 14:166-169, 1964.
8. Nelson, Robert S.: *Radioactive Phosphorus in the Diagnosis of Gastrointestinal Cancer.* Springer-Verlag, Berlin, Heidelberg, New York, 1967.
9. Oka, S., and Sugiura, M.: Polarization gastrocamera (in Japanese). *Gastrointest Endosc,* 10:224-231, 1968.
10. Tasaka, S., Oki, I., and Associates: A study on the temperature of the gastric mucosa (in Japanese). *Gastrointest Endosc,* 12:259-266, 1970.
11. Suzuki, T., Miyake, T., and Associates: Microgastrofiberscope—a new device in diagnosis of gastric cancer based on dissecting microscope findings. *Japanese Archives of Internal Medicine,* 17:27-39, 1970.
12. Namiki, M., Kochi, H., and Associates: Treatment of peptic ulcer by local injections (in Japanese). Shindan to Chiryo, 53:831-837, 1971.

PERITONEOSCOPY IN GASTROENTEROLOGY

CHAPTER 35

HISTORY, ANATOMY, INDICATIONS CONTRAINDICATIONS, PERITONEOSCOPIC TECHNICS, NORMAL FINDINGS, COMPLICATIONS

FERNANDO VILLA

INTRODUCTORY REMARKS

THIS IS NOT INTENDED to be an extensive anatomical description of the abdomen; instead, it is only to point out the organs that could be analyzed by peritoneoscopy* as well as the important structures that could be damaged at the moment of the pneumoperitoneum development or the time of trocar insertion into the abdominal wall.

HISTORY

Peritoneoscopy[1] is a relatively new endoscopic procedure, if we consider that it was started in a very rudimentary way by Ott[2] (1901), who called it celioscopy. He used a vaginal speculum inserted through an abdominal incision. Ott was followed by Kelling[3] in the same year, using a cystoscope.

The development of peritoneoscopy has thus spanned the past seventy

---

* The words Peritoneoscopy and Laparoscopy are used interchangeably in this section.

539

TABLE 35-I
HISTORY

Author	Year	Country	Event
Ott	1901	Russia	
Kelling	1901	Germany	
Jacobaeus	1910	Sweden	
Bertram, Bernheim	1911	U.S.A.	
Renon	1913	France	
Meirelles	1913	Argentina	
Roccavilla	1914	Italy	
Orndoff	1920	U.S.A.	Introduced O_2 for pneumoperitoneum
Follikoffer	1924	Germany	First to report a large number of cases Introduced CO_2 for pneumoperitoneum
Short	1925	England	
Korbsch & Kalk	1927	Germany	First atlas of laparoscopy
Kitayama	1929	Japan	
Ruddock	1934	U.S.A.	Designed instrument which took biopsies and controlled bleeding by electrocoagulation
Lee	1942	U.S.A.	Aspirated gallbladder and injected contrast material for cholecystography

years. Among the different authorities who have contributed to its use throughout the world, some have developed new instruments or modifications of them, others have pioneered various technics, with modifications in the use of different gases for pneumoperitoneum. To avoid an extensive review of the history, the following table has been prepared to give the most relevant events in the development of this interesting diagnostic method.

ANATOMY

The abdominal cavity is bordered by the diaphragm at the uppermost part, by the anterior and posterior abdominal walls, respectively, at the sides, and by the pelvic floor inferiorly. The diaphragm communicates with the thoracic cavity by means of two main hiatuses, the esophageal and the aortic. Occasionally a congenital incomplete closure of the Bochdalek and Morgagni orifices occurs. Diaphragmatic hernias may be found in any of the aforementioned hiatuses; however, pneumoperitoneum, pneumothorax, or mediastinal emphysema usually will not develop, because the diaphragm is covered with the parietal peritoneum and this prevents air from getting into the chest cavity.

The anterior abdominal wall constitutes the most important area for peritoneoscopy, because through this area the pneumoperitoneum development as well as the trocar insertion into the abdominal cavity must be carried out.

The superficial epigastric artery and vein in the subcutaneous tissue as well as the inferior epigastric artery and veins running behind the rectus abdominis muscle are parallel to each other. These vessels can usually be found extending from the intersection of the middle third and inner third of an imaginary line from the symphysis pubis to the anterior superior iliac spine. They run in an oblique course within 2cm of the umbilicus, then continue directly up, keeping 2cm away from the midline until they reach the thorax where they merge with the thoracic arteries and veins.

The rectus abdominis extends from the costal margin to the pubis where it is attached to the anterior and posterior margin and is the main support for the middle part of the anterior abdominal wall. This muscle is highly vascular and, in order to avoid damage, it is preferable to use the midline as the site for incision and insertion of the trocar.

When the midline cannot be used as the site for the incision (e.g. because of a previous midlaparotomy scar), then a lateral approach should be utilized. Lateral approaches to be used as site areas are: (1) 3cm away from the costal margin and the liver edge, (2) 3cm away from the iliac bone, (3) 4cm away from the midline, or 2cm away from the lateral border of the rectus abdominis, and (4) 2cm inward from the extension of the prolongation of the anterior axillary line.

On the posterior surface of the anterior wall is the falciform ligament which extends from the diaphragm to the umbilicus. This falciform ligament runs obliquely to the right because it is displaced by the ligament of the umbilical vein (round ligament). This ligament is useful for the location of the right and left lobes of the liver. Except for rare cases (Baumgarten's syndrome), the umbilical vein stays closed. In portal hypertension, the paraumbilical veins, which run along with the umbilical ligament, are dilated.

Extending from the umbilicus to the urinary bladder are the urachus and vesicoumbilical veins. Sometimes the urachus separates itself from the abdominal wall, forming a true ligament. Originating in the umbilicus and spreading out toward the inguinal region are the ligaments of the umbilical arteries which can be used as a good reference point to locate the annulus inguinalis.

INDICATIONS

It is preferable to apply this procedure as a diagnostic method,[4, 5] after several other investigations have been carried out. However, in some instances, if the process of investigation may cause the patient's condition to deteriorate, then diagnosis of the suspected clinical problem may be aided by peritoneoscopy. The procedure can be used safely, and its use may reduce expense and length of hospitalization. Indications are quite different from those for exploratory laparotomies. Most of the latter are done with the idea of removing part or all of an organ, and most are usually carried out on a therapeutic basis. When laparotomies are done as a diagnostic approach, their value becomes less significant. The risk is higher than in peritoneoscopy, and the final results, diagnostically, are equal or less than in similar conditions approached by peritoneoscopy.

Use of peritoneoscopy is recommended because of the many conditions that can be analyzed in patients by this technic. Once some clinical impression is established, peritoneoscopy is useful in finding pathological manifestations in the abdominal cavity. Biopsies, as well as quality photographs, can also be taken with this method.

Some of the common indications are as follows:

1. Proficiency of the examiner
2. Failure of other diagnostic tests and procedures in probable abdominal disease
3. When laparotomy should be avoided
4. For research purposes with informed consent of patient
5. For direct cholangiography and splenoportography
6. Diseases of the peritoneum, especially those associated with ascites
7. Diseases of the liver, with or without jaundice
8. Diseases of the spleen
9. Diseases of the gallbladder and bile ducts, especially in the presence of jaundice
10. Diseases of the stomach and intestines
11. Diseases of the pancreas or kidneys, for detecting an enlargement due to tumor or cyst
12. Diseases of the pelvic organs
13. Indefinite abdominal masses
14. Evaluating liver scans of lesions
15. For staging of lymphoma
16. To biopsy intra-abdominal organs and peritoneum involved in pathological processes (e.g., granuloma, carcinoma, other tumors) under direct vision
17. To obtain photographs[5] of normal and abnormal conditions at the time of peritoneoscopic examination
18. In cases of chronic ascites during peritoneal dialysis or hemodialysis
19. In certain pancreatic disorders (e.g., pseudocyst, carcinoma, etc.)

CONTRAINDICATIONS

Whenever a procedure is considered we must always weigh the indications against the contraindications. However, as the examiner gains experience in the procedure, the relative contraindications are narrowed and riskier operations may be attempted. It is advisable for the beginner to follow the group of contraindications given here.

A. Absolute
   1. Acute diseases, whether in brain, lung, heart, or abdomen
   2. Chronic diseases, if the degree of health deterioration is such that any procedure may precipitate death
   3. Blood dyscrasias in which improvement does not follow the usual therapeutic measures

B. Relative
   1. Adhesions, when there is a history of generalized peritonitis or previous surgical interventions (sometimes these adhesions are absolute contraindications)
   2. Large inguinal, umbilical, or hiatus hernia
   3. Eventrations of the abdominal wall (diaphragmatic)
   4. Mental illness

PERITONEOSCOPIC TECHNICS

The peritoneoscopic technic has certain basic steps which are listed below (included are some personal variations). Fundamental steps include:
   1. Clinical evaluation of the patient
   2. Psychological preparation of the patient
   3. Period of fasting (eight to twelve hours prior to the procedure)
   4. Preanesthesia, the method to be decided by the operators. We use Demerol and atropine sulfate and may add either Benadryl, or Valium
   5. Preparation of the abdomen is similar to preparation for laparotomy
   6. Anesthesia, either general or local. We prefer the latter. For a local anesthetic, carbocaine 1 per cent or lidocaine 1 per cent is preferred. However, it may vary with the operator and the new anesthetics being developed.
   7. *a)* Pneumoperitoneum
      b) Incision and insertion of peritoneoscope trocar

Pneumoperitoneum

The pneumoperitoneum is initiated before inserting the trocar. Selection of the area in which to inject the gas varies. One of the most common is in the left lower quadrant, at a point on an imaginary line drawn between the umbilicus and the anterior iliac spine, at the junction of the outer third and the middle third of that line. (This area is preferable because there is less danger of puncturing important vessels, such as the epigastric arteries.) Areas such as the right lower quadrant or above and below the midline at the umbilicus can also be used.

For this step several needles have been developed. One frequently used is the Verres needle; this has a soft, rounded, hollow probe within the sharp-ended needle which penetrates the peritoneal cavity. We use a spinal tap needle, gauge #8, because this is less traumatic. Once the needle is considered to be in the peritoneal cavity the pneumoperitoneum is developed, using either oxygen, carbon dioxide, nitrous oxide, or air. Air is not often used due to the nitrogen content and possible embolization. Oxygen is frequently used if no cauterization or electrical devices are to be utilized, since a spark may produce a gas explosion. Carbon dioxide is a safe gas, and electrical manipulation may be done without danger of explosion. Nitrous oxide may be of some potential danger because some nitric gas can be produced around sparks.

Insertion of Peritoneoscope Trocar

Again the area of inserting the trocar may vary with the operator and the condition of the abdomen. Usually the midline either above or below the umbilicus is preferable. If the procedure is done under local anesthesia, a circumference of 3cm should be anesthetized. Then a 1cm incision is made and, with the pneumoperitoneum present, the trocar is forced through the abdominal cavity. When the trocar is removed, very little gas will leak from the trocar sleeve left in. The rest of the field is covered with sterile towels to isolate it from contamination. If the pneumoperitoneum is induced with a pneumo-apparatus, adjusting the automatic pressure (around 15mm of Hg) will keep the abdominal cavity distended to a comfortable degree for examining the intra-abdominal organs (see Fig. 35-1).

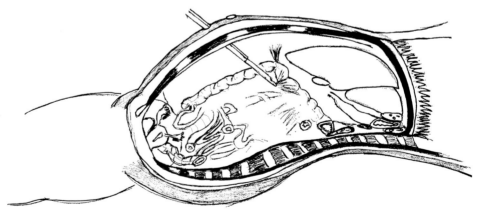

Figure 35.1. Diagrammatic sketch of sagittal section through abdomen, showing pneumoperitoneum and relative position of organs.

NORMAL PERITONEOSCOPIC FINDINGS

The parietal and visceral peritoneum is normally smooth, shiny, and soft. When thick or rough surfaced, it represents an abnormal condition (peritonitis).

The omentum appears yellow due to the presence of fat. The amount of fat is variable in relation to body build. Examples of abnormal findings are lipomas (fat accumulation), cirrhosis, and cachexia (depletion of omentum).

A negligible amount of fluid can also be seen.

The size of the liver is judged proportionately to height and body build. The liver has a smooth surface, a smooth, thin, soft edge and a brown-mahogany color (Plate 98). Glisson's capsule is transparent, except when it has been affected by previous inflammatory disease. The right and left hepatic ligaments are seen, except in cases of congenital absence.

The fundus of the gallbladder is normally seen; on lifting up the liver, the entire gallbladder may be visible, as well as part of the cystic duct (Plate 99). The gallbladder is usually greenish in color; however, when filled with bile, it may be a greenish blue. If the gallbladder is partially emptied, the color may be a yellowish white. On the surface are many arteriolar and venuolar ramifications. Different ligaments can also be detected, such as the cholecystoduodenal and/or the cholecystocolonic. Sometimes the gallbladder may appear collapsed. This is due to contraction and does not necessarily mean it is diseased.

The spleen has the same color as the liver but is slightly darker. The size is calculated by the area scanned by the optical piece over the organ. Another method of determining the size of the spleen is to use points of reference for comparison. For example, I have observed from experience that when the spleen rests on the parietocolic ligament, located below the spleen, it is twice its normal size; when it overlaps the ligament, it is more than twice normal size. The splenic capsule is transparent but is seen more frequently than the liver capsule; it has a tendency to become thick, and in many instances it changes the color of the organ to a more grayish tone.

The stomach is well visualized from the intra-abdominal esophagus to the pyloric area. The anterior wall and both curvatures are also visible, but the posterior wall cannot be seen. Upon lifting the left lobe of the liver, the lesser omental sac and the quadratus lobe of the liver become visible. This area is significant for detection of pancreatic pseudocyst.

The small bowel is easily seen. However, the difference between jejunum and ileum cannot be distinguished except for loops close to the stomach and terminal ileum. The wall is smooth and shiny. The mesenterium can be well seen.

TABLE 35-II

SIGNIFICANT DATA REGARDING COMPLICATIONS

	Incidence (%)
Air discomfort	1 to 3
Perforations	0.32 to 1.6
Subcutaneous emphysema	0.05 to 1.9
Mediastinal emphysema	0.26
Air embolism	Very rare
Perforation of a vessel	Rare
Biliary peritonitis	One case
Mortality	0.0012 to 0.1

The teniae coli is a good identifying feature to help find the colon. Once the colon is recognized, the appendix can also be distinguished (Plate 100). When the appendix cannot be seen in the standard position, the left lateral decubitus is advised.

During examination the right and left parietal colic ligament can be observed as well as the appendix epiploica. Diverticula of the colon can also be recognized.

Finally, by placing the patient in the Trendelenburg position, the sigmoid, upper rectum, urinary bladder, and cul-de-sac can be seen. The uterus, tubes, round ligaments, and ovaries can be observed in female patients.

COMPLICATIONS

From the very beginning of the procedure, complications should be kept in mind. To avoid complications the operator must first be well trained in the manipulations of the instruments. He must know the criteria for the proper selection of the site of puncture for pneumoperitoneum. He must also have the knowledge required to properly select the site and to safely introduce the trocar. It is mandatory that the operator be aware of the patient's condition, so that he may give proper consideration to indications and contraindications. At the time of the procedure, he must consider the local abdominal characteristics (scars, for example).

These steps must be considered before peritoneoscopy is done in order to minimize the number of complications. Complications which may arise during the procedure are listed in Table 35-II.

REFERENCES

1. Villa, F. and Steigmann, F.: Peritoneoscopy. Moses Paulson: *Gastroenterologic Medicine*. Baltimore, Lea & Febiger, 1969.
2. Otto, D.: Illumination of the Abdomen (Ventroscopy) J. Akush.: *Zhensk, Boleg*, 15:1045, 1901.

3. Kelling, G.: Ubber Oesophagoskopie, Gastroskopie Kolloiskopie, *Munchen Med. Wenschr, 49*:21, 1902.
4. Ruddock, J. C.: Peritoneoscopy. *South Surgeon, 8*:113, 1939.
5. Wittman, I.: Peritoneoscopy. Akadinia Kiado, Budapest, 1966.
6. Kalk, H. and Wildhirt, E.: Lehrbuch und Atlas der Laparoskopie und Leberpunktion. G. Thieme Stuttgart, 1962.

CHAPTER 36

PHOTO PERITONEOSCOPY, HEPATITIDES, METABOLIC LIVER DISEASES, PERITONEAL DISEASES

HERWARTH LENT

HISTORY AND DEVELOPMENT OF PHOTO PERITONEOSCOPY

THE NATURAL HISTORY OF viral hepatitis has remained an unsolved problem in spite of numerous statistical and clinical investigations. Day by day, however, the question arises: When has a hepatitis healed completely? Does it smoulder over years as chronic persistent or chronic aggressive hepatitis underneath? Has the process at this stage perhaps come to a standstill or does it eventually change into a more or less active cirrhosis? These questions must be answered critically in every single case in any investigation. This is not often possible by clinical, serologic, immunologic and puncture findings alone, as there are locally different appearances in all hepatic disorders and varying combinations with fatty degenerations—metabolic or nutritional—which may not show themselves in sufficient significance.

In an attempt to solve these questions in Europe, laparoscopy (peritoneoscopy) was introduced into the clinic by Kalk[1] in 1929. Since 1943, this procedure, mostly combined with the aimed biopsy technic, has established itself very well.[2-5] Therewith the "two-dimensional" intravital morphologic diagnostics of the liver began. The visual laparoscopic findings alone, however, had not yet been generally accepted in the absence of genuine documentation, being too subject to the judgment of the examiner. Above all the findings did not display sufficient weight, equivalent to that of the histologic specimen, even taking into consideration that a small liver specimen gives only a localized, not always representative, area of the liver for examination and is at best a snapshot of the biologic happening. Therefore, comparisons between visual laparoscopy and histologic findings showed discrepancies of 12-60 per cent, depending on statistical interpretation as well as the experience of the investigators.[6] Especially, cirrhosis often did not come into full account in the specimen.[2, 7-9]

Laparoscopy reached an essential revolution with the introduction of the electronic flash, improvements of the optical system and lighting installation[10, 11] permitting accurate documentation of the visual findings. The diagnostic gain is more satisfying, the nearer one comes to the pathologic location. However, in the diagnostically important close-up, a sharp reproduction of findings differing in size is not possible with a fixed focus optic. Because of the blurred depth penetration, two photolaparoscopes were developed in cooperation with the firm R. Wolf/Knittlingen. One was intended for a summary view with an optic angle of 65 degrees (Figs. 36-1b and 2a) and an object distance of 4cm and with a copy scale, from object to film level, of 1.1:1. The second was for a close-up view (Figs. 36-1c and 2b) with an object distance of 2cm and a copy scale of 2:1 from object to film level. As source of light, the intra-abdominal electronic flash was chosen, with a view to better illumination of the object.[12]

This is not possible in a comparable measure with the proximal electronic flash reflected over a fibered bundle of rays, as for instance in the also strong-lighted rod lens optic after Hopkins. With its large optic angle of 85 degrees and an object distance of 4 to 7cm it certainly supplies useful photographs on a large scale with relatively sharp depth penetration, but also gives distortions. Also, there is not enough information about its use in close-up views.

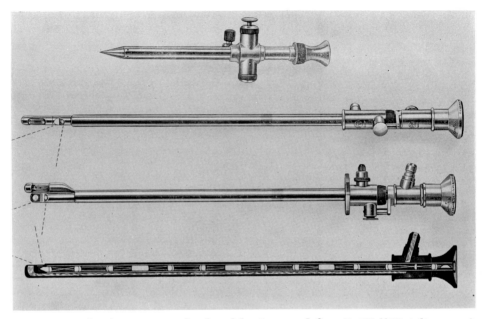

Figure 36.1. Photolaparoscopes developed by Lent and firm R. Wolf/Knittlingen: a) Trocar and cannula. b) Optic for summary view with cold light source in ringlike arrangement in laparoscope-mantle. Electronic flash distal to the entering optical lens system. c) Optic with cold light source distal to the entering optical lens system. Electronic flash lateral to it. d) Way of ray bundle and lighting arrangement.

A main problem of close-up photography with strong-light optics is the equal illumination, free of reflection, of the visual field. The optic described by me attains this because the electronic flash is not fixed in front of the endoscope objective, where its point would touch the liver and the visual field cannot be illuminated sufficiently, but is mounted lateral to it (Fig. 36-1). Therewith the visual direction of the optic coincides with the illumination of the visual field through the flash.

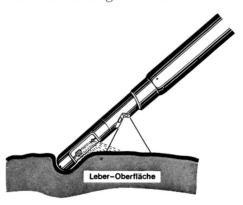

Leber–Oberfläche

Figure 36-2a. Way of ray bundle and lighting arrangement in closeup optic.

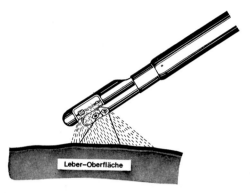

Figure 36-2b. Closeup optic with cold light source distal to the entering optical lens system. Electronic flash lateral to it.

The second problem concerns the depth penetration. According to physical law, it decreases with increasing brightness of the optic, enlarging of the copy scale, and prolongation of the focal distance of the photographic objective. It amounts to 10 to 7mm with object distance of 40mm, but only 2.5 to 4mm with object distance of 20mm. Essential for sharp reproduction therefore is the visual object distance corresponding to the object distance calculated for the optic. Unfortunately the latter cannot be measured accurately during the examination, as the human eye adapts itself to various layers of depth penetration, exact focusing aids not being employable because of the nearly parallel ways of rays behind the ocular and its large loss of light. This minute adjustment demands therefore skill and experience. It is performed by turning the optical direction of view at first vertical to the object. Now the source of illumination represents itself in the center of the visual field as reflection, more marked on smooth than on uneven surfaces. Photographs in this geometrical true position, however, do not supply useful information because of the interfering light reflex in the center of the picture. Therefore this reflex is shifted just outside the visual field by slight turning, that is, tilting of the optic and in this slightly tangential illumination, throwing the object into relief, the exposition in suitable object distance is performed.

ROLE OF PERITONEOSCOPY IN ACUTE AND CHRONIC LIVER DISEASE

With the improvements in photolaparoscopy discussed above, a reproducibility of finer liver structures up to the order of magnitude of lobules and periportal fields was made possible in addition to a visualization of characteristic changes of vessel systems on the surface of the liver. Subsequently further morphologic and—for the first time—intravital pathophysiologic aspects of the liver were offered.[13] At an increasing rate laparophotographs proved significant for better judgment of the actual process in the liver, mainly in follow-up observations. Even the pathologists appreciated it as a supplement in essential points to the histologic findings.

In our comparisons of photolaparoscopic and puncture findings, complete discrepancies in detailed diagnosis were noted in only 6 per cent and partial discrepancies in 22 per cent, despite the different dimensions of observation and criteria of judgment in histology compared with endoscopy. Eighteen per cent of histologic diagnoses were wrong, as ascertained by long-time observations of the process, as against 10 per cent wrong interpretations with laparoscopy.[14]

The reason for improved results of the laparoscopic finding was a comprehensive survey of the entire liver with close-up photographs even in diffuse inflammatory and metabolic diseases. The interpretation of photolaparoscopic findings, however, requires as much experience as does judgment of histologic puncture specimens which also form constellations of findings.

By reason of these perceptions, in Germany the opinion prevails to use primarily photolaparoscopy combined with the aimed biopsy in the differential diagnosis of liver diseases, especially since some contradictions to biopsy, e.g. cysts, hemangioma, beginning primary liver carcinoma, and circumscribed cholestasis, can only be ascertained laparoscopically. For follow-up investigations the percutaneous liver biopsy can be employed, after the hepatic disorder has been ascertained as a diffuse process by laparoscopy.[8]

PERITONEOSCOPIC PATHOLOGY OF HEPATITIDES

A convincing survey of this subject can only be obtained by extensive picture material, not demonstrable here, and hence the descriptive representation will have to be incomplete.

Acute Hepatitis

Acute hepatitis in general is no indication for laparoscopy. It will only be observed where differential diagnostic considerations give reason for it. The so-called big red liver[2] is marked by edema of the glossy, bright red organ with slight rounding of the lower edge and mostly or completely vanished lobular marking. There are a diffuse increase of thin transparent lymph vessels, stagnation of valve bearing, segmented main lymph vessels, and fine arterial vascularization.

The fine lymph vessels can often be made visible only with magnifying lenses and slight underexposure. While lymph channels under normal conditions run alongside the big intrahepatic vessels to the liver hilus and in adults hardly appear on the capsular surface, in the presence of inflammatory processes, they are conspicuously evident through increase of the lymph volume, probably as a result of opening anastomoses between deep and peripheral lymph systems. They help to remove the increased albuminous fluid and express therewith the macroscopic mesenchymal activity, which otherwise can only be comprehended histologically.

Subsiding Acute Hepatitis

This more often represents an indication for laparoscopy, in order to obtain a clear morphologic print for follow-up investigations that may become necessary later, e.g. in transitions of the process to the chronic stage, thereby gaining an insight to the pathogenesis. The findings on the surface are similar to those of acute hepatitis, only markedly less severe.

In healing, fibrosis occurs, with deposits mostly of regularly arranged, gray-white connective tissue in the periportal fields, resulting in fine lobular granulation of surface clearly differentiating it by brown lobules differing in size caused by lipofuscin deposits. Sometimes more deeply situated periportal fibrosis shimmers through the most superficial parenchymal layer, indicating the intrahepatic site (Plate 101). In the instance of thorotrastosis, the Thorotrast is mainly deposited in the periportal fields, appearing laparophotographically in the form of fine, silvery white, reticular structures. The extent of periportal fibrosis usually shows better in a picture of the surface, but its etiology can be determined by a puncture specimen. Increase of the peripheral lymph stream cannot be seen after the development of inactive fibrosis.

Retarded Progressing Acute Hepatitis

There is frequently an exudation of albuminous fluid to the surface from the fine network of stagnated, and therefore more permeable, lymph vessels. In due course, capsular fibrosis develops. The capsule can be a diffuse, delicate gray and may just be transparent or, occasionally, may be compact and white, the underlying liver tissue thus escaping examination. This is more often the case on the upper than the undersurface and is extremely rare on the whole liver. With the confirmation of such capsular fibrosis in the presence of sometimes unobstrusive puncture findings, a former hepatitis without symptoms may be detected.

Capsular fibrosis can nevertheless not be judged without criticism as healed hepatitis, as it can smoulder continuously. Here the minute representation of a place not involved with capsular fibrosis is as important as the histologic finding.

When an acute hepatitis runs protractedly, with serologic signs of cholestasis, a laparoscopy is always indicated. In these cases one often finds that, in contrast to the usual picture of acute hepatitis, there is a more or less heavy intrahepatic cholestasis, with gray-brown-green lobules sharply limited against each other because of a distinctly marked periportal fibrosis. The protracted process of a hepatitis with cholestatic distinction finds its anatomic explanation as a recessive hepatitis on the ground of a posthepatitis periportal fibrosis. This, however, cannot be called a chronic hepatitis, as it can turn clinically, serologically and morphologically into fibrosis (Plate 102).

Chronic Hepatitis

Chronic hepatitis as a group of etiologically as well as morphologically different, more or less progressive, disease processes of the liver was described first in 1947 by Kalk.[15] Comparative laparoscopic and histologic follow-up studies in their varying courses included their possible ending in cirrhosis.

The subdivision into chronic persistent and chronic aggressive hepatitis based on pathologic-anatomic criteria was undertaken in 1968 within the European Association Study of the Liver (EASL). This has proved valuable in practice on the whole, so long as the classification was based on all the morphologic findings along with the clinical symptomatology, and not on the histologic findings alone. After all, there are forms of progress which cannot simply be forced into this subdivision.

Chronic Persistent Hepatitis

This is a mild form of a covert or nonjaundiced hepatitis, often with a prolonged course, and because of its trifling, uncharacteristic symptoms is usually discovered only by chance. It has generally a tendency to complete restoration and a favorable prognosis. However, it can also turn into a chronic aggressive hepatitis. It is distinguished histologically by chronic portal inflammatory infiltration without disturbances of the lobular architecture and slight fibrosis.[16] Probably it is identical with chronic portal hepatitis.[17]

The appearance of the surface bears a likeness to that in acute hepatitis. The liver, however, is generally less swollen, the lower edge mostly sharp, the lobular marking partly faded, partly more pronounced than normal, due to delicate portal fibrosis (Plate 103). Essential are an ubiquitous increase of the peripheral lymph current and a distinct enlargement and swelling of the spleen, sometimes with small prolapses of splenic tissue. As splenomegaly always exists, the spleen might not be unimportant in the continuance of the inflammatory process. Whether the splenic enlargement is due to an immunologic mechanism or to a persistent splenitis due to the underlying process in the liver, must be reserved to further investigations.

Merely from the result of a puncture a differentiation between chronic persistent and nonspecific reactive hepatitides proves difficult and can be reached only through follow-up biopsies. If there are corresponding clinical and serologic findings and laparoscopic and histologic criteria of a chronic persistent hepatitis, a stronger suspicion in this direction is more justified than with findings based on a single puncture specimen alone.

In practice, occasionally an assertion in this sense is necessary, based on laparoscopic findings and clinical symptomatology, even in the presence of a largely normal histology. This may need to be verified in follow-up studies.

Chronic Aggressive Hepatitis

This condition is pathologic-anatomically defined roughly by chronic inflammatory infiltration of the periportal fields, extending over the basal sections of the lobules to the neighboring ones, penetrating into them by producing active partitions and disturbing thereby the lobular architecture in all stages up to complete transformation of parenchyma in the sense of a cirrhosis.[16, 18] Laparoscopically it offers a varied, many-colored picture of the surface, often with completely different deviations on the same organ. Generally the liver is enlarged noticeably and the consistency increased, recognizable by the lower edge of the liver reaching far into the abdomen as well as the stronger pulsations imparted by the aorta. The lobular marking is partly nonexistent. In places lobules of uneven size and arranged irregularly with different red coloring are more dissociated through widened gray-red to gray-white periportal fields. By viewing on a tangential level, delicate, slightly irregular granulations, also shallow wavings with more or less marked streaky or plain capsular fibrosis on the upper as well as under surface are found.

To these morphologic findings changes of the capsular vessels are added. In areas with intensive reddening, most delicate arterial vascularization, often with small sanguineous extravasation, can be seen. Also impressive is a considerable increase in the lymph stream, with a heavy stagnation of the main lymph channels which, often tightly filled, set themselves against the surface and flow into large collecting vessels to the ligamentum falciforme, over the lateral lower edge, the undersurface of the liver, to the liver hilus or from the convexity of the right and left lobes to the diaphragm (Plate 104). Such lymphangiectases correspond completely with anatomic and lymphographic findings, i.e. increasing dilation and varicosity of hilar lymph channels and of the ductus thoracicus.[19-22] The functional significance of the morphologic appearances is therefore mainly distinguished by an alteration of these two vessel systems, which otherwise in their behavior cannot be directly observed intravitally. The increase of the visible lymph stream regularly correlates well with the extent of the inflammation and the mesenchymal activity, and its accurate consideration forms an essential part of the laparoscopic judgment of activity. Even without morphologic indications for a beginning transformation of liver tissue, small stagnated, dichotomously branching, blue-red capsular veins in places, with venous stagnation in places along the ligamentum falciforme, sometimes point to a beginning portal hypertension.

Within the chronic aggressive hepatitis, recent necrosis may be seen either in the form of multiple, small, yellowish, slightly sunken groups with irregular arrangement, or as outspread sunken areas with multiple petechial hemorrhages. More frequently, one observes their residues in the form of multiple, smaller sunken scars with localized capsular fibroses on the bottom. Following widespread necrosis, shallow scars sharply set against the remaining liver tissue are seen. Deeply situated, finely granulated, gray-white areas with delicate nutritive arterial vascularization may also be seen, sometimes with regeneration in the surroundings. Finally as a consequence of necrosis it may come to form deep furrows and further to subdivide the left lobe into a small rest of connective tissue.

Besides this short sketch of the multiform picture of the surface, in practice different changes on the same organ may be observed, together with corresponding histology of a chronic aggressive hepatitis. For instance, in some patients chronic aggressive hepatitis and chronic persistent hepatitis can be seen side by side. In other patients localized capsular fibrosis with smooth surfaces, stagnation of lymph vessels in places and a finely granular change of the undersurface may be seen. In still other patients, besides symptoms of the chronic aggressive hepatitis, irregular nodules are seen in places with complete change of all vessel systems due to constriction in the area of the portal vein, e.g. portal hypertension. The new formation of thin arteries and increasing insufficiency of lymph channels as they discharge into the main channels make the essential component of the hemodynamics of cirrhosis obvious (Plate 105). In some patients a morphologically pronounced active cirrhosis with much fatty degeneration, for instance, through abuse of alcohol, is noted; the histology may reveal as the primary disease—in agreement with immunologic results—not the abuse of alcohol, but a chronic aggressive hepatitis with fatty degeneration and processes of changing liver structure.

Finally there are chronic hepatitides which can, through clinical, immunologic, and histologic criteria, in the course of many years neither be described as persistent nor as already aggressive, even though future development in the direction of cirrhosis is beginning to show, macroscopically confirmed by local pseudolobulation and commencing changes of structure of the vessel system.

Thus, again and again photolaparoscopy reveals, in contrast to biopsy alone, morphologically and functionally variable aspects of different manifestations of hepatitis, with many transitional stages leading to cirrhosis on the same organ. The problem of hepatitis does not become easier through this extensive "bioptical" morphologic view, but perhaps may become clear gradually by follow-up investigations, as discussed.

METABOLIC LIVER DISEASE

In laparophotograms metabolic disorders reveal themselves to begin with by characteristic color shades. Presupposition for their comparable representation is, however, the use of the same optic, the same working distance, a similar line of sight and the same flash energy.

Lipofuscinosis

Lipofuscinosis is clinically unimportant, often being observed in periportal fibrosis of younger patients in the form of central lobular brown coloring. This is seen also in siderosis, where it is diffuse and mainly appears as a fine, regular granulation on the surface.

Idiopathic Hemochromatosis

This condition is usually discovered in the stage of cirrhosis with an almost regular, fine nodulation. In comparison with other forms of cirrhosis, however, it is characterized by an intensive rusty brown color and, on palpation, by such hard consistency as is met with only in advanced primary carcinoma of the liver (Plate 106).

Acute Intermittent Porphyria

The surface of the liver shows irregularly arranged, bizarre, dark blue-violet patches. In addition, the picture of the surface is associated with nearly obligatory changes of an accompanying hepatitis. The actual proof of porphyria is the red fluorescence of the specimen under the Wood lamp. This is not the case in Wilson's disease which also shows blue patches due to deposits of copper pigments mainly on top of the cirrhotic nodules.[3]

Dubin-Johnson Syndrome

This rare disorder primarily represents a contraindication for percutaneous biopsy because of its biochemically evident cholestasis and a disturbance of excretory function for cholescytographic contrast medium and sulfobromophthalein. One is impressed with the dark gray-black coloring of distinctly definable, regularly arranged lobules, due to deposits of melanin.

Fatty Degeneration of Liver

In practice most fatty degeneration of the liver of various degrees is caused by chronic alcohol abuse, diabetes mellitus, or disturbances of fat metabolism. Some years ago it seemed impossible to judge the extent correctly by laparoscopy, the bioptic finding being the decisive dimension.

With the help of improved optics and photography with magnifying lenses, this second dimension of viewing became effective. A comparative judgment, though, should only follow the synthesis of both kinds of investigations, as the extent of fat dispersion in pathologic-anatomic as well as laparoscopic views becomes more differentiated regionally due to increasing fatty degeneration, and a correct assertion about the grade of fatty degeneration of the whole organ is impossible from one puncture specimen, but only by the average of specimens from six different segments of the liver.[23] This however not being practical, the laparoscopic assessment of the extent of fatty degeneration side by side with the finding in the puncture specimen has an additional significance.

Distinct Fatty Degenerations

Slight fatty degenerations of liver cells can hardly be differentiated by laparoscopy, but are of little clinical importance. In distinct fatty degenerations an enlarged liver is visible, with a rounded undersurface, a soft consistency palpable through puncture—whereby the surrounding area turns into an intensive yellow—and a distinct lobular bound, pale red-orange-yellow speckled, smooth surface. Additionally as a functional criterion multiple stagnated capsular veins appear (Plate 107). In fatty degeneration these are observed more regularly and earlier than a corresponding coloring of the organ, which appears with pronounced increase of fatty degeneration. Corresponding to biochemical findings of a slight intrahepatic cholestasis, interlobular branches of the portal vein are compressed through hepatic lobules, having become voluminous by fatty degeneration. Even these slight degrees of portal hypertension become important through communication of interlobular veins as well as normally invisible capsular veins on the surface, in the form of short dichotomous blue-red veins.

Uncomplicated Fatty Degenerations, Degrees I and II

Here the orange-yellow irregular speckles on the more stagnated organ with distinctly rounded undersurface become more conspicuous. Only in uniform fatty degeneration of all parts of the liver is the surface a diffuse orange-yellow. More often one observes—analogic to differing distribution of fat within the hepatic lobules—areas of heavier deposits of fat in uneven distribution, differing in size and intense yellow, set off hazily against pale red areas with less severe fatty degeneration. Lobular separation cannot be seen anymore. Stagnation of the capsular veins is more pronounced; often perivenous hemorrhages are seen, superficial lymph vessels being absent.

When the process is due to alcohol intoxication resulting in reactive mesenchymal proliferation, as in *Fettleber* hepatitis,[16] and thus to a finding of pathologic value, irregular orange-yellow granulations, more stagnated capsular veins and—as an indication of the mesenchymal activity—a heavy increase of the peripheral lymph stream are observed. The suppositions being the same further on, the development of an active cirrhosis with heavy fatty degeneration, i.e. a fatty cirrhosis with every morphologic and hemodynamic sign of complete change of liver tissue, sometimes speedily results.

DISEASES OF THE PERITONEUM

Another indication for laparoscopy is the differential diagnosis of ascites, further abdominal diseases of unknown origin, which cannot be diagnosed clearly by other means of examination. Often the more troublesome exploratory laparotomy may be avoided, especially since the laparoscopic survey over the peritoneum and large abdominal areas is usually better. Acute peritonitis, being a contraindication, is not observed.

Peritonitis Tuberculosa

Peritonitis tuberculosa may be seen with or without ascites as a part of miliary tuberculosis. In these cases the otherwise glossy, smooth, transparent, nearly avascular peritoneum—parietal and visceral—thickens showing fine vascularization and is seen speckled with millet-seedlike, yellowish white, glossy nodules of equal size and distribution, soft to touch. In addition delicate recent vascular adhesions appear, especially between loops of small intestine. In spite of some distinctive criteria, the differentiation from peritonitis carcinomatosis remains difficult, histology and culture being decisive. The ileocecal tuberculosis has become just as rare, an indication being the conglomeration in the loops of the small intestine, mesentery, and ascending colon forming a mass with recent dense injections of the vessels.

Acute Pancreatitis

Acute pancreatitis that has receded for a long period leaves necrosis of fatty tissue on the peritoneum and the mesentery. This is visible as yellow-white, irregular, sharply limited groups without any reaction in the surrounding.

Peritonitis Carcinomatosa

The appearance here is similar to that in peritonitis tuberculosa, being speckled, with slightly raised, yellowish white solid groups. It differs however, in size and shape, is more often confluent, is never transparent—apart from metastases of the partly transparent, mucous, and thereby characteristic Gallert carcinoma (Plate 108)—is dense and hard to touch with the optic or on palpation with a rod, and bleeds easily. In the surrounding area often a very fine, atypical arterial vascularization is observed, sometimes being diffuse. Differentiation between peritonitis tuberculosa and carcinomatosa is possible macroscopically with knowledge of the presentation of the primary tumor, but it may sometimes be extremely difficult so that the histology holds the decisive position.

In the manner discussed, the laparoscopic examination with extensive photographic documentation, and with that alone, has reached a clinical importance, comparable in its value only to x-ray films. Thereby it does not compete with the puncture findings, but together with them forms one of the aids necessary in synthesis for a correct judgment of the often multiform progress of diseases of the liver.

REFERENCES

1. Kalk, H., Bruhl, W., and Sieke, E.: Die gezielte Leberpunktion. *Deutsche med Wschr*, 69:693, 1943.
2. Kalk, H., and Wildhirt, E.: *Lehrbuch und Atlas der Laparoskopie und Leberpunktion.* Stuttgart, Thieme, 1962.
3. Beck, K.: *Atlas der Laparoskopie.* Stuttgart. Schattauer, 1968.
4. Siede, W., and Schneider, H.: *Leitfaden und Atlas der Laparoskopie.* München, Lehmann, 1962.
5. Wildhirt, E.: *Bedeutung und Wert der Laparoskopie und gezielten Leberpunktion.* Stuttgart, Thieme, 1964.
6. Lent, H., and Jansen, H. H.: Die Beobachtung der Leberoberflache mit dem Photolaparoskop und ihre Bedeutung fur die klinische praxis. *Deutsche med Wschr*, 83:24, 1958.
7. Lindner, H.: Grenzen und Gefahren der perkutanen Leberbiopsie mit der Menghini Nadel. *Deutsche med Wchnschr*, 92:1751, 1967.
8. Lindner, H.: Zur Frage der diagnostischen Sicherheit der Laparoskopie und perkutanen Leberbiopsie mit der Menghini Nadel. In Demling, L., and Ottenjann, R.: *Endoscopie, Methoden und Ergebnisse.* München, Werk Verlag Dr. Banaschewski, 1969, pp. 130-139.
9. Vido, J., and Wildhirt, E.: Korrelationen zwischen makroskopischen und mikroskopischen Befunden bei der Leberbiopsie. In Demling, L., and Ottenjann, R.: *Endoskopie, Methoden und Ergebnisse.* München, Werk Verlag Dr. Banaschewski, 1969, pp. 128-129.
10. Caroli, J.: La laparophotographie en couleurs par l'endographe de A. Foures. *Rev med chir mal foie*, 31:15, 1955.
11. Lent, H.: Die Entwicklung der Photolaparoskopie mit dem Electronenblitz. *Acta hepatosplen*, 9:195, 1962.
12. Lent, H.: Diagnostische Möglichkeiten mit modernen Laparoskopoptiken. In Ottenjann, R.: *Fortschritte der Endoskopie.* Stuttgart, Schattauer, 1970, vol. II, pp. 273-284.
13. Lent, H.: Feinstrukturen der Leberoberflache bei laparoskopischer Lupenbetrachtung. In *Endoscopy of the Digestive System.* Proceedings 1st European Congress Digestive Endoscopy, Basel, Karger, 1969, pp. 102-103; *Endoscopy 1*:107, 1969.

14. Lent, H.: Vergleichende photolaparoskopisch histologische Untersuchungen bei diffusen Lebererkrankungen. *Acta hepatosplen, 16*:174, 1969.
15. Kalk, H.: Die chronischen Verlaufsformen der hepatitis epidemica in Beziehungen zu ihren anatomischen Grundlagen. *Deutsches med Wschr, 72*:308, 1947.
16. Thaler, H.: *Leberbiopsie.* Heidelberg, Springer, 1969.
17. Popper, H., and Schaffner, F.: The vocabulary of chronic hepatitis. *New Engl and J Med, 284*:1154, 1971.
18. Wepler, W., and Wildhirt, E.: *Klinische Histopathologie der Leber.* Stuttgart, Thieme, 1968.
19. Baggenstoss, A. H., and Cain, J. C.: The hepatic hilar lymphatics of man: Their relation to ascitis. *New Engl and J. Med, 256*:531, 1957.
20. Beltz, L., Esser, G., and Grenzmann, M.: Zur Lymphdynamik bei der portalen Hypertension. *Fortschr Geb Röntgenstrahlen, 111*:1, 1969.
21. Dumont, A. E., and Mullholland, J. H.: Hepatic lymph in cirrhosis. In Popper, H., and Schaffner, F.: *Progress in Liver Diseases.* New York, 1955, vol. II.
22. Rusznyak, I., Foldi, M., and Szabo, G.: *Lymphologie, Physiologie und Pathologie der Lymphgefasse und des Lymphkreislaufes.* Stuttgart, Fischer, 1969.
23. Kremer, G. J., Katzenbach, G., Mevissen, H., Hegner, J., and Netter, P.: Zur regionalen Verteilung des Triglyzeridund Phospholipoidgehaltes in normalen und verfetteten menschlichen Lebern. *Leber Magen Darm, 1*:125, 1971.

CHAPTER 37

HEPATIC CIRRHOSIS AND MALIGNANT LIVER DISEASES, PERITONEOSCOPIC FINDINGS

Jacques Caroli and Leonidas H. Berry

INTRODUCTORY STATEMENT

PERITONEOSCOPY IS VERY USEFUL for the study of liver diseases. By this method it is possible to make complete, nonoperative, *in vivo* anatomic diagnoses. Direct biopsies from suspicious areas of the liver done under peritoneoscopic control are far superior to percutaneous blind biopsies, and much safer. In this article we will limit our discussion to the results of our own experience with various types of hepatic cirrhosis and malignant tumors of the liver and will include a brief description of hepatic involvement in lymphoreticular malignancies.

HEPATIC CIRRHOSIS OF VIRAL ORIGIN

Without laparoscopy, one may miss the diagnosis of postnecrotic cirrhosis of viral origin in a typical case.

CASE HISTORY

A 35-year-old woman had viral hepatitis five years ago. She was treated with corticosteroids and was followed up at two week intervals. A mild transaminase elevation persisted. A blind liver biopsy was normal. The possibility of transaminitis of Popper was considered. At peritoneoscopy, however, she had typical postnecrotic, macronodular cirrhosis.

ALCOHOLIC CIRRHOSIS

In our experience the macronodular type of cirrhosis, in which the nodules are more than 1 to 5cm in diameter associated with splenomegaly, is rarely of alcoholic origin and may be of viral etiology. When a liver is markedly enlarged and has a butter yellow coloration, and beside lesions of sclerosis, contains fat vesicles in 70 to 90 per cent of the liver cells, alcohol can be considered the only or almost only cause of such structural and morphological changes.[1] When histologically a cirrhotic liver shows more or less well preserved Mallory bodies in large quantities, one can be sure that whether it is nodular or not, atrophic or hypertrophic, the cellular reconstruction and regeneration are of alcoholic origin, even if the patient denies any alcoholic excess.

When a nodular cirrhosis shows the rusty color of hemochromatosis and the characteristic tattoo of iron is found in the hepatic cells, and when the sclerosis is confirmed by histology, an alcoholic etiology is the rule and posthepatic etiology is the exception.

LATE POSTHEPATITIC CIRRHOSIS

It is not rare that ten or twenty years after a catarrhal icterus of severe degree, a macronodular cirrhosis is discovered even though the patient appears to be doing well and to be cured for a long time. Biologically this cirrhosis may be silent and a minimal retention rate of bromsulfalein may only be present. In such patients systematic endoscopy will permit the discovery of this macronodular cirrhosis that is very well compensated. This study may be made before any surgery is contemplated.[2, 3] A slight retention of bromsulfalein is sufficient evidence for intervention.

CRYPTOGENIC CIRRHOSIS

So-called cryptogenic cirrhosis,[2, 3] especially anicteric hepatitis, is frequently found in the Mediterranean area. The endoscopic aspect, in general, is that of a postnecrotic macronodular cirrhosis. Very often there is, in addition, a capsulitis, reminiscent of sugar-icing liver. We must add here that Curschmann's disease can be diagnosed *in vivo* only by endoscopy.

LAENNEC'S CIRRHOSIS

When endoscopy reveals a true Laennec's cirrhosis, an alcoholic etiology is the rule, whereas hepatitis as a cause is the exception. But these cirrhoses must have the following features, namely, a complete hardening of the liver, decrease in size, reddish discoloration, and nodules not over 2mm in diameter.

The liver size as assessed by the endoscopic technic has an important prognostic value. The hepatomegaly can be the best or the worst thing. In the former, it affects a patient in a good state of nutrition. The surface of the liver may be smooth or sometimes nodular, and histologic sections show that the areas of sclerosis are less extensive than the areas of normal parenchyma. The enormous liver carries a poor prognosis in young women with temperature elevations. The French writers at the end of the nineteenth century called these "malignant cirrhoses." Endoscopy reveals a hard liver with a smooth surface which cuts easily; no subcapsular nodule is visible, and color is lighter than normal, sometimes like butter.

Finally, endoscopy may reveal over the liver, the spleen and the peritoneum, numerous granulations whose acid-fast etiology can be ascertained only by biopsy. The evolution of these lesions was constantly fatal until antibiotics, antituberculous therapy and anabolic agents came into use.

WILSON'S DISEASE

Peritoneoscopy with biopsy[2, 4] may assist in the diagnosis of Wilson's disease. This is a type of postnecrotic macronodular cirrhosis, but its true peritoneoscopic feature is the presence of bluish spots and discolored nodules. In some instances the color may be metallic grey.

Cutanea Tardiva Porphyria

This type of lesion sometimes occurs as a part of the picture of alcoholic cirrhosis of the liver. In this disease, the appearance of bluish spots has been described in the literature; however, we have seen only one case of this type. Biopsy in this instance revealed red fluorescence with ultraviolet light.

PRIMARY BILIARY CIRRHOSIS

The diagnosis of this disease, peritoneoscopically, is based upon the following features: The liver has a very smooth edge and a firm consistency. There is seldom any abnormal change in pigmentation except in the late stages of severe disease with biliary retention. Usually there are no nodules. The gallbladder appears soft and translucid as a rule, although in 10 per cent of cases, primary biliary cirrhosis[2] may be associated with cholelithiasis. In contrast, in obstructive biliary cirrhosis[5] there is *tattooing* of the hepatic surface proportional to the degree of jaundice. This picture is considerably exaggerated when the obstruction is caused by a carcinoma of the head of the pancreas, ampulla of Vater or an impacted stone in the ampulla. In these cases, the gallbladder is seen to be greatly distended.

In obstructive cirrhosis due to stones,[6, 7] the biliary tree which can be seen is very different from that described in association with carcinoma. In the former, the gallbladder is often small and retracted. When the stones are contained in the gallbladder, their hard consistency can be palpated through the peritoneoscope.

Recently, Doniach reported the development of a test based upon her researches with antimitochondrial antibodies. She found a positive reaction in the presence of primary biliary cirrhosis and a negative reaction with obstructive biliary cirrhosis. These findings are not always consistent with those observed by peritoneoscopy.

Duodenoscopy with papilla cannulation has been used in the differential diagnosis of primary biliary cirrhosis and obstructive biliary cirrhosis. By this method, it has been found that in primary biliary cirrhosis, the common bile duct is normal and the intrahepatic ducts are deformed. In obstructive biliary cirrhosis, attempts at diagnosis with this method have given poor results. It is a moot question whether duodenoscopy with cannulation of the papilla of Vater will supercede the use of laparoscopy and laparophotography as used in the past.

BANTI'S SYNDROME

This syndrome is remarkable. Palpation of the abdomen is diagnostic, because of the considerable splenomegaly present, while the liver is barely palpable.

Endoscopy reveals that the liver is small, with a thin border and firm consistency. The liver may, however, be macronodular. Despite this observation, in these forms, which after all are juvenile diseases, there is a good prognosis when the spleen is removed. The spleen may weigh more than 3kg. A successful splenorenal anastomosis is desirable.

In summary, the earlier the nodules observed during endoscopy are formed, the better is the prognosis. With the same clinical and biologic aspects (jaundice, ascites, hepatic insufficiency), two different anatomic lesions evolve. One involves a collapse and a diffuse necrosclerosis; this is generally fatal. The other consists of giant regeneration nodules developed early; the prognosis is relatively good. Due to the mass of hepatic parenchyma functionally healed, this cirrhosis is relatively well tolerated and can last several decades.

GIANT ADENOMATOUS HYPERPLASIA
CASE HISTORY[2, 3]

A child, 6 years old, was hospitalized in 1956 because of jaundice of three months' duration. The biologic signs at this time included: hyperpositive flocculation test, elevation of gamma-globulin and a disturbance of coagulation contraindicating biopsy. The liver was slightly enlarged and the spleen was palpable.

Endoscopy revealed considerable changes. More than half the left lobe of the liver, at the level of the edge of the organ was transformed into a sclerosed, thin plaque wall around itself. Biopsy at this level, if done, would have shown only the lesion of fibronecrosis without any remnant of hepatic parenchyma. In contrast, the right segment of the left lobe showed a massive hyperplasia and appeared to be made of normal parenchyma. If biopsy were done at that level, it would have shown more or less normal liver tissue. The entire inferior aspect of the right lobe of the liver was transformed by a nodular hyperplasia of massive proportion divided by deep grooves.

This patient was seen again fifteen years later and was in perfect health. She has refused all followup examinations, but the hypertrophied spleen is still there to show that the cirrhosis is still in evidence.

COMPENSATORY MACRONODULAR HYPERTROPHY

Despite the fact that the beginning of an illness had predicted a catastrophic evolution, one can witness a complete disappearance of all alarming symptoms, including jaundice and ascites in the absence of any kind of treatment. In these cases, endoscopy revealed that a favorable prognosis usually is observed in compensatory macronodular hypertrophy. The following case is an example.

A woman, aged 55, when examined for the first time, had rather marked icterus, with nervous symptoms, edema, ascites and elevation of the cholesterol level. Spontaneous clearing of the jaundice and the anasarca came as a surprise. Since that time, her general condition has been satisfactory despite intolerance for Delta-cortisone (diabetes, hypertension, duodenal ulcer).

Laparophotography, done only six months after the onset of jaundice, revealed the presence of a voluminous projection the size of a nut. This probably represented hyperplasia which occurred very early and permitted an unexpected survival. This endoscopy corrected the impression obtained from the examination of the histologic slides because the tissue sample represented only a small fragment from a limited area involved with cirrhosis, and showed no hyperplastic tissue.

If the endoscopic observation of macronodule, regardless of its biologic significance, is a favorable sign, this is only so if the condition is controlled because those cases of postatrophic macronodular cirrhosis remain a dangerous sequela. These patients really are exposed to the possibility of hepatic insufficiency in a progressive manner, with many complications such as septicemia due to enterobacter organisms and hemorrhage due to rupture of esophageal varices. One must add also eventual malignant degeneration.

When, in the opposite case, in the middle of icteric phase a cirrhosis of the liver without nodule develops, with a marked granular atrophy, one must consider the prognosis is very poor.

CHRONIC ACTIVE HEPATITIS AND PERSISTING HEPATITIS

The cirrhoses we have just reviewed—macronodular, adenomatous, atrophic, subacute and Banti types—are really complications of viral hepatitis. This was brought into evidence more than twenty-five years ago in the thesis of Saladin. It is rather curious to observe that Groote and Desmets, who work in Louvain, see this type of lesion only exceptionally. Others, on the contrary, think it is only a question of persistent hepatitis or chronic active hepatitis. This would be one of the commonest forms of this sequela of hepatitis.

Of 140 cases recently studied, in 75 per cent the onset was marked by icterus. In statistics produced by Belgian, Scandinavian and English writers, most of the patients showed no icterus at the beginning, the principal manifestations being anorexia, nausea, and asthenia.

We would not insist on the extrahepatic syndromes (arthralgia, glomerulonephritis, arteritis nodosa), as does one observer, and we will not insist either on the immunologic sign (anti-DNA, anti-mitochondrial, anti-smooth tissue antibody). The reaction to Australian antigen may be positive if anti-smooth fiber and antibodies are missing. The problem here is to know whether endoscopy may contribute to the diagnosis. With considerable reservation, we will say that peritoneoscopy may sometimes reveal very early the existence of small cirrhotic nodules on the edge of the liver or scattered on its surface. Similar consultation must lead one to accept this evidence of cirrhosis even before a puncture biopsy is able to bring the proof. For the rest, when the liver is hard, cirrhosis is extensive and disseminated. The liver scarred with plaques indicates the role of inflammatory manifestations with much more clarity. In reality, this disease must especially be followed biologically and by repeated puncture biopsy; there is little room for peritoneoscopic investigation.

SUBACUTE ATROPHY WITH NECROSCLEROSIS— DIFFUSE WITHOUT REGENERATION

CASE HISTORY

A man, 56 years old, at onset of illness had asthenia, anorexia, and loss of weight. Itching started one month before jaundice. There was no history of alcoholism or infectious contact and no treatment by injection. The jaundice became so marked without collateral circulation, ascites, or enlarged spleen, the first thought was neoplastic obstruction. This diagnosis seemed to be confirmed by considering the bilirubinemia, which was marked, and the negative result of the flocculation test. However, cholesterol and gamma globulin levels remained very high. Diagnosis was made only during laparoscopy and laparophotography,[2, 3] giving not only the diagnosis but also the prognosis. Despite the severe jaundice, the liver was of a light color, with a severe collapse affecting the right liver; otherwise, the liver was of increased consistency. Although of recent onset, there is already a collateral circulation at the level of the epiploon and the round ligament. Corticosteroid treatment did not prevent coma, and ACTH therapy led to ascites and edema. Gross photography of the liver at necropsy revealed a pale, sclerotic, atrophic parenchyma.

In our experience, patients showing subacute atrophy without jaundice or with jaundice after apparent recovery are fairly numerous. After two or three months of evolution, the transaminase activity becomes normal, which reassures the physician, the patient, and his family. The spleen is no longer palpable and there is but little ascites. Only histoendoscopy reveals the gravity of the situation. One must take into consideration fundamentally the following facts: (1) bilobar atrophy of the liver; (2) smooth not nodular atrophy; (3) the liver may be whitish in color or may be greenish, especially in biliary retention of a severe degree; (4) the edge of the liver is always thin, though it may be rounded. Puncture biopsy shows the intensity of this sclerotic process, the trabecular division, the absence of signs of regeneration, and the hepatocellular alterations. Sclerosis, if in the foreground, is much more pronounced than the cellular infiltration.

MALIGNANT TUMORS

Primary Cancer of the Liver

Without reaching the proportions found in Black Africa or the Far East, hepatoma has become more frequent in occurrence, mainly in France. But, dealing with a cancer associated with a cirrhosis or a malignant abdominal tumor, laparoscopy is not a good method of investigation. It gives a correct answer in only half the cases.

A large number of investigation methods, in addition to puncture biopsy, has been made available in recent years, and the majority of cases now can be diagnosed *in vivo*. Gold scintillography completed by selemethionine, gold scintillography completed by bleomycin, determination of the D-fetoproteins, and selective arteriography, are among the methods used.

Endoscopy in Primary Cancer Developing in Healthy Livers

The neoplastic mass in primary liver cancer is intrahepatic and is covered for a long time with almost thick, healthy liver. It is usual that the tumor is not seen even at laparostomy. During laparoscopy at the level of the right or left lobe, the hepatic gland looks deformed and swollen. When the deformation affects the anterior edge of the gland, the latter loses its habitual thinness and presents a more or less voluminous hump. When the tumefaction affects the caudate lobe, even if superficially, the liver appears normal; it pushes the gallbladder to the right and the round ligaments to the left. As the tumor first develops, the liver modifies and at the point of invasion ulcerates. Sometimes over a large zone it becomes whitish, then necrotic. These foci are the source of intraperitoneal hemorrhages, often lethal. It is not unusual in patients with malignant hepatoma, during severe abdominal pains, to see in laparoscopy a mass of clots around the liver.

Endoscopy in Primary Cancer Following Liver Cirrhosis

In France, Africa, and the Far East, most of the malignant hepatomas are associated with liver cirrhosis. In France, most are alcoholic in origin, but outside of that country, macronodular atrophic cirrhosis is the commonest. The latter is without doubt viral in origin, as are numerous post-cirrhotic malignant hepatomas with positive reaction to Australian antigen. The data of endoscopy, according to our own statistics, are valuable in only 59 per cent of cases. A study was done with 120 observations, but for which only forty-three endoscopies were performed. In only 29 per cent of patients has cancer been diagnosed by this means.

When several cirrhotic nodules coalesce, they take on a whitish tint and look like bacon. By their color and size they can be differentiated from the rest of the gland. Rarely this carcinomatous transformation is unique. Most often it is multilocular. It is rare, however, that this carcinomatous nodule becomes difficult to recognize. When there is suspicion of neoplastic degeneration, every single nodule of the cirrhosis must be inspected; when one is mainly congested, it must be considered suspect. Puncture biopsy is done at this level, taking good care to avoid consecutive hemorrhages.

Endoscopic diagnosis often gives negative results and is not always easy. The scintillographic gaps filled by selemethionine or bleomycin[3] have more value. The same holds true about hypervascularization and arterial tufts seen after selective opaque injections.

Metastatic Cancer

Peritoneoscopy with biopsy remains a very effective method for the diagnosis of malignancies of the liver. In the early stages, it is relatively easy to differentiate between metastatic carcinoma of the liver and primary carcinoma of the liver. However, in late stages, it may be difficult or impossible by peritoneoscopy and biopsy to make the differentiation. Peritoneoscopy with guided liver biopsy in malignant liver disease is much more effective than percutaneous blind liver biopsy. This is particularly true in a typical case where the clinical picture begins with acute symptoms and high fever, and the differentiation from acute cholecystitis has to be made. In our experience, laparoscopy with guided biopsy has been particularly effective because of the frequency with which the malignant nodules tend to be superficial and are often easily reached on the superior and inferior surfaces of the liver.

Peritoneoscopic Findings in Metastatic Malignancy in the Liver

The laparoscopist usually sees whitish hard patches or nodules in varying degrees of dissemination at the liver surface. This varies from a few nodules to the advanced phase in which the gross picture is that of a cauliflower. Regardless of the size and number of the nodules, most are surrounded by a zone of congestion. When there is bile retention, there is also a zone of greenish discoloration.

Melanoma of the Liver

The laparoscopic appearance of liver metastases from melanosarcoma presents a striking and characteristic color. The melanin pigment is easily seen as black patches on the surface of the liver. Necrotic ulcerations will eventually occur on these surfaces. The best characteristics are so classic that it is usually unnecessary to carry out guided biopsies of the lesion. Furthermore, biopsy in these cases is particularly likely to be followed by hemorrhage due to necrosis. This occurrence may be exceptional but when hemorrhage occurs, it is often profuse. Such an attitude on biopsy has the following counterpart: A skillful endoscopist may make the mistake of assessing, on the laparoscopic examination alone, the existence of liver metastasis when there is none.

In hydatid cyst of tenia granulosarcoma, this mistake has been made in a considerable number of cases, twelve of thirty-four. This is a very significant figure because in such cases one cannot perform the exploratory puncture. Fortunately, immunoelectrophoresis has solved this sometimes difficult problem in recent years.

HODGKIN'S DISEASE AND LEUKEMIAS

Endoscopy seems not often useful in the diagnosis of these conditions. However, occasions arise when there are no palpably enlarged peripheral lymph nodes and when one has to determine the etiology of a mediastinal mass. The best indication for endoscopy is in the case of febrile evolution, often undulating. In about 50 per cent of patients the examination of the liver is diagnostic.[1, 7] This makes unnecessary other procedures such as lymphography, which may be distressing. Lymphoreticular malignancies in endoscopy sometimes look like tuberculous granulomas except that, in general, the elements are too small or too large. There may sometimes be whitish patches. In other cases the appearance is more tumorous. The whitish patches are larger in size and look like alveolar echinococcosis. In certain observations the endoscopic appearance may be misleading and may be that of a large cauliflower tumor which may be diagnosed as malignant epithelial metastasis.

The guided puncture in these cases is indispensible for diagnosis. The fragments show all the histologic characteristics of Hodgkin's disease, also recognizable because of the inflammatory infiltration, the eosinophilic cells with polymorphonuclears and Sternberg cells, whose details are known to everyone.

We consider that leukemic diseases are much more in the field of puncture biopsy than of endoscopy, because the liver, normal in gross appearance, may on puncture biopsy reveal foci of white, characteristic elements. Lymphosarcomas can manifest themselves by monstrous hepatomegaly, with rapid evolution. Endoscopy is difficult because of the size of the liver and the variegated appearance. One could only do a puncture biopsy which reveals neoplastic cells of lymphocytic origin.

REFERENCES

1. Caroli, J., Mainguet, P., et Ricordeau, P.: Contribution a l'etude des cirrhoses alcooliques. *Dtsch Ges Verd Stoffw krkh, 20,* Tag. Kassel. Okt 1959 paru In Gastroenterologia, Suppl. ad vol. 95:94-114, 1961.
2. Foures, A., Ricordeau, P., and Caroli, J.: La laparoscopie en pathologie hepatique. *Arch Mal App Digestif, 40:*1342, 1951.
3. Caroli, J. and Ricordeau, P.: Value of peritoneoscopy and peritoneoscopic photographic in color and of scintillography in the diagnosis of liver diseases. In Popper, H. and Schaffner, F.: *Progress in Liver Diseases,* New York, Grune & Stratton, 1961, Chapter 21, pp. 296-314.
4. Caroli, J. et Ricordeau, P.: Valeur diagnostique comparative de la ponction-biopsie dans les affections hepatobiliaires de l'adulte. In *Libro de Actas del IV Congreso Internacional de Patologia Clinica,* Madrid, 1960.
5. Caroli, J.: La laparophotographie en couleurs par l'endographe de A. Foures. Sa valeur diagnostique dans les maladies du foie et des voies biliaires. Revue Medicochirurgicale des Maladies du foie, de la Rate et du Pancreas 30, 3, 15, 1955.
6. Caroli, J. et Ricordeau, P.: Etape laparoscopique dans le diagnostic des icteres par retention. In Caroli, J.: *Les icteres par retention. Diagnostic medico-chirurgical.* Paris, Masson, 1956, pp. 163-226.
7. Caroli, J. et Eteve, J.: Etape histologique dans le diagnostic des icteres par retention. In Caroli, J.: *Les icteres par retention. Diagnostic medico-chirurgical.* Paris, Masson, 1956, pp. 227-263.

CHAPTER 38

PERITONEOSCOPIC TECHNICS IN JAPAN, DIRECT CHOLECYST-CHOLANGIOGRAPHY, POSTPUNCTURE REPAIR, PATHOLOGY

Hiroshi Tadaki and Kiyomi Miura [*]

HISTORY

Peritoneoscopy was introduced in Japan by Kitayama[1] in 1929. After application to clinical situations, the accumulated clinical experience was reported in 1936.[2]

[*] We acknowledge the cooperation and assistance of the Medical Department of Professor S. Yamagata, Tohoku University School of Medicine, Japan.

In 1957, Yamagata brought the Henning-Sass-Walf type instrument from Germany to Japan. Numerous modifications were made and, with the technical assistance of Machida Company, a series of new instruments, known as Yamagata-Machida type instruments, became available.

In 1959, color motion pictures were taken, using the Yamagata-Machida water-cooling peritoneoscope.[3] In 1960, the Tohoku University type W80, with a visual angle of 80 degrees, was introduced to replace the previous instrument, which had a visual angle of 60 degrees. In 1963, endoscopic color television was introduced by Yamagata and Miura; clinical experience with this instrument was reported at the first Japanese Congress of Endoscopy.[4] With the introduction of glass fiber, application of glass fiber to the endoscopic instrument became popular. In 1968, a light-guiding peritoneoscope was made by Machida Company with a 500w Xenon short lamp as the light source. This instrument gave greater illumination and a more detailed view of the lesion. This is the most widely used instrument in Japan at present (Fig. 38-1).

A survey made in 1970 revealed that peritoneoscopic examination was then used in approximately 400 institutions all over Japan. Reports were obtained from 132 (33%) of these institutions, which showed that a total of 24,133 patients had been subjected to the peritoneoscopic examination

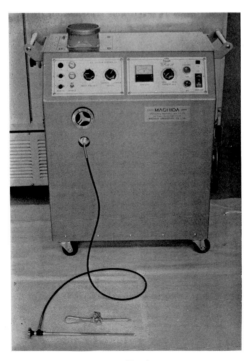

Figure 38-1. SLC type peritoneoscopic set. Peritoneoscope is connected to the external light source. Trocar is properly placed.

TABLE 38-I

CASES EXAMINED BY PERITONEOSCOPY IN JAPAN
UP TO 1970 (NATIONWIDE SURVEY)

		%
Diseases of the liver	17,195	71.2
Diseases of the gallbladder and bile ducts	3,131	12.9
Diseases of the stomach	} 605	2.5
Diseases of the intestine		
Diseases of the pancreas	570	2.4
Diseases of the peritoneum	1,022	4.2
Diseases of the blood	588	2.4
Diseases of the retroperitoneum (except pancreas)	210	0.9
Diseases of the female organ	407	1.7
Miscellaneous	405	1.7
Total	24,133	

Enquete sent to 400 inst.; return obtained from 132 inst. (1970).

(Table 38-I). This is a marked increase, compared to the 3,319 examinations in thirty-five institutions reported in 1961 by Yamakawa.

Patients subjected to the peritoneoscopic examination included 17,195 cases (71.2%) with various hepatic diseases; 3,313 cases (12.9%) with various biliary tract diseases; and 1,022 cases (4.2%) with various peritoneal diseases. Hepatic and biliary tract diseases appear to be the diseases most often subjected to the examination.

An analysis of 2,410 peritoneoscopic examinations over a 14-year period at Dr. Yamagata's medical department at the Tohoku University School of Medicine showed a high percentage of cases with liver disease. A majority of them had morbus Banti, reflecting the investigative interest of the department in this area (Table 38-II).

TABLE 38-II

CASES EXAMINED BY LAPAROSCOPY IN OUR MEDICAL DEPARTMENT

		%
Diseases of the liver	1,135	47.2
Diseases of the gallbladder and bile ducts	342	14.2
Diseases of the stomach	265	11.0
Diseases of the intestine	77	3.2
Diseases of the pancreas	175	7.3
Diseases of the peritoneum	219	8.6
Diseases of the blood	144	6.4
Diseases of the retroperitoneum (except pancreas)	15	0.6
Diseases of the female organ	7	0.3
Miscellaneous	31	1.2
Total	2,410	

Peritoneoscopic examination cannot be disregarded when determining the feasibility of surgery in patients with malignant diseases. Operability can be decided by the presence or absence of a metastasis in an intra-abdominal organ, which can be determined by peritoneoscopic examination. Periodic peritoneoscopic examination also helps in judging effectiveness of cancer chemotherapy. Because of these facts, the percentage of patients with gastrointestinal tract diseases subjected to peritoneoscopy is greater at Tohoku University than the percentage shown in the nationwide survey. The majority of patients with peritoneal diseases subjected to the examination were patients with peritoneal carcinomatosis. In most of them, the primary lesion was found in either the gastrointestinal tract or the pancreas. In short, in this medical department, a wider variety of cases were subjected to peritoneoscopic examination, partly because of the different interest but mainly because of the development of accessory tests that were combined with the peritoneoscopic examination, which will be discussed later.

PROCEDURE

Instruments are sterilized by formalin vapor or ethylene-oxide gas. The examining room is equipped with appropriate window shutters so the room may be darkened. A multipurpose operating table, which facilitates changes in position of the patient, is recommended. X-ray television equipment or x-ray apparatus is needed, and space, location, and equipment of the examination room should be designed accordingly. Examination is done with the patient in a fasting state. A normal saline enema is routinely given twice, three and two hours before the examination. Patient is asked to void and defecate before the examination. No premedication as described by Kalk[5] is given, except for pentobarbital which is given one hour before and again thirty minutes before the examination. In general, no other medications are given. Only local anesthesia with 0.5 per cent procaine is given during the procedure. Needless to say, all investigations to rule out possible hemorrhagic diathesis should be finished a day before the examination. Some institutions in Japan use Isomytal or a tranquilizer as the basic anesthetic medication; in other institutions, narcotics are prescribed. Only two institutions report routine use of general anesthesia for peritoneoscopic examination.

For air insufflation, a three-way cock with an attached self-regulating valve is connected with a 100ml syringe. Approximately 2,000-3,000ml of air is insufflated. Wittmann[6] reports the use of a manometer, but we are satisfied with the above-mentioned method. Some workers advocate the use of carbon dioxide or oxygen to prevent air embolism and to enhance the absorption of insufflated gas. However, we have not experienced any particular hazards attributable to the use of air. For details of other technics of air insufflation, the reader is referred to textbooks on peritoneoscopic examination. In general, observation, taking color pictures of the observed findings for future reference, and biopsy under direct observation conclude the examination. In some instances, special examinations, which will be discussed presently, will be performed if indicated.

DISEASES OF BILIARY TRACT AND PERITONEOSCOPY

Peritoneoscopic diagnosis of cholelithiasis, cholecystitis, pericholecystitis, gallbladder cancer, and extrahepatic biliary obstruction, is based on peritoneoscopic findings, which will be discussed next.

Cholelithiasis

No definite peritoneoscopic evidence of cholelithiasis exists. The diagnosis is made through deductive inference from observation of the gallbladder wall. In some instances, hypertrophy or inflammatory atrophy of the gallbladder wall may be found. If the stone is embedded in the wall, the wall may show surface irregularity (ruggedness). If the stone is impacted in the cystic duct, dilatation of the duct occurs, and a part of the dilated duct can be glimpsed through the peritoneoscope, giving the impression of a double gallbladder. If the stone occupies almost all of the gallbladder, by judicial use of a probe, the stone can be palpated through the gallbladder wall as a solid, hard mass. All these will help in reaching the diagnosis of cholelithiasis. However, when the gallbladder wall is intact and normal, the diagnosis cannot be made through peritoneoscopic examination alone.

Cholecystitis and Pericholecystitis

Cholecystitis and pericholecystitis are seen, in most cases, as the inevitable consequence or complication of cholelithiasis. However, they are seldom seen in the acute stage. We reach the diagnosis of cholelithiasis in most patients with cholecystitis or pericholecystitis. Peritoneoscopic examination of the gallbladder wall will reveal a turbid, gray-yellowish surface color, with hypertrophied wall, proliferation of fine superficial small vessels on the surface, and dilatation and abnormal course of these blood vessels. If pericholecystitis is present, adhesion with the caudal surface of the liver, omentum major, intestine, and/or visceral peritoneum occurs. A single glimpse would be enough to recognize these findings, and the inference is that inflammation in that area existed previously.

Gallbladder Cancer

Early detection of gallbladder cancer is difficult. Although with peritoneoscopic examination detection of gallbladder cancer has shown some improvement, and diagnosis can be made relatively earlier than previously, most gallbladder cancers seen by peritoneoscopic examination are far advanced. Therefore, the information regarding gallbladder cancer is usually limited to the findings of an advanced cancer. A cancerous gallbladder shows an opaque and thickened surface, unevenly distributed red spots, and disfigurement. Blood vessels decrease in number and the wall is hardened, forming a mass with an opaque, yellowish, marble-like appearance. In some instances, adhesions with the omentum occur, forming a large mass. In this situation, direct observation of the gallbladder surface may not be possible. Sometimes a part of the gallbladder is observed with a marble-like, opaque appearance, giving the impression of a whitish deposit. In most cases, contiguous metastatic infiltration to the right hepatic lobe will be observed. In some instances, these metastases form a mass. The tumefaction alone, however, is not indicative of malignant process. Conditions of surrounding organs and the appearance of the covering peritoneum (omentum major) should be carefully examined before reaching a final conclusion.

Extrahepatic Obstruction

Obstruction of the extrahepatic biliary tract is caused by stones, malignant processes, etc., located either in the hepatic ducts, cystic duct, common bile duct, or head of the pancreas. Therefore, depending upon the location of the lesion, peritoneoscopic findings will differ. It is possible to estimate the location of the lesion from peritoneoscopic findings, with the most important landmark being the grade of distention of the gallbladder, as was reported by Kalk.[5] However, this does not help in deciding the nature of the lesion.

RESULTS OF PERITONEOSCOPIC EXAMINATION; DIAGNOSTIC ACCURACY

In cases with cholelithiasis, due to the fact that the diagnosis of the cholelithiasis is based on the presence of pericholecystitis and cholecystitis, correct diagnosis was made in 114 of 151 cases (75.5%),[6] but by peritoneoscopic examination the diagnosis was made in 114 of 126 cases, the tendency of *overreading* can be seen in this situation. In twenty-six cases, a diagnosis of normal gallbladder was made, and in five cases, there was a diagnosis of gallbladder cancer.

In cases of carcinoma of gallbladder, twenty-four of thirty-three cases were correctly diagnosed, and of thirty-six cases of carcinoma of the common bile duct, twenty were correctly diagnosed, showing a relatively lower diagnostic rate. It may be noted that in twenty cases, only a diagnosis of obstructive jaundice was made, but no further delineation was possible. In eighty-eight patients with pancreatic cancer, the diagnosis was reached because they were all advanced cases with large tumefaction.

DIRECT CHOLECYSTOGRAPHY AND CHOLANGIOGRAPHY UNDER PERITONEOSCOPIC CONTROL—POSTPUNCTURE REPAIR TECHNICS

As with any diagnostic method, peritoneoscopic examination has its limitations. The diagnostic yield can be increased, however, by combining peritoneoscopy with other, accessory methods. This is especially true in patients with biliary tract diseases. In cases of obstructive jaundice, location of the lesion can be determined rather easily, but the nature of the lesion is difficult to establish. The best method, in our opinion, of detecting the nature of the lesion is direct cholangiography under peritoneoscopic observation. The method was first reported by Kalk[7] in 1933; however, since peritoneoscopic examination was not popular at that time, its use was limited. Royer[8] reported the use of this method in diagnosis of dyskinesia of the biliary tract, but because of the possibility of biliary leakage, the method was not widely used. With the development of newer puncture technics and instruments to prevent biliary leakage, this method became one of the routine examinations.

Methods

At first, the gallbladder is directly observed through the peritoneoscope, and its size, location of adherence, tonicity, adhesions to other organs, etc., are evaluated. If the gallbladder cannot be directly visualized, it may be brought into the visual field by raising it with forceps. One of the following puncture methods then can be decided upon, according to the status of the gallbladder.

1. Method P: Specially made instruments are used.
2. Method A: Insertion of needle into intrahepatic bile canal.
3. Method B: Transhepatic gallbladder puncture method.
4. Method C: Direct gallbladder puncture method.
5. Methods A + C and A + B.

After deciding which method is to be used, the needle is inserted (Fig. 38-2) under direct vision through the peritoneoscope. The needle is connected to an extension tube that, in turn, is connected to a syringe. The contents are aspirated. If the needle is inserted in the lumen, either bile is aspirated or mandrel is stained by bile. If either of these do not happen, it may mean either that the needle is inserted in the bladder wall or stone per se, or that the lumen of the needle is obstructed by highly viscous contents of particles. In these situations, change of the direction of insertion, reinsertion of mandrel, or an injection of a small quantity of saline will clarify the situation. After making sure that the needle is properly inserted into the lumen, contrast medium is injected and x-ray pictures are taken, depending on the visualization by the contrast medium. After taking the x-ray pictures, the contents are aspirated, antibiotics are injected to pre-

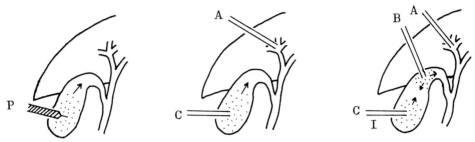

Figure 38-2. Direct-vision cholecyst-cholangiography under peritoneoscopic control. Various approaches are: P. Specially made instrument; I. Gallbladder puncture needle used; A. Direct puncture of intrahepatic bile duct; B. Transhepatic puncture of gall-bladder; C. Direct puncture of gallbladder; A + C. Combined A and C.

vent infection, and the needle is gradually withdrawn, after making sure that all of the contents are aspirated. After withdrawing the needle, a drain is placed under the gallbladder.

As this entire procedure is done under direct vision through the perito-neoscope, the presence or absence of biliary leakage can be observed both during and after the procedure. Necessary corrective measures, therefore, can be taken immediately. Aspirated bile is examined bacteriologically, bio-chemically, and cytologically.

Selection of Puncture Method

Method P

The special instruments used in this method were devised by Yamagata et al. in 1966[9] and were reported at the first Congress of the International

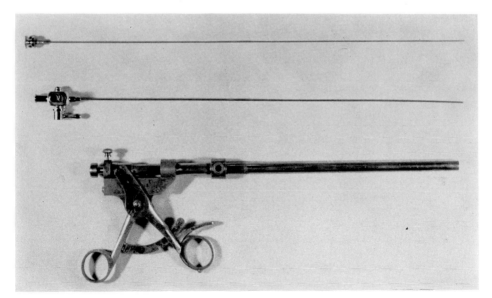

Figure 38-3. Yamagata peritoneoscopy instruments for gallbladder puncture and repair.

Society of Endoscopy. The details of the instruments are shown in Figure 38-3. They are inserted percutaneously into the peritoneal cavity and guided to the surface of the gallbladder under direct observation through the peritoneoscope. On reaching the gallbladder wall, the tip of the instrument is placed tightly against the wall and a portion of the wall is aspirat-

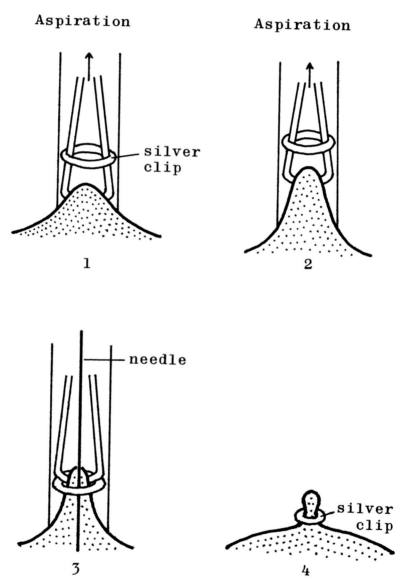

Figure 38-4. Technic of gallbladder puncture and repair under peritoneoscopic control. 1. A part of gallbladder wall is aspirated into the instrument tube, and a silver clip is applied at that part. 2. Aspiration is continued with gentle pressure, and clip is gradually tightened. 3. Needle is inserted into gallbladder lumen. After removal of needle, silver clip is closed tightly. 4. Shows silver clip tightened at the puncture site.

ed into the instrument and fixed by forceps attached inside the instrument. This portion of the bladder wall is punctured by inserting a needle of 1mm diameter through the instrument, thus reaching the lumen of the bladder. The locus of the puncture in the gallbladder wall can be closed by the application of a silver clip, which slides down over the tip of the forceps, thus preventing biliary leakage. After the procedure, the silver clip is crushed to close the puncture (Fig. 38-4). The method can be applied in all cases where part of the gallbladder wall can be observed. It is especially effective in patients with empty gallbladders. On the other hand, it is not indicated in patients with greatly thickened gallbladder walls or highly distended gallbladders. In these conditions the fixation of the wall by forceps is difficult (Plate 109).

Plate 109, Figure 38-4 demonstrates a distended gallbladder with a silver clip applied. This is a case of a 60-year-old male with cancer of the hepatic duct. The gallbladder was not originally distended. Complete aspiration of contrast medium after the procedure is unnecessary in this type of situation because the cystic duct and common bile duct are intact.

Method A

This method is indicated in patients with obstructive jaundice where a distension of the intrahepatic biliary tree can be expected. This is a percutaneous method, and the actual procedure is relatively easy. The method can also be used in patients who have had previous cholecystectomy. Kubota[10] reported recently that by carefully selecting the location of needle insertion, percutaneous insertion of the needle into the intrahepatic biliary duct can be done without much difficulty, even in cases without biliary duct expansion.

Method B

This is the percutaneous insertion method. The needle, which is inserted from the surface of the skin into the peritoneal cavity, is directed by peritoneoscopic observation to the gallbladder through the liver. The method was first reported by Kalk[7] and Nagai.[11] The liver acts to seal the locus of puncture. Therefore, the method is indicated when there are adhesions between gallbladder and liver. It is necessary that the adhesions should be observed by peritoneoscopic examination. However, the degree of the exposure of the gallbladder from the edge of the liver, the relation between the location of the edge of the liver and the costal arch, and tonicity of the gallbladder appear to play an important role in the actual performance of this method. Although the method enjoys the highest rate of success, there are instances when it cannot be applied even in the presence of the aforementioned adhesions.

Method C

This is the method of direct puncture of the free wall of the gallbladder. The method was originally reported by Royer[12] and by Henning et al.[13] The probability of biliary leakage is the highest with this method. The method is indicated when there is empyema of the gallbladder, a moderate to high degree of gallbladder thickening, well-developed perivesicular adhesions, etc. Because of the high risk of biliary leakage, it is advisable to inject solutions containing antibiotics into the gallbladder wall to cause local swelling, thereby closing off the locus of needle insertion and preventing leakage.

Methods A + C and A + B

When Methods A, B, or C fail to show the expected lesion in the field of the respective biliary duct system as demonstrated by injecting contrast media, any two of these methods may be combined (Fig. 38-5).

The needles used in each of Methods A, B, and C are identical. The

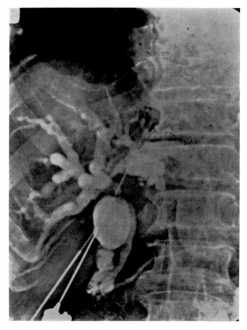

Figure 38-5. Combined intrahepatic (A) cholangiogram and peritoneoscope-controlled (C) cholecyst-pancreatogram demonstrates actual use of A + C method. Note the location of lesion in the hepatic duct. Above that lesion, intrahepatic bile ducts were dilated. However, as shown, the gallbladder can be well distended and show no abnormality. Common bile duct is clear. Also shown is a part of the pancreatic ducts. A part of the duodenum is filled with contrast medium. Patient is a 60-year-old male.

length of the needle is 62mm, with a diameter of 1.8mm at the top taper-ing down to 1mm. This makes needle handling much easier.

Cytologic Examination of Bile

Cytologic examination of the aspirated bile is important not only in es-tablishing qualitative diagnosis of the lesion but also in early diagnosis of malignant diseases. Henning[13] has already pointed out this possibility. In our experience with 116 cases, cancer cells were found in ten out of twelve patients with gallbladder cancer (83.3%), in four of eleven patients with common bile duct cancer (36.3%), in five of eleven patients with hepatic bile duct cancer (45.5%), and in one of sixteen patients with cancer of the pancreas (6.2%). The rate of detection is higher in cases of gallbladder cancer and cancer of the hepatic bile duct (Table 38-III). This fact was thought to be due to the closeness of the location of biliary puncture and sampling to the location of the lesion. However, in one patient with can-cer of the hepatic bile duct, although the location of bile sampling was far from the location of the lesion, cancer cells were found in the aspirat-ed bile. This might imply that the stream of bile carried the cancer cells to the location of the sampling. According to the report made by Akashi et al.,[14] there seems to be no relationship between the location of bile sampling and the location of the lesion to the yield of positive cytology. This does not agree with our finding; furthermore, the detection rate is higher than in our experience. Some modification of the sampling method may be necessary to increase the rate of cancer cell detection in bile.

TABLE 38-III

RESULTS OF CYTOLOGIC EXAMINATION OF THE BILE OBTAINED
AT THE TIME OF DIRECT CHOLANGIOGRAPHY

Diseases	Cases Examined	Positive for Cancer Cystic Bile	Ductal Bile	Positive %	Duodenal Juice (%)
Cancer of biliary bladder	12	10 (1)	0 (1)	83.3	33.3
Cancer of common bile duct	11	1 (5)	3 (2)	36.3	
Cancer of hepatic bile duct	11	0 (1)	5 (5)	45.5	41.6
Pancreatic Cancer	16	1 (6)	0 (9)	6.2	31.8
Total	50	12 (13)	8 (17)	40.0	35.6
Biliary tract stones	36	0 (36)	0 (0)	0	0.6
Cholecystopathia	11	0 (11)	0 (0)	0	false
Others	19	0 (19)	0 (0)	0	positive
Total	66	0 (66)	0 (0)	0	
Grand Total	116	12 (79)	8 (17)		

No. of cases (Negative for cancer cell).

The early detection of gallbladder cancer and cancer in the biliary tract is, as is well known, difficult. Most of them are detected at a stage when surgical cure can no longer be effective. At present, with improvements that make direct cholangiography less hazardous, peritoneoscopic examination combined with direct cholangiocholecystography and cytologic examination of the aspirated bile is thought to be the most potentially successful method of early detection of malignant diseases of the biliary system.

SPLENOPORTOGRAPHY UNDER PERITONEOSCOPIC EXAMINATION

Splenoportography is an important method in detecting the presence or absence and location of extrahepatic portal obstruction and stenosis, in diagnosing esophageal varices through the findings of the coronary vein of the stomach, in obtaining supportive evidence of liver cirrhosis and fibrosis through findings of inflammation of the intrahepatic part of the portal vein, in diagnosing liver tumors and abscesses, and in obtaining accessory findings in cases with common bile duct cancer and pancreatic cancer through the detection of stenosis or distortion of the extrahepatic portal vein or splenic vein. However, the percutaneous method is hazardous, for splenic puncture is always associated with the danger of bleeding. Splenoportography under peritoneoscopic examination will facilitate early dis-

TABLE 38-IV

PERITONEOSCOPES IN JAPAN

Type	Length (mm)	Diameter (mm)	Angle of Lens	Field of Vision	Size of Lens (F.mm)	Picture (mm)	Camera
Tohoku Univ. type standard ..	335	7.0	120°	60°	51 54–8	6–	Olimpus penF 51.6mm
Tohoku Univ. type W 80	335	8.0	120°	80°	72–9 54	8	Olimpus penF 75.0mm
Tohoku Univ. type LA	404	8.0	180°	60°		11	Olimpus penF 75.0mm
Tohoku Univ. type LC	320		180°	–45° + 5°		17	Kowa medical
Tohoku Univ. type SL-C	345	8.5	120°	60°		17	Kowa medical
Juntendo Univ. type (Takei)..	290	7.0	90°	55°	50	9	Olimpus penF
Juntendo Univ. type (Shinko)	340	7.5	120°	60°	50	12	Olimpus penF
Yamakawa: Aramaki cine type Takei	290	9.5	120°	60°	25	7	Bolex
Yamakawa: Aramaki cine type Shinko	340	8.5	120°	60°	25	7	Bolex
Shinko Opt. wide type	340	8.0	135°	90°	50		Asahipentax
Shinko Opt. Osaka Univ. type	340	7.5	120°	90°	50	12	Olimpus penF
Shinko Opt. standard type ...	340	7.5	120°	60°	50	12	Olimpus penF
Shinko SL type	266	7.5	120°	60°			

TABLE 38-V

ACCIDENTS IN PERITONEOSCOPIC EXAMINATION IN 24,133 CASES

Accidents	Cases	%
Subcutaneous emphysema	260	1.343
Shock	78	0.403
Bleeding	16	0.083
Mediastinal emphysema	6	0.031
Puncture of intestine	3	0.015
Intraperitoneal hematoma	1	0.005
Hypersensitivity reaction to procaine	1	0.005
Immediate death	4	0.021

covery of the bleeding and, depending upon the status of bleeding, appropriate treatment can be taken without unnecessary delay.

PERITONEOSCOPES IN JAPAN

Many types of peritoneoscopes are currently used in Japan (Table 38-IV). They all have their advantages and disadvantages. Like all medical precision instruments, the peritoneoscope is as good as and not better than the skill and efficiency of the operator.

ACCIDENTS IN PERITONEOSCOPY

Peritoneoscopy is an excellent adjuvant to the diagnostic study of abdominal disease. It should always be evaluated as a supplement to other methods of study, such as biochemistry and x-ray. Its indications and the evaluation of its results must always be assessed by the well-trained clinician, for, without clinical judgment, the peritoneoscopist is merely a technician.

Peritoneoscopy in the major institutions of Japan is well controlled and supervised, but even in the very best hands the procedure is not without its dangers. Responses to a recent survey of accidents associated with peritoneoscopy are shown here in tabular form (Table 38-V). Among 24,133 examinations, four were associated with immediate fatality, a percentage of 0.021. The major complications associated with fatality are not identified. It is noteworthy that of the complications that occurred, only three out of 24,133 were intestinal puncture, and while sixteen accidents are listed under bleeding, only one is listed under intraperitoneal hematoma. Care in selection of patients and skill in carrying out the procedure must be the ever-present watchwords in the prevention of accidents.

REFERENCES

1. Kitayama, K.: Pleuro-peritoneoscopie. *Acta med Okayama, 41*:1427-1429, 1926.
2. Kanai, I., and Iwasaki, H.: Experience of the peritoneoscopy. *Bull Naval M A, 25*:2, 130, 1936.

3. Yamagata, S.: Studies on the endoscopic examination. *Jap J Gastroenterol,* 58:6, 645, 1961.
4. Yamagata, S., and Miura, K.: Now and future of the endoscopic examination. *Jap Gastroenterol Endo,* 6:3, 142, 1964.
5. Kalk, H., and Bruhl, W.: *Leitfaden der laparoskopie und gastroskopie.* Stuttgart, Thieme, 1951.
6. Wittmann, I.: Peritoneoscopy. *Akad Kiadó Budapest,* 25: 1966.
7. Kalk, H.: Laparoskopische cholecysto-cholangiographie. *Deutsche med Wchnschr,* 77:590-591, 1952.
8. Royer, M., Mazune, P., and Koban, S.: Biliary dyskinesia studied by means of peritoneoscopic cholangiography. *Gastroenterology,* 16:83-90, 1950.
9. Yamagata, S., Miura, K., Tadaki, H., and Komatsu, K.: A new instrument for peritoneoscopic cholangiography. *Proceedings of the First Congress of the International Society of Endoscopy,* 516-519, 1966.
10. Kubota, H.: On percutaneous cholangiography. *Stomach & Intestine,* 5:423, 1970.
11. Nagai, T.: Studies on the laparoscopic cholecysto-cholangiography. *Jap J Gastroenterol,* 52:1-18, 1955.
12. Royer, M.: Die laparoskopische cholangiographie. *Fortschr Geb Röntgenstrahlen,* 77:690-705, 1952.
13. Henning, J., Demling, L., and Giggalberger, H.: Über die Laparoskopische cholecysto-cholangiographie. *München med Wchnschr,* 94:830-834, 1952.
14. Akashi, M., Hirai, S., Trukawa, M., Sugihara, Y., and Uchimura, M.: Studies on the cytologic examination of bile for definitive diagnosis of cancer of the gallbladder and biliary tract. *Stomach & Intestine,* 6:12, 1611-1616, 1971.

CHAPTER 39

PART I: PARASITIC LIVER DISEASES: FASCIOLA HEPATICA, HYDATID CYSTS, HEPATIC AMEBIASIS

Arturo D. Jorge

INTRODUCTION

IN OUR CLINIC, LAPAROSCOPY is usually performed to investigate liver disease such as acute or chronic hepatitis, cirrhosis, and the reticuloses. The diagnosis of neoplastic conditions has an important place in our work. Parasitic disease of the liver is seen less frequently but our usual findings are hydatid cysts, hepatic fascioliasis, and amebiasis; these present clinically as hepatomegaly, a mass in the liver, obstructive jaundice, or sometimes mimic chronic hepatitis. Laparoscopy is helpful on occasion by facilitating liver biopsy under vision, which allows a precise diagnosis.

FASCIOLA HEPATICA

Fasciola hepatica is a trematode worm of widespread distribution, found in all five continents. The adult parasite is flat, is shaped like a leaf, and is 30mm long and 13mm wide.

Animals and man become infected by eating plants, most often watercress leaves, to which is attached the encysted worm. On entering the duodenum, the organisms pass through the intestinal wall and make their way to the peritoneal cavity and thence to the liver. There they traverse Glisson's capsule, enter the liver substance and end up attached posteriorly in the bile ducts where they develop to maturity.[1]

Clinical Features

Clinical features are usually protean. Abdominal pain localized to the right hypochondrium with or without hepatomegaly, nausea, vomiting, diarrhea and meteorism are common. Marked weakness, diaphoresis, and weight loss may occur in some patients. Respiratory symptoms and sometimes pleural effusions[2] are not unusual in the invasive stage of the illness. Obstructive jaundice may complicate the picture in the later stages, due to irritation of the biliary passages by parasites.

Laboratory Findings

Laboratory findings usually show a leukocytosis of up to 16,000 to 18,000 with an eosinophilia of up to 60 per cent. The erythrocyte sedimentation rate is raised to between 20 and 100mm in the first hour. As for the liver function tests, the oxalic and pyruvic transaminase levels are always slightly raised. The alkaline phosphatase level is abnormal in 80 per cent of patients, and we have noted that gammaglutamyltranspeptidase is usually raised to about 500IU. Gamma globulin is raised in nearly 90 per cent. Diagnosis is confirmed by finding eggs of the parasite in either feces or bile.

Radiology

Chest x-rays sometimes show pleural effusion, foci of bronchopneumonia, or infiltrations similar to those found in Löffler's syndrome, which may develop in the course of illness. Oral cholecystograms and intravenous cholangiograms may show chronic cholecystitis without gallstones but with considerable loss of tone. The bile duct is sometimes dilated and there may be evidence of defects in its lumen, which raises the suspicion of the presence of gallstones. When exploration of the bile duct is performed, one or more Fasciola hepatica may be discovered.

Liver Scan

Serial scans using Au^{198} or I^{131} that are performed during the invasion phase show moving gaps which correspond to the migration of the parasite through the liver substance.[3]

Laparoscopic Pathology

We use the Lumina laparoscope with modern magnifying equipment. This instrument has an electronic flash apparatus built in on the distal side which facilitates photography. We use an Exacta Varex 11a camera with Riwo lenses of 75, 95 and 110mm and 35mm Agfa CT films of 18 DIN and 50 ASA. Using a specially adapted Polaroid camera we can get four laparoscopic views on a plate. For making films a 16mm Beaulieu camera with Kodak Ektachrome film of 22 DIN and 125 ASA is used.

During the invasion phase the liver is deep red in color, and there are small yellow or orange-yellow nodules on the surface which have the appearance of microabscesses. The extent of the lesions depends on the amount of infection present. Sometimes multiple lesions are found in both right and left lobes. In the stationary phase, when fasciola is localized in the bile ducts, the only finding may be a moderate degree of capsular fibrosis (Plate 110).

When colonization of the bile ducts by the parasite occurs, it causes bile duct obstruction. The liver then appears dark green in color. The surface is smooth and there may be a fine, reticular fibrosis of the capsule. The presence of the parasite in the bile duct causes the gallbladder to be distended and tense, whereas its presence above the junction of the cystic and hepatic ducts causes the gallbladder to be flaccid and small.

The walls of the gallbladder are sometimes thickened (Plate 111), fibrous and pearly white as in a true chronic cholecystitis. After treatment with emetine, dihydroxyemetine, and chloroquine the liver appears light red in color with patchy capsular fibrosis (Plate 112).

HYDATID CYST OF THE LIVER

Hydatid cysts are the larval stage of the tapeworm Echinococcus granulosus. The definitive hosts of the parasite are the dog, the wolf, or the jackal. Cattle, sheep, goats, and man are the intermediate hosts. The adult parasite lives in the small intestine of the definitive host. The parasite segments are excreted in the feces and the eggs are liberated, contaminating the water and plants in the immediate vicinity. Transmission is by ingestion of contaminated material. Spread is also possible by direct contact between dogs and man.

On ingestion of the eggs by the intermediate host, the embryos are liberated in the small intestine. They pass through the villi and may travel either through the portal system, with localization in the liver, or through the lymphatics and thoracic duct into the general circulation with secondary localization to the liver. Children comprise 10 to 20 per cent of cases while the remaining 80 to 90 per cent of cases occur in the second decade of life. Anatomical localization to the liver was seen in 60 per cent of 16,-000 cases reported in Argentina and summarized by Ivanissevich.[4]

Clinical Features

Hydatid cysts frequently reach the stage of calcification without giving rise to symptoms and diagnosis is often made as a finding during x-ray examination or autopsy.

The usual symptoms of these uncomplicated cysts are heaviness in the epigastrium or right hypochondrium and distention or a feeling of displacement of something in the abdomen. Frequently the patient has noticed the presence of swelling in the right hypochondrium. Sometimes there is typical biliary colic, which is thought to be due to anaphylactic phenomena since there is no communication with the biliary tract. The usual complications of hydatid cysts are (1) calcification,[5] which is actually a form of cure in 10 per cent of the cases, (2) infection and (3) in rare instances, perforation into the peritoneal cavity, causing true hydatid peritonitis. The infection has been known to pass through the diaphragm and enter a bronchus. This can result in vomiting of hydatid material[6] or in the infection reaching the pleura, causing pleural effusions.

Laboratory Findings

When a hydatid cyst communicates with the biliary tract it is possible to ascertain the presence of the parasite by examination of bile or feces.

A positive Cassoni test using sterile hydatid fluid implies present or past hydatid disease but a negative result does not absolutely rule out the disease.[7, 8] Blood films show varying degrees of eosinophilia; when biliary colic is associated with the cysts. Abnormalities of liver function suggesting obstructive jaundice may be seen.

Radiology

Plain x-rays of the abdomen may show elevation of the right diaphragm, which may occasionally be paralyzed. When calcification is present the cyst may be discerned as a round calcified shadow which may have clear or irregular outlines. Barium meal examination shows displacement of the neighboring organs when the cyst is large enough.

Oral cholecystograms and intravenous cholangiograms[9] sometimes show direct communication between the biliary tract and the cavity of the cyst.

Angiograms of the splenic and portal veins and selective hepatic arteriograms show displacement of the vascular network and may demonstrate very well a filling defect which corresponds to the cavity of the cyst.[10, 11]

Liver Scan

Liver scans done with Au[198] or I[131] show typical filling defects when the cysts are more than 2cm in diameter (Fig. 39 I-2). The main use of liver scans is to localize those cysts deep in the liver substance which are not amenable to diagnosis by other methods of investigation.[12–14]

Laparoscopic Pathology

It is possible by this technic to see hydatid cysts perfectly, except for those which are within the liver substance and make no impression on the surface of the liver. Cysts may be single or multiple; 65 to 70 per cent are found in the right lobe, 12 per cent in the left lobe, and the remainder are in both lobes. Single cysts sometimes give the appearance of a pearly white swelling (Plate 113), but at other times they have a flat aspect which is distinguished from the rest of the liver by the gray-white or pearly white color (Plate 114). Sometimes, however, there are multiple, small white nodules which occupy most of the liver, and we have even seen cysts occupying almost the whole right lobe, which was composed of numerous small white protuberances. In every case there is a marked increase in the lymphatics and in hyperemia around the cysts. In certain cases the greater omentum covers all or part of the area (Plate 115). The uninfected areas of the liver may appear entirely normal, or there may be capsular fibrosis of moderate or marked degree and may be either complete or partial over one or both lobes. There is sometimes compensatory hypertrophy of the healthy liver substance, giving rise to the mistaken suspicion that there are hydatid cysts within it.

Laparoscopy has enabled us on several occasions to diagnose splenic hydatid, some of which were primary in nature. Their incidence in Argentina is from 1.57 to 2.30 per cent.[15, 16] The other splenic hydatids were secondary. We have noted that splenic hydatids are violet-blue and are usually located at one or the other pole of the spleen (Plate 117). The rest of the spleen may be normal in appearance or there may be capsular fibrosis. The cysts must not be ruptured, for this causes spread in the peritoneum or serious anaphylaxis.

HEPATIC AMEBIASIS

Entamoeba histolytica is a protozoon with three stages of development, the trophozoite, the precyst, and the cyst. When conditions are unfavorable the parasite takes on its resistant, cystic form. The cyst at first has one nucleus and on maturing, has four. The normal habitat of Entamoeba histolytica is the mucosa of the large bowel. Both trophozoites and cysts are excreted in feces. Man becomes infected by ingesting the cysts, which particularly contaminate water and foodstuffs. Once in the intestine the cyst sheds its wall and develops into the trophozoite.

Entamoeba histolytica is a world-wide parasite but occurs more frequently and causes more disease in tropical countries. The fact that it was first described by Lösch in St. Petersburg in 1875 serves to remind us of its universal distribution.

Clinical Features

The lesions in the liver by Entamoeba histolytica are the amebic abscess and what is called chronic amebic hepatitis.[17-27] Patients with abscesses present with pain in the right hypochondrium. Fever, sweating, and shivering are common symptoms. Palpation reveals a tender, enlarged liver and guarding of the abdominal muscles. The movements of the right diaphragm are reduced. Laboratory tests show a marked neutrophil leukocytosis. The transaminase levels progress from a slight to a marked elevation. Alkaline phosphatase and gammaglutamyltranspeptidase values are abnormal. Usually there is a lowered serum albumin level and a slight increase in gamma- and a_2-globulins.

Patients with chronic amebic hepatitis complain of weakness, debility, anorexia, and a feeling of heaviness in the right hypochondrium. Doxiades has described the presence of ascites in some cases. Those who write on the subject state that palpation of the abdomen always reveals hepatomegaly and sometimes splenomegaly.

Laboratory Findings

The diagnosis of amebic abscess can be confirmed by puncture and seeing the chocolate-like fluid and the presence of the ameba. The diagnosis of chronic amebic hepatitis is made from the typical features of the disease and the presence of any of the forms of the ameba. Schaffer considers that growing amebas from liver tissue in culture media is conclusive evidence of chronic amebic hepatitis but this has not yet been achieved.[28]

Radiology

When there is an amebic abscess in the right lobe, the right diaphragm is raised or paralyzed, and sometimes there is pleural effusion. Angiograms of the splenic and portal veins show the site, size, and shape of the abscess. In chronic amebic hepatitis splenoportal angiography shows slight displacement of the smaller vessels.

Liver Scans

Liver scans with Au^{198} or I^{131} show areas which do not take up the radioactive material, and these indicate the position of the amebic abscess.[29]

Laparoscopic Pathology

We have had the opportunity to examine patients with chronic hepatitis, some of whom gave a history of amebic dysentery and some of whom had parasites present in feces. However, we could not be certain whether we were dealing with chronic amebic hepatitis or the coexistence of amebiasis and chronic hepatitis. In these cases laparoscopy revealed hepatomegaly. The edge of the liver was blunt and was 3 to 4cm below the right costal margin. The surface of the liver was pink-red with some areas of deeper red (Plate 118) and had some slight roughening and some patches of capsular fibrosis. In other cases there was marked capsular fibrosis. The gallbladder was normal.

We have never seen evidence of portal hypertension. Sometimes the spleen was 2cm below the left costal margin, scarlet in color and firmer than usual.

REFERENCES

1. Faust, E. C., Russel, P. F., and Jung, R. C.: *Craig and Faust's Clinical Parasitology,* 8th ed. Philadelphia, Lea & Febiger, 1970.
2. Crinquette, J., Becquet, R., and Vilain, B.: Les manifestations respiratoires au cours de la distomatose a Fasciola hepatica. *J franc med et chir thorac,* 19:529, 1965.
3. Albot, G., Lunel, J., Barbe, J., and Brouant, J. F.: Distomatose hepatique observee au stade hepatitique; donnees de la gammagraphie avant et apres le traitment. *Presse med,* 70:1564, 1962.
4. Ivanissevich, O., and Rivas, C. I.: Equinococosis hidatidica. *Min ed y just* Buenos Aires, 1961.
5. Casiraghi, J. C.: El tratamiento del quiste hidatidico del higado y sus complicaciones. Buenos Aires, Trigesimo Congr. Argent. de Cirug. 1959, fasc. I, p. 528.
6. Armand Ugon, C. V.: Tratamiento de la hidatidosis pulmonar. Buenos Aires, Trigesimitercer Congr. Argent. de Cirug. 1962, fasc. II, p. 520.
7. Grana, A.: El diagnostico biologico de la hidatidosis. *El dia med. Buenos Aires* 17:306, 1946.
8. Perez Fontana, V.: Alergia hidatidica. *Arch internat hidat,* 20:30, 1961.
9. Manos, A.: Diagnostic de la rupture intrabiliaire des kystes hydatique du foie par la ch olecistographie. *Arch internat hidat* 16:241, 1957.
10. Malenchini, M., Braiero, M., and Leva, A.: La esplenoportografia en enfermos con quistes hidaticos del higado. *El dia med Buenos Aires,* 29:2370, 1957.
11. Tourinho, O. B.: Spleno-porto-graphie transparietal. *Rev brasil de cir,* 36:425, 1957.
12. Caroli, J., and Bonneville, B.: Valeur diagnostique de la scintillographie hepatique. *Arch mal app digest,* 51:55, 1962.
13. Gomez Lopez, J., Hernandez Madariaga, R., and Lopez Gonzalez, A.: La gammagrafia en el estudio de las enfermedades hepaticas. *Rev espan enferm ap digest,* 20:115, 1961.
14. Touya, J. J., Muxi, F., Traibel, J., Lapido, F., Oehninger, C., and Ferrari, M.: Importancia de la gammagrafia en el diagnostico de la hidatidosis hepatica no complicada. *Arch internat hidat,* 21:561, 1963.
15. Garat, R., and Echevarria, O.: Hidatidosis del bazo y fosa subfrenica. *Arch internat hidat,* 21:427, 1963.

16. Loyarte, H., Ferro, A., Curutchet, J. L., Fernandez Tasende, D., and Cereseto, P. L.: Los quistes hidaticos del bazo y de la celda Esplenica. *Arch internat hidat, 21*:202, 1963.

17. Appert, O., and Middendorp, U. G.: Der Amobe Leberabzess. *Praxis 58*:1260, 1969.

18. Bhaskara Reddy, D., Sumathikumari, C., and Maharajsaran, B.: Hepatic amoebiasis: Amoebic hepatitis and amoebic abscess with particular reference to connective tissue reaction and distribution of amoebae. *J Path Bact, 12*:104, 1969.

19. Doxiades, Th.: Chronische Amobenhepatitis. *Munchen med wchnschr, 104*:1431, 1962.

20. Doxiades, Th.: *Akute und Chronische Lebererkrankungen.* Stuttgart, Thieme, 1966, p. 152.

21. Doxiades, Th., and Candreviotis, N.: Ascite amibienne et ambiase hepatique. *Bull et mem soc med Paris, 113*:654, 1962.

22. Doxiades, Th., Candreviotis, N., Yiotsas, Z. D., and Smyniotis, F. E.: Chronic amebic hepatitis, *Arch int Med, 111*:219, 1963.

23. Doxiades, Th., Candreviotis, N., and Yiotsas, Z.: *Chronic amoebic hepatitis as a distinct clinicopathological entity.* Proc. World Congress, Gastroenl. p. 130, 1962.

24. Keeley, K. J., Schaman, A., and Scott, A.: Definitive diagnosis of amebic liver abscess: Value of liver biopsy. *Brit M J*, Vol. II 2nd half of year: 375, 1962.

25. Ochsner, A., and DeBakey, M.: Amebic hepatitis and hepatic abscess: An analysis of 181 cases with review of the literature. *Surgery, 13*:460, 1943.

26. Paul, M.: New concepts of amebic abscess of liver. *Brit J Surg, 47*:502, 1960.

27. Vakil, B. J., Metha, A. J., and Desai, H. N.: Atypical manifestations of amoebic abscess of liver, *J Trop Med Hig, 73*:63, 1970.

28. Steinitz, H.: Amoebiasis und chronische Hepatitis. In *Aktuelle Hepatologie*, Stuttgart, Thieme, 1969, p. 81.

29. Salah Ibrahim, M., and Abdel Wahab, M. F.: Detection of amebic liver by isotope scanning. *Brit M J*, :1325, 1963.

PART II:
TUBERCULOMA OF THE LIVER,
AMEBIC ABSCESS,
SCHISTOSOMIASIS JAPONICUM

SOL Z. ALVAREZ

TUBERCULOMA OF THE LIVER

PATIENTS WITH HEPATOBILIARY TUBERCULOSIS as seen in the Philippines can be divided into two main groups: those with a chronic recurrent obstructive jaundice and those with an enlarged hard nodular liver simulating cancer of the liver but without jaundice[1] (tuberculoma). It is in the latter group that peritoneoscopy has great value in establishing the diagnosis. While blind aspiration liver biopsy may yield the diagnosis, the lesion can also be missed and a normal tissue obtained. A guided liver biopsy under direct vision during peritoneoscopy would be more accurate.

Peritoneoscopic Findings

In most instances, both lobes of the liver are enlarged and are dark brown or dark gray in color. The granulomatous lesions (tuberculoma) appear as cheesy white, sometimes chalk-white, irregular nodules of varying sizes, some of them resembling tumor masses (Plates 119 and 120). Some lesions are confluent and form larger lesions. The lesion may be localized to one lobe, but in most cases both lobes are involved.

595

Inflammatory reactions with adhesions to the parietal peritoneum may be seen surrounding some of the lesions. Tubercles may sometimes be seen at the parietal peritoneum overlying the lesions at the areas of adhesions and sometimes at the falciform ligament. Occasionally the granulomatous lesions may be found on a cirrhotic liver.

The spleen may be found to be enlarged, and small, whitish granulomatous lesions may at times be seen at the surface.

If there is an accompanying tuberculous peritonitis, then one sees the parietal peritoneum to be thickened and studded with tubercles. The serosa of the bowels and falciform ligament may also be involved.

Differential Diagnosis

The gross appearance of tuberculoma of the liver at peritoneoscopy may simulate primary cancer of the liver and sometimes metastatic cancer of the liver.

In contrast to primary cancer of the liver, which in the Philippines is associated with cirrhosis of the liver in 80 per cent of cases,[2] tuberculoma of the liver usually occurs on a previously normal liver. The tumor nodules of primary cancer of the liver appear more elevated or bulging and have a yellowish white hue (Plate 121). The lesions of tuberculoma appear less elevated, sometimes almost flat and are cheesy white and sometimes chalk white in appearance (Plates 122 and 123).

The lesions of metastatic cancer of the liver appear umbilicated; the lesions in tuberculoma of the liver show no central depression or umbilications.

A guided liver biopsy under direct vision will definitely establish the diagnosis histologically.

One characteristic feature of tuberculoma of the liver is that it gives a gritty and stony hard sensation during the liver biopsy. On the other hand, neoplastic lesions give a soft sensation during the needle biopsy.

We have recently reviewed our experience on the use of peritoneoscopy in tuberculoma of the liver and liver cancer. Twenty-five cases were diagnosed as tuberculoma of the liver on the basis of peritoneoscopic findings. Six turned out to be liver cancer on biopsy, giving a 24 per cent error on gross diagnosis.[2, 3] On the other hand, of eighty-three cases given a peritoneoscopic diagnosis of primary cancer of the liver, eighty-two were confirmed histologically as cancer. One turned out to be tuberculoma of the liver, giving an error of 1.2 per cent. These errors on gross diagnosis may, however, be corrected by doing a guided liver biopsy during peritoneoscopy.

AMEBIC ABSCESS OF THE LIVER

In suspected cases of amebic abscess of the liver, we seldom resort to peritoneoscopy since most of the lesions occur at the superior and posterior aspects of the right lobe and a blind liver puncture will usually yield abscess material. Prior to the liver puncture, a liver scan usually helps determine the site for puncture. However, there are instances wherein peritoneoscopy is of value in the diagnosis of liver abscess. These are:

1. When the abscess involves the left lobe, so that blind liver puncture is dangerous and usually not done.
2. When the differential diagnosis includes primary cancer of the liver, in which there is a fluctuant tender mass.

Peritoneoscopic Findings

The lobe of the liver involved is usually enlarged and swollen and the surface, while smooth, gives a *stretched* appearance. The main abscess as it points to the surface is seen as a localized bulging (Plate 124). This is reddish orange in color, compared to the grayish color of the liver at the periphery of the abscess. Palpation of the bulging area with a palpating rod or from the abdominal wall shows its fluctuant character. Usually a solitary abscess is seen, but sometimes more than one abscess may be seen. Adhesions from the abscess area to the parietal peritoneum are usually present, denoting the inflammatory nature of the lesion.

Differential Diagnosis

The lesion of amebic abscess may simulate a big hepatoma nodule, especially if the malignancy undergoes hemorrhagic and cystic degeneration.

The presence of an associated cirrhosis usually favors the diagnosis of hepatoma. Puncture of the bulging lesion under direct vision gives chocolate-colored or anchovy-saucelike material if due to amebic abscess, blood and necrotic material if due to hepatoma.

SCHISTOSOMIASIS JAPONICUM

Patients with schistosomiasis at the third stage show evidence of portal hypertension, such as huge splenomegaly, ascites, and esophageal varices. The liver may be enlarged or small. The value of peritoneoscopy in these patients is to rule out other causes of ascites and to see whether the liver is grossly cirrhotic in appearance or just shows periportal fibrosis.

Peritoneoscopic Findings

The liver may be seen to be enlarged or to be small. It may appear grossly cirrhotic (usually coarsely nodular) or may appear pale gray with few scars but show scattered flat oval or elongated, whitish lesions at the surface (Plate 125) which on biopsy reveal a granuloma with schistosoma ova (Plate 126).

The spleen is usually large and grayish in color; the surface shows fibrinous exudate. However, at times, whitish granulomatous lesions are also seen at the surface. These are similar to those seen in the liver, the characteristic lesion seen in schistosomiasis.

REFERENCES

1. Alvarez, S. Z., and Fabra-Coronel, R.: The clinical features of hepatobiliary tuberculosis in the Philippines. Abstract. Fourth World Congress of Gastroenterology, Copenhagen, 1970.
2. Alvarez, S. Z., Perez, J. Y., Roman, F. J., and Sagad-Angeles, D.: Primary cancer of the liver in the Philippines: A study of 300 cases (in press).
3. Alvarez, S. Z., and Perez, J. Y., Jr.: Clinical experience with Machida fibreoptic laparoscope. Proc. Fourth Asian-Pacific Congr. Gastroenterology, Manila, 1972.

AUTHOR INDEX

SUBJECT INDEX

COLOR SECTION

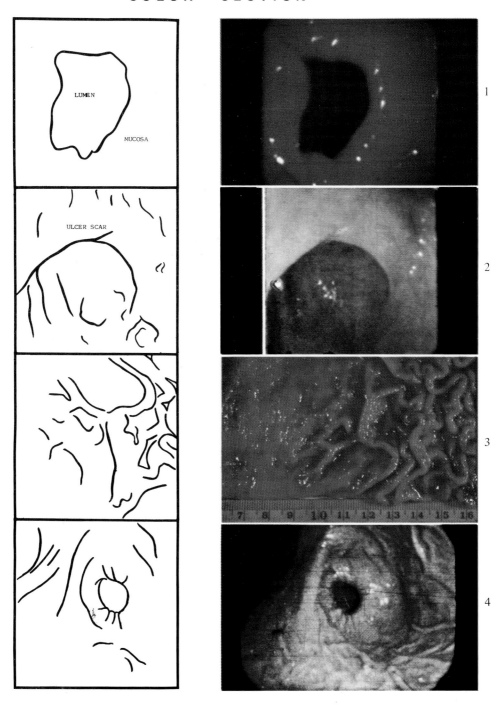

Plate 1. Normal mucosa, view from high body.
Plate 2. Normal antrum and angulus except tiny ulcer scar easily overlooked.

Plate 3. Tortuous folds, greater curvature. Surgical specimen.
Plate 4. Antrum – "no blind spot."

ALL COLOR PHOTOGRAPHS ARE IDENTIFIED WITH CORRESPONDING CHAPTERS, SO THAT THE COLOR SECTION MAY BE STUDIED SEPARATELY WITH PERIODIC REFERENCE TO CHAPTERS.

5'

7'

9'

11'

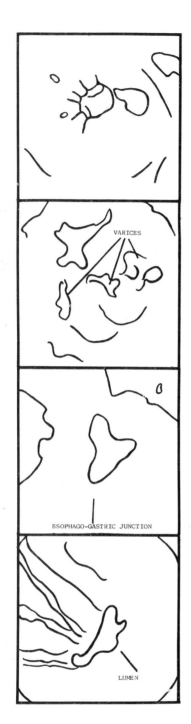

VARICES

ESOPHAGO-GASTRIC JUNCTION

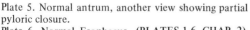
LUMEN

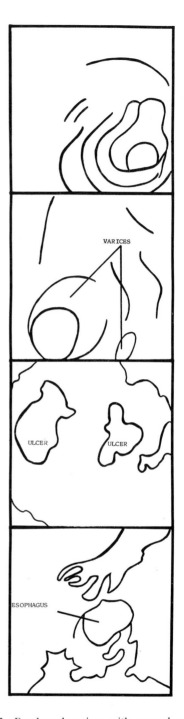

ESOPHAGUS

VARICES

ULCER   ULCER

Plate 5. Normal antrum, another view showing partial
pyloric closure.
Plate 6. Normal Esophagus. (PLATES 1-6, CHAP. 2)

Plate 7. Esophageal varices with normal mucosal
coloration.
Plate 8. Esophageal varices with bluish coloration.

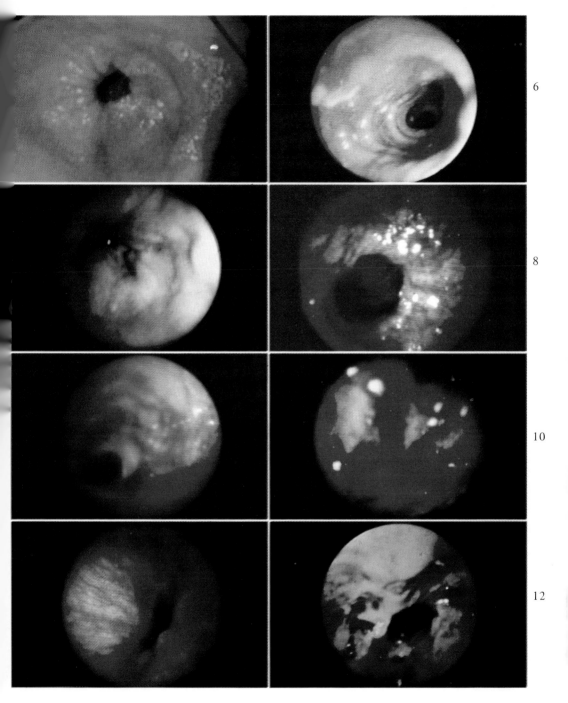

Plate 9. Esophageal-gastric junction — early esophagitis.
Plate 10. Mid-esophageal superficial ulcers.

Plate 11. Esophagitis with mild esophageal stenosis. (PLATES 7-11, CHAP. 8)
Plate 12. Acute peptic esophagitis with benign stricture. (Courtesy of Dr. Richard McCray)

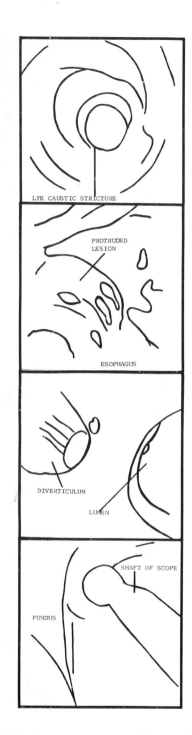

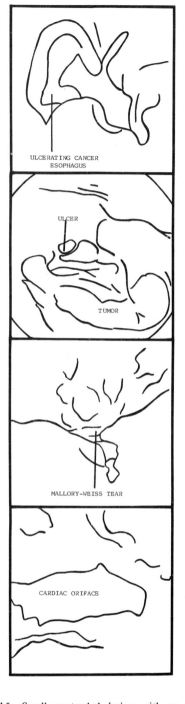

Plate 13. Endoscopic appearance of lye caustic stricture 19 days after ingestion, showing smooth tapering of esophagus. (PLATES 12-13, CHAP. 9)

Plate 14. Almost the entire circumference of the esophagus is involved in ulcerating carcinoma.

Plate 15. Small protruded lesion with an uneven surface, proven to be cancerous by esophagoscopic biopsy.

Plate 16. Posterior wall ulcerating tumor. Smooth margin not so high with regard to size of tumor.

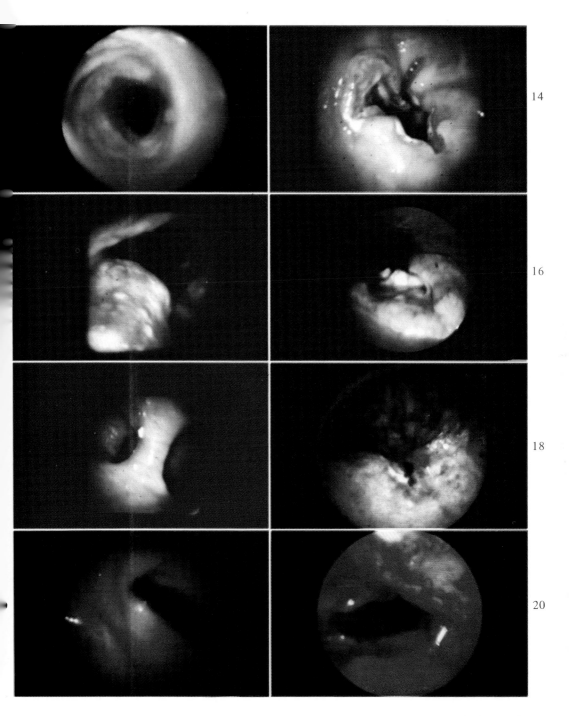

14

16

18

20

Esophagoscopic biopsy showed non-epitheleal malignant tumor. Post-op histological section revealed leiomyosarcoma.

Plate 17. Large saccular diverticulum of esophagus to the left of lumen. Thirty-nine (39cm.) centimeter from incisor teeth. (PLATES 14-17, CHAP. 11)

Plate 18. Linear tear of gastric cardia (Mallory-Weiss lesion) in patient with esophageal hiatus sliding hernia.

Plate 19. Retroflexed view of esophageal hiatus and of gastric fundus.

Plate 20. Carcinoma narrowing the cardiac orifice. (PLATES 18-20, CHAP. 13)

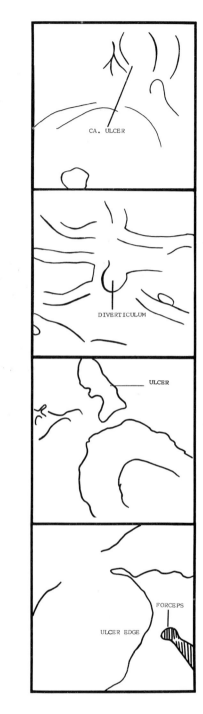

21′

23′

25′

27′

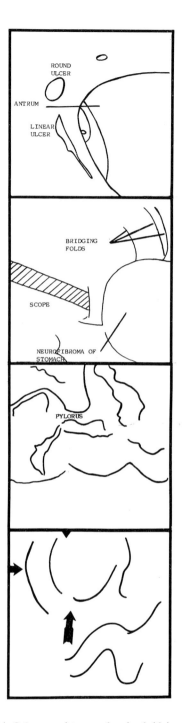

2

Plate 21. Type II (Borrmann) Ca ulcer on lesser curvature of antrum. Blind gastrocamera photograph.
Plate 22. Round ulcer on lesser curvature and linear ulcer on posterior wall of lower body.
Plate 23. Orifice of diverticulum, on greater curvature of mid-body. Blind gastrocamera photograph.

Plate 24. Submucosal tumor showing bridging folds at cardiac orifice. Surgery revealed neurofibroma. Retroflexed photograph, blind gastrocamera. (Courtesy S. Ashizawa) (PLATES 21-24, CHAP. 14)
Plate 25. Benign gastric ulcer on angulus. (Side viewing instrument): Note elliptical shape, smooth edges and clean white base. (Courtesy L. Berry)

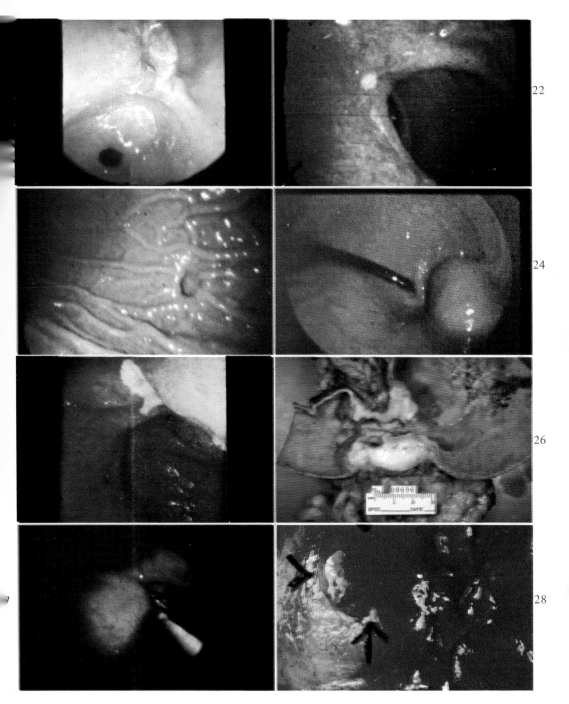

Plate 26. Gross surgical specimen of an ulcerated pyloric channel tumor. Note the normal mucosal mantle covering the proximal edge.

Plate 27. Biopsy of gastric ulcer – correct: Note forceps lying across edge of ulcer.

Plate 28. Close-up view of surgical specimen of a small (11mm) grossly benign ulcer. Note the rectangular "moist" plaque (arrows) extending from only one edge which is intramucosal carcinoma.

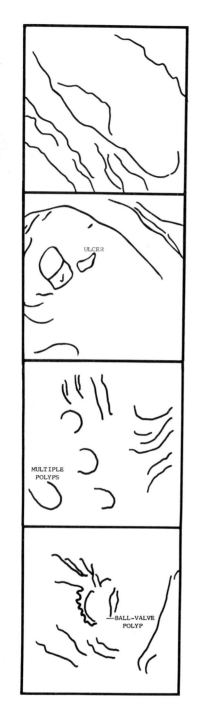

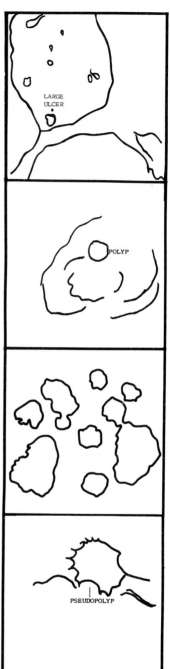

Plate 29. Suspicious benign gastric ulcer: Edema makes ulcer appear to be in tumor mass.
Plate 30. Steroid ulcer, lesser curvature. Note tiny clots at probable site of gross hemorrhage 4 hours before. (Courtesy L. Berry)
Plate 31. Healing benign prepyloric ulcer. Not seen on X-ray side viewing scope left side. (Courtesy L. Berry) (PLATES 25-31, CHAP. 15)

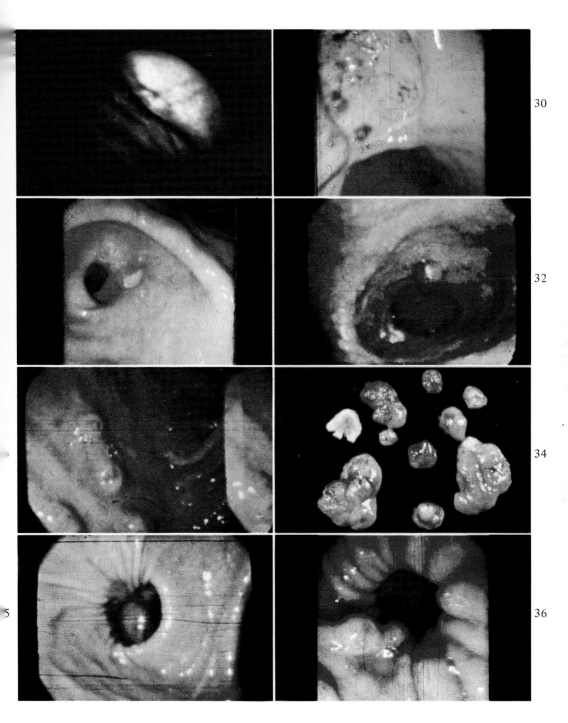

30

32

34

36

5

Plate 32. Single Benign Adenomatous polyp hanging from anterior wall of antrum.
Plate 33. Multiple discrete adenomatous polyps on greater curvature and anterior wall.

Plate 34. Benign polyps removed in a case of "polyadenomes polypeux".
Plate 35. "Ball-Valve" polyp at the pylorus.
Plate 36. "Knuckle" defect on rugal fold with vigorous peristalsis simulating polyp.

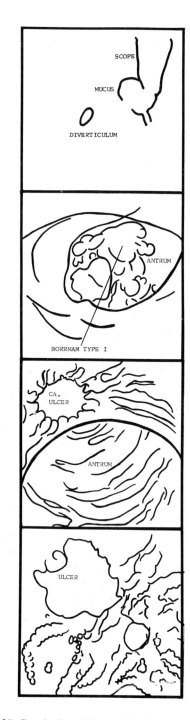

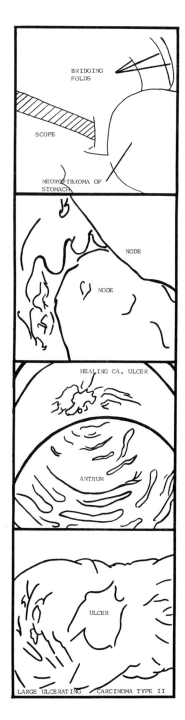

Plate 37. Gastric diverticulum in fundus, and mucus at G-E junction seen by retroflexion.

Plate 38. Submucosal tumor showing "bridging" folds at cardiac orifice. ery revealed neurofibroma. Retroflexed photograph, blind gastrocamera.

tesy S. Ashizawa) (PLATES 32-38, CHAP. 16)

Plate 39. Polypoid carcinoma of antrum (Courtesy S. Ashizawa)

Plate 40. Polypoid carcinoma, Borrmann Type I

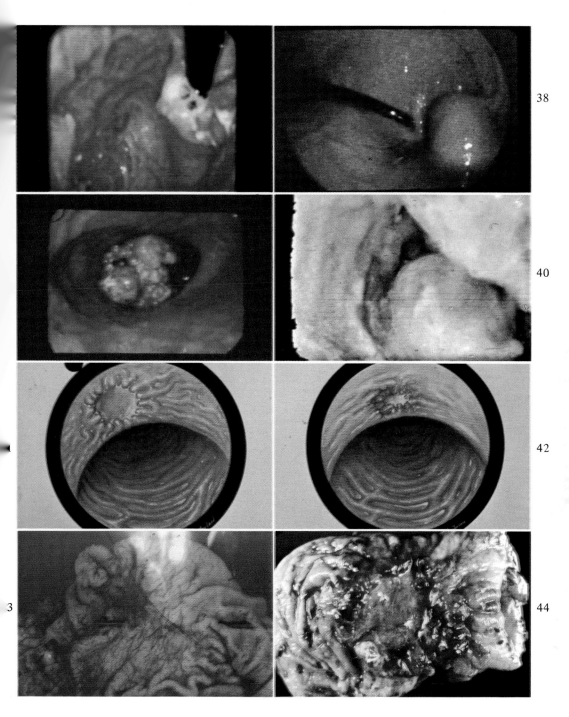

Plate 41. Non-infiltrating carcinomatous ulcer, Borr-mann Type II before "healing." (drawing)
Plate 42. Non-infiltrating carcinomatous ulcer, Borr-mann Type II after "partial healing." (drawing)

Plate 43. Carcinomatous ulcer, Borrmann Type II resected stomach (23 yr. survival)
Plate 44. Large ulcerating carcinoma Type II high cardia − posterior wall missed in three x-ray examina-tions. Seen repeatedly by endoscopy.

45'

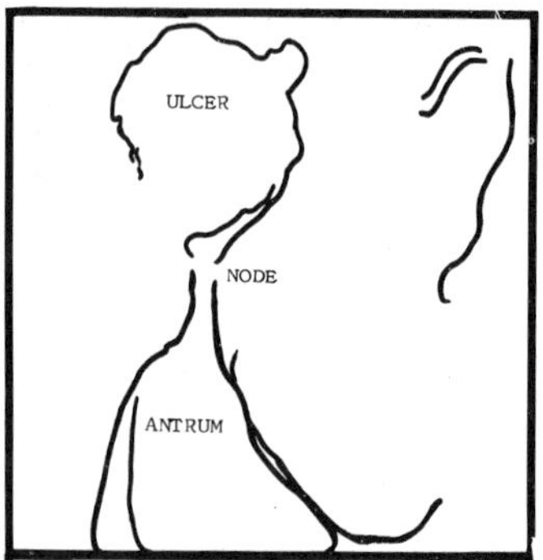

ULCER

NODE

ANTRUM

NODOSE WALL

ULCER

CA ULCER
TYPE III

47'

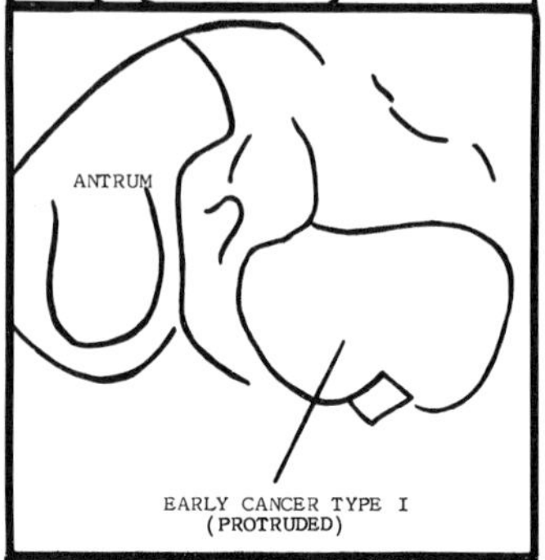

ANTRUM

EARLY CANCER TYPE I
(PROTRUDED)

(SUPERFICIAL ELEVATED)

49'

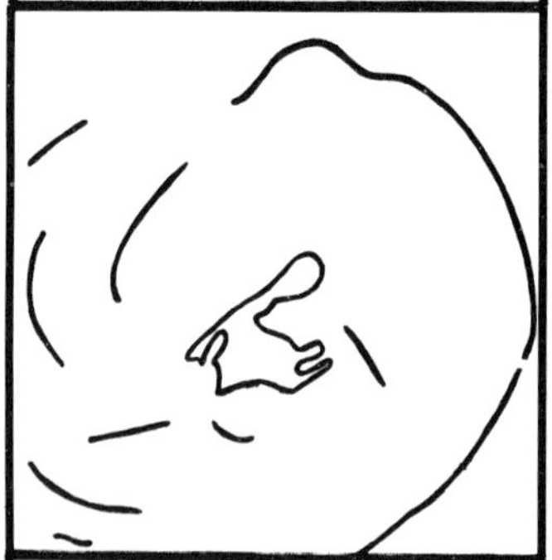

(SUPERFICIAL
FLAT) TYPE

51'

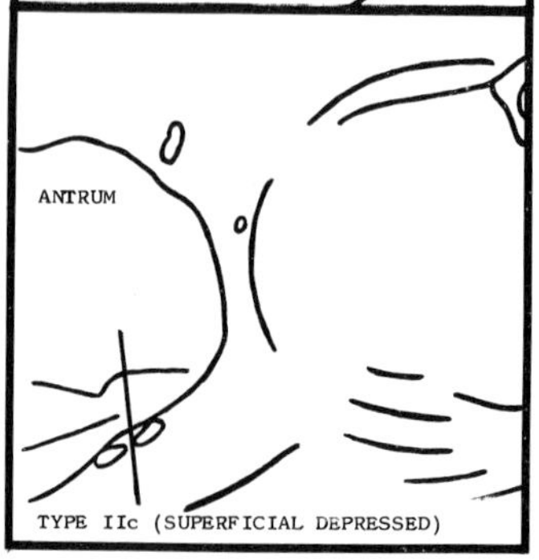

ANTRUM

TYPE IIc (SUPERFICIAL DEPRESSED)

ANTRUM

TYPE III (EXCAVATED)

5

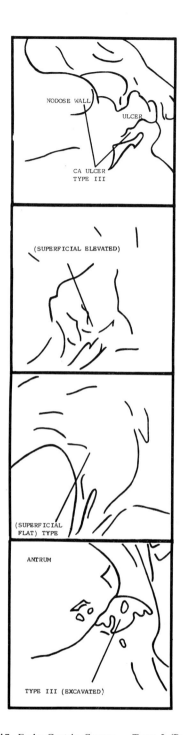

Plate 45. Infiltrating carcinomatous ulcer with poly-
poid wall, Borrmann Type III.
Plate 46. Infiltrating carcinomatous ulcer Borrmann
Type III (Courtesy S. Ashizawa) (PLATES 39-46,
CHAP. 17)

Plate 47. Early Gastric Cancer – Type I (Protruded
type).
Plate 48. Early Gastric Cancer – Type IIa (Superficial
Elevated type).

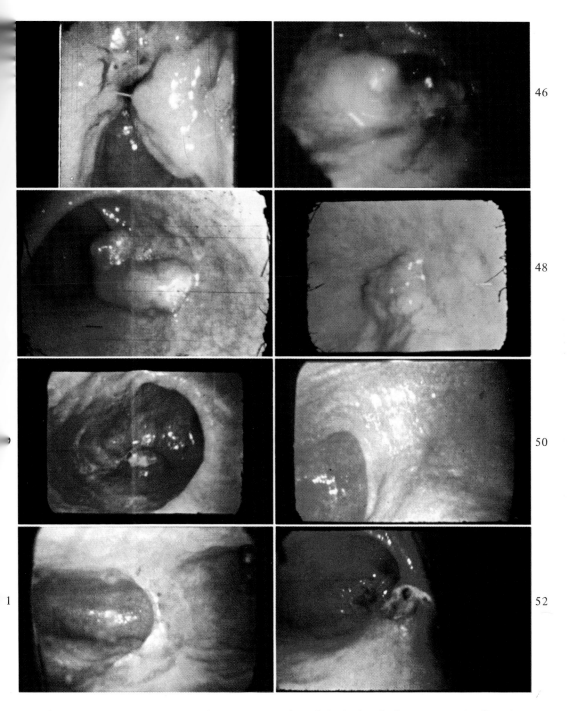

Plate 49. Early Gastric Cancer – Combined type IIa plus IIc (Low Elevation Plus Central Depression).
Plate 50. Early Gastric Cancer – Type IIb (Superficial Flat type).

Plate 51. Early Gastric Cancer – Type IIc (Superficial Depressed type).
Plate 52. Early Gastric Cancer – Type III (Excavated type).

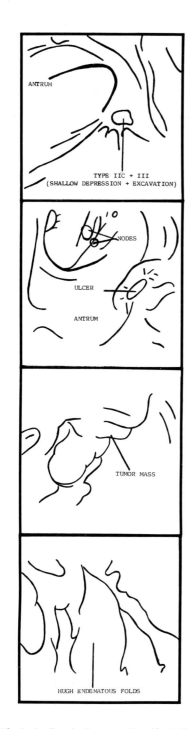

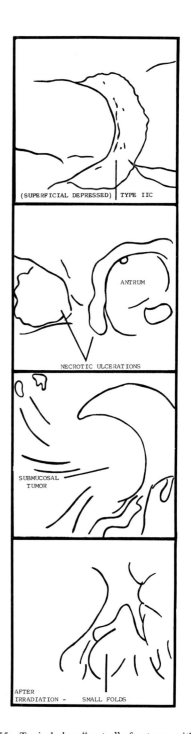

Plate 53. Early Gastric Cancer – Combined Type IIc Plus III (Shallow Depression plus Excavation).
Plate 54. Early Gastric Cancer – Type IIc (Superficial Depressed). (PLATES 47-54, CHAP. 18)

Plate 55a. Typical ulcer "crater" of antrum, with small nodular masses. Reticulum cell sarcoma.
Plate 55b. "Crater" ulcer, reticulum cell sarcoma after therapy.

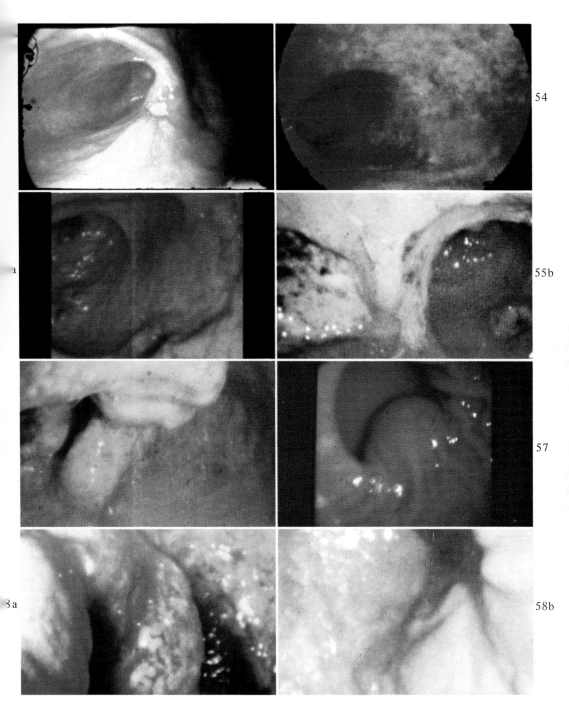

54

55b

57

58b

Plate 56. Ulcerating gastric mass, probably carcinoma. Biopsy showed lymphoreticular hyperplasia.
Plate 57. Smooth, submucosal mass with "bridging folds." Leiomyoma.

Plate 58a. Huge edematous folds. Case of multiple myeloma.
Plate 58b. Multiple myeloma after irradiation, fold diminished. (PLATES 55A-58B, CHAP. 19)

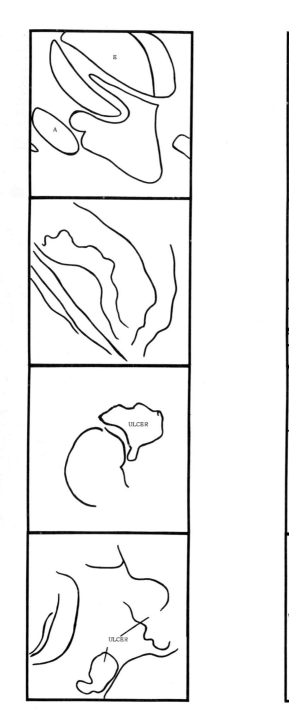

59'

61'

63'

65'

6

66

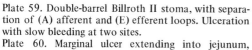

Plate 59. Double-barrel Billroth II stoma, with separation of (A) afferent and (E) efferent loops. Ulceration with slow bleeding at two sites.
Plate 60. Marginal ulcer extending into jejunum,

Billroth II. (Courtesy R. McCray)
Plate 61. Jejunum immediately distal to Billroth stoma with exudation, friability, edema and ulceration.
Plate 62. Parallel Kerckring folds of jejunum.

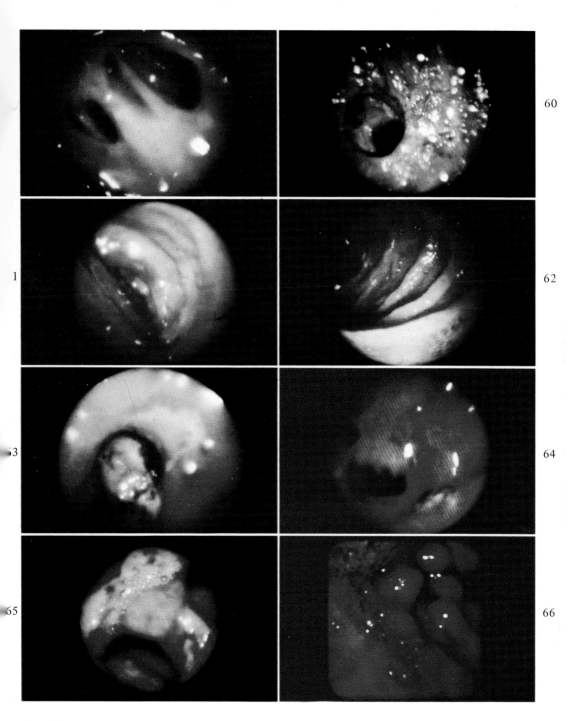

60

62

64

66

Plate 63. Large jejunal ulcer after gastric resection.
Plate 64. Duodenal ulcer four weeks after pyloroplasty, ulcer with recurrent bleeding.

Plate 65. Double barrel Billroth II stoma. Ulceration and bleeding on jejunal bridge and margin. (PLATES 59-65, CHAP. 20)
Plate 66. Giant gastric folds and hypertrophic gastropathy.

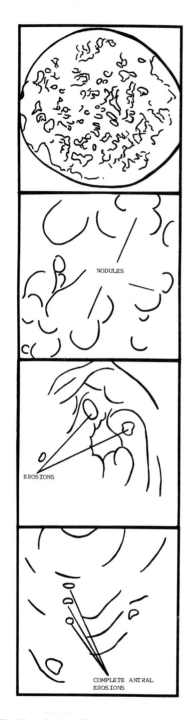

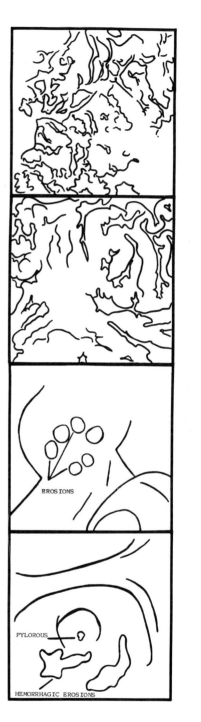

Plate 67. Chronic superficial gastritis anterior wall in an alcoholic with severe liver disease (Courtesy Mc-Cray).

Plate 68. Extensive chronic atrophic gastritis, anterior wall.

Plate 69. Hypertrophic gastropathy, posterior wall.

Plate 70. Surgical specimen removed for duodenal ulcer, hypertrophic gastropathy. (PLATES 66-70, CHAP. 21-I)

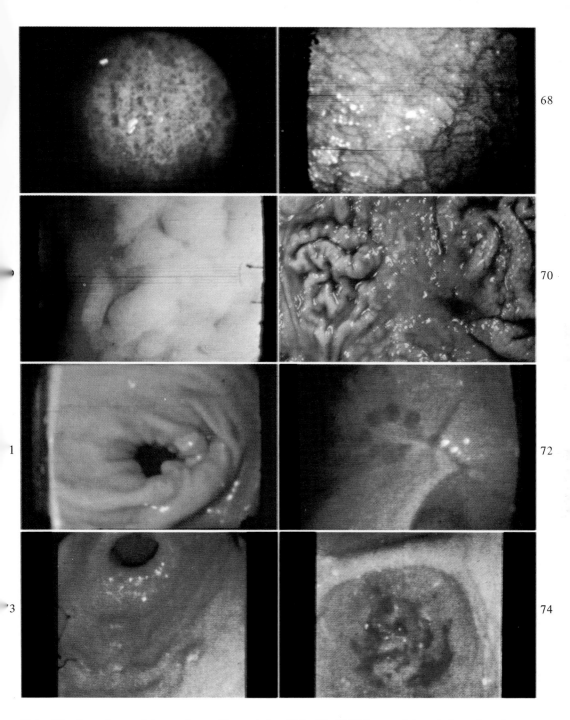

68

70

72

74

Plate 71. Several complete erosions with central fibrinoid necrosis.
Plate 72. Histamine-induced erosions ten minutes after intravenous injection.

Plate 73. Multiple complete antral erosions (proven Crohn's disease of the stomach)
Plate 74. Bleeding antral erosions due to secondary amyloidosis of mucosal blood vessels. (PLATES 71-74, CHAP. 22)

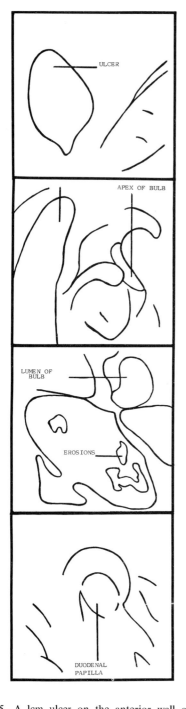

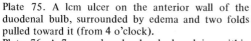

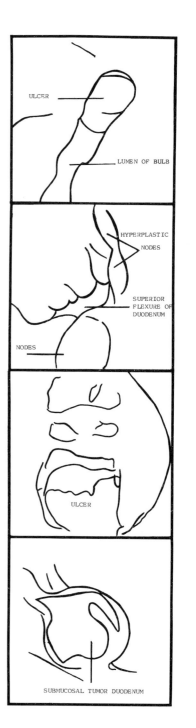

Plate 75. A 1cm ulcer on the anterior wall of the duodenal bulb, surrounded by edema and two folds pulled toward it (from 4 o'clock).

Plate 76. A 7mm pyloroduodenal ulcer lying within the duodenum seen through the pylorus.

Plate 77. Scar from old ulcer disease with folds distally due entirely to peristalsis.

Plate 78. "Hyperplastic" duodenitis. Large hyperemic folds and mummilations are present.

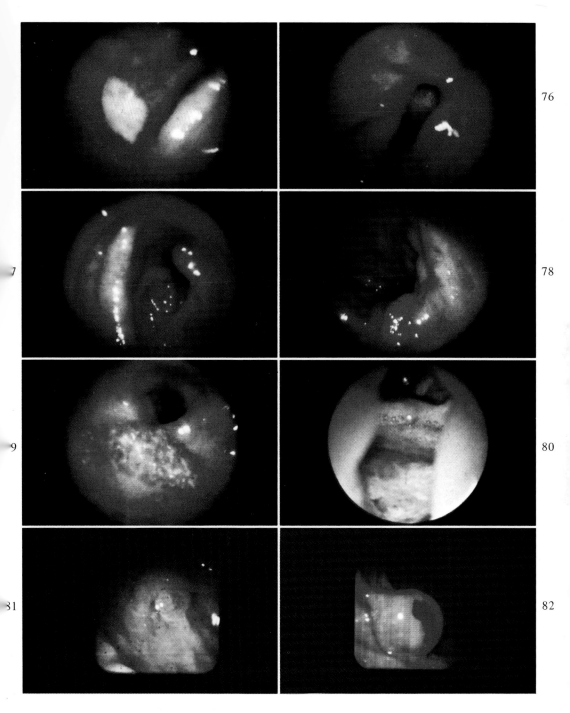

76

78

80

82

Plate 79. "Pepper and salt" acute duodenitis. The distal portion of the duodenal bulb shows partial stenosis.
Plate 80. Acute duodenal ulcer. (Courtesy McCray)
(PLATES 75-80, CHAP. 23)

Plate 81. Duodenal papilla.
Plate 82. Submucosal tumor at the superior flexure. Bleeding from top of the tumor is result of biopsy.

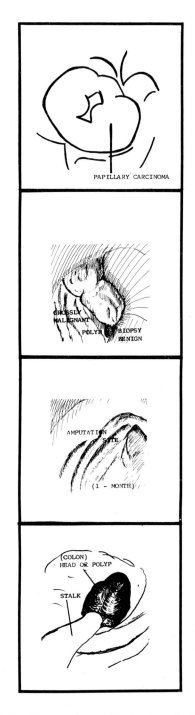

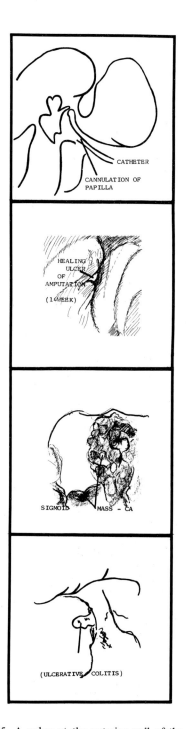

Plate 83. Papillary carcinoma. Duodenal papilla is seen as an irregular localized tumor with the granular eroded orifice.
Plate 84. Cannulation of the duodenal papilla. (PLATES 81-84, CHAP. 24)

Plate 85. A polyp at the anterior wall of the gastric angle of stomach.
Plate 86. The condition of the amputation site one week later, represented by a shallow ulcer.

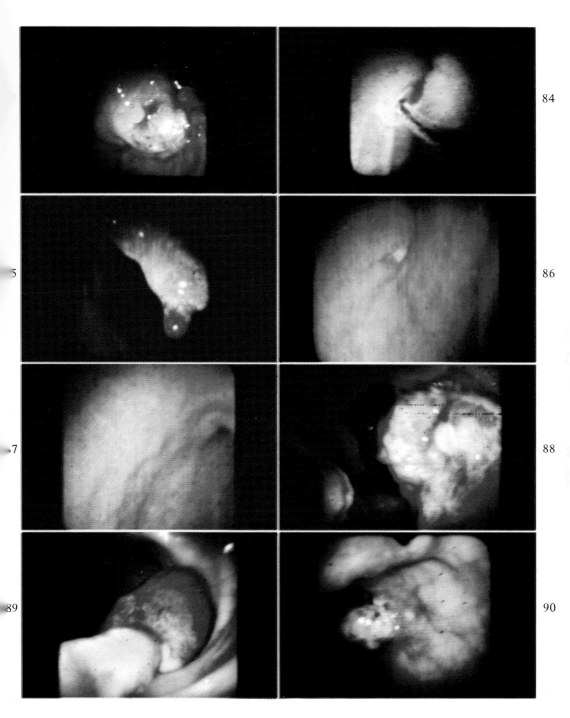

84

86

88

89

90

Plate 87. The condition of the amputation site one month later, showing complete healing of the ulcer. (PLATES 85-87, CHAP. 28II)

Plate 88. Fungating and Ulcerated Carcinoma of Sigmoid.
Plate 89. Pedunculated Polyp-Descending Colon.
Plate 90. Chronic Ulcerative Colitis with Pseudopolyp.

91'

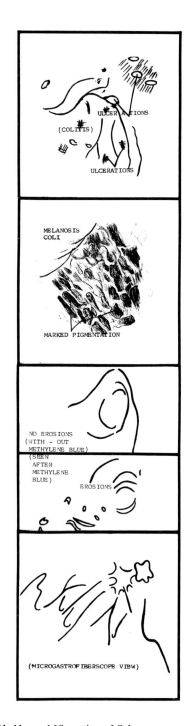

93'

95'

97'

(COLITIS)

CYST

CYST

CYST

CYST

POLYP

THERMISTER

9

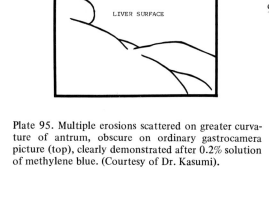

LIVER SURFACE

98

Plate 91. Mucosal Ulceration of Colon.
Plate 92. Colitis Cystic Profunda.
Plate 93. Melanosis Coli.
Plate 94. Pneumotosis Cystoides. (PLATES 88-94, CHAP. 30)

Plate 95. Multiple erosions scattered on greater curvature of antrum, obscure on ordinary gastrocamera picture (top), clearly demonstrated after 0.2% solution of methylene blue. (Courtesy of Dr. Kasumi).

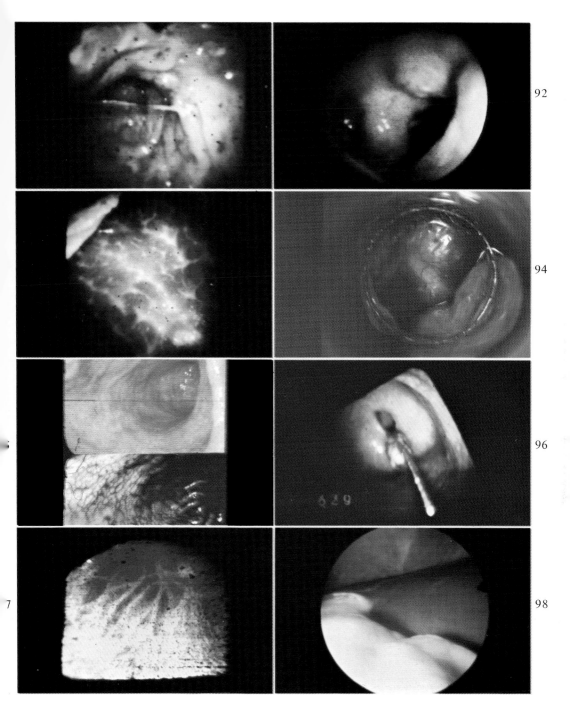

92

94

96

98

Plate 96. A gastric polyp projected on a color TV screen for endoscopy. The temperature of the polyp is measured with a thermister.

Plate 97. Thirteen times magnification of regenerating epithelium around an ulcer photographed with micro-gastrofiberscope. (Courtesy of Dr. Miyake) (PLATES 95-97, CHAP. 34)

Plate 98. Surface of Normal Liver and Gallbladder

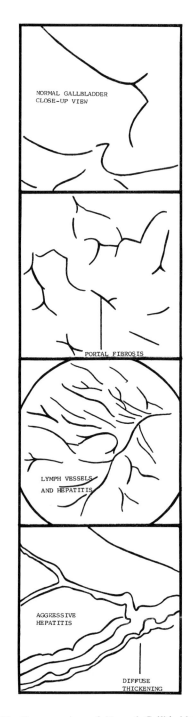

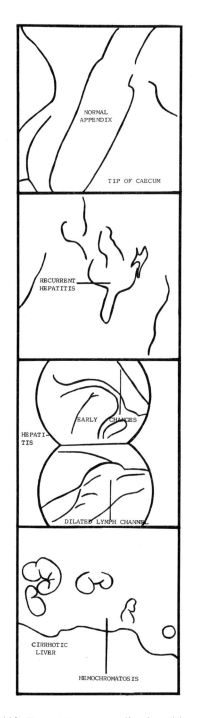

Plate 99. Close-up view of Normal Gallbladder and Portion of Liver

Plate 100. Normal Appendix and Tip of Normal Caecum (PLATES 98-100, CHAP. 35)

Plate 101. Inactive periportal fibrosis with finely granulated surface, connective tissue-like whitish deposits in the periportal fields and a few very short stagnated capsular veins. Also some periportal fibroses more deeply situated, shimmer through the most peripheral parenchymal layer. (Object distance 20mm).

Plate 102. Recurrent, now receding hepatitis on the ground of periportal fibrosis, with development of a more recent relatively dense capsular fibrosis in the area of a very delicate net of lymph vessels. (Object distance 20mm).

Plate 103. Chronic persistent hepatitis with proper lobular marking, finest periportal fibrosis in places, distinct increase of thin lymph vessels and a segmented lymph vessel of medium size. Also beginning, translucent capsular fibrosis. (Object distance 20mm).

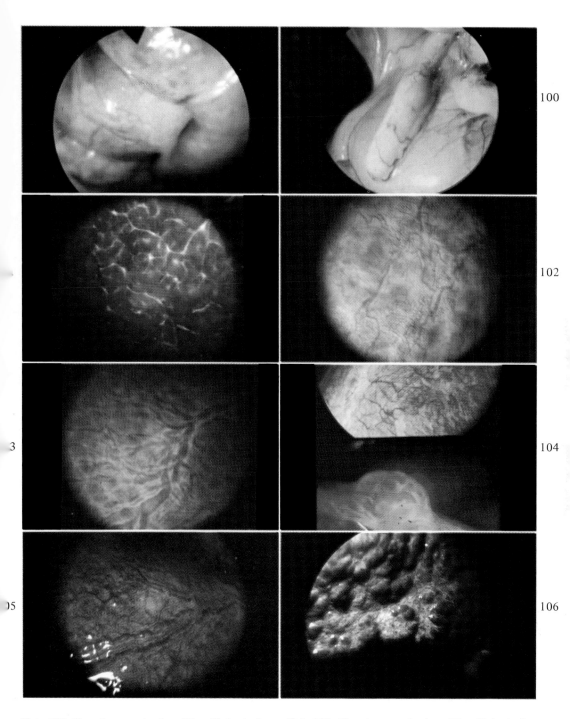

Plate 104. Chronic aggressive hepatitis with beginning change of liver tissue, shallow waving of the surface, distinct stagnation of a main lymph channel, fine lymph vessels flowing into it and heavier arterial vascularization (Object distance 35mm). Below, a varicose dilation of a main lymph channel on the lower edge of the right lobe above the gallbladder (Object distance 20mm).

Plate 105. Chronic aggressive hepatitis with beginning change of liver tissue, icteric coloring of isolated nodules, slight diffuse capsular thickening, stronger stagnation of two segmented main lymph channels with icteric-colored contents and heavy arterial vascularization between main lymph channels.

Plate 106. Cirrhosis of the liver with irregularly noduled, rusty brown surface in hemochromatosis. In the valleys between nodules run tightly bundled, very thin lymph vessels. (Object distance 40mm).

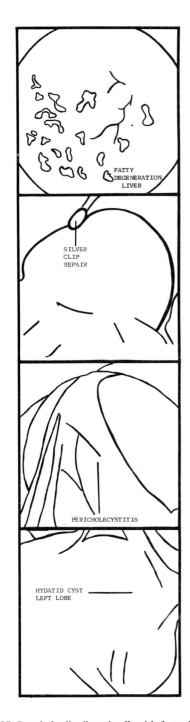

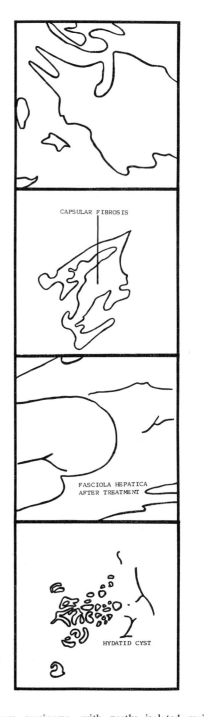

Plate 107. Regularly distributed yellowish fatty degen-eration of the liver without recognizable lobular marking. (Object distance 20mm).

Plate 108. Peritoneal carcinomatosis in presence of mammary carcinoma, with partly isolated mainly confluent, whitish raised groups and distinctly in-creased arterial vascularization. (Object distance 30mm). (PLATES 101-108, CHAP. 36)

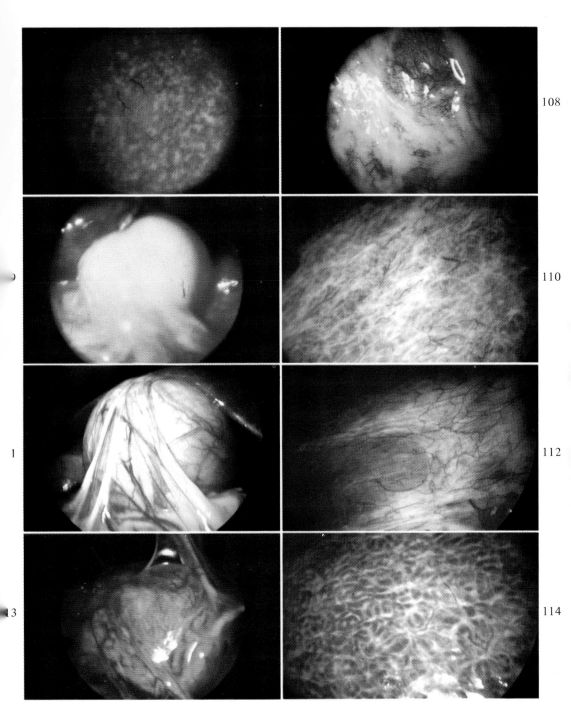

108

110

112

114

Plate 109. Distended gallbladder with silver clip applied at the upper center. (PLATE 109, CHAP. 38)
Plate 110. Moderate capsular fibrosis in Fasciola hepatica.
Plate 111. Chronic cholecystitis with pericholecystitis in Fasciola hepatica.
Plate 112. The liver after treatment with emetine and chloroquine in Fasciola hepatica.
Plate 113. Single hydatid cyst in left hepatic lobe.
Plate 114. Single hydatic cyst, a flat aspect.

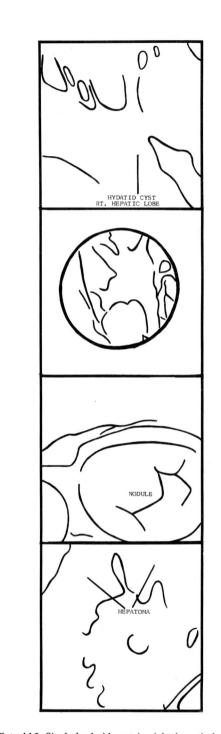

115′

117′

119′

121′

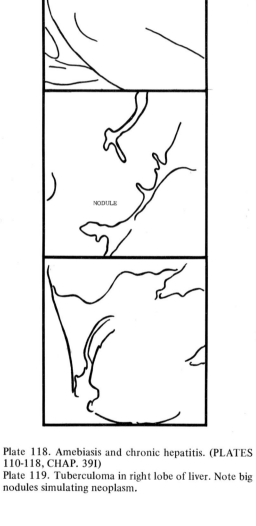

1

1

12

Plate 115. Single hydatid cyst in right hepatic lobe in communication with the biliary tract.
Plate 116. Primary splenic hydatid.
Plate 117. Secondary splenic hydatid.

Plate 118. Amebiasis and chronic hepatitis. (PLATES 110-118, CHAP. 39I)
Plate 119. Tuberculoma in right lobe of liver. Note big nodules simulating neoplasm.

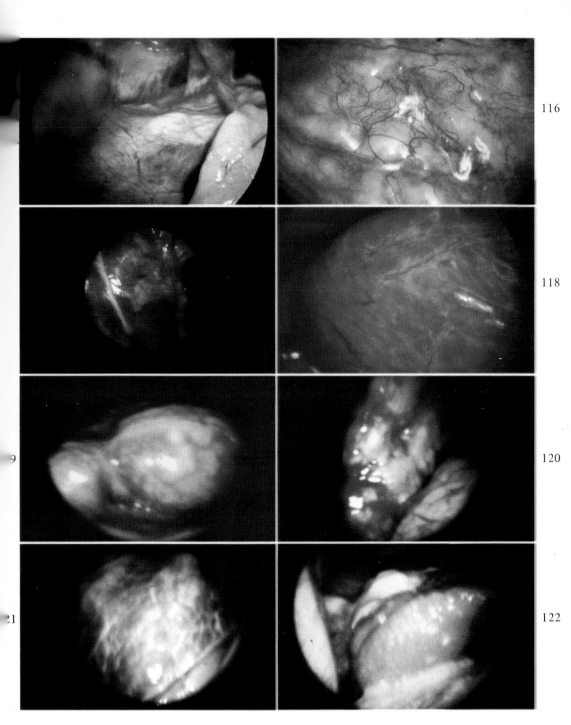

116

118

120

122

Plate 120. Tuberculoma. Undersurface of right lobe of liver shows large, whitish nodules simulating tumor neoplasm.

Plate 121. Hepatoma, right lobe of liver. Note the yellowish hue of the two tumor nodules and the associated cirrhosis.

Plate 122. Tuberculoma. Left lobe of liver shows large, cheesy-white lesions at the surface.

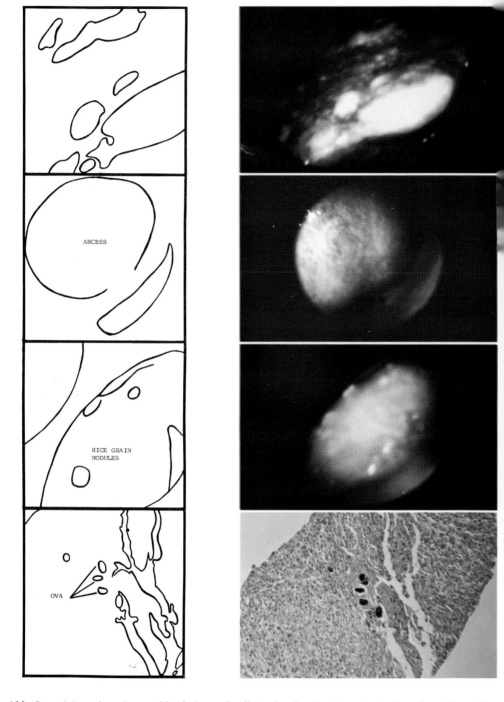

123'

124'

ABCESS

125'

RICE GRAIN
NODULES

126'

OVA

Plate 123. Several irregular, cheesy-white lesions of tuberculoma are seen at the surface of the right lobe.
Plate 124. Amebic abscess, right lobe of liver. Note the bulged appearance and the inflammatory reaction at the inferior surface.
Plate 125. Schistosomiasis japonica in right lobe of the liver, showing the rice-grain sized, oval nodules at the surface.
Plate 126. Histological section of the needle biopsy specimen taken under direct vision over one of the whitish nodules seen in Figure 6. Note the presence of several Schistosoma japonicum ova. (PLATES 119-126, CHAP. 39II)